Epstein–Barr Virus

INFECTIOUS DISEASE AND THERAPY

Series Editor

Burke A. Cunha

Winthrop-University Hospital
Mineola, and
State University of New York School of Medicine
Stony Brook, New York

Additional Volumes in Preparation

Epstein–Barr Virus

edited by

Alex Tselis
Wayne State University
Detroit, Michigan, U.S.A.

Hal B. Jenson
Baystate Health
Springfield, Massachusetts, U.S.A.
and
Tufts University School of Medicine
Boston, Massachusetts, U.S.A.

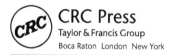

CRC Press
Taylor & Francis Group
Boca Raton London New York

CRC Press is an imprint of the
Taylor & Francis Group, an **informa** business
A TAYLOR & FRANCIS BOOK

CRC Press
Taylor & Francis Group
6000 Broken Sound Parkway NW, Suite 300
Boca Raton, FL 33487-2742

First issued in paperback 2019

© 2006 by Taylor & Francis Group, LLC
CRC Press is an imprint of Taylor & Francis Group, an Informa business

No claim to original U.S. Government works

ISBN-13: 978-0-8247-5425-9 (hbk)
ISBN-13: 978-0-367-39106-5 (pbk)
Library of Congress Card Number 2005054882

Library of Congress Cataloging-in-Publication Data

Epstein-Barr virus / edited by Alex Tselis, Hal B. Jenson.
    p. ; cm. -- (Infectious disease and therapy ; v. 38)
  Includes bibliographical references and index.
  ISBN-13: 978-0-8247-5425-9 (alk. paper)
  ISBN-10: 0-8247-5425-5 (alk. paper)
  1. Epstein-Barr virus diseases. 2. Epstein-Barr virus. I. Tselis, Alexandros Constantine, 1956- II. Jenson, Hal B. III. Series.
  [DNLM: 1. Epstein-Barr Virus Infections. 2. Epstein-Barr Virus Infections--virology. 3. Herpesvirus 4, Human. 4. Lymphoproliferative Disorders. WC 571 E64 2006]

QR201.E75E64 2006
616.9'101--dc22   2005054882

Visit the Taylor & Francis Web site at
http://www.taylorandfrancis.com

and the CRC Press Web site at
http://www.crcpress.com

To Polly, my wife, and LiAnne, our daughter, who make my life's work possible and meaningful.

Hal B. Jenson

To my wife, Carol, and our children, Zachary, Benjamin, and Genevieve, who provide love, encouragement, and a zest for living.

I am grateful to Robert Lisak, John Booss, Robert DeLong, Francisco Gonzalez-Scarano, Omar Khan, Robert McKendall, and Howard Lipton for their teaching, encouragement, and discussions over the years.

Alex Tselis

Finally, we thank Jinnie Kim of Taylor & Francis for her patient and gentle prodding of authors and editors alike.

Foreword

Viruses that infect and cause disease in humans might be classified into three broad groups based on their epidemiologic behavior. The members of the first group are agents such as measles virus, poliovirus, and influenza viruses—ancient human pathogens that are transmitted in epidemic waves. These viruses do not persist after human infection; they must be periodically reintroduced into the human population in order to provoke an epidemic. The susceptibility of the human population to disease is, in part, related to the extent of preexisting immunity to the virus, so called "herd immunity." The second group consists of viruses that have reached humans directly or indirectly from an animal reservoir. Recent examples are the SARS coronavirus, HIV, and Ebola virus, although rabies virus is an ancient example. Since humans have not evolved in parallel with these viruses, they are naïve hosts; therefore, humans are uniquely susceptible to devastating diseases caused by these viruses. The natural hosts and reservoirs, horseshoe bats for SARS coronavirus or nonhuman primates in the case of HIV, are likely to be asymptomatic when infected. Disease in humans induced by these agents is an example of "cross-species virulence." The third group is comprised of viruses that establish life-long persistence once humans are infected. Infection is nearly universal in the human population. These viruses can be transmitted perpetually from person to person, even in isolated tribes having no contact with the outside world. Epstein–Barr virus and many other members of the herpesvirus family are examples of this group. Epstein–Barr virus has coevolved for millions of years with humans and their nonhuman primate ancestors. Both humans and the virus have developed intricate strategies to maintain this coexistence.

The current volume explores many aspects of the biology and disease-inducing potential of this remarkable ancient denizen of the human population. Epstein–Barr virus has developed unique strategies to attach to and penetrate cells, and for its genome to persist in the cell nucleus, to partition when the cells divide, and to switch from a latent state, with limited gene expression, to a fully replicative state in which mature viruses can be synthesized in order to spread among cells and individuals. Each of these phases of the viral life cycle parasitizes specific host cellular functions. For example, the virus uses host cell surface proteins as receptors for entry and host chromosomal proteins as machines for partitioning the viral genome to daughter cells. Host transcriptional activators and repressors and host encoded epigenic mechanisms such as DNA methylation and histone modification play essential roles in the control of Epstein–Barr viral gene expression.

The virus is large and complex. Despite considerable heroic efforts of many laboratories investigating the cellular and molecular biology of Epstein–Barr virus infection, a number of specific details of the viral life cycle at the cellular level remain to be unraveled. For example, what physiologic signals trigger the virus to leave latency and begin to replicate? Which cellular functions are needed for the virus to replicate its DNA? What is the nature of the host cell environment that is favorable for the manufacture of mature viruses? In what way does the differentiation state of the cell, for example, lymphoid versus epithelial, favor latency versus lytic replication?

There are those who say that the immune system evolved to control microbial infection, particularly infection by viruses such as Epstein–Barr virus. Epstein–Barr virus confronts a broad array of effective host immune responses: antibodies, innate immunity, such as NK cells and the interferon system, and adaptive T cellular immunity. These immune responses control Epstein–Barr virus replication and the proliferation of B cells infected by Epstein–Barr virus. However, once the virus gains a foothold in the human host, the immune system never completely eradicates the virus. Thus, the virus has evolved an elaborate strategy of immune evasion that facilitates persistence after infection. Epstein–Barr virus modulates its gene expression program so that highly antigenic viral proteins are not expressed during the latent phase of the life cycle. Some viral proteins antagonize the interferon system and others prevent antigen presentation via the immunoproteosome. Thus, in healthy individuals, Epstein–Barr virus and the host immune system have reached a standoff.

Many diseases discussed in this book can be understood as manifestations of the battle between Epstein–Barr virus and the immune system. For example, infectious mononucleosis is an exuberant immune response to an initial encounter with the virus. Some Epstein–Barr virus–associated diseases such as demyelinating central nervous system disease (see Chapter 8), and possibly other autoimmune disease, may represent bystander consequences of the antiviral immune response. Epstein–Barr virus may induce autoantibodies and self-reactive T cells through the process of molecular mimicry. Epstein–Barr virus–associated lymphoproliferative disease is the result of inadequate host immune surveillance contingent on genetic (X-linked lymphoproliferative disease, see Chapter 16), acquired (AIDS, see Chapter 9), or iatrogenic (posttransplant, see Chapter 12) immunodeficiency. A dramatic translational application to medicine of understanding the interactions between Epstein–Barr virus and the immune system has now made it possible to prevent or treat Epstein–Barr virus–induced lymphoproliferative disease by adoptive transfer of Epstein–Barr virus–specific immune cells (Chapter 18).

The history of Epstein–Barr virus is closely linked to its association with the most common childhood malignancy in Africa, the B-cell lymphoma discovered by Denis Burkitt during his "tumor safaris" in East Africa. Epstein–Barr virus was first visualized in electron micrographs of this tumor, but its mere presence in the tumor did not prove that it was the cause. Epstein–Barr virus is the first human virus to fulfill the Koch–Henle postulates for a human cancer virus. Epstein–Barr virus is regularly, if not invariably, associated with certain cancers, such as endemic Burkitt lymphoma in Africa (see Chapter 10), nasopharyngeal cancer in Asia (see Chapter 14), and Hodgkin's disease (see Chapter 11). The virus can immortalize B cells in culture. It can induce lymphomas in nonhuman primates and SCID mice. Certain viral oncogenes, such as LMP1, can promote lymphomagenesis in transgenic mice. All of these are properties that are consistent with, and expected of, a cancer virus.

Many Epstein–Barr virus–associated cancers are relatively common, with incidence rates as high as 10 per 10^5 persons per year. Yet, even in areas of the world with a high incidence of Epstein–Barr virus–associated cancer, the majority of individuals infected with the virus do not develop cancer. Thus, those interested in the link between Epstein–Barr virus and cancer have struggled to provide an explanation for why the virus is capable of inducing cancers only in a few individuals. In the majority of infected individuals, viral persistence is not accompanied by clinically significant signs or symptoms. Many theories have postulated that essential environmental cofactors (e.g., holoendemic malaria in Burkitt lymphoma; exposure of weaning infants to salt-cured fish in nasopharyngeal cancer), age of infection with the virus, host cell genetic factors, genetic or acquired immune deficiency, or somatic cell mutations are crucial variables that promote carcinogenesis by Epstein–Barr virus. Only in the case of the chromosomal translocations involving the Ig and c-myc genes that are invariable in Burkitt lymphoma do we have clearly defined unique genetic events in the host that can account for the occurrence of cancer only in some Epstein–Barr virus–infected individuals. There is little doubt that immunodeficiency predisposes to certain cancers such as malignant lymphoproliferative diseases. The benign and malignant smooth muscle cancers are detected especially in children with AIDS (see Chapter 15). Nonetheless, patients with Burkitt lymphoma, which occurs within the first decade after viral infection, or patients with nasopharyngeal cancer, which is usually detected in the third decade of life and after, are not globally immunodeficient.

The readers of this volume will encounter it as the first book largely devoted to the explication and exploration of the clinical features and pathogenesis of the wide spectrum of Epstein–Barr virus–associated diseases. The reader will be informed by more than 40 years of intensive research about the epidemiology, virology, molecular biology, immunopathogenesis, and pathology of these diseases. Yet a careful reading will stimulate the reader to continue to ponder and attempt to unravel the many unresolved questions about the behavior of Epstein–Barr virus in the cell, in the human, its natural host, and in human populations. Foremost among these crucial unanswered questions is how the interplay between virus and host determines the occurrence of the striking array of diverse diseases that follow infection with Epstein–Barr virus.

George Miller, MD
John F. Enders Professor of Pediatric Infectious Diseases
Professsor of Epidemiology, and Molecular Biophysics and Biochemistry
Yale University, New Haven, Connecticut, U.S.A.

Preface

Epstein–Barr virus is an important and fascinating human pathogen. A member of the herpesvirus family, Epstein–Barr virus infects almost all humans worldwide. It is the direct cause of or a contributing factor to a wide variety of human diseases, ranging from subacute febrile illness to classic infectious mononucleosis to acute complications such as encephalitis and, perhaps most intriguing, to several forms of cancer. There have been numerous recent advances along many lines of investigation in our understanding of this ubiquitous virus and its myriad pathogenic effects. The time has come to summarize them in a single monograph.

The story of the discovery of Epstein–Barr virus and its associated diseases is an epic tale that continues to evolve. The first chapter of the book lays the foundations, beginning with the story of the discovery of the virus and links to human disease. An exposition follows of the molecular biology of the virus by Jeffrey Cohen. A comprehensive chapter by Warren Andiman details the epidemiology of the virus and its many associated diseases. These clinical and epidemiological observations were crucial to the discovery of Epstein–Barr virus and its relationship to disease. Gerald Niedobitek and Hermann Herbst authoritatively discuss the distinctive pathogenesis and pathology of Epstein–Barr virus disease in a chapter that includes the characterization of persistent and latent infection. The interaction between the virus and the immune system is an important, indeed crucial, aspect of Epstein–Barr virus disease that is detailed in a chapter by Scott Burrows and Andrew Hislop.

The next two chapters discuss many of the general clinical aspects of acute infection. Jan Andersson details the quintessential clinical form of Epstein–Barr virus infection, infectious mononucleosis, including the differential diagnosis and the diagnostic criteria. Atypical presentations, clinical complications, and therapy of the acute infection are included. Greg Storch, Joseph Merline, and Alex Tselis review the methods of laboratory diagnosis, including characterization of the serologic response to Epstein–Barr virus, which is an important means of differentiating recent from remote infection. This chapter also reviews the specific application of many newer diagnostic methods, including direct detection of viral antigens by immunohistochemistry and of the viral genome by polymerase chain reaction.

The manifestations of specific organ involvement of Epstein–Barr virus form the core of the book, beginning with a chapter by Alex Tselis and Kumar Rajamani detailing the acute neurological complications of Epstein–Barr virus infection, which have a very broad spectrum of clinical manifestations and can be fatal. The long-term consequences of Epstein–Barr virus infection are increasingly significant in this era of immunosuppressed populations. Complications of Epstein–Barr virus,

including oral hairy leukoplakia, are prominent among persons with acquired immu-
nodeficiency syndrome and are surveyed in the chapter by Richard Ambinder. Many
of the lifelong risks of Epstein–Barr virus infection entail development of Epstein–
Barr virus–associated tumors. Discussions of the oncologic aspects of Epstein–Barr
virus infection are covered in separate chapters, including Burkitt lymphoma by
Jeffery Sample and Ingrid K. Ruf, Hodgkin's disease by Gerald Niedobitek and
Hermann Herbst, posttransplant lymphoproliferative disease by Lode Swinnen,
T-cell lymphomas by James Jones, nasopharyngeal carcinoma by Sai Wah Tsao
and colleagues, and leiomyosarcoma by Hal Jenson. The intriguing X-linked lym-
phoproliferative disease is thoroughly reviewed by Thomas Seemayer and colleagues.

The remainder of the book addresses issues that are less well understood and
remain to be clarified and conquered. Because Epstein–Barr virus infection involves
so many organ systems in a chronic and sometimes unsuspected, often unpredictable
manner that makes it difficult to distinguish the contribution of persistent Epstein–
Barr virus infection to disease, a number of illnesses are postulated to have a
complete or partial etiologic relationship to Epstein–Barr virus. This has given rise
to some controversy. The issue of how to ascribe the cause of a disease to Epstein–
Barr virus is taken up in a chapter by James Jones, and a number of such diseases
are cataloged. A comprehensive survey of the available and potential therapies of
Epstein–Barr virus disease appears in the chapter by Cliona Rooney and Patrizia
Comoli. This includes not only conventional antiviral medications, but also newer
modes of immunotherapy, particularly adoptive therapy with human leukocyte anti-
gen-matched, Epstein–Barr virus–specific T-cell immunotherapy. The last chapter of
the book, by Andrew Morgan and A. Douglas Wilson, discusses the prevention of
Epstein–Barr virus infection by vaccination, presenting the case for the development
of a vaccine, possible vaccine strategies, and the status of vaccine research.

The book is a broad and comprehensive survey for both clinicians and basic
researchers with sufficient detailed information to serve as a springboard for further
basic and clinical studies, including studies of pathogenesis. The basic science and
molecular virology necessary to understand the manifold manifestations of Epstein–
Barr virus infection are emphasized throughout to facilitate the understanding and
foster further investigations of this important and intriguing human pathogen.

Alex Tselis
Hal B. Jenson

Contents

Contributors

Richard F. Ambinder   Department of Oncology, Johns Hopkins School of Medicine, Baltimore, Maryland, U.S.A.

Jan Andersson   Division of Infectious Diseases, Karolinska University Hospital, Huddinge, Stockholm, Sweden

Warren A. Andiman   Departments of Pediatrics, Epidemiology, and Public Health, Yale University School of Medicine, New Haven, Connecticut, U.S.A.

Scott R. Burrows   Cellular Immunology Laboratory, Queensland Institute of Medical Research, Herston, Brisbane, Australia

Jeffrey I. Cohen   Medical Virology Section, Laboratory of Clinical Infectious Diseases, National Institutes of Health, Bethesda, Maryland, U.S.A.

Patrizia Comoli   Laboratorio Sperimentale di Immunologia e Trapianti, U.O. di Oncoematologia Pediatrica, IRCCS Policlinico S. Matteo, Pavia, Italy

Thomas G. Gross   Department of Pediatrics, Ohio State University, and Division of Hematology/Oncology/BMT, Children's Hospital, Columbus, Ohio, U.S.A.

Hermann Herbst   Gerhard-Domagk-Institut für Pathologie, Westfälische Wilhelms-Universität, Münster, Germany

Andrew D. Hislop   Cancer Research U.K., Institute for Cancer Studies, University of Birmingham, Edgbaston, Birmingham, U.K.

Dolly P. Huang[†]   Sir Y. K. Pao Centre for Cancer, The Chinese University of Hong Kong, Prince of Wales Hospital, Shatin, N.T., Hong Kong Special Administration Region, P.R. China

Hal B. Jenson   Baystate Health, Springfield, and Tufts University School of Medicine, Boston, Massachusetts, U.S.A.

[†]Deceased.

James F. Jones Viral Exanthems and Herpesvirus Branch, Centers for Disease Control and Prevention, Atlanta, Georgia, and Department of Pediatrics, National Jewish Medical and Research Center, Denver, Colorado, U.S.A.

Arpad Lanyi Department of Pathology/Microbiology and Center for Human Molecular Genetics, University of Nebraska Medical Center, Nebraska Medical Center, Omaha, Nebraska, U.S.A.

Kwok Wai Lo Department of Anatomical and Cellular Pathology, The Chinese University of Hong Kong, Shatin, N.T., Hong Kong Special Administration Region, P.R. China

Joseph R. Merline DMC University Laboratories and Department of Pathology, Wayne State University, Detroit, Michigan, U.S.A.

Andrew J. Morgan Department of Cellular and Molecular Medicine, School of Medical Sciences, University of Bristol, Bristol, U.K.

Gerald Niedobitek Institut für Pathologie, Friedrich-Alexander-Universität, Erlangen, Germany

Kumar Rajamani Department of Neurology, Wayne State University, Detroit, Michigan, U.S.A.

Cliona Rooney Department of Pediatrics, Center for Cell and Gene Therapy, Baylor College of Medicine, Houston, Texas, U.S.A.

Ingrid K. Ruf Department of Molecular Biology and Biochemistry, University of California, Irvine, California, U.S.A.

Jeffery T. Sample Department of Biochemistry, St. Jude Children's Research Hospital, Memphis, Tennessee, U.S.A.

Thomas A. Seemayer Department of Pathology/Microbiology, University of Nebraska Medical Center, Nebraska Medical Center, Omaha, Nebraska, U.S.A.

Gregory A. Storch Department of Pediatrics, Washington University School of Medicine, St. Louis Children's Hospital, St. Louis, Missouri, U.S.A.

Janos Sumegi Division of Hematology/Oncology, Children's Hospital Medical Center, Cincinnati, Ohio, U.S.A.

Lode J. Swinnen Department of Oncology, Division of Hematologic Malignancies, Johns Hopkins School of Medicine, Baltimore, Maryland, U.S.A.

Sai Wah Tsao Department of Anatomy, The University of Hong Kong, Pokfulam, Hong Kong Special Administration Region, P.R. China

Alex Tselis Department of Neurology, Wayne State University, Detroit, Michigan, U.S.A.

A. Douglas Wilson Department of Cellular and Molecular Medicine, School of Medical Sciences, University of Bristol, Bristol, U.K.

1

The History of Epstein–Barr Virus

Alex Tselis

Department of Neurology, Wayne State University, Detroit, Michigan, U.S.A.

The history of the discovery of Epstein–Barr virus (EBV) and its associated diseases is arguably one of the great medical detective stories of the 20th century. It is a tale of astute observations and serendipitous stumbles. It begins with the recognition of a febrile illness affecting affluent young people in the Western Hemisphere, proceeds to the observations by a missionary surgeon in East Africa of a bizarre facial tumor among young children, to a chance attendance of a lecture by a young British virologist, to the isolation of a hitherto unknown virus from tumor cell lines, to a young woman's case of infectious mononucleosis (IM) in Philadelphia, and culminates in the identification of a ubiquitous virus that causes an array of illnesses. The range of outcomes includes asymptomatic infection, temporary but debilitating illness, encephalitis, lethal lymphoproliferative syndrome, and several malignancies including lymphoma affecting jaws and viscera, Hodgkin's disease, nasopharyngeal carcinoma, posttransplant lymphoproliferative syndrome, and leiomyosarcoma.

The syndrome of fatigue, malaise, fever, sore throat, and cervical lymphadenopathy with splenomegaly was first described in the late 1800s by several groups in Russia, Germany, France, Britain, and the United States (1).

The syndrome was clinically heterogeneous, with much controversy about the precise characteristics and clinical spectrum of the disease. In fact, it was not even clear that only one disease was being described. A number of other diseases resembled the illness very closely, including streptococcal pharyngitis, diphtheria, various childhood enanthems, acute leukemia, Hodgkin's and non-Hodgkin's lymphoma, and disseminated tuberculosis. Indeed, there were reports in the early part of the 20th century of spontaneously resolving leukemia. But, as experience accumulated, a distinct clinical entity with characteristic clinical and laboratory findings gradually emerged (1).

The first formal descriptions of IM were apparently by Filatov in 1885 and by Pfeiffer in 1889. They noted that the febrile illness was accompanied by a sore throat, posterior cervical lymphadenopathy, and hepatosplenomegaly. They described some pathological findings, such as mediastinal and mesenteric lymphadenopathy. Pfeiffer noted the possibility of chronic cases of the disease, and possible spread in the household (1). Other descriptions were published in the late 1800s and early 1900s (1). Tidy and Morley (2) in 1921 described the leukocytosis seen in one of their patients and reviewed the literature, although they did not identify the important observations of atypical lymphocytes noted later by Sprunt and Evans. The uncertain nature of the disease is illustrated by the occasional confusion with acute leukemia and other diseases. Downey and McKinlay noted that some cases of spontaneously improving leukemia were really examples of "acute lymphadenosis" (3). The credit to Filatov and Pfeiffer for the original descriptions has been disputed, however, by Hoagland, who pointed out that the illnesses they described were atypical in some ways (4).

The next important observation that helped in defining the disease associated with primary EBV infection occurred in 1920, when Sprunt and Evans introduced the term "IM" and described the characteristic hematological finding of "atypical lymphocytes" in patients with febrile lymphadenopathy and eventual spontaneous recovery. Sprunt and Evans differentiated IM from acute leukemia, which the illness—with the atypical cells—resembled. They correctly concluded that "the six cases presented in this paper exhibited a mononuclear leukocytosis in reaction to acute infection," although they were unable to decide whether this was an idiosyncratic reaction to any of a number of pathogens or whether it was due to a particular pathogen (Fig. 1) (6).

An important turning point in characterizing and diagnosing IM was the serendipitous observation that antibodies that coincidentally agglutinated sheep red blood cells occurred acutely in high titer during primary EBV infection. These antibodies are "heterophile antibodies" because they cross-react with antigens occurring among several species that do not correspond to the phylogenetic relationships.

It has been known since the work of Forssman in 1911 (7) that human serum normally contains heterophile antibodies that agglutinate sheep red blood cells. The antigen on sheep red cells to which these antibodies are directed is the Forssman antigen, which is a pentahexosyl ceramide. It is widely distributed on sheep and horse erythrocytes, guinea pig kidney cells, and on cells from certain human malignancies. Most human sera contain antibodies to the Forssman antigen. Hanganutziu in 1924 (8) and Deicher in 1926 (9) observed that patients with serum sickness also had heterophile antibodies that agglutinated sheep red cells. The antigen on the

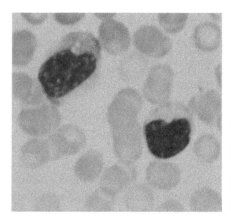
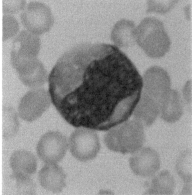

Figure 1   Atypical mononuclear cells in a case of IM. These are large irregular pleomorphic cells, with a resemblance to neoplastic leukocytes. *Abbreviation*: IM, infectious mononucleosis. *Source*: From Ref. 5.

sheep erythrocytes to which these antibodies react is called the Hanganutziu–Deicher (H-D) antigen, which is associated with sialic acid groups on gangliosides and glycoproteins. The H-D antigen is different from the Forssman antigen.

In an interesting aside, when Hoagland in the early 1960s referred to the heterophile antibody as the Paul–Bunnell (PB) antibody, he was quickly corrected:

> Several years ago, I used the latter term (PB test). I received a letter from Dr. Hanganutziu informing me that *he* had discovered the heterophile antibody reaction, in 1924 . . . (4).

Although Hanganutziu and Deicher discovered the presence of sheep agglutinins in serum sickness, the observation that IM also gave rise to heterophile antibodies was made by Paul and Bunnell in 1932 (10). These authors investigated the specificity of the observation that sheep cell agglutinins occurred in serum sickness and studied patients with rheumatic fever, which clinically resembled serum sickness. They tested a number of control sera. One of these, from a patient with IM, gave extremely high titers of agglutinating activity, as described below:

> In the course of this study a number of controls from individuals suffering from serum sickness and a variety of other clinical conditions were assembled. Quite by accident it was discovered that heterophile antibodies (demonstrable in the form of sheep cell agglutinins) were present in a specimen of serum from a patient, ill with IM, in much higher concentration than has been described in serum sickness or in any other clinical condition which we have studied (10).

The authors extended their testing by comparing the sheep cell–agglutinating ability of serum from patients with IM with that of normal controls as well as from patients with various other infectious and neoplastic diseases. The titers were consistently greater among the patients with IM, although there was some overlap with patients with serum sickness.

These heterophile antibodies also agglutinate horse and goat erythrocytes, and cause lysis of bovine red cells in the presence of a complement. These so-called PB antigens on sheep, horse, goat, and beef cells are not necessarily identical. This observation gave rise to the modern monospot test for EBV-associated IM (see Chapter 7). The question of how much of the agglutinating activity was nonspecific (i.e., Forssman antibody) was settled by the observation that incubation with guinea pig kidney cells removed this nonspecific reactivity, and the agglutinin that was left was due to heterophile antibodies. Finally, Bailey and Raffel (12) showed that beef erythrocytes specifically removed IM-associated heterophile antibodies, so that if the agglutinins left after guinea pig kidney absorption were removed by beef cells, it confirmed that these were IM-associated antibodies. This was the basis of the Davidsohn differential absorption test (Fig. 2) (13).

Thus, with the heterophile test, which served as a confirmatory marker of IM, the clinical spectrum of IM was broadened to include multiple manifestations of the disease. Various epidemiologic studies provided greater insight about the illness. A study noting that cadets at a military academy tended to suffer from IM during the month or two after returning from leave eventually led to the idea of human-to-human spread. In fact, Hoagland speculated about the transmission of the disease by deep kissing and exposure to saliva (14). The initial attempts to isolate the etiologic agent were hampered by the primitive state of virology at the beginning of the 20th century. From the 1940s to the 1960s, further attempts to study the disease by inoculating experimental animals or human volunteers were generally unsuccessful,

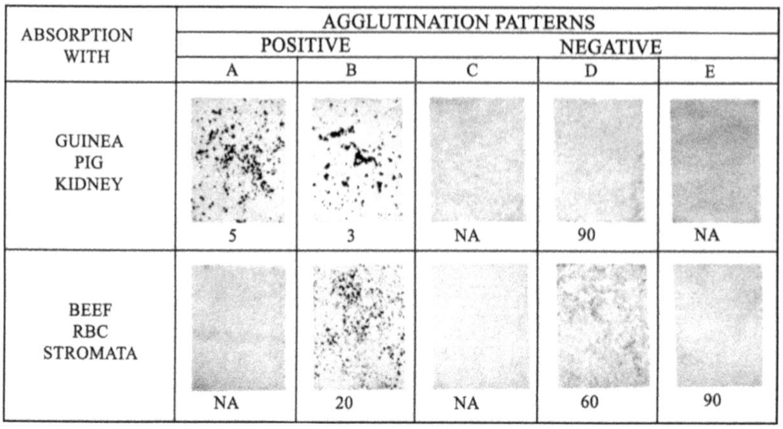

ABSORPTION WITH	AGGLUTINATION PATTERNS				
	POSITIVE			NEGATIVE	
	A	B	C	D	E
GUINEA PIG KIDNEY	5	3	NA	90	NA
BEEF RBC STROMATA	NA	20	NA	60	90

Figure 2 Heterophile antibody serology of IM showing agglutination of sheep red cells by positive but not negative sera, with abolition of agglutinin activity by beef red cell stromata. *Abbreviation*: IM, infectious mononucleosis. *Source*: From Ref. 11.

probably because many of the subjects had already been exposed to EBV and were therefore immune to the acute disease (15). Further subsequent searches for the etiologic agent remained frustratingly fruitless, despite the accumulation of suggestive epidemiologic facts from the meticulous observations of Hoagland, and others, about the illness in military personnel (4,16).

One of Hoagland's contemporaries was a missionary surgeon working with the British Colonial service in East Africa, named Denis P. Burkitt. As a postwar colonial service surgeon, Burkitt was assigned to Lira, Uganda, in 1946, where with the help of one other physician, he served a population of more than 250,000 (17). He became experienced in tropical medicine and studied the effect of climate and geography on the distribution of hydroceles, a process he called "doing geographical pathology." He was able to connect this condition with infection by *Filaria bancrofti* (18). This experience prepared him well for his work on the tumor that was to be named after him.

In 1948, Burkitt was reassigned to the Mulago Hospital in Kampala, Uganda, where he shared the surgical duties with another surgeon. He occasionally noticed and attempted to remove fatal jaw tumors from children, but these did not make any special impression on him at the time.

One day in 1957, Burkitt was asked by Dr. Hugh Trowell, who had performed some of the original investigations on kwashiorkor, to see a young boy named "Africa" who had tumors on both sides of the upper and lower jaws. This was apparently different from what Burkitt had seen before. He examined the patient carefully but was unable to conclude as to whether the illness was due to a tumor or infection. He was "totally baffled" (18). Several weeks later, while visiting a colleague at the Jijoya Hospital, he saw another small child with the same striking appearance in the hospital courtyard (Fig. 3). The coincidence was astonishing, and Burkitt returned to Mulago Hospital with a determination to systematically look for further cases of this illness. He reviewed the medical records of children with jaw tumors and other cancers, and began to keep track of children coming into the hospital with similar diseases. The accumulated pathologic data clearly showed that the jaw tumors were associated with multiple visceral tumors, particularly of the

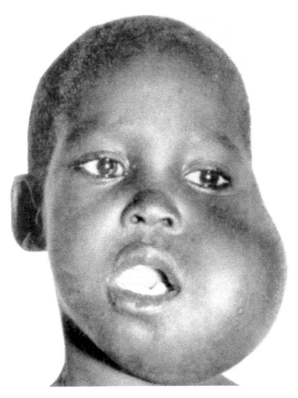

Figure 3 Burkitt lymphoma presenting as a mandibular tumor in a five-year-old boy. *Source*: From Ref. 19.

kidneys, ovaries, liver, lungs, epicardium, and brain (Figs. 4–8). Many such cases with unusual tumors were noted, and gradually, the idea of a single underlying neoplastic process took shape. This scenario is reminiscent of the gradual realization that all those apparently different febrile cervical lymphadenopathies were the result of a single underlying disease—IM (Fig. 9).

To quote Burkitt:

> The seminal observation made at the outset of the Burkitt lymphoma (BL) investigation was that two or more tumours that had hitherto been considered totally different in nature often occurred together in the same patients. This observation demanded an explanation, and a common cause seemed a reasonable possibility. Previously, orbital manifestations had been viewed as retinoblastoma, those in the kidneys or adrenals as neuroblastoma, those involving the ovaries as granulosa cell tumours, and so on—all these tumours being composed of small round cells. Subsequently they were shown to be related in the shared but distinctive age distribution of each tumour, and later still their geographical distribution was shown to be identical . . . (23).

> We had to define a clinical syndrome and for this we needed to apply logic. All the results of a common cause occur together. Different diseases can occur in the same individuals and in the same communities if they share the same cause. If you smoke cigarettes, you get bronchitis, lung cancer and stained fingers. That is not to say that stained fingers cause lung cancer. Through association, however, they are an index of the disease (24).

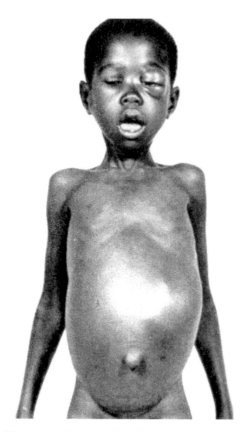

Figure 4 Five-year-old girl with Burkitt lymphoma presenting as an abdominal mass and left orbital tumor. *Source*: From Ref. 20.

In 1958, Burkitt published his first paper on the tumor in a surgical journal (25). Papers describing additional clinical manifestations and the pathology of the tumor followed several years later (26,27), and kindled great interest regarding the tumor in the scientific world.

At about the time Burkitt published his first paper, he described these cases to George Oettle, director of the Cancer Research Unit of the South African Institute for Medical Research, who had considerable experience with unusual tumors. Oettle remarked, "This tumor does not occur in South Africa." This made Burkitt consider the geographical distribution of the disease, its "geographical pathology," and the factors affecting its incidence. On a minimal budget, he designed a survey for the disease for African physicians (17).

Over the next three years, Burkitt received 300 to 400 replies and gradually mapped out a rough geographic distribution of the tumor. The resulting "lymphoma belt" had to be investigated in more detail. Burkitt recruited two medically qualified friends (Williams and Nelson) to go on a "safari" for the disease.

In 1961, Burkitt obtained a £150 grant to buy a used station wagon and supplies, and set off with Williams and Nelson on the first of three safaris, during which they visited various clinics. The 10,000-mile "Long Safari," from October 7 to December 17, 1961, took a north–south route through areas of both high and low incidence. Two other later safaris went through specific areas of high and low incidence.

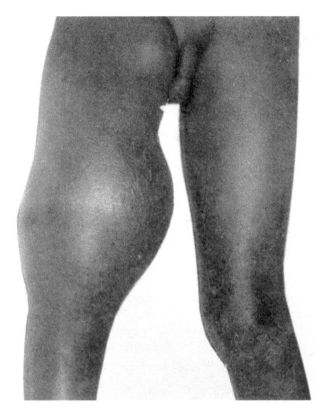

Figure 5 Tumor in the right femur in a five-year-old boy. *Source*: From Ref. 20.

During the safaris, Burkitt and his colleagues noted that the tumor was not seen in areas above a certain elevation, and that this elevation was lower as they went farther away from the equator. Prof. Haddow, director of the East Africa Virus Research Institute at Entebbe, Uganda, pointed out that these "height barriers" really corresponded to a (average) temperature barrier of about 60°F. A side safari to West Africa revealed areas with constant temperature but variable disease prevalence. The geographically astute Haddow noted that areas of low disease incidence

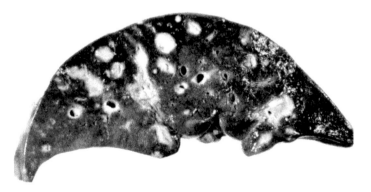

Figure 6 Burkitt lymphoma involving the liver, with scattered tumor nodules, some of which are centered on veins. *Source*: From Ref. 21.

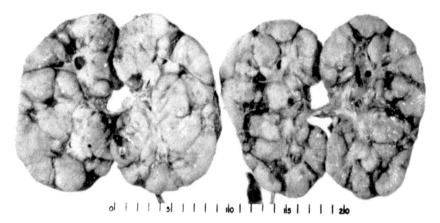

Figure 7 Burkitt lymphoma involving the kidneys, most of the parenchyma of which has been replaced by tumor nodules. *Source*: From Ref. 21.

corresponded to areas of low rainfall, thus defining a "rainfall barrier." The paper describing the results of the safari was published in 1962 (Fig. 10) (28).

Haddow observed that the distribution of the disease followed that of the tsetse fly, which suggested the involvement of an insect vector. Furthermore, an epidemic in 1959 of o'nyong nyong fever, which is caused by a mosquito-transmitted

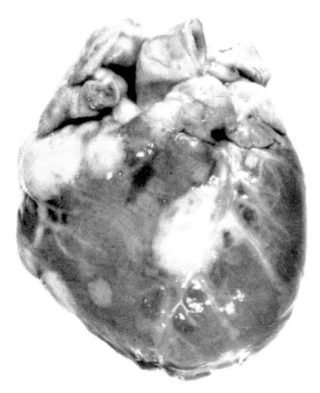

Figure 8 Burkitt lymphoma involving the heart. Note the subepicardial tumor deposits along the coronary arteries and the atrioventricular groove. *Source*: From Ref. 21.

(A)

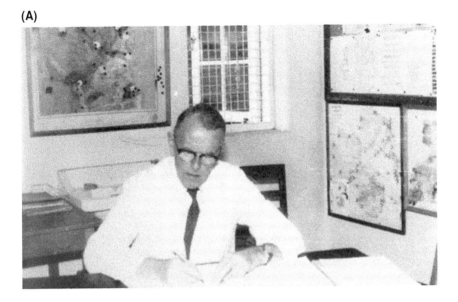

(B)

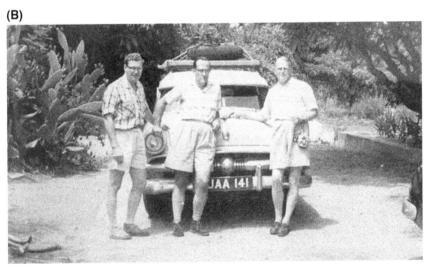

Figure 9 (**A**) Denis Burkitt. (**B**) (*From left to right*): Clifford Nelson, Williams, and Burkitt about to embark on the Long Safari. *Source*: From Ref. 22.

alphavirus, occurred in the same places as BL. The map of BL closely followed that of yellow fever, which is also transmitted by mosquitoes. These findings suggested a viral or other infectious etiology, possibly vectorborne, of BL.

In March 1961, Burkitt returned to England on leave and gave a lecture to the medical students at the Middlesex Hospital in London about his experiences in Africa. M. Anthony (aka M.A.) Epstein, a virologist at the Bland Sutton Institute, who had an interest in oncogenic chicken viruses (Rous sarcoma virus) (30,31), happened to be sitting in the audience. Epstein understood the implications of Burkitt's work immediately and arranged to have biopsy specimens sent to him after the talk (Fig. 11).

Burkitt sent samples of tumor tissue to Epstein, in London, who was able to establish cell lines from the tumor (32). One of the first shipments contained a cloudy

The "Lymphoma Belt"

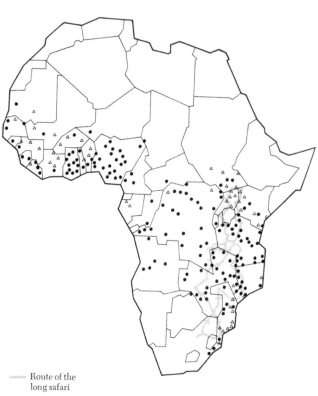

Route of the
long safari

● Areas where there are several cases.

△ Areas where the tumour is known to be common but where there is no
specific documentation.

Figure 10 The lymphoma belt in Africa. *Source*: From Ref. 22.

fluid bathing the tumor sample, which Epstein thought was contaminated with bacteria (33).

> On Friday 5 December 1963, a biopsy sample delayed en route by fog arrived late in the afternoon. The tissue was floating in transit fluid made cloudy by what was assumed to have been heavy bacterial contamination, and was therefore judged useless for culture, especially with the week-end break just about to begin. Nevertheless, the cloudy fluid was examined by wet-film microscopy and surprisingly it was found that no bacteria were evident, but instead that clouds of round viable tumor cells had been shaken free from the cut surfaces of the lymphoma sample in transit. This BL-cell suspension appeared remarkably similar to the malignant lymphoid cells of mouse lymphomas grown as ascites tumours, with which Fisher had successfully established continuous suspension cultures. Accordingly, the free BL biopsy cells were cultured in suspension for the first time, and the first BL-derived line ("EB1") readily grew out (33).

In 1964, electron microscopy showed herpes-like viral particles in the cells (Fig. 12) (35).

However, the virus could not be isolated by any conventional means, and Epstein turned to Werner and Gertrude Henle, a husband and wife team of

A COMBINED MEDICAL AND SURGICAL STAFF MEETING

will be held

on Wednesday, 22nd March, 1961 at 5.15 p.m.

IN THE COURTAULD LECTURE THEATRE.

Mr. D.P.Burkitt from Makerere College,

Uganda will talk on "The Commonest Children's

Cancer in Tropical Africa. A Hitherto

unrecognised Syndrome".

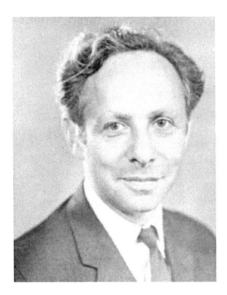

Figure 11 (*Top*) Announcement of Burkitt's talk at the Middlesex Hospital, London. (*Bottom*) M. A. Epstein. *Source*: From Refs. 22, 29.

virologists working at the Children's Hospital of Philadelphia (CHOP), who also had an interest and expertise in the virology etiology of tumors. At that time, they were trying to detect tumor viruses in clinical samples supplied by C. Everett Koop, a pediatric surgeon at CHOP. They investigated for a virus by determining if tumor cells from a tissue sample were resistant to superinfection by vesicular stomatitis virus, which would imply viral interference by a putative cancer virus. Koop told the Henles about BL after a trip to Africa, where he had learned about the disease (Fig. 13).

> When Chick Koop returned in 1963 from a conference in Africa, he told us about Burkitt's lymphoma and urged us to work on it because the epidemiology of this most frequent tumor of African children strongly suggested that it was caused by a virus (36).

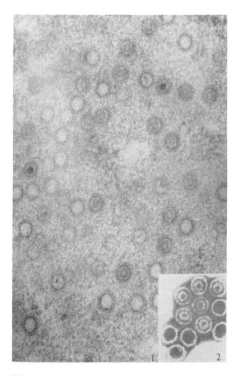

Figure 12 Immature Epstein–Barr virus virions in an EB1 line cell ×127,500. (*Inset*): EBV virions in an EB3 cell line ×127,500. Note that some of the virions are empty, but others contain central nucleoids. *Source*: From Ref. 34.

Serum samples were sent to the Henles' laboratory for further investigation and, hopefully, identification of the virus. Using an immunofluorescence assay (see chap. 7), they found that antibodies to the virus were present in sera from patients with BL, but also from many others, including healthy laboratory staff (37). The first hint connecting the virus to acute disease came when one of the Henles' laboratory technicians, Elaine Hutkin, whose serum was used as a negative control for antibodies to EBV, developed IM (38). Her serum then became strongly positive for EBV antibodies (Fig. 14).

Epidemiologic studies stimulated by this observation established the etiologic link between EBV and IM. The Henles turned to James Niederman, at Yale, who had collected sera from incoming freshman college students and had data concerning their subsequent health status. In their cohort of 29 college students who developed IM during their college years, none had antibodies to the virus before becoming ill, and all had antibodies afterwards (39). Multiple other such epidemiologic studies (see Chapter 3) established the etiological relationship between EBV and IM.

Further studies of subjects infected by EBV showed that specific antibodies persisted indefinitely (40), the virus was shed in saliva both during acute IM and long after recovery (41), and receptors for the virus were present on B-lymphocytes (42). The virus was shown to transform B-lymphocytes, which normally do not survive more than a few days in vitro, leading to outgrowth of cells that grew in perpetuity ["lymphoblastoid cell lines" (LCLs)] (43,44)—a process that was termed immortalization by Miller (45). The immortalized cell lines synthesized polyclonal immunoglobulins (46). The implications for the study of viral oncogenesis were obvious, but this

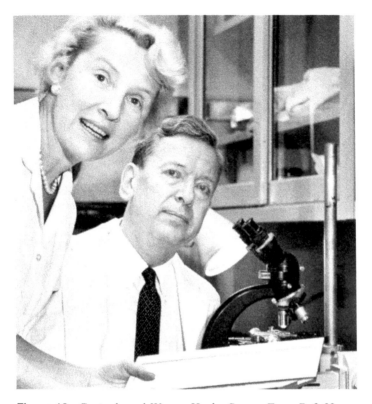

Figure 13 Gertrude and Werner Henle. *Source*: From Ref. 22.

ability of EBV to transform B-lymphocytes has been widely exploited. For example, in population genetic studies, B-cells obtained from individuals of various populations are transformed by EBV to generate sufficient DNA to allow sequencing and detection of DNA polymorphisms (47).

The question regarding the nature of the persistence of EBV is of considerable clinical and biological interest. The intermittent presence of EBV in saliva implied that there is not only active replication but also latent infection from a viral reservoir. That B-lymphocytes (or their progenitors) form such a reservoir is implied by the observation that in two individuals who underwent bone marrow transplants, exogenous EBV (in one case from the patient's husband and in the other from the donor) replaced the patients' pretransplant EBV, as detected by immunoblotting detection of EBV nuclear antigens (EBNAs) from the patients' pre- and posttransplant LCL (48). Sixbey et al. showed that lytic replication of EBV probably occurs in oropharyngeal squamous epithelial cells, thus providing a route of transmission of the virus (49).

The antibody response to EBV infection was dissected by several groups, including the Henles in Philadelphia and George Klein in Sweden. When different EBV-infected cell lines were used as substrates and samples from the acute and convalescent phases of IM and other EBV diseases were tested, distinct antibody patterns were observed. Antibodies to viral capsid antigens (VCAs) were identified by their ability to coat and agglutinate purified virus (50). Other sera had high titers of antibody that stained cells, such as Raji and Roswell Park Memorial Institute (RPMI) 64–10 cells, that were abortively infected with no virion production (51). These antibodies were distinct from anti-VCA antibodies. The viral antigen is synthesized "early" in the

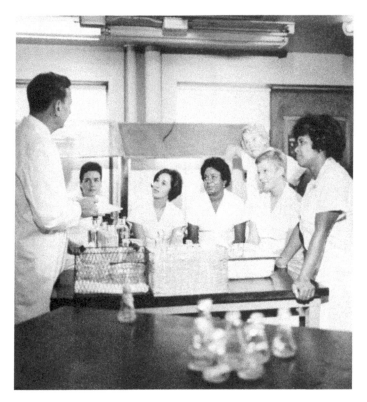

Figure 14 The Henles' laboratory staff. Werner Henle is at the left, Gertrude Henle is in the background, and Elaine Hutkin, the first person who was demonstrated to Epstein–Barr virus seroconvert during an attack of infectious mononucleosis, is seated third from left. *Source*: From Ref. 22.

course of cellular infection, before virions are produced (52). Antibody to early anti-gen (EA) is not typically present in sera with the highest titers of anti-VCA antibodies, and is usually momentarily present only in patients with IM (39). When searching for complement fixing antibodies, Reedman and Klein found that antibodies to EBNA stained the nuclei of EBV latently infected cell lines and Burkitt-derived cell lines (53).

While the involvement of EBV in IM was investigated, the relation of the virus to BL was more clearly elucidated. In 1964, Epstein et al. identified EBV in BL cells (35), but this was not considered proof of causality. After all, the presence of virus in the lymphoma cells is also compatible with the notion that the tumor cells were especially susceptible to infection with a ubiquitous virus, with the virus as a mere passenger. Thus, it was possible that the tumor occurred first, and viral infection of tumor cells followed. This was tested in a heroic study conducted by Guy de The (54) in 1978 in which sera from 42,000 children in the West Nile district of Africa were obtained, tested for EBV antibodies, and the children followed prospectively for the development of BL. The (geometric mean) titers of anti-VCA antibodies in subjects who eventually developed BL were much higher than those of the controls, by a ratio of 4:1. Titers to the other antigens—EA and EBNA—were no different between pre-BL and control subjects.

In a 1968 survey of various cancers, Old et al. examined the prevalence of EBV seropositivity and found that, along with the expected high prevalence of EBV antibodies in patients with BL, there was an even higher prevalence in patients with primary nasopharyngeal carcinoma (55). A study published in the next year confirmed this and showed that elevated EBV antibodies were not seen in geographic controls who were healthy or had other types of head and neck cancers (56). Finally, zur Hausen et al. showed the presence of EBV DNA in nasopharyngeal carcinoma and BL cells by in situ hybridization in 1970 (57). Thus, EBV was established as the first virus to be directly associated with human cancers.

Over the next several decades, more and more diseases were shown to be associated with EBV. In immunosuppressed populations, EBV-related neoplasms achieved prominence. As stem cell and solid organ transplants became common so did posttransplant lymphoproliferative syndrome. The increased incidence of lymphomas in transplant patients was noted fairly early (58), and the evidence of an association with EBV followed soon after (59). Starzl et al. added to the evidence by showing that reversing immunosuppression by discontinuing (or reducing) immunosuppressive therapies often resulted in the reduction or resolution of the lymphomas, in most of which EBV DNA or EBNA could be detected (60). Ho et al. demonstrated the presence of EBV DNA in posttransplant lymphomas by DNA–DNA

Historical Milestones in Epstein–Barr Virus

Year	Milestone
1885	Filatov describes subacute febrile illness which is thought to be IM
1889	Pfeiffer describes subacute febrile illness (Drüsenfieber or glandular fever), which is thought to have been IM
1911	Forssman reports on the presence of sheep cell agglutinins in human serum
1920	Sprunt and Evans publish their observation of atypical lymphocytes in glandular fever and introduce the term "IM"
1924	Hanganutziu identifies sheep cell agglutinins in humans with serum sickness
1926	Deicher also identifies sheep cell agglutinins in humans with serum sickness
1932	Paul and Bunnell publish observations of heterophile antibodies in IM
1937	Introduction of the Davidsohn differential absorption test
1958	Burkitt publishes first paper on jaw sarcomas in African children
1961	Burkitt and O'Conor publish detailed clinical and pathologic report of "Malignant Lymphoma in African Children"
1962	Burkitt publishes report of "Long Safari"
1964	Epstein, Achong, and Barr identify herpesvirions by electron microscopy in BL tissue
1967	Technician in Henles' laboratory seroconverts to EBV after developing IM
1968	Henle and Henle identify EBV as the etiology of IM
1968	Old identifies high EBV titers in nasopharyngeal carcinoma patients
1970	Zur Hausen et al. report detection of EBV DNA in BL and NPC tissue
1973	Jondal and Klein identify the EBV receptor on lymphocytes
1975	Purtillo et al. describe X-linked lymphoproliferative syndrome
1978	De The et al. publish epidemiologic evidence that EBV causes BL
1988	Jones et al. report EBV-driven T-cell lymphomas arising in patients with chronic active EBV infection
1994–1995	Prevot et al., McClain et al., and Lee et al. report EBV in association with leiomyosarcomas among immunocompromised persons with HIV infection or following organ transplantation

Abbreviations: BL, Burkitt lymphoma; HIV, human immunodeficiency virus; IM, infectious mononucleosis; NPC, nasopharyngeal carcinoma.

hybridization as well as by detection of EBNA in the nuclei of the tumor cells using anticomplement immunofluorescence (59).

In 1975, Purtilo et al. reported (61) the case of a boy who died from a fulminant form of IM characterized by extensive lymphoproliferation. He described the presence of similar illnesses in many of his male relatives, thus demonstrating that the disease was X linked. They suggested that the "fatal proliferation of lymphocytes" was likely triggered by EBV, and that the "immunological shutoff mechanisms for controlling the proliferation of lymphocytes... were inadequate." Further evolution of our understanding of X-linked lymphoproliferative syndrome is found in chapter 16.

In 1988, Jones et al. reported fulminant T-cell lymphomas arising in three patients with chronic active EBV infection, and found that the neoplastic T-cells were EBV infected, clonally arising from a single EBV-infected T-cell (62).

The AIDS epidemic has generated an immunosuppressed population which is particularly susceptible to the development of EBV-related lymphoproliferative disease. An unusually large number of B-cell lymphomas in AIDS patients were seen early on in the epidemic in San Francisco, Los Angeles, Houston, and New York (63). Primary brain lymphoma, a very rare neoplasm, was noted in about 5% of an HIV clinic population in San Francisco early on in the AIDS epidemic (64). Other EBV-related lymphomas are not uncommon in this group of patients (see Chapter 9). The most recent human cancer to be associated with EBV is leiomyosarcoma (see Chapter 15), but is limited to immunocompromised persons, including persons with AIDS (61,62) and organ transplant recipients (63).

The story of how EBV was discovered and its causal connections is a fascinating and dynamic one, continuing to shed light on viral pathogenesis and oncogenesis, with new disease manifestations evolving almost from decade to decade.

REFERENCES

1. Carter R, Penman H. The early history of infectious mononucleosis and its relation to "glandular fever". In: Carter R, Penman H, eds. Infectious Mononucleosis. Oxford: Blackwell Scientific Publications, 1969:1–18.
2. Tidy H, Morley E. Glandular fever. Br Med J 1921; 1(452).
3. Downey H, McKinlay C. Acute lymphadenosis compared with acute lymphatic leukemia. Arch Intern Med 1923; 32:82–112.
4. Hoagland R. Infectious Mononucleosis. New York: Grune and Stratton, 1967.
5. Finch SC. Laboratory findings in infectious mononucleosis. In: Carter RL, Penman HG, eds. Infectious Mononucleosis. Oxford: Blackwell Scientific Publications, 1969; (chap. 3).
6. Sprunt T, Evans F. Mononuclear leukocytosis in reaction to acute infections ("infectious mononucleosis"). Johns Hopkins Hospital Bull 1920; 357:410–416.
7. Forssman J. Die Herstellung hochwertiger spezifischer Schafhamolysine ohne Verwendung von Schafblut. Biochem Ztschr 1911; 37:78.
8. Hanganutziu M. Hemagglutinines heterogenetiques apres injection de serum de cheval. C R Soc Biol 1924; 91:1457–1459.
9. Deicher H. Uber die Erzeugung heterospezifischer Hemagglutinine durch Injektion artfremden Serums I. Mitteilung. Ztschr Hyg Infektionskr 1926; 106:561–579.
10. Paul J, Bunnell W. The presence of heterophile antibodies in infectious mononucleosis. Am J Med Sci 1932; 183:191–194.
11. Davidsohn I, Lee CL. The clinical serology of infectious mononucleosis. In: Carter RL, Penman HG, eds. Infectious Mononucleosis. Blackwell Scientific Publications, 1969; (chap. 11).

12. Bailey G, Raffel S. Hemolytic antibodies for sheep and ox erythrocytes in infectious mononucleosis. J Clin Invest 1935; 14:228–244.
13. Davidsohn I. Serologic diagnosis of infectious mononucleosis. JAMA 1937; 108:289–295.
14. Hoagland R. The transmission of infectious mononucleosis. Am J Med Sci 1955; 229:262–272.
15. Niederman J, Scott R. Studies on infectious mononucleosis: attempts to transmit the disease to human volunteers. Yale J Biol Med 1965; 38:1–10.
16. Evans A. Infectious mononucleosis in University of Wisconsin students: Report of a five-year investigation Am J Hyg 1960; 71:342–362.
17. Glemser B. Mr Burkitt and Africa. Cleveland, OH: World Publishing Company, 1970:236.
18. Burkitt D. The discovery of Burkitt's lymphoma. Charles S Mott Award Lecture. Cancer 1983; 51:1777–1786.
19. Burkitt DP. General features and facial tumours. In: Burkitt DP, Wright DH, eds. Burkitt's Lymphoma. Edinburgh: E & S Livingstone, 1970:236; (chap. 2).
20. Burkitt DP. Lesions outside the jaws. In: Burkitt DP, Wright DH, eds. Burkitt's Lymphoma. Edinburgh: E & S Livingstone, 1970:236; (chap. 3).
21. Wright DH. Gross distribution and hematology. In: Burkitt DP, Wright DH, eds. Burkitt's Lymphoma. Edinburgh: E & S Livingstone, 1970.
22. Glemser B. Mr Burkitt and Africa. New York: World Publishing Company, 1970.
23. Burkitt D. The beginnings of the Burkitt's lymphoma story. IARC Sci Publ 1985; 60:11–15.
24. Burkitt D. Discovering Burkitt's lymphoma: a special address to the second international symposium on the Epstein–Barr virus and associated diseases. In: Levine P, Ablashi D, Nonoyama M, Pearson G, Glaser R, eds. Epstein–Barr Virus and Human Disease. Clifton, New Jersey: Humana Press, 1987:xxi–xxxi.
25. Burkitt D. A sarcoma involving the jaws in African children. Br J Surg 1958; 46:218–223.
26. Burkitt D, O'Conor G. Malignant lymphoma in African children 1. A clinical syndrome. Cancer 1961; 14:258–269.
27. O'Conor G. Malignant lymphoma in African children 2. A pathological entity. Cancer 1961; 14:270–283.
28. Burkitt D. Determining the climatic limitations of a children's cancer common in Africa. Br Med J 1962; 2:1019–1023.
29. Epstein MA. Long term tissue culture of Burkitt lymphoma cells. In: Burkitt DP, Wright DH, eds. Burkitt's Lymphoma. Edinburgh: E & S Livingstone, 1970:xxi–xxxi; (chap. 13).
30. Epstein M. The identification of the Rous virus; a morphological and biological study. Br J Cancer 1956; 10:33–48.
31. Epstein M. Composition of the Rous virus nucleoid. Nature 1958; 181:1808.
32. Epstein M, Barr Y. Cultivation in vitro of human lymphoblasts from Burkitt's malignant lymphoma. Lancet 1964; 1:252–253.
33. Epstein M. Historical background; Burkitt's lymphoma and Epstein–Barr virus. IARC Sci Publ 1985; 60:17–27.
34. Epstein MA, Achong BG. The EB virus. In: Burkitt DP, Wright DH, eds. Burkitt's Lymphoma. Edinburgh: E & S Livingstone, 1970:xxi–xxxi; (chap. 22).
35. Epstein M, Achong B, Barr Y. Virus particles in cultured lymphoblasts from Burkitt's lymphoma. Lancet 1964; 1:702.
36. Henle G, Henle W. Epstein–Barr virus: past, present and future. In: Levine P, Ablashi D, Pearson G, Kottaridis S, eds. Epstein–Barr Virus and Associated Diseases. Dordrecht: Martinus Nijhoff Publishing, 1985.
37. Henle G, Henle W. Immunofluorescence in cells derived from Burkitt's lymphoma. J Bacteriol 1966; 91:1248–1256.
38. Henle G, Henle W, Diehl V. Relation of Burkitt's tumor-associated herpes-type virus to infectious mononucleosis. Proc Natl Acad Sci USA 1968; 59:94–101.

39. Niederman J, McCollum R, Henle G, Henle W. Infectious mononucleosis. Clinical manifestations in relation to EB virus antibodies. JAMA 1968; 203:139–142.
40. Neiderman J, Evans A, Subrahmanyan M, McCollum R. Prevalence, incidence and persistence of EB virus antibody in young adults. N Engl J Med 1970; 282:361–365.
41. Gerber P, Lucas S, Nonoyama M, Perlin E, Goldstein L. Oral excretion of Epstein–Barr virus by healthy subjects and patients with infectious mononucleosis. Lancet 1972; 2: 988–989.
42. Jondal M, Klein G. Surface markers on human B and T lymphocytes II. Presence of Epstein–Barr virus receptors on B-lymphocytes. J Exp Med 1973; 138:1365–1378.
43. Pope J. Establishment of cell lines from peripheral leucocytes in infectious mononucleosis. Nature 1967; 216:810–811.
44. Pope J, Horne M, Scott W. Transformation of foetal human leukocytes in vitro by filtrates of a human leukaemic cell line containing herpes-like virus. Int J Cancer 1968; 3:857–866.
45. Miller G. Epstein–Barr virus—immortalization and replication. N Engl J Med 1984; 310:1255–1256.
46. Rosen A, Gergely P, Jondal M, Klein G, Britton S. Polyclonal Ig production after Epstein–Barr virus infection of human lymphocytes in vitro. Nature 1977; 267:52–54.
47. Bowcock A, Kidd J, Mountain J, et al. Drift, admixture, and selection in human evolution: a study with DNA polymorphisms. Proc Natl Acad Sci USA 1991; 88: 839–843.
48. Gratama J, Oosterveer M, Zwaan F, Lepoure J, Klein G, Ernberg I. Eradication of Epstein–Barr virus by allogeneic bone marrow transplantation: implications for sites of viral latency. Proc Natl Acad Sci USA 1988; 85:8693–8696.
49. Sixbey J, Nedrud J, Raab-Traub N, Hanes R, Pagano J. Epstein–Barr virus replication in oropharyngeal epithelial cells. N Engl J Med 1984; 310(19):1225–1230.
50. Henle W, Hummeler K, Henle G. Antibody coating and agglutination of virus particles separated from the EB3 line of Burkitt lymphoma cells. J Bacteriol 1966; 92:269–271.
51. Henle W, Henle G, Zajac B, et al. Differential reactivity of human sera with EBV-induced "early antigens." Science 1970; 169:188–190.
52. Hampar B, Derge J, Martos L, et al. Sequence of spontaneous Epstein-Barr virus activation and selective DNA synthesis in activated cells in the presence of hydroxyurea. Proc Natl Acad Sci USA 1972; 69:2589–2593.
53. Reedman B, Klein G. Cellular localization of an Epstein–Barr virus-associated complement-fixing antigen in producer and non-producer lymphoblastoid cell lines. Int J Cancer 1973; 11:499–520.
54. de The G, Geser G, Day N, et al. Epidemiological evidence for causal relationship between Epstein-Barr virus and Burkitt's lymphoma from Ugandan prospective study. Nature 1978; 274:756–761.
55. Old L, Boyse E, Geering G, Oettgen H. Serologic approaches to the study of cancer in animals and in man. Cancer Res 1968; 28:1288–1299.
56. de Schryver A, Friberg S, Klein G, et al. Epstein-Barr virus-associated antibody patterns in carcinoma of the post-nasal space. Clin Exp Immunol 1969; 5:443–459.
57. zur Hausen H, Schulte-Holthausen H, Klein G, et al. EBV DNA in biopsies of Burkitt tumours and anaplastic carcinomas of the nasopharynx. Nature 1970; 228:1056–1058.
58. Starzl T. Discussion of Murray JE, Wilson RE, Tilney NL, et al. Five years experience in renal transplantation with immunosuppression: survival, function, complications and the role of lymphocyte depletion by thoracic duct fistula. Ann Surg 1968; 168:416–435.
59. Ho M, Miller G, Atchison RW, et al. Epstein–Barr virus infections and DNA hybridization studies in post-transplantation lymphoma and lymphoproliferative lesions: the role of primary infection. J Infect Dis 1985; 152:876–886.
60. Starzl T, Nalesnik M, Porter K, et al. Reversibility of lymphomas and lymphoproliferative lesions developing under cyclosporin-steroid therapy. Lancet 1974; 1:583–587.

61. Purtilo D, Yang J, Cassel C, et al. X-linked recessive progressive combined variable immunodeficiency (Duncan's disease). Lancet 1975; 1:935–940.
62. Jones J, Shurin S, Abramowsky C, et al. T-cell lymphomas containing Epstein–Barr viral DNA in patients with Epstein-Barr virus infections. N Engl J Med 1988; 318:733–741.
63. Ziegler JL, Beckstead J, Volberding P, et al. Non-Hodgkin's lymphoma in 90 homosexual men. Relation to generalized lymphadenopathy and the acquired immunodeficiency syndrome. N Engl J Med 1984; 311:565–570.
64. So Y, Beckstead J, Davis R. Primary central nervous system lymphoma in acquired immune deficiency syndrome: a clinical and pathological study. Ann Neurol 1986; 20:566–572.

2

Virology and Molecular Biology of Epstein–Barr Virus

Jeffrey I. Cohen
Medical Virology Section, Laboratory of Clinical Infectious Diseases,
National Institutes of Health, Bethesda, Maryland, U.S.A.

INTRODUCTION

Epstein–Barr virus (EBV), or human herpesvirus 4, is a member of the herpesvirus family. EBV is the sole human member of the lymphocryptovirus or gamma 1 herpesvirus subfamily, while Kaposi's sarcoma–associated herpesvirus (human herpesvirus 8) is a member of the rhadinovirus or gamma 2 herpesvirus subfamily. A number of simian homologs of EBV have been found including rhesus, African green monkey, chimpanzee, and baboon viruses (1). The rhesus homolog of EBV contains the identical repertoire of lytic and latent genes that are present in EBV (2). Thus, it is likely that EBV evolved from a simian counterpart.

VIRUS STRUCTURE AND GENOME

Like other members of the herpesvirus family, EBV DNA is surrounded by an icosahedral nucleocapsid composed of 162 capsomeres. There are three major capsid proteins. The nucleocapsid is in turn enclosed by a protein tegument, which is surrounded by the viral envelope that consists of multiple viral glycoproteins.

The EBV genome consists of a linear, doubled-stranded DNA that is 184 kilobase pairs in length (3,4). The genome consists of terminal repeats (TR), unique long domains, and internal repeats (IR) (Fig. 1). The genome encodes nearly 100 proteins. While many of the genes expressed during lytic infection have homologs in the other human herpesviruses, genes expressed during latent infection are not present in other human viruses.

Two types of EBV infect humans. They differ primarily in the sequences of the latent genes. B-cells transformed with EBV-1 arise more rapidly in vitro than cells transformed with EBV-2; the viral protein predominantly responsible for these differences is EBV nuclear antigen (EBNA)-2 (6). In addition, different strains of EBV can be distinguished by differences in the number of repeats within the genome. Over 95% of EBV isolates in the United States, Europe, and Southeast Asia are

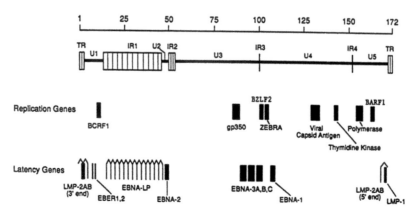

Figure 1 Map of EBV genome. The genome of EBV (B95-8 strain) contains 184 kilobase pairs of DNA (*top line*) consisting of TR, IR, and U regions (*second line*). The genome encodes about 90 replication proteins, a few of which are shown (*third line*) and eight proteins expressed during latency (*fourth line*). *Abbreviations*: EBV, Epstein–Barr virus; TR, terminal repeats; IR, internal repeats; U, unique. *Source*: From Ref. 5.

EBV-1. Patients with HIV in the United States and Europe have a much higher frequency of EBV-2. In HIV-positive homosexuals the frequency of EBV-2 is about 30%, while in HIV-positive hemophiliacs the frequency is 10% (7). EBV-1 and EBV-2 are present in similar frequencies in equatorial Africa and New Guinea (8). Patients with HIV may be coinfected with more than one strain of EBV-1 or EBV-2, with both EBV-1 and EBV-2, or with intertypic recombinants (9,10).

VIRUS REPLICATION

EBV infects epithelial cells in the oropharynx (11) and resting B-cells. Infection of epithelial cells results in a lytic effect with replication of the virus and release of virions from the cell. During lytic replication, the viral genome is copied by the viral DNA polymerase and therefore is sensitive to the action of acyclovir.

In contrast, infection of primary B-cells usually results in a latent infection with expression of only eight proteins without production of virions. These latently infected B-cells, termed lymphoblastoid cells, are transformed or immortalized and can replicate indefinitely. The viral genome circularizes to form an episome and the TR at the ends of the genome join together. There is a fixed number of TR in a given cell. Analysis of the number of TR in EBV-associated malignancies has been used to ascertain whether the tumors arose from a single EBV-infected cell and, therefore, are clonal for EBV. Only a small fraction of latently infected B-cells subsequently undergo lytic infection. During latent infection the viral genome is replicated by a cellular polymerase and therefore is insensitive to the action of acyclovir.

Other cells can also be infected with EBV, although the efficiency of infection is markedly reduced. Burkitt lymphoma B-cells, T-cells, and natural killer (NK) cells can become latently infected with EBV. The EBV genome can persist as an episome or become integrated in the chromosome of virus-infected Burkitt lymphoma cells. In addition, certain epithelial cell lines including gastric and colon carcinoma cells can be infected.

The receptor for EBV in B-cells is CD21, also known as the C3d complement receptor (12). The major virus glycoprotein, gp350, binds to this receptor to enter into B-cells. In addition, the major histocompatibility complex (MHC) class II molecule serves as a coreceptor for EBV, and the viral glycoprotein gp42 binds to MHC class II (13). Epithelial cells lack CD21, and therefore another receptor, that has not yet been identified, is presumably present in these cells.

EBV can be obtained from saliva of infected persons or from latently infected B-cells that have been induced to replicate EBV by treatment with butyrate, azacytidine, phorbol ester, cross-linking of surface immunoglobulin (Ig), or lethal irradiation. Marmoset cell lines infected with EBV, such as B95–8 cells, are a useful source of infectious virus. Infection of epithelial cell lines usually results in very low levels of virus production.

LATENT INFECTION

Only a few of the nearly 100 EBV genes are expressed during latent infection. These latent genes are the six EBNAs, two latent membrane proteins (LMPs), two EBV encoded RNAs (EBERs), and transcripts from the BamHI A region of the genome (Table 1). Only two of these genes, EBNA-1 and LMP-1, are expressed during lytic infection. Genetic studies have shown that five of these genes are essential for B-cell transformation by EBV in vitro.

Patterns of Latent Infection

Four different patterns of latency have been associated with EBV infection (Table 2) (14). In latency 1, EBNA-1 is the only protein expressed in addition to the EBERs and BamHI A transcripts. This is the pattern of gene expression seen in tissues from patients with Burkitt lymphoma. In latency 2, EBNA-1, LMP-1, and LMP-2 are expressed with the EBERs and BamHI A RNAs. This pattern is seen in tissues from patients with Hodgkin's disease, peripheral T-cell lymphomas, and nasopharyngeal carcinoma. In latency 3, all of the EBV-associated latency proteins are expressed as well as the EBERs and BamHI A RNAs. Latency 3 is seen in EBV-associated

Table 1 EBV Latency Proteins

Protein	Required for transformation	Functions
EBNA-1	Yes	Episomal maintenance
		Upregulates viral genes
EBNA-2	Yes	Upregulates viral and cellular genes
EBNA-3	-A, -C: yes; -B: no	Inhibits EBNA-2 activity; upregulates cellular genes
EBNA-LP	Probably	Augments EBNA-2 activity
LMP-1	Yes	CD40 signaling
		Activates NF-κB, c-jun terminase kinase
		Upregulates multiple cellular genes
		Oncogene
LMP-2	No	Prevents EBV reactivation from latency

Abbreviations: EBNA, Epstein–Barr virus nuclear antigen; EBNA-LP, Epstein–Barr nuclear antigen leader protein; EBV, Epstein–Barr virus; LMP, latent membrane protein.

Table 2 Patterns of Latent Infection

Latency type	EBER	EBNA-1	EBNA-2	EBNA-3	LMP-1	LMP-2	BARTs	Site expressed
1	+	+	−	−	−	−	+	Burkitt lymphoma
2	+	+	−	−	+	+	+	Nasopharyngeal carcinoma; Hodgkin's disease
3	+	+	+	+	+	+	+	Infectious mononucleosis; lymphoproliferative disease
Other	+	±	−	−	−	+	?	Peripheral blood B-lymphocytes

Abbreviations: EBER, Epstein–Barr virus-encoded ribonucleic acid; EBNA, Epstein–Barr virus nuclear antigen; LMP, latent membrane protein; BARTs, *Bam*HI A rightward transcripts.

lymphoproliferative disease, infectious mononucleosis, and in EBV-transformed B-cells in vitro (lymphoblastoid cell lines). In the fourth latency program, present in B-cells circulating in the peripheral blood, LMP-2 transcripts and, in some cases, EBNA-1 transcripts are expressed (15,16).

EBNA-1

EBNA-1 is expressed during latent and lytic infection and the protein is present in all EBV-associated tumors. EBNA-1 is essential for transformation of B-cells by EBV. Transgenic mice expressing EBNA-1 develop B-cell lymphomas in some (17) but not all (17a) strains of mice.

EBNA-1 binds to a sequence on the EBV genome termed oriP (18) and associates with mitotic chromosomes (19). The oriP sequence is the origin for viral DNA replication and consists of a number of repeated elements that form the binding site for EBNA-1. Binding of EBNA-1 to oriP and its association with chromosomes allows the viral genome to be maintained during division of the cell. The crystal structure of EBNA-1 has been determined, both alone and bound to DNA (20,21). EBNA-1 contains a core domain that does not bind DNA even though its structure resembles that of the DNA-binding domain of the papillomavirus E2 protein and a flanking domain that binds DNA. The human origin recognition complex (ORC) is associated with oriP, and replication from oriP requires ORC and is reduced by geminin, an inhibitor of the replication initiation complex (22,23).

EBNA-1 also transactivates gene expression. EBNA-1 upregulates its own expression, through its Cp or Wp promoters. EBNA-1 can activate transcription from episomal DNA, but not from integrated DNA (24).

EBNA-1 can be expressed from one of four promoters (25). These are named for the *Bam*HI fragments of the EBV genome on which they are located. The Qp promoter is used in cells that are infected with a latency type 1 or 2 program, the Cp or Wp promoters [which also drive expression of EBNA-2, EBNA leader protein

Table 3 EBV Proteins That Modulate the Immune Response

Protein	Cellular homolog	Function
EBNA1	None	Inhibits degradation by proteosomes
LMP-1	CD40	Inhibits apoptosis
BZLF1	None	Inhibits interferon gamma activity
BHFR1	bcl-2	Inhibits apoptosis
BALF1	bcl-2	Modulates apoptosis
BARF1	CSF-1R	Inhibits interferon alpha
BCRF1	IL-10	Inhibits interferon gamma and IL-12

Abbreviations: CSF, colony stimulating factor; EBNA, Epstein–Barr virus nuclear antigen; IL, interleukin; LMP, latent membrane protein.

(EBNA-LP), and EBNA-3] are used in cells infected with a latency type 3 program, and the Fp promoter is used during lytic infection.

EBNA-1 contains a glycine–alanine repeat region that acts in *cis* to inhibit protein degradation in the ubiquitin–proteosomal pathway (Table 3) (26). This pathway is important for cleavage of proteins into small peptides for presentation with MHC class I molecules to cytotoxic T-cells. The ability of EBNA-1 to inhibit its own degradation is thought to allow cells expressing the protein to avoid destruction by class I restricted cytotoxic T-cells. Transfer of the glycine–alanine repeats to other proteins allows the latter to avoid degradation in proteosomes (27).

EBNA-2

EBNA-2 is required for B-cell transformation by the virus (28,29). EBNA-2 upregulates expression of both viral and cellular proteins. EBNA-2 upregulates EBNA-1 through the Wp and Cp promoters. EBNA-2 also stimulates expression of LMP-1 and LMP-2 (30). EBNA-2 upregulates expression of CD21, CD23, c-fgr, and c-myc (31–33). CD21 is the EBV receptor and CD23 is expressed on the surface of EBV-transformed B-cells. A soluble form of CD23 may act as a growth factor for EBV-infected cells (34) and, therefore, CD23 may act as an autocrine stimulator of B-cell growth. c-fgr is a tyrosine kinase that may be important for growth of B-cells, while dysregulation of c-myc is associated with the unregulated B-cell proliferation in Burkitt lymphoma.

EBNA-2 interacts with a number of cellular proteins to mediate its transactivating function. EBNA-2 binds to Jκ, also termed C-promoter binding factor (CBF-1), to activate the EBNA Cp, LMP-1, LMP-2, and CD23 promoters (35). Jκ recognizes a DNA sequence, GTGGGAA, on EBV and cellular promoters to activate gene expression. In this regard EBNA-2 is functionally similar to the Notch receptor which also binds to Jκ to activate genes during development (36,37). EBNA-2 also binds PU-1, a DNA-binding protein, to upregulate the LMP-1 promoter (30) and AUF1 to activate the EBNA Cp promoter (38).

EBNA-2 contains an acidic domain that is critical for transcriptional activation (39). This domain associates with components of the transcription complex including transcription factor (TF)IIB, TFIIH, TATA binding protein (TBP) associated factor (TAF)40, RPA70, p100, and cAMP-response element–binding protein (CREB) binding protein (CBP)/p300 (40–43).

EBNA-LP

EBNA-LP is the 5' gene encoded in a transcript with the EBNA–2 gene. While EBNA-LP has not been proven to be essential for transformation, deletion of the carboxy terminus of the protein markedly reduces the ability of the virus to transform B-cells (44).

EBNA-LP augments the ability of EBNA-2 to activate expression of LMP-1, LMP-2 (45), and cellular proteins (46). While EBNA-LP has been shown to bind to p53 and the retinoblastoma protein (47), it is unclear what significance these interactions have for the role of EBNA-LP in B-cell transformation. In addition, EBNA-LP binds to a number of other cellular proteins including heat shock protein 70, DNA protein kinase catalytic subunit, HA95 (a nuclear protein that may be involved in mitosis), and α and β tubulin (48).

EBNA-3

There are three EBNA-3 proteins, EBNA-3A, EBNA-3B, and EBNA-3C, which show weak homology to each other and are present in tandem in the viral genome. EBNA-3A and EBNA-3C are required for B-cell transformation by the virus, while EBNA-3B is dispensable (49,50).

The EBNA-3 proteins bind to Jκ with a higher efficiency than EBNA-2. Binding of the EBNA-3 proteins to Jκ prevents the latter from binding to DNA and inhibits the ability of EBNA-2 to upregulate gene expression (51).

The EBNA-3 proteins also upregulate expression of cellular and viral genes. EBNA-3C increases the expression of CD21 and LMP-1 (52,53), and EBNA-3B upregulates expression of CD40 and bcl-2 (54). EBNA-3C interacts with the human metastatic suppressor protein Nm23-HI and inhibits the ability of the latter to suppress the migration of Burkitt lymphoma cells (55).

LMP-1

LMP-1 is expressed in both latently and lytically infected B-cells. LMP-1 is required for transformation of B-cells by EBV (56). LMP-1 functions as an oncogene for the virus. Rodent fibroblasts expressing LMP-1 show a transformed phenotype with loss of anchorage dependence, markedly reduced requirements for serum, loss of contact inhibition, and the ability to grow as colonies in agar. Injection of these fibroblasts into nude mice results in the formation of tumors (57). Transgenic mice expressing LMP-1 in B-cells develop B-cell lymphomas (58). Transgenic mice expressing LMP-1 in the skin develop epithelial hyperplasia with increased expression of keratin 6 (59). LMP-1 has transmembrane domains that are located in lipid rafts on the membrane of the cell, and the protein is associated with the cell cytoskeleton (60).

LMP-1 is a functional analog of a constitutively activated form of CD40 and can complement the activity of CD40 in transgenic mice (61). CD40 is a member of the tumor necrosis factor (TNF) receptor family. Interaction of CD40 in B-cells with its ligand results in oligomerization of CD40, binding of the protein to TNF-associated factors (TRAFs), and B-cell activation and proliferation. LMP-1 binds to TRAFs 1, 2, 3, and 5, TNF receptor-associated death domain (TRADD), receptor interacting protein (RIP), and Janus-activated kinase 3 (62–65). These interactions result in activation of nuclear factor kappa B (NF-κB), c-jun N-terminal kinase, signal transducers and activators of transcription, B7 costimulatory protein, the p38 mitogen activated protein (MAP) kinase pathway, and stress activated kinases (66–69). The resultant effect is constitutive B-cell proliferation. LMP-1 also interacts with TRAFs in epithelial cells resulting in increased expression of epidermal growth factor (70). EBV-associated B-cell lymphomas in humans show activation of NF-κB, and LMP-1 colocalizes with TRAF-1 and TRAF-3 (71). Thus, LMP-1 is critical for B-cell proliferation and development of lymphomas in vivo.

Expression of LMP-1 in cells upregulates a large number of proteins and results in multiple phenotypic changes. LMP-1 stimulates expression of intracellular adhesion molecules (ICAM)-1, lymphocyte function associated antigen-1 (LFA)-1, and LFA-3. LMP-1 also upregulates expression of Fas, CD23, CD40, and MHC class II (52,72). LMP-1 induces secretion of IgM and interleukin (IL)-6 (73,74) and upregulates expression of matrix metalloproteinase-9 (75). LMP-1 expression in epithelial cells inhibits their differentiation (76) and alters the morphology of keratinocytes (77). Expression of LMP-1 in lymphoma cells induces clumping of the cells and increases formation of villous projections (52). LMP-1 can also inhibit the ability of EBNA-1 to transactivate the EBNA Cp and LMP-1 promoters (78) and inhibits BZLF1 transcription and induction of lytic replication (79).

LMP-1 has several antiapoptotic effects on the cell. LMP-1 upregulates expression of A20, myeloid cell leukemia (mcl)-1, bcl-2, and bfl-1, all of which inhibit apoptosis (80–83). Both bcl-2 and A20 are upregulated in transgenic mice expressing LMP-1 (58). LMP-1 also inhibits expression of c-myc and thereby further protects cells from apoptosis (84).

LMP-2

Two forms of LMP-2 are expressed in EBV-infected B-cells. LMP-2A and LMP-2B are colinear, except that they differ in their 5′ exons. The resultant proteins are identical except that LMP-2A is predicted to have an additional 119 amino acids at its amino terminus compared with LMP-2B. LMP-1 and LMP-2 colocalize in the membrane of B-cells, and both are present in lipid rafts (60,85). LMP-2 is not required for B-cell transformation (86).

LMP-2 functions to prevent EBV reactivation in latently infected B-cells. Cross-linking of immunoglobulin on the surface of EBV-transformed B lymphoma cells in the absence of LMP-2 can induce lytic replication of the virus. However, expression of LMP-2 on the surface of the cell blocks this effect. LMP-2 binds to fyn and lyn, members of the B-cell src family of protein tyrosine kinases, and to syk. Binding of LMP-2 to these proteins results in constitutive low level phosphorylation of the proteins. This, in turn, is thought to inhibit their ability to activate phospholipase C, mobilize calcium, and induce lytic replication of EBV in response to external signals (87–89). LMP-2 is also phosphorylated by the src family of protein tyrosine kinases.

Expression of LMP-2 in B-cells of transgenic mice allows the cells to survive in the absence of normal B-cell receptor signaling (90). Expression of LMP-2 in epithelial cells results in transformation of the cells with anchorage-independent growth, the ability to form colonies in agar, and induction of tumors when inoculated into nude mice (91). LMP-2 also inhibits differentiation of epithelial cells and activates the Akt serine–threonine protein kinase.

EBERs

Two polyadenylated, nontranslated RNAs, EBER-1 and EBER-2, are expressed in latently infected EBV-transformed B-cells. They are the most highly expressed EBV RNAs in latently infected cells, and probes to these transcripts have been used extensively for detection of EBV in tissues.

Both EBERs are dispensable for B-cell transformation by the virus (92). However, expression of the EBERs in EBV-negative lymphoma cells enhances their malignant phenotype with the ability to grow in soft agar and induce tumors when inoculated into severe combined immunodeficient (SCID) mice (93). In addition, expression of EBERs upregulates the bcl-2 gene and enhances the resistance of cells to apoptosis. Transfection of EBERs into EBV-negative B-cells upregulates expression of IL-10 and may function as an autocrine growth factor for the cells (94).

The EBERs interact with interferon-inducible oligoadenylate synthetase and with double-stranded RNA-activated protein kinase (95,96). EBER-1 also inhibits the protein kinase in vitro (97). Wild-type EBV expressing the EBERs shows no difference in its ability to block the effects of interferon compared with an EBV mutant lacking the EBERs (98). The EBERs also bind to the nuclear proteins La and EAP (EBER-associated protein) (99,100).

Other Latency-Associated Genes

A number of EBV transcripts encoded in the rightward direction from the *Bam*HI A region of the genome have been detected in EBV-infected B-cells and nasopharyngeal carcinomas (101). These *Bam*HI A rightward transcripts include the BARF0 and RPMS1 genes. Transcripts corresponding to the BARF0 gene have been detected in latently infected B-cells (102). At present BARF0 protein has not been detected in latently infected cells, although antibodies to the protein have been found in patients with nasopharyngeal carcinoma (103). An alternatively spliced form of BARF0, termed RK-BARF0, can upregulate expression of LMP-1 in the absence of EBNA-2, and RK-BARF0 interacts with Notch (104). RPMS1 transcripts are present in B-cells that are latently infected with EBV and in Hodgkin's disease tissue. RPMS1 protein interacts with Jκ to interfere with EBNA-2 mediated upregulation of proteins (105).

Table 4 Selected Epstein–Barr Virus Lytic Proteins

Protein	Expression class	Function
BZLF1	IE	Transcriptional activator
BRLF1	IE	Transcriptional activator
BALF5	E	DNA polymerase
BXLF1	E	Thymidine kinase
BcLF1	L	Viral capsid antigen
gp350	L	Major viral glycoprotein, binds CD21 on B-cells
gp85	L	Important for fusion of virus to B-cells
gp42	L	Binds to MHC class II molecules on B-cells

Abbreviations: E, early; IE, immediate early; L, late; MHC, major histocompatability complex.

LYTIC INFECTION

EBV encodes approximately 90 proteins that are expressed during lytic virus replication (Table 4). By analogy with other herpesviruses, these are classified as immediate-early, early, and late proteins. Immediate-early genes are transcribed after infection in the presence of protein synthesis inhibitors. Early genes are expressed in the presence of viral DNA synthesis inhibitors, while late genes are not transcribed when these inhibitors are present. In general, immediate-early genes are important for regulating gene expression in the virus, early proteins encode enzymes that are important for viral DNA replication, and late proteins encode structural proteins of the virion. EBV lytic genes are named by the *Bam*HI fragment in which they are located, whether they are expressed in a leftward (L) or rightward direction (R), and the number of their position in the *Bam*HI fragment. For example, BZLF1 is the first transcript expressed in the leftward direction in the *Bam*HI Z fragment of EBV.

Immediate-Early Proteins

The major immediate-early proteins of EBV are encoded by BZLF1 and BRLF1. BZLF1 protein is also termed Z Epstein–Barr replication activator (ZEBRA) or Zta, while BRLF1 protein is also known as Rta. BZLF1 and BRLF1 proteins activate transcription of viral early genes (106,107). BZLF1 protein inhibits transcription from the EBNA Cp promoter and may facilitate the switch from latent to lytic infection (108). Binding of NF-κB or p53 to BZLF1 protein inhibits the ability of the viral protein to transactivate viral gene expression (109,110). BZLF1 protein also downregulates the interferon gamma receptor and inhibits the ability of interferon gamma to activate its target genes including IRF-1, CIITA, and MHC class II (111).

Early Proteins

EBV early proteins include enzymes that are important for viral DNA replication, inhibitors of apoptosis, a soluble cytokine receptor, and proteins that activate expression of other early genes. Six viral proteins have been identified as replication proteins using an in vitro assay to amplify plasmids containing the lytic origin of replication (ori-lyt) (112). These replication proteins are the viral DNA polymerase (encoded by BALF5), the DNA polymerase processivity factor (encoded by BMRF1), the single-stranded DNA-binding protein homolog (encoded by BALF2), the primase homolog (encoded by BSLF1), the helicase homolog (encoded by BBLF4), and the helicase-primase homolog (encoded by BBLF2/3). The viral thymidine kinase (encoded by BXLF1) phosphorylates acyclovir and results in activation of the drug with inhibition of the viral DNA polymerase and viral DNA replication. Other early viral proteins important for viral DNA replication are the ribonucleotide reductase proteins encoded by BORF2 and BaRF1 and the uracil DNA glycosylase encoded by BKRF3.

BHRF1 and BALF1 are homologs of bcl-2, a cellular protein that inhibits apoptosis. Both proteins have been shown to protect cells from apoptosis. BHRF1 colocalizes with bcl-2 in the mitochondria and inhibits apoptosis in both B-cells (113) and epithelial cells (114), while BALF1 has been shown to modulate the effect of BHRF1 in epithelial cells (115).

BARF1 protein acts as a soluble colony stimulating factor (CSF)-1 receptor. Although BARF1 has very limited amino acid homology to the CSF-1 receptor, the viral protein blocks the activity of CSF-1 (116). CSF-1 stimulates expression of interferon alpha by monocytes, and BARF1 blocks the ability of CSF-1 to enhance secretion of the cytokine (117). Because interferon alpha activates NK cell cytotoxicity, BARF1 may inhibit the ability of NK cells to control virus-infected cells.

The BSMLF1 and BMRF1 proteins activate expression of other early genes (118). These two proteins make up part of the early antigen–diffuse complex, because the antigens are found to be present in both the nucleus and the cytoplasm on immunofluorescence staining. BHRF1 and BORF2 comprise part of the early antigen–restricted complex because they are restricted to the cytoplasm.

Late Proteins

EBV late proteins include the viral glycoproteins, nucleocapsid proteins, and a viral cytokine. Most of the viral capsid antigen (VCA) is comprised of the major nucleocapsid protein, which is encoded by BcLF1. Antibodies to the VCA are used in the diagnosis of virus infection.

EBV encodes several glycoproteins including gp350, gp110, gp85, gp42, and gp25. gp350, encoded by BLLF1, is the major viral envelope protein and binds to its receptor, CD21, on B-cells. Deletion of gp350 from the virus markedly reduces, but does not eliminate, infectivity of the virus (119). Purified recombinant gp350 is being studied as a vaccine candidate (120).

EBV gp110, encoded by BALF4, is the homolog of herpes simplex virus (HSV) glycoprotein B, which is required for HSV entry into cells. Three EBV glycoproteins, gp85, gp42, and gp25, form a trimolecular complex. EBV gp85, encoded by BXLF2, is the homolog of HSV glycoprotein H (gH). gp85 is important for fusion of the virus to B-cells and absorption to epithelial cells. gp85 is essential for infection of B-cells and epithelial cells (121–123). gp25, the product of BKRF2, is a homolog of HSV gL and acts as a viral chaperone to transport gp85 to the cell membrane (124). The third component of the complex, gp42 (encoded by BZLF2), binds to MHC class II molecules (125) and functions as a coreceptor for virus entry in B-cells (13). In contrast, gp42 is not required for EBV infection of epithelial cells (126). gp85 and gp25 can also form a heterodimer. EBV also encodes homologs of HSV gN (encoded by BLRF1) and gM (encoded by BBRF3) that are important for egress of virus from the cell (127).

BCRF1 protein, also termed viral IL-10, shares over 80% amino acid identity with human IL-10 (128). Viral IL-10 inhibits interferon gamma secretion by peripheral blood mononuclear cells and release of IL-12 from macrophages (92,129). These activities may serve to protect virus-infected cells from cytotoxic T-cells. Viral IL-10 also stimulates growth of B-cells (130) and inhibits the activity of dendritic cells (131). The viral cytokine has less activity than its cellular homolog for stimulating expression of MHC class II and for inhibiting expression of IL-2.

CONCLUSIONS

EBV is a highly infective virus that infects over 95% of humans. The virus encodes a limited number of proteins during latent infection that allow the virus to activate B-cell proliferation and immortalize B-cells in vitro while avoiding apoptosis. Many of these viral proteins upregulate cellular gene expression and engage pathways that normally occur during B-cell activation. EBV markedly limits expression of viral proteins during latent infection to minimize the number of targets for destruction by cytotoxic T-cells. During lytic infection, a large number of viral genes are expressed. In addition to proteins required for viral DNA replication and for assembly of virions, the virus expresses several proteins that modulate the immune response. These proteins block apoptosis and inhibit the activity of interferon alpha and interferon gamma.

REFERENCES

1. Wang F, Rivailler R, Rao P, Cho Y-G. Simian homologues of Epstein–Barr virus. Philos Trans R Soc Lond B 2001; 356:489–497.
2. Rivailler P, Jiang H, Cho Y-g, Quink C, Wang F. Complete nucleotide sequence of the rhesus lymphocryptovirus: genetic validation for an Epstein–Barr virus animal model. J Virol 2002; 76:421–426.
3. Baer R, Bankier AT, Biggin MD, et al. DNA sequence and expression of the B95-8 Epstein–Barr virus genome. Nature 1984; 310:207–211.
4. Hatfull G, Bankier AT, Barrell BG, Farrell PJ. Sequence analysis of Raji Epstein–Barr virus DNA. Virology 1988; 164:334–340.
5. Cohen JI. Molecular biology of Epstein–Barr virus and its mechanism of B-cell transformation. In: Straus SE, ed. Epstein–Barr virus infections: biology, pathogenesis and management. Ann Intern Med 1993; 118:45–48.
6. Rickinson AB, Young LS, Rowe M. Influence of Epstein–Barr virus nuclear antigen EBNA-2 on the growth phenotype of virus-transformed B-cells. J Virol 1987; 61: 1310–1317.
7. Yao QY, Croom-Carter D, Tierney RJ, et al. Epidemiology of infection with Epstein–Barr virus types 1 and 2: lessons from the study of a T-cell immunocompromised hemophiliac cohort. J Virol 1998; 72:4352–4363.
8. Abdel-Hamid M, Chen JJ, Constantine N, Massoud M, Raab-Traub N. EBV strain variation: geographical distribution and relation to disease state. Virology 1992; 190: 168–175.
9. Yao QY, Tierney RJ, Croom-Carter D, et al. Frequency of multiple Epstein–Barr virus infections in T-cell immunocompromised individuals. J Virol 1996; 70:4884–4894.
10. Yao QY, Tierney RJ, Croom-Carter D, et al. Isolation of intertypic recombinants of Epstein–Barr virus from T-cell immunocompromised individuals. J Virol 1996; 70: 4895–4903.
11. Sixbey JW, Nedrud JG, Rabb-Traub N, Hanes RA, Pagano JS. Epstein–Barr virus replication in oropharyngeal cells. N Engl J Med 1984; 310:1225–1230.
12. Fingeroth JD, Weiss JJ, Tedder TF, Strominger JL, Biro PA, Fearon DT. Epstein–Barr virus receptor of human Bs is the C3d receptor CR2. Proc Natl Acad Sci USA 1984; 81:4510–4516.
13. Li Q, Spriggs MK, Kovats S, et al. Epstein–Barr virus uses HLA class II as a cofactor for infection of B lymphocytes. J Virol 1997; 71:4657–4662.
14. Kerr BM, Lear AL, Rowe M, et al. Three transcriptional distinct forms of Epstein–Barr virus latency in somatic cell hybrids: cell phenotype dependence of viral promoter usage. Virology 1992; 187:189–201.
15. Tierney RJ, Steven N, Young LS, Rickinson AB. Epstein–Barr virus latency in mononuclear cells: analysis of viral gene transcription during primary infection and in the carrier state. J Virol 1994; 68:7374–7385.
16. Qu L, Rowe DT. Epstein–Barr virus latent gene expression in uncultured peripheral blood lymphocytes. J Virol 1992; 66:3715–3724.

17. Wilson JB, Bell JL, Levine AJ. Expression of Epstein–Barr virus nuclear antigen 1 induces B-cell neoplasia in transgenic mice. EMBO J 1996; 15:3117–3126.

17a. Kang MS, Lu H, Yasui T, et al. Epstein–Barr virus nuclear antigen-1 does not reduce lymphoma in transgenic FVB mice. Proc Natl Acad Sci USA 2005; 102:820–825.

18. Yates J, Warren N, Reisman D, Sugden B. A cis-acting element from the Epstein–Barr viral genome that permits stable replication of recombinant plasmids in latently infected cells. Proc Natl Acad Sci USA 1984; 81:3806–3810.

19. Harris A, Young BD, Griffin BE. Random association of Epstein–Barr virus genomes with host cell metaphase chromosomes in Burkitt's lymphoma-derived cell lines. J Virol 1985; 56:328–332.

20. Bochkarev A, Barwell JA, Pfuetzner RA, Bochkareva E, Frappier L, Edwards AM. Crystal structure of the DNA binding domain of the Epstein–Barr virus origin-binding protein, EBNA-1, bound to DNA. Cell 1996; 84:791–800.

21. Bochkarev A, Barwell JA, Pfuetzner RA, Furey W, Edwards AM, Frappier L. Crystal structure of the DNA binding domain of the Epstein–Barr virus origin-binding protein, EBNA-1. Cell 1995; 83:39–46.

22. Chaudhuri B, Xu H, Todorov I, Dutta A, Yates JL. Human DNA replication initiation factors, ORF and MCM, associate with oriP of Epstein–Barr virus. Proc Natl Acad Sci USA 2001; 28:10085–10089.

23. Dhar SK, Yoshida K, Machida Y, et al. Replication from oriP of Epstein–Barr virus requires human ORC and is inhibited by geminin. Cell 2001; 106:287–296.

24. Kang M-S, Hung SC, Kieff E. Epstein–Barr virus nuclear antigen 1 activates transcription from episomal but not integrated DNA and does not alter lymphocyte growth. Proc Natl Acad Sci USA 2001; 98:15233–15238.

25. Deacon EM, Pallesen G, Niedobitek G, et al. Epstein–Barr virus and Hodgkin's disease: transcriptional analysis of virus latency in the malignant cells. J Exp Med 1993; 177: 339–349.

26. Levitskaya J, Shapiro A, Leonchiks A, Ciechanover A, Masucci MG. Inhibition of ubiquitin/proteosome-dependent protein degradation by the Gly-Ala repeat domain of the Epstein–Barr virus nuclear antigen 1. Proc Natl Acad Sci USA 1997; 94:12616–12621.

27. Shapiro A, Imreh M, Leonchiks A, Imreh S, Masucci MG. Minimal glycine-alanine repeat prevents the interaction of ubiquinated IKB-alpha with the proteosome: a new mechanism for selective inhibition of proteolysis. Nat Med 1998; 4:939–944.

28. Cohen JI, Wang F, Mannick J, Kieff E. Epstein–Barr virus nuclear protein 2 is a key determinant of lymphocyte transformation. Proc Natl Acad Sci USA 1989; 86: 9558–9562.

29. Hammerschmidt W, Sugden B. Genetic analysis of immortalized functions of Epstein–Barr virus in human B lymphocytes. Nature 1989; 340:393–397.

30. Johannsen E, Koh E, Mosialos G, Tong X, Kieff E, Grossman S. Epstein–Barr virus nuclear protein 2 transactivation of the latent membrane protein 1 promoter is mediated by Jk and PU. 1. J Virol 1995; 64:253–262.

31. Knutson JC. The level of c-fgr RNA is increased by EBNA-2, an Epstein–Barr virus gene required for B-cell immortalization. J Virol 1990; 64:2530–2536.

32. Kaiser C, Laux G, Eick D, Jochner N, Bornkamm GW, Kempkes B. The proto-oncogene c-myc is a direct target gene of Epstein–Barr virus nuclear antigen 2. J Virol 1999; 73:4481–4484.

33. Wang F, Gregory CD, Rowe M, et al. Epstein–Barr virus nuclear antigen 2 specifically induces expression of B-cell activation antigen CD23. Proc Natl Acad Sci USA 1987; 84:3452–3456.

34. Swendeman S, Thorley-Lawson DA. The activation antigen BLAST-2, when shed, is an autocrine BCGF for normal and transformed B-cells. EMBO J 1987; 6:1637–1642.

35. Henkel T, Ling PD, Hayward SD, Peterson MG. Mediation of Epstein–Barr virus EBNA-2 transactivation by recombination signal-binding protein Jkappa. Science 1994; 265:92–95.

36. Sakai T, Taniguichi Y, Tamura K, et al. Functional replacement of the intracellular region of the Notch 1 receptor by Epstein–Barr virus nuclear antigen 2. J Virol 1998; 72:6034–6039.
37. Gordadze AV, Peng R, Tan J, et al. Notch IIC partially replaces EBNA2 function in B-cells immortalized by Epstein–Barr virus. J Virol 2001; 75:5899–5912.
38. Fuentes-Panana EM, Peng R, Brewer G, Tan J, Ling PD. Regulation of the Epstein–Barr virus C promoter by AUF1 and the cyclic AMP/protein kinase A signaling pathway. J Virol 2000; 74:8166–8175.
39. Cohen JI. A region of herpes simplex virus VP16 can substitute for a transforming domain of Epstein–Barr virus nuclear protein 2. Proc Natl Acad Sci USA 1992; 89: 8030–8034.
40. Tong X, Wang F, Thut CJ, Kieff E. The Epstein–Barr virus nuclear protein 2 acidic domain can interact with TFIIB, TAF40, and RPA70 but not with TATA-binding protein. J Virol 1995; 69:585–588.
41. Tong X, Drapkin R, Reinberg D, Kieff E. The 62- and 80-kDA subunits of transcription factor IIH mediate the interaction with Epstein–Barr virus nuclear protein 2. Proc Natl Acad Sci USA 1995; 92:3259–3263.
42. Tong X, Drapkin R, Yalamanchili R, Mosialos G, Kieff E. The Epstein–Barr virus nuclear protein 2 acidic domain forms a complex with a novel coactivator that can interact with TFIIE. Mol Cell Biol 1995; 15:4735–4744.
43. Wang L, Grossman SR, Kieff E. Epstein–Barr virus nuclear protein 2 interacts with p300, CBP, and PCAF histone acetyltransferases in activation of the LMP1 promoter. Proc Natl Acad Sci USA 2000; 97:430–435.
44. Mannick JB, Cohen JI, Birkenbach M, Marchini A, Kieff E. The Epstein–Barr virus nuclear protein encoded by the leader of the EBNA RNAs is important in B lymphocyte transformation. J Virol 1991; 65:6826–6837.
45. Harada S, Kieff E. Epstein–Barr virus nuclear protein LP stimulates EBNA-2 acidic domain-mediated transcriptional activation. J Virol 1997; 71:6611–6618.
46. Sinclair AJ, Palmero JI, Peters G, Farell PJ. EBNA-2 and EBNA-LP cooperate to cause G_0 to G_1 transition during immortalization of resting human B lymphocytes by Epstein–Barr virus. EMBO J 1994; 13:3321–3228.
47. Szekely L, Selivanova G, Magnusson KP, Klein G, Wiman KG. EBNA-5, an Epstein–Barr virus-encoded nuclear antigen, binds to the retinoblastoma and p53 proteins. Proc Natl Acad Sci USA 1993; 90:5455–5459.
48. Han I, Harada S, Weaver D, et al. EBNA-LP associates with cellular proteins including DNA-PK and HA95. J Virol 2001; 75:2475–2481.
49. Tomkinson B, Robertson E, Kieff E. Epstein–Barr virus nuclear proteins (EBNA) 3A and 3C are essential for B lymphocyte growth transformation. J Virol 1993; 67: 2014–2025.
50. Tomkinson B, Kieff E. Use of second-site homologous recombination to demonstrate that Epstein–Barr virus nuclear protein 3B is not important for lymphocyte infection or growth transformation. J Virol 1992; 66:2893–2903.
51. Robertson ES, Lin J, Kieff E. The amino-terminal domains of Epstein–Barr virus nuclear proteins 3A, 3B, and 3C interact with RBPJκ. J Virol 1996; 70:3068–3074.
52. Wang F, Gregory C, Sample C, et al. Epstein–Barr virus latent membrane protein (LMP-1) and nuclear proteins 2 and 3C are effectors of phenotypic changes in B lymphocytes: EBNA-2 and LMP-1 cooperatively induce CD23. J Virol 1990; 64: 2309–2318.
53. Allday MJ, Crawford DH, Thomas JA. Epstein–Barr virus (EBV) nuclear antigen 6 induces expression of the EBV latent membrane protein and an activated phenotype in Raji cells. J Gen Virol 1993; 74:361–369.
54. Silins SL, Sculley TB. Modulation of vimentin, the CD40 activation antigen and Burkitt's lymphoma antigen (CD77) by the Epstein–Barr virus nuclear antigen EBNA-4. Virology 1994; 202:16–24.

55. Subramanian C, Cotter MA, Robertson ES. Epstein–Barr virus nuclear protein EBNA-3C interacts with the human metastatic suppressor Nm23-HI: a molecular link to cancer metastasis. Nat Med 2001; 7:350–355.

56. Kaye KM, Izumi KM, Kieff E. Epstein–Barr virus latent membrane protein 1 is essential for B-lymphocyte growth transformation. Proc Natl Acad Sci USA 1993; 90:9150–9154.

57. Wang D, Liebowitz D, Kieff E. An EBV membrane protein expressed in immortalized lymphocytes transforms established rodent cells. Cell 1985; 43:831–840.

58. Kulwichit W, Edwards RH, Davenport EM, Baskir JF, Godfrey V, Raab-Traub N. Expression of the Epstein–Barr virus latent membrane protein 1 induces B-cell lymphoma in transgenic mice. Proc Natl Acad Sci USA 1998; 95:11963–11968.

59. Wilson JB, Weinberg W, Johnson R. Expression of the BNLF-1 oncogene of Epstein–Barr virus in the skin of transgenic mice induces hyperplasia and aberrant expression of keratin 6. Cell 1990; 61:1315–1327.

60. Higuchi M, Izumi KM, Kieff E. Epstein–Barr virus latent-infection membrane proteins are palmitoylated and raft-associated: protein 1 binds to the cytoskeleton and through TNF receptor cytoplasmic factors. Proc Natl Acad Sci USA 2001; 98:4675–4680.

61. Uchida J, Yasui T, Takaoka-Shichijo Y, et al. Mimicry of CD40 signals by Epstein–Barr virus LMP-1 in B lymphocyte responses. Science 1999; 286:300–303.

62. Mosialos G, Birkenbach M, Yalamanchili R, VanArsdale T, Ware C, Kieff E. The Epstein–Barr virus transforming protein LMP1 engages signalling proteins for the tumor necrosis factor receptor family. Cell 1995; 80:389–399.

63. Devergne O, Hatzivassiliou E, Izumi KM, et al. Association of TRAF1, TRAF2, and TRAF3 with an Epstein–Barr virus LMP1 domain important for B-lymphocyte transformation: role in NF-KB activation. Mol Cell Biol 1996; 16:7098–7108.

64. Izumi KM, Kieff ED. The Epstein–Barr virus oncogene product latent membrane protein 1 engages the tumor necrosis factor receptor-associated death domain protein to mediate B lymphocyte growth transformation and activate NF-κB. Proc Natl Acad Sci USA 1997; 94:12592–12597.

65. Izumi KM, McFarland EC, Ting AT, Riley EA, Seed B, Kieff ED. The Epstein–Barr virus oncoprotein latent membrane protein 1 engages the tumor necrosis factor-associated proteins TARDD and receptor-interacting protein (RIP), but does not induce apoptosis or require RIP for NF-κB activation. Mol Cell Biol 1999; 19:5759–5767.

66. Eliopoulos AG, Blake SMS, Floettmann JE, Rowe M, Young LS. Epstein–Barr virus-encoded latent membrane protein 1 activates the JNK pathway through its extreme C terminus via a mechanism involving TRADD and TRAF2. J Virol 1999; 73:1023–1035.

67. Eliopoulos AG, Gallagher NJ, Blake SM, Dawson CW, Young LS. Activation of the p38 mitogen-activated protein kinase pathway by Epstein–Barr virus encoded latent membrane protein 1 coregulates interleukin-6 and interleukin-8 production. J Biol Chem 1999; 274:16085–16096.

68. Hatzivassiliou E, Miller WE, Raab-Traub N, Kieff E, Mosialois G. A fusion of the EBV latent membrane protein-1 (LMP-1) transmembrane domains to the CD40 cytoplasmic domain is similar to LMP1 in constitutive activation of epidermal growth factor, nuclear factor-KB, and stress-activated protein kinase. J Immunol 1998; 60:1116–1121.

69. Gires O, Kohlhuber F, Kilger E, et al. Latent membrane protein 1 of Epstein–Barr virus interacts with JAK3 and activates STAT proteins. EMBO J 1999; 18:3064–3073.

70. Miller WE, Cheshire JL, Raab-Traub N. Interaction of tumor necrosis factor receptor-associated factor signaling proteins with the latent membrane protein 1 PXQXT motif is essential for induction of epidermal growth factor receptor expression. Mol Cell Biol 1998; 18:2835–2844.

71. Liebowitz D. Epstein–Barr virus and a cellular signaling pathway in lymphomas from immunosuppressed patients. N Engl J Med 1998; 338:1413–1421.

72. Devergne O, McFarland EC, Mosialos G, Izumi KM, Ware CF, Kieff E. Role of the TRAF binding site and NF-κB activation in Epstein–Barr virus latent membrane protein 1-induced cell gene expression. J Virol 1998; 72:7900–7908.

73. Kilger E, Kieser A, Baumann M, Hammerschmidt W. Epstein–Barr virus-mediated B-cell proliferation is dependent upon latent membrane protein 1, which stimulates an activated CD40 receptor. EMBO J 1998; 17:1700–1709.

74. Busch LK, Bishop GA. The EBV transforming protein, latent membrane protein 1, mimics and cooperates with CD40 signaling in B lymphocytes. J Immunol 1999; 162: 2555–2561.

75. Yoshizaki T, Sato H, Furukawa M, Pagano JS. The expression of matrix metalloproteinase 9 is enhanced by Epstein–Barr virus latent membrane protein 1. Proc Natl Acad Sci USA 1998; 95:3621–3626.

76. Dawson CW, Rickinson AB, Young LS. Epstein–Barr virus latent membrane protein inhibits human epithelial cell differentiation. Nature 1990; 344:777–780.

77. Fahraeus R, Rymo L, Rhim KS, Klein G. Morphologic transformation of human keratinocytes expressing the LMP gene of Epstein–Barr virus. Nature 1990; 345: 447–449.

78. Sandberg ML, Kaykas A, Sugden B. Latent membrane protein 1 of Epstein–Barr virus inhibits as well as stimulates gene expression. J Virol 2000; 74:9755–9761.

79. Adler B, Schaadt E, Kempkes B, Zimber-Strobl U, Baier B, Bornkamm GW. Control of Epstein–Barr virus reactivation by activated CD40 and viral latent membrane protein 1. Proc Natl Acad Sci USA 2002; 99:437–442.

80. Fries KL, Miller WE, Raab-Traub N. Epstein–Barr virus latent membrane protein 1 blocks p53-mediated apoptosis through the induction of the A20 gene. J Virol 1996; 70:8653–8659.

81. Wang S, Rowe M, Lundgren E. Expression of the Epstein–Barr virus transforming protein LMP1 causes a rapid and transient stimulation of the bcl-2 homologue Mcl-1 levels in B-cell lines. Cancer Res 1997; 56:4610–4613.

82. Henderson S, Rowe M, Gregory CD, et al. Induction of bcl-2 expression by Epstein–Barr virus latent membrane protein 1 protects infected B-cells from programmed cell death. Cell 1991; 65:1107–1115.

83. D'Souza B, Rowe M, Walls D. The bfl-1 gene is transcriptionally upregulated by the Epstein–Barr virus LMP1, and its expression promotes the survival of a Burkitt's lymphoma cell line. J Virol 2000; 74:6652–6658.

84. Kawanishi M. Expression of Epstein–Barr virus latent membrane protein 1 protects Jurkat T-cells from apoptosis induced by serum deprivation. Virology 1997; 228: 244–250.

85. Dykstra ML, Longnecker R, Pierce SK. Epstein–Barr virus targets lipid rafts to block the signaling and antigen trafficking function of the BCR. Immunity 2001; 14:57–67.

86. Longnecker R, Miller CL, Tomkinson B, Miao XQ, Kieff E. Deletion of DNA encoding the first five transmembrane domains of Epstein–Barr virus latent membrane proteins 2A and 2B. J Virol 1993; 67:5068–5074.

87. Miller CL, Burkhardt AL, Lee JH, Stealey B, Longnecker R. Integral membrane protein 2 of Epstein–Barr virus regulates reactivation from latency through dominant negative effects on protein-tyrosine kinases. Immunity 1995; 2:155–166.

88. Miller CL, Lee JH, Kieff E, Longnecker R. An integral membrane protein (LMP2) blocks reactivation of Epstein–Barr virus from latency following surface immunoglobulin crosslinking. Proc Natl Acad Sci USA 1994; 91:772–776.

89. Miller CL, Longnecker R, Kieff E. Epstein–Barr virus latent membrane 2A blocks calcium mobilization in B lymphocytes. J Virol 1993; 67:3087–3094.

90. Caldwell RG, Wilson JB, Anderson SJ, Longnecker R. Epstein–Barr virus LMP2A drives B-cell development and survival in the absence of normal B-cell receptor signals. Immunity 1998; 9:405–411.

91. Scholle F, Bendt KM, Raab-Traub N. Epstein–Barr virus LMP2A transforms epithelial cells, inhibits cell differentiation, and activates Akt. J Virol 2000; 74:10681–10689.

92. Swaminathan S, Hesselton R, Sullivan J, Kieff E. Epstein–Barr virus recombinants with specifically mutated BCRF1 genes. J Virol 1993; 67:7406–7413.

93. Komano J, Maruo S, Kurozumi K, Oda T, Takada K. Oncogenic role of Epstein–Barr virus-encoded RNAs in Burkitt's lymphoma cell line Akata. J Virol 1999; 73: 9827–9831.

94. Kitagawa N, Goto M, Kurozumi K, et al. Epstein–Barr virus-encoded poly(A)(-) RNA supports Burkitt's lymphoma growth through interleukin-10 induction. EMBO J 2000; 19:6742–6750.

95. Sharp TV, Raine DA, Gewert DR, Joshi B, Jagus R, Clemens MJ. Activation of the interferon-inducible (2′-5′) oligoadenylate synthetase by the Epstein–Barr virus RNA, EBER-1. Virology 1999; 257:303–313.

96. Clarke PA, Schwemmle M, Schickinger J, Hilse K, Clemens MJ. Binding of the Epstein–Barr virus small RNA EBER-1 to double-stranded RNA-activated protein kinase. Nucleic Acids Res 1991; 19:243–248.

97. Clarke PA, Sharp NA, Clemens MJ. Translational control by the Epstein–Barr virus small RNA EBER-1. Reversal of the double stranded RNA-induced inhibition of protein synthesis in reticulocyte lysates. Eur J Biochem 1990; 193:635–641.

98. Swaminathan S, Huneycutt BS, Reiss CS, Kieff E. Epstein–Barr virus-encoded small RNAs (EBERs) do not modulate interferon effects in infected lymphocytes. J Virol 1992; 66:5133–5136.

99. Lerner MR, Andrews NC, Miller G, Steitz J. Two small RNAs encoded by Epstein–Barr virus and complexed with protein are precipitated by antibodies from patients with systemic lupus erythematosus. Proc Natl Acad Sci USA 1981; 78:805–809.

100. Toczyski DP, Steitz JA. EAP, a highly conserved cellular protein associated with Epstein–Barr virus small RNAs (EBERs). EMBO J 1991; 10:459–466.

101. Smith PR, deJesus O, Turner D, et al. Structure and coding content of CST (BART) family RNAs of Epstein–Barr virus. J Virol 2000; 74:3082–3092.

102. Kienzle N, Buck M, Greco S, Krauer K, Sculley TB. Epstein–Barr virus-encoded RK-BARK protein expression. J Virol 1999; 73:8902–8906.

103. Gilligan KJ, Rajadurai P, Lin J-C, et al. Expression of the Epstein–Barr virus BamHI A fragments in nasopharyngeal carcinoma: evidence for a viral protein expressed in vivo. J Virol 1991; 65:6252–6259.

104. Kusano S, Raab-Traub N. An Epstein–Barr virus protein interacts with Notch. J Virol 2001; 75:385–395.

105. Zhang J, Chen H, Weinmaster G, Hayward SD. Epstein–Barr virus BamHI—a rightward transcript-encoded RPMS protein interacts with the CBF1-associated corepressor CIR to negatively regulate the activity of EBNA2 and NotchIC. J Virol 2001; 75:2946–2956.

106. Chevallier-Greco A, Manet E, Chavrier P, Mosnier C, Daillie J, Sergeant A. Both Epstein–Barr virus (EBV)-encoded trans-acting factors, EB1 and EB2, are required to activate transcription from an EBV early promoter. EMBO J 1986; 5:3243–3249.

107. Feederle R, Kost M, Baumann M, et al. The Epstein–Barr virus lytic program is controlled by the co-operative functions of two transactivators. EMBO J 2000; 19: 3080–3089.

108. Sinclair AJ, Brimmell M, Farrell PJ. Reciprocal antagonism of steroid hormones and BZLF1 in switch between Epstein–Barr virus latent and productive cycle gene expression. J Virol 1992; 66:70–77.

109. Gutsch DE, Holley-Guthrie EA, Zhang Q, et al. The bZIP transactivator of Epstein–Barr virus, BZLF1, functionally and physically interacts with the p65 subunit of NF-κB. Mol Cell Biol 1994; 14:1939–1948.

110. Zhang Q, Gutsch D, Kenney S. Functional and physical interaction between p53 and BZLF1: implications for Epstein–Barr virus latency. Mol Cell Biol 1994; 14:1938–1939.

111. Morrison TE, Mauser A, Wong A, Ting JP-Y, Kenney SC. Inhibition of interferon-gamma signaling by an Epstein–Barr virus immediate-early protein. Immunity 2001; 15:787–799.

112. Fixman ED, Hayward GS, Hayward SD. Trans-acting requirements for replication of Epstein–Barr virus ori-lyt. J Virol 1992; 66:5030–5039.

113. Henderson S, Huen D, Rowe M, Dawson C, Johnson G, Rickinson A. Epstein–Barr virus-coded BHRF1 protein, a viral homolog of bcl-2, protects human B-cells from programmed cell death. Proc Natl Acad Sci USA 1993; 90:8479–8483.

114. Dawson CW, Dawson J, Jones R, Ward K, Young LS. Functional differences between BHRF1, the Epstein–Barr virus-encoded bcl-2 homologue, and bcl-2 in human epithelial cells. J Virol 1998; 72:9016–9024.

115. Bellows DS, Howell M, Pearson C, Hazlewood SA, Hardwick JM. Epstein–Barr virus BALF1 is a BCL-2 like antagonist of the herpes virus antiapoptotic BCL-2 proteins. J Virol 2002; 76:2469–2479.

116. Strockbine LD, Cohen JI, Farrah T, et al. The Epstein–Barr virus BARF1 gene encodes a novel soluble CSF-1 receptor. J Virol 1998; 72:4015–4021.

117. Cohen JI, Lekstrom K. Epstein–Barr virus BARF1 protein is dispensable for B-cell transformation and inhibits alpha interferon secretion from mononuclear cells. J Virol 1999; 73:7627–7632.

118. Ruvolvo V, Wang E, Boyle S, Swaminathan S. The Epstein–Barr virus nuclear protein SM is both a post-translational inhibitor and activator of gene expression. Proc Natl Acad Sci USA 1998; 95:8852–8857.

119. Janz A, Oezel M, Kurzeder C, et al. Infectious Epstein–Barr virus lacking major glycoprotein BLLF1 (gp350/gp220) demonstrates the existence of additional viral ligands. J Virol 2000; 74:10,142–10,152.

120. Jackman WT, Mann KA, Hoffmann HJ, Spaete RR. Expression of Epstein–Barr virus gp350 as a single chain glycoprotein for EBV subunit vaccine. Vaccine 1999; 17:660–668.

121. Miller N, Hutt-Fletcher LM. A monoclonal antibody to glycoprotein gp85 inhibits fusion but not attachment of Epstein–Barr virus. J Virol 1998; 62:2366–2372.

122. Molesworth SJ, Lake CM, Borza CM, Turk SM, Hutt-Fletcher LM. Epstein–Barr virus gH is essential for penetration of B-cells but also plays a role in attachment of virus to epithelial cells. J Virol 2000; 74:6324–6332.

123. Oda T, Imai S, Chiba S, Takada K. Epstein–Barr virus lacking glycoprotein 85 cannot infect B-cells and epithelial cells. Virology 2000; 276:52–58.

124. Yaswen LR, Stephens EB, Davenport LC, Hutt-Fletcher LM. Epstein–Barr virus glycoprotein gp85 associates with the BKRF2 gene product and is incompletely processed as a recombinant protein. Virology 1993; 195:387–396.

125. Spriggs MK, Armitage RJ, Comeau MR, et al. The extracellular domain of the Epstein–Barr virus BZLF2 protein binds the HLA-DR beta chain and inhibits antigen presentation. J Virol 1996; 70:5557–5563.

126. Wang X, Kenyon WJ, Li Q, Mullberg J, Hutt-Fletcher LM. Epstein–Barr virus uses different complexes of glycoproteins gH and gL to infect B lymphocytes and epithelial cells. J Virol 1998; 72:5552–5558.

127. Lake CM, Hutt-Fletcher LM. Epstein–Barr virus that lacks glycoprotein gN is impaired in assembly and infection. J Virol 2000; 74:11,162–11,172.

128. Moore KW, Vieira P, Fiorentnio DF, Trounstine ML, Khan TA, Mosmann TR. Homology of cytokine synthesis inhibitory factor (IL-10) to the Epstein–Barr virus gene BCRF1. Science 1990; 248:1230–1234.

129. Hsu D-H, de Waal Malefyt R, Fiorentino DF, et al. Expression of interleukin-10 activity by Epstein–Barr virus protein BCRF1. Science 1990; 250:830–832.

130. Miyazaki I, Cheung RK, Dosch H-M. Viral interleukin 10 is critical for the induction of B-cell growth transformation by Epstein–Barr virus. J Exp Med 1993; 178:439–447.

131. Takayama T, Nishioka Y, Lu L, Lotze MT, Tahara H, Thomson AW. Retroviral delivery of viral interleukin-10 into myeloid dendritic cells markedly inhibits their allostimulatory activity and promotes the induction of T-cell hyporesponsiveness. Transplantation 1998; 66:1567–1574.

3

Epidemiology of Primary Epstein–Barr Virus Infection and Infectious Mononucleosis

Warren A. Andiman

Departments of Pediatrics, Epidemiology, and Public Health,
Yale University School of Medicine, New Haven, Connecticut, U.S.A.

INTRODUCTION

The Epstein–Barr virus (EBV) is a ubiquitous pathogen. It causes infection throughout the world in all populations. In general, the younger the age at which the primary infection occurs, the more likely it is to be mild and clinically insignificant. In many developing countries, almost all infections caused by EBV occur early in life and are either unaccompanied by symptoms or associated with only minor, nonspecific illnesses, such as low-grade fever or sore throat. In the more industrialized countries of the world in which substantial portions of the population enjoy higher socioeconomic status, primary infection is often delayed until adolescence or early adulthood. Among older adolescents and adults, significant numbers of individuals become ill during infection, which often takes the form of classic, heterophile antibody–positive infectious mononucleosis (IM).

EBV infections are not highly contagious, certainly significantly less so than influenza, measles, or chicken pox; intimate contact is necessary for transmission to occur. It is usually not possible to trace the links among sequential cases. Asymptomatic virus shedders, individuals experiencing either a primary infection or a recurrence, are the major sources of infection in the community. Saliva and oropharyngeal secretions represent the principal vehicles responsible for transmission of infection from person-to-person. Rarely, infection is transmitted by blood transfusion.

SOURCES OF EPIDEMIOLOGIC DATA

Morbidity and Mortality Associated with IM

Data concerning the epidemiology of IM are obtained almost entirely from special research projects that have focused on particular and well-circumscribed populations, such as college health services, community health care providers, military populations, and laboratories serving these communities. Prevalence and incidence data, when analyzed in toto, provide a generally clear portrait of the manifestations of IM in the population at large. However, some of the data are no doubt flawed as a result of questions about "the numerator," i.e., how well the strict diagnostic criteria for IM are actually met among reported cases, and about "the denominator," i.e., how well the groups of persons being surveyed are a true reflection of much larger population tracts. Information suggesting that clinical case reports, at least in the past, were frequently incorrect is available from a study in which as many as one-third of the serum samples from patients believed to have IM, and sent to a state laboratory for heterophile antibody tests, were negative (1).

In most countries and in most states in the United States, IM is not a reportable disease. Exceptions are the State of Connecticut, where the disease had been reportable for a number of decades (but is no longer a reportable disease), and the U.S. Armed Forces, but from data collected only on hospitalized cases. Furthermore, because IM is so rarely fatal, a comprehensive analysis of the mortality associated with the disease has not been undertaken. A review of fatal complications of IM was published by Evans in 1967 (2).

Serologic Surveys

Before 1968, the heterophile antibody test was the sole serologic tool available for confirming the diagnosis of the acute infection, especially in its incarnation as classical IM. However, the heterophile antibody response is transient and primarily comprises immunoglobulins of the immunoglobulin M (IgM) class. Furthermore, heterophile antibody is much less commonly present in younger children with atypical forms of the disease. Hence, heterophile antibody testing is only useful for providing incidence (not prevalence) data concerning the more classical infection as it occurs in adolescents and young adults, and usually only in the course of prospective studies. The test has great specificity if performed well, utilizing differential absorptions and preserved horse erythrocytes or beef hemolysins. In the past three decades, the heterophile antibody test has been frequently adapted for use in physicians' offices and clinics in the form of various rapid "spot" tests. There is often little quality control in the use of such tests. In addition, the use of office-based rapid tests has resulted in much less frequent confirmatory testing by state or reference laboratories. Therefore, an increasing dearth of data are being collected from specialized laboratories in which quality control is significantly better.

The discovery in 1968 that EBV was the etiologic agent of IM heralded an era in which viral-specific antigen tests could be used for diagnosis of IM, as well as for those subclinical or atypical primary infections that are also caused by EBV. Because IgG antibody persists for years, serosurveys based exclusively on the presence of IgG antibody to viral capsid antigen (VCA) in blood samples describe accurately the overall prevalence of EBV infections in various age groups and populations. In time, other viral-specific antigens were discovered, including early antigen (EA) and EBV nuclear antigen (EBNA). When measured in combination with one another, antibody responses to these antigens have allowed epidemiologists to more accurately establish the relationship between atypical forms of mononucleosis and EBV and to define the prevalence in given populations of current, recent, or past infection. Tests for measuring IgM antibody responses to VCA and antibodies to EBNA (or various components thereof) have helped greatly in this regard.

The seroepidemiologic studies that have yielded the greatest insights into the incidence of EBV infection and the diseases associated with EBV have been those that have focused on defined populations followed over time. Sera collected at baseline establish the number of subjects who are either susceptible or immune at the study's onset. Antibody measurements made during the course of such studies help to define the incidence of infection. When such serologic measurements are combined with careful descriptions of intercurrent illnesses, it becomes possible to delineate more clearly the spectrum of clinical events and syndromes associated with seroconversion to the virus. Such studies have proven that many seroconversion events are associated with only minor illnesses, especially in younger children, and that even among adolescents, primary EBV infection is accompanied by classical manifestations of IM in only about 50% of instances.

Contribution of Virus Isolation Techniques to Epidemiologic Studies

The transformation assay, which is the basis of the diagnostic method for detecting infectious EBV in blood or body secretions, is labor intensive and tedious. Therefore, it has not been used extensively in large epidemiologic studies. Nevertheless, the unusual capacity of EBV to transform quiescent human umbilical cord lymphocyte into rapidly growing clumps of cells that can be subcultured indefinitely ("immortalized") has been used as a research method. It has been used in well-circumscribed, smaller studies that were designed to explore in detail aspects of person-to-person transmission, patterns of oropharyngeal excretion and reactivation in both normal and specialized hosts (e.g., patients who are either naturally or iatrogenically immunosuppressed or patients with autoimmune diseases), and viral persistence in blood and lymphoid tissues.

DESCRIPTIVE EPIDEMIOLOGY

Prevalence and Incidence: Primary Infection

Measuring antibody to the VCA of EBV is the principal method by which the prevalence of infection has been assessed in populations throughout the world (3). In developing countries, many of which are tropical, the great majority of children ($\geq 75\%$) between the ages of four and six years have antibodies to VCA in the blood, demonstrating that they have previously been infected. Because antibody to VCA is, for all intents and purposes, a marker of lifelong immunity, recurrent or recrudescent infections due to EBV do not occur in these groups and IM is virtually unknown as a clinical entity. Conversely, in the countries of Western Europe and in the United States, only 30% to 50% of children in the early school age years have antibodies to VCA. However, within these countries, acquisition of infection occurs at higher rates in certain specific childhood populations. For example, a study was conducted by Chang et al. (4) in a Washington, D.C., "nursery" that provided domiciliary care for children who were temporary wards of the state. The nursery housed approximately 50 children, of ages 6 months to 35 months, and was considered crowded but sanitary. Of the 115 children tested for EBV antibody on admission, 37% were seropositive, and 63% of those who were initially seronegative seroconverted prior to discharge. The proportion of EBV seropositive children increased from 19% at the age of six months to 68% at the age of 19 to 24 months, an overall seroconversion rate of 9% per month. These rates are as high as those observed in many nonindustrialized countries of the world. The only identifiable variable that correlated significantly with EBV seroconversion was the duration of time the children remained in the nursery. Children residing in the nursery for up to 4.4 months and children residing at home for an equal length of time had similar seroconversion rates, but for children residing in the nursery for up to 7.4 months, the seroconversion rates were considerably higher. Neither the age of the children and their sex nor the season of the year appeared to influence the rate of seroconversion. Another study performed prospectively in an orphanage in Chicago showed similar rates of seroconversion, but it took as long as a year for the pace of seroconversion in the institutionalized child nursery to increase (5). Too little is known about the orphanage environment to explain these differences.

Serosurveys of antibody prevalence to VCA have also been performed among young adults in many parts of the world; military recruits and college students have been the groups most commonly studied. Among young soldiers in parts of South America and the United States and among some groups of college freshmen in Asia, over 80% of subjects were found to have been previously infected. In the undergraduate and first-year medical students of the University of the Philippines, antibody prevalence rates hovered around 75% (6). In contrast, among young college students in the United States, New Zealand, and England, EBV antibody prevalence ranged from 26% to 64%. Similarly, in a large survey undertaken in English colleges and universities in 1969, antibodies to EBV were present in 57% of serum samples from freshmen (7,8). Depending on location, such data indicate that approximately one-third to three-quarters of these students were susceptible to primary infection at the time they entered college; it also means that many such students were liable to develop IM. In some college surveys, the broadening of admission criteria in the late 1960s and early 1970s to permit the matriculation of young adults from a greater variety of minority and socioeconomic groups was reflected in a greater proportion of EBV seropositives in the freshman classes of such schools.

Among adults in England and Scandinavia who reach the middle years, approximately 85% are seropositive (9–11). In contrast, only 60% to 65% of similarly aged adults in Melbourne, Australia, were found to be seropositive (9). The authors of the Australian study attributed these lower rates to the lower population densities found in Australia compared to those in other industrialized countries. Even in the large cities of Australia, a greater predominance of single-unit dwellings over tenements and flats, the absence of the extremes of poverty and overcrowding, and the much greater frequency of outdoor activities for much of the year may account for these differences in the prevalence rate.

Prevalence and Incidence: IM

In most countries and in most states in the United States, IM is not a reportable disease. Nevertheless, a number of attempts have been made to quantify disease rates in a few "open" populations in the United States and Western Europe. In the decades prior to 1975, recorded incidence rates were 45, 48, 60, and 200 cases per 100,000 populations per year in Atlanta, Georgia; Connecticut; Denmark; and Olmstead County, Minnesota (which includes the Mayo Clinic), respectively (12–14). In the 15- to 19-year-old age group in metropolitan Atlanta, Georgia, a rate of 345 cases per 100,000 per year was ascertained (15). However, the rate of IM in blacks was only one-thirtieth as high as in whites. During periods when active surveillance was undertaken, sometimes in combination with simplified reporting forms, the rate of IM in Connecticut increased to as many as 70 cases per 100,000 persons per year.

A comprehensive population-based study was performed in Rochester, Minnesota, over a period of two decades (1950–1969) (16). A unique data resource made it possible to review all diagnosed cases of IM. Although the total number of "recorded cases" during the 20 years was 1818, only 776 met the combined criteria of residency, clinical features, reactive heterophile antibody, and peripheral lymphocytosis. Thus, the number of "diagnosed cases" or "reported cases" was approximately twice as high as the average annual incidence of "accepted" cases—99 per 100,000 persons. The higher incidence rates reported from Rochester, Minnesota, when compared to other sites probably reflect better ascertainment as well as a population which, in the years of the study, was almost entirely white and of relatively high socioeconomic status. In both males and females, the highest incidence occurred among persons aged 16 to 19 years. Few cases occurred below the age of five years or above the age of 35 years. No seasonal pattern was ascertained. Contact of a patient with another known case was reported in only a handful of cases. More specifically, in 769 of the 772 families involved, only a single case of IM occurred prior to the reported case. All four secondary cases (one intrafamilial and three extrafamilial) were diagnosed within 10 weeks of the index case.

The Centers for Disease Control and Prevention has undertaken surveys of the incidence of IM in colleges in the United States. Such surveys produced incidence rates as high as 840 cases per 100,000 students in the years 1971 and 1972 (17).

Occurrence of Mononucleosis in Special Settings

Colleges and Universities

IM is a prominent and commonly observed disease on the college campus. In some studies, IM is second only to acute respiratory diseases as a cause of admission to the infirmary (18). The most complete and informative studies of the epidemiology, incidence, and clinical manifestations of mononucleosis are those derived from surveys and prospective analyses conducted at schools of higher learning in the United States and Western Europe. Studies of these kinds benefit from the careful clinical records kept by many student health services of a population that is nonmobile ("captive") for most of the year and an age group that reflects the peak incidence of the disease.

During the late 1960s and early 1970s, a system of IM case surveillance was established in nearly a score of American colleges and universities by the American College Health Association and the Centers for Disease Control and Prevention (19). The number of undergraduates at the various schools ranged from small ($N = 743$) to large ($N = 32{,}277$). Specific inclusion criteria were stipulated to define cases. During the 1969 to 1970 academic year, an overall incidence of 1112 cases per 100,000 students (range: 110–2235 per 100,000) per school year was reported. This rate was approximately three times higher than that found in similar age groups in the general population. Rates for blacks were less than one-tenth that for whites. As in other studies, no definite seasonal pattern was discovered, although the number of cases declined at the time of school breaks and holidays. No rebound of cases following school breaks was discovered as had been described in the classic studies by Hoagland (20). Also, less than 15% of patients gave a history of contact with other IM cases. However, among all patients who did report contact with a known case, acquisition of infection from roommates was much less frequent than that from "dates" or close friends. Attack rates for each academic class could be calculated for most of the 19 schools included in the study: overall, incidence declined from approximately 1600 cases per 100,000 freshmen to 750 cases per 100,000 seniors, undoubtedly reflecting an ever-diminishing pool of susceptibles among each successive class of students. Incidence rates in females exceeded that in the males among freshmen and sophomores, but were lower among juniors and seniors.

The most well-executed prospective study to examine the incidence of inapparent and apparent infection (including IM) in college students was performed at Yale University by Niederman et al. (6) between 1958 and 1968. Baseline serum specimens and histories of past infection were obtained from all entering students over a five-year period. Subsequently, acute and convalescent phase sera were obtained from many students when diseases consistent with IM developed. Matched blood specimens were also obtained from 150 students four to eight years after the first (freshman) sample was taken. Only 2 of the 150 students had a history of IM before they entered Yale; both had antibodies to EBV-VCA and they neither developed IM while in college nor had changes in their antibody titers. Of the 150 students, 34% had antibodies to VCA at the time of the baseline blood-draw despite having a history negative for IM; all retained antibody reactivity and none developed IM. The remaining 65% of the students ($N = 97$) were both seronegative and had no history of IM. During the next four to eight years, 28 of these students experienced clinically apparent IM associated with elevations of both heterophile and EBV-specific antibody; 15 other subjects seroconverted without signs or symptoms of IM. Hence, in these college students, the ratio of apparent to unapparent infection was approximately 2:1. The total incidence of primary EBV infection in the course of college life was 44%, or approximately 11% per year, and the prevalence of EBV capsid antibody reactivity rose from 35% at 17 to 18 years of age to 64% at four to eight years later. A progressive yearly increase in the number of cases was noted during the four years of college life; four additional cases occurred after graduation. A clinical attack rate of 4.4 per 100 person-years of life occurred in 365 EBV antibody–negative students, whereas no cases developed in 147 EBV antibody–positive students. In general, antibody levels were well maintained during this period; over 75% whose sera were examined one to four years following apparent illness maintained titers of VCA antibody of 1:40 or greater, and none lost detectable antibody. Students who experienced subclinical primary infections also maintained VCA antibody responses throughout the period of follow-up. This study proved incontrovertibly that antibody to EBV is consistently absent before IM, regularly appears in the course of the illness, and persists for years after both clinical and subclinical infections. EBV infections have a spectrum of biologic expression that range from unapparent to clinically overt and classical. The ratio between overt and unapparent disease is conditioned by geography, socioeconomic condition, and the age at which the primary infection occurs.

A study similar to the one performed at Yale was conducted over a period of four years in a single class at the United States Military Academy at West Point (7). In the freshman class of 1401 cadets that matriculated in July 1969, 64% had antibody to EBV-VCA on entry and 36% lacked such antibody. The rate of antibody prevalence varied in relation to the geographic area within the United States from which the cadet originated—those from the west, north central, and New England states had an antibody prevalence of about 50% whereas those from the west, south central, and east south central states had an antibody prevalence that exceeded 75%. Antibody prevalence also varied with economic status, with rates averaging 77% in cadets from families with incomes under $6000, in contrast to rates of 59% in cadets from families with incomes above $30,000.

Among the 890 cadets who had antibody on entering the Academy, none developed IM during college (of these, only 5.6% had a prior history of IM). Among 437 cadets without antibody on entry, 54 (12.4%) seroconverted (were infected) in the freshman year—27 had illnesses compatible with or highly suggestive of IM and 39 had no IM-like illness. These data are similar to those obtained at Yale. The calculated annual infection rates were somewhat higher than that observed at Yale, ranging from 15 to 31 infections per 100 susceptibles per year. Overall, the incidence of EBV infection was 46% over the four-year period (201 infections in 437 cadets). Of these, only 26% had heterophile-positive clinical IM, a proportion smaller than that observed at Yale. As had been observed in multiple other studies, the EBV infection rate among exposed and susceptible roommates was no higher than in susceptible roommates not similarly exposed. No clustering in particular dormitory or military units was apparent.

Viewed in toto, the prospective college studies all support the concept that EBV is the sole cause of heterophile-positive IM and that in young adults, IM is the predominant and most widely recognized host response to primary infection. The presence of antibody to EBV is the most predictable measure of immunity (or susceptibility) to infection. None of the students who had antibody at the time of entering college acquire IM. In all studies, the rate of infection in the freshman year has been remarkably similar, ranging around 12% to 13% per year. The studies differ in their findings regarding the ratio of apparent to unapparent infection—these ratios have ranged from 3:1 to 1:3. These differences may reflect the rate at which students seek medical care, differences in the intensity of clinical surveillance, or unknown population-specific host factors. The consistent lack of evidence for the spread among roommates, in light of the known intermittent presence of EBV in oropharyngeal secretions of many immune individuals, supports strongly the thesis that the virus is not casually transmitted and requires intense exposure to virus-laden body fluids.

IM in the Armed Forces

IM is not generally regarded as a characteristic disease of the new military recruit, among which are commonly included diseases caused by *Neisseria meningitidis*, adenoviruses, influenza virus, and *Mycoplasma pneumoniae*. Nevertheless, IM does occur and at rates about three times higher than in the general population. Data made available from surveys undertaken in the Army, Navy, and Air Force in the 1950s and 1960s indicate that 140 to 228 IM-associated hospital admissions occur per 100,000 persons per year (21). During these decades, the rates were remarkably steady from year to year. For reasons not explained, the rates were higher still among U.S. Army personnel based in the Pacific and Far East, when compared to those at home, in Alaska, or in Europe (21). In the Marine Corps, IM ranked behind acute upper respiratory diseases, cellulitis and abscesses, pneumonia, and rubella (in the late 1960s) as the fifth most common diagnosis reported on "sick lists." IM was also a major cause of "lost time," principally because of the need for hospitalization. Among infections reported in Air Force personnel between 1966 and 1970, IM ranked behind streptococcal infections (including scarlet fever) and rubella and ahead of mumps and "infectious hepatitis" as the third most common infectious disease, with an incidence of 178 cases per 100,000 persons per year.

Geographic and Temporal Distribution

Infection with EBV as assessed by measurements of antibody to the capsid antigen of the virus has been detected in all parts of the world, including remote areas of Brazil and Alaska (5,22).

Clinical IM occurs most often in those countries where exposure to the virus is delayed until adolescence and young adulthood. The nations where this epidemiologic phenomenon has been most notably expressed include the countries of Western Europe, Canada, the United States, New Zealand, and Australia. In contrast, IM is rarely seen in the developing and nonindustrialized countries of the world. For example, one study conducted at the University of the Philippines in the late 1960s revealed a very high prevalence of pre-existing antibody to EBV, which was associated with a complete absence of cases of IM among thousands of admissions of students to the college infirmary. As noted previously, the prevalence of VCA antibody also varied significantly among freshman cadets entering the U.S. Military Academy, depending on the part of the country from which the student originated (7).

There is no evidence of temporal fluctuations in the incidence either of asymptomatic primary infections caused by EBV or of IM. No changes in the incidence of IM could be ascertained either at Yale University between the years 1963 and 1967 or in a population-based study in the midwestern United States conducted over a 20-year period. However results from two studies have shown rises in incidence over periods varying from two to three decades during the mid-part of the 20th century. A Swedish study showed a nearly 10-fold increase in hospitalizations with IM over approximately 20 years (23). A study from Connecticut also demonstrated a slightly greater than 10-fold increase, from 3.9 cases to 46.7 cases per 100,000 persons (13). It is likely that such increases reflect a combination of better reporting and the use of more accurate diagnostic criteria. Unfortunately, the Swedish study did not present data (the "denominator") regarding the total number of hospitalizations per year.

A number of studies conducted in the United States have come to different conclusions regarding a seasonal or annual peak in cases of IM. Early studies of students at the University of Wisconsin and at West Point showed yearly peaks in February, four to six weeks after the winter break (18,24). It was hypothesized that these cases occurred at the end of the known incubation period of IM, exposure having occurred during winter break when more avid exchange of saliva among good friends would likely have taken place. A report from Atlanta showed a smaller peak in early fall and a large one in late winter to early spring; no explanation for these peaks was presented (15). No seasonal peaks were reported from a surveillance study of 19 colleges and universities (17) or from the longitudinal study undertaken in Rochester, Minnesota (16).

Socioeconomic Status, Gender, and Race

EBV infections occur in all ethnic groups without evidence of explainable differences in antibody prevalence among those from varying genetic or cultural origins. Although one study in Hawaii reported higher prevalence rates among native Hawaiians and Filipinos than among whites of the same age, it was reasoned that levels of hygiene, socioeconomic status, and a host of disparate cultural and domestic practices could not be separated from the facts of pure ethnicity.

In most studies it has been difficult to separate the effects of race and socioeconomic status on the prevalence of infection or the incidence of IM. Although the incidence of IM among whites in Atlanta, Georgia, was approximately 30 times higher than among blacks, this is now known to reflect the earlier acquisition of the primary infection among African Americans rather than any differential susceptibility for developing the disease (15). These differences in rates of antibody prevalence have also been noted at West Point where positive serostatus among blacks was higher (85%) than that observed in Caucasians (65%) (7).

In studies of antibody prevalence in large populations, no differences have been found when females are compared to males. A few studies suggest that girls develop IM at a somewhat younger age (about 16 years) when compared to boys (about 18 years) (15,16).

Age

Primary infection occurs much earlier in life in the poorer and less industrialized countries of the world than in the more affluent and more industrialized countries. Within industrialized nations, primary infection occurs at an earlier age among those in the more socioeconomically compromised sectors of society than in the more upwardly mobile and wealthy sectors.

When age-specific antibody acquisition to EBV was examined by Evans (3) and by Jennings (25), there were striking differences among three of the populations studied. At the age of four years, antibody prevalence was approximately 20%, 45%, and 80% among children in Connecticut, Hawaii, and Barbados, respectively. By the age of 10 years, the prevalence rates had risen to 58%, 65%, and 90%, respectively, in the same three populations. In two prospective studies done in Ghana by Biggar et al. over 80% of toddlers had acquired antibody before their second birthdays and none developed signs of IM later (26,27).

IM has a peak incidence in the age group 15 to 25 years. Data on incidence of IM have been garnered from surveys of hospitalized patients in Western Europe and the United States (15,28,29) and from reports prepared by state public health laboratories (1,30,31). Information collected from the Wisconsin State Laboratory revealed rates of approximately 300 cases of IM per 100,000 persons in the age group 15 to 19 years and half that number of cases in the age group 20 to 24 years. Only several dozen cases occurred in the age group of five to nine years, and less than five cases in the age group zero to four years. When the peak age frequencies of positive heterophile tests are recorded, only about 10% of positive reactions occur in serum samples obtained from five- to nine-year-old children and about 6% from those in the age group 65 to 69 years.

The entire spectrum of ages at which one is likely to encounter true cases of IM and bonafide positive heterophile antibody reactions is shifted downward in developing countries. For example, in one study from Brazil, the average age at which heterophile-positive cases of IM was encountered was about 13 years; the oldest case was 15 years (32).

EBV Infections in Childhood

Numerous children from poor environments are known to acquire antibodies to EBV at an early age. Such children rarely develop classical IM in association with their early seroconversion events and they fail to develop the disease later in life, at a time when their more advantaged peers traditionally show signs of the disease. These observations have led investigators to attempt to answer a number of questions concerning early childhood infection: (i) Are early antibody conversions associated with specific illnesses? (ii) How early in life might some seroconversion events occur? (iii) How durable and protective are the antibodies that develop early in life? (iv) How readily and by what means do early infections spread within families? Answers to the first and fourth questions can only be obtained successfully in the context of prospective, longitudinal cohort studies.

Using serum specimens and detailed clinical data collected over a number of years as part of the Cleveland Family Study, Gertrude and Werner Henle observed that none of the early, primary EBV infections ascertained by seroconversion was accompanied by obvious signs and symptoms suggestive of a diagnosis of IM (33). It was further determined that among the frequent occurrences of nonbacterial tonsillitis and pharyngitis in children aged three to five years, EBV accounts for no more than approximately 2% of cases. Thus, most EBV infections in childhood remain silent or are accompanied, at most, by mild discomfort of the throat or upper respiratory tract. It appeared from this dataset that primary EBV infections occur mainly during two periods, either under the age of six years or over the age of 10 years. Because many of the children in this study came from the higher socioeconomic strata, they escaped infection in the first decade of life and sometimes longer. Further analysis of the data derived from the Cleveland Family Study reaffirmed that, following primary infection, antibodies to EBV tend to persist at readily detectable and nearly constant levels for as long as 14 years. Whether the durability of the antibody responses could be accounted for, in some instances, by superinfections or recrudescent infections could not be determined. Finally, limited data indicated that introduction of the virus into a family generally did not lead to its spread to susceptible young siblings of the patient.

Some of these earlier findings were confirmed in a comprehensive seroepidemiologic study of a semirural community of sugarcane farmers and petrochemical workers in southern Louisiana (34). Among 209 children assessed, 13 children (6.2%) were found to be experiencing a current or recent primary EBV infection. The frequency of these infections was highest in the first decade of life and were almost always asymptomatic. IM-like illnesses did not occur and heterophile antibody responses were not detected. The occasional association of primary infection with minor illnesses has been recorded in three other studies: Tischendorf et al. (5) described a number of minor febrile episodes associated with upper respiratory tract infections, pharyngitis, tonsillitis, and otitis media in a group of young orphans; Shapiro et al. (35) found that two of nine infants experienced upper respiratory tract infections in association with seroconversion events; and Joncas et al. (36) noted that a small number of antibody conversions occurred in association with poorly differentiated respiratory and enteric syndromes in 10% of 60 children aged zero to three years.

Joncas et al. (36) also made a concerted effort to attempt to identify EBV infections in the neonatal period; they studied 112 newborn infants and their mothers, 25 neonates undergoing exchange transfusion, and a convenience sample of 114 hospitalized infants (36). Immortalized cell lines could be established from the blood of two infants following transfusion. Although both seroreverted (i.e., lost antibody) by six months of age, the possibility of an abortive infection unaccompanied by an active antibody response could not be excluded. The finding of significantly higher newborn than maternal EBV antibody titers in three cases was also suggestive of abortive congenital infections. In a related study undertaken by Visintine et al. (37), evidence was sought for the possibility that EBV might be responsible for some instances of congenital infection. A lymphocyte-transforming agent (LTA) was recovered from the oropharynx of one 16-day-old premature newborn who developed transient hepatosplenomegaly. It is not clear whether this infant was infected in utero, intrapartum, or as a neonate. However, LTA could not be found in the oropharyngeal secretions of 82 healthy term infants, 28 infants with cardiac or other congenital defects, or infants suspected of having the "toxoplasmosis, other agents, rubella, cytomegalovirus, herpes simplex (TORCH) syndrome." Also, LTA could not be found in the cervixes of 125 pregnant or postpartum women. In contrast, as in previous studies, EBV was recovered from the oral secretions of 14 of 68 (21%) children with a variety of minor illnesses.

Two studies indicate that, occasionally, either fully or partly expressed IM occurs in young children. Tamir et al. (38) focused attention on 22 children in whom atypical mononuclear cells appeared in the peripheral blood, sometimes associated with splenomegaly, lymphadenopathy, tonsillitis, or hepatomegaly. Of these children, 21 had rising titers of EBV antibodies. In contrast, of those in a control group, only 5 of 27 children were seropositive. It was concluded that in children with febrile illnesses in whom atypical lymphocytosis occurs, incomplete manifestations of IM should be suspected even in the absence of a Paul–Bunnell heterophile antibody response. Ginsburg et al. (39) measured antibodies to EBV in 43 consecutive pediatric patients with signs and symptoms of IM and a positive monospot test. Three-quarters of such patients showed clear-cut evidence of primary EBV infections. In specimens from the 13 patients whose virus-specific serologic tests did not confirm acute infection with EBV, further testing proved that the initial monospot tests were incorrectly interpreted (i.e., false positives). The study demonstrates that classical, heterophile antibody–positive IM occurs in young children (in this case in those 2 to 13 years of age; mean, 7.2 years) and, in these instances, the disease is often indistinguishable from cases in adolescents and young adults.

EBV Infection and IM in Older Adults

Seroepidemiologic studies have demonstrated that 90% to 100% of adults over 60 years of age are seropositive for EBV (40–44). Therefore, up to 10% of older individuals are susceptible to primary infection. Schmader et al. (45) performed a computer search for reports in the literature on EBV infection in the elderly host and also reviewed serology reports at the Duke University Medical Center for heterophile antibody–positive patients greater than 60 years of age. It was discovered that geometric mean antibody titers to EBV and the proportion of persons with high antibody titers to EBV increased with age. These serologic changes were usually not associated with clinical illness and were thought to reflect recrudescent or repeat infections with the virus. Twenty-nine reports of IM in elderly adults were uncovered in the literature search. In general, these reports revealed that elderly persons with IM have significantly fewer occurrences of pharyngitis, lymphadenopathy, and splenomegaly, but more episodes of jaundice when compared with adolescents and young adults. Such patients present primarily with constitutional symptoms, including fevers, fatigue, arthralgias, myalgias, and weakness, among others. The development of atypical lymphocytosis is often the first clue to the diagnosis, although the appearance of these abnormal cells in the peripheral blood is sometimes delayed for weeks. In a handful of instances, lymphoproliferative diseases ("atypical mononuclear cell infiltration," "malignant lymphoma," and "monocytic leukemia") have been reported in association with serologically confirmed episodes of primary EBV infection in elderly adults, but in no such instance has EBV genome material or EBV-associated antigen been sought in the affected tissues (46,47).

Some of these findings have been confirmed in another review of the literature that focused on the manifestations of EBV infection in adults over 40 years of age (48). Although fever (sometimes prolonged), anorexia, headache, fatigue, and non-specific pain were somewhat more common in this group, older patients experiencing infection were less likely to present with lymphadenopathy, pharyngitis, spleno-megaly, or atypical lymphocytosis. It was suggested that among older patients in whom localized lymphadenopathy, "unusual" blood smears, or thrombocytopenia dominate the clinical picture, lymphoma and leukemia have to be systematically "ruled out." Liver involvement (especially hepatomegaly, jaundice, and hyperbiliru-binemia) appears to be more common in those over 40 years of age than in younger patients, frequently leading to diagnostic considerations other than IM (e.g., extra-hepatic biliary obstruction). As in young children, conventional heterophile antibody tests or "spot" tests tend to be negative in older adults, even though IgM antibodies to the capsid antigens of the virus can be measured (49).

Finally, in some instances in older adults, neurologic signs and symptoms either dominate the clinical picture or precede the other more usual manifestations of the dis-ease. (This sometimes occurs in younger patients too.) The more common neurologic presentations of EBV infection that have been reported in the elderly include Bell's palsy, acute optic neuritis, distal limb paresthesias, and Guillain–Barré syndrome (45,50–53).

Epidemics, Outbreaks, and Pseudo-Outbreaks of IM

There is no clear evidence that true epidemics or major outbreaks of mononucleosis have occurred in the last five decades. In earlier times, significant outbreaks of "glandular fever" were reported, as for example in the United States in the latter part of the 19th century (54) and in the first part of the 20th century (55) and from the Falkland Islands in 1930 (56). Two possibly legitimate hospital outbreaks were reported in the British Medical Journal in 1943 and in 1958 (57,58); the first of these two occurred in an emergency medical hospital during World War II. A very high incidence of IM was reported in Army posts and military camps; these "quasi-outbreaks" are likely explained by the high and rapid turnover of men in military installations under adverse conditions.

Under some circumstances, IM may be more contagious than expected. Ginsburg et al. (59) reported nine current or recent cases of primary EBV infection, all occurring in females, among 29 staff members of an obstetrics–gynecology clinic on an Air Force base. Five affected individuals displayed classical signs and symp-toms of IM, and all developed antibody responses consistent with a primary infec-tion. The remaining four had mild symptoms or were asymptomatic. All but one had a positive monospot test. Three other persons experienced milder, concurrent ill-nesses but none could be ascribed to EBV. Only two of the involved staff were room-mates. It was hypothesized that poorly washed coffee cups or airborne dissemination of virus might be possible sources for this unusual outbreak.

Despite these reports, a considerable body of epidemiologic evidence collected in the past 40 years weighs heavily against the notion that epidemics of IM can occur. In many populations, primary infection occurs in a majority of individuals in the youngest age groups in sporadic fashion; such individuals are not susceptible to IM later in life. Furthermore, in those age groups and segments of society in which the incidence of mononucleosis is highest (e.g., on military installations, in college dormitories, among teenagers living at home, etc.), there is little evidence of person-to-person spread within the confines of the domiciliary unit.

Several pseudo-outbreaks of IM have been reported and investigated. In these instances, a combination of inappropriate ordering of diagnostic tests for mononucleosis and poor laboratory technique accounted for the misdiagnoses and faulty reports. Two such outbreaks were reported by Armstrong et al. (60). One involved nine children attending a daycare center, all of whom were tested in physicians' offices for heterophile antibody using rapid differential slide tests. The tests were later discovered to have been done incorrectly. The second pseudo-outbreak involved nearly 300 college students. The diagnosis of infection was inappropriately attributed to the presence of IgG antibody to the VCA of EBV; heterophile antibody tests and other viral-specific serologic tests were not done.

A third pseudo-outbreak occurred in 1990 among 57 persons (including outpatients, inpatients, and staff) at a community hospital in Puerto Rico (61). An investigation determined that during the period when reported cases were at their peak, 50% or more of all blood specimens submitted for heterophile agglutination tests were interpreted as positive. The false reading of the tests as positive was attributed to a few newly hired, inexperienced technicians. The findings in this investigation revealed that reported cases were neither consistent with the incubation period of IM nor its mode of spread; that the epidemiologic characteristics of persons with negative tests were similar to those with positive tests; and, most importantly, that no person had both the clinical and hematologic findings consistent with IM. The health care professionals who arrived at these diagnoses incorrectly assumed that a positive test alone meant that their patients had IM, beginning a cycle in which, as more tests were reported as positive, more tests were ordered. Appropriate clinical criteria were not applied when ordering and interpreting the diagnostic tests.

Lastly, an epidemic of IM was reported in an Army post in 1946; 556 persons were admitted or examined over a 14 month period (62). Review of the evidence indicates that Davidsohn absorption tests were performed in only a small proportion of cases, "abnormal" blood smears were reported in nearly every patient admitted to the hospital during the period, an unexpectedly large number of cases were reported in blacks, and many patients who were "counted" as cases presented with skin eruptions, meningitic signs, and pneumonia, clinical manifestations rarely associated with the classical syndrome of IM as we now know it.

Transmission

As first suggested by Hoagland in his landmark study of the mid-1950s, exchange of saliva and other oropharyngeal secretions during kissing is almost certainly the principal activity which leads to transmission of EBV among adolescents and young adults (20). A later five-year study conducted by Evans at the University of Wisconsin confirmed the earlier findings (18). In infants and toddlers, contamination of the environment and its objects (e.g., toys, cups, and eating surfaces) with saliva and activities such as kissing, fondling, and mouth-to-mouth transfer of food lead to transmission of infection to seronegative youngsters by their parents and adult caregivers as well as by already-seropositive playmates and peers.

Personal household contact is not sufficient to produce secondary infections or cases of IM. The Henles assessed data collected as part of the Cleveland Family Study, whose subjects were comprised principally of closed, Western-style nuclear family groups (33). In these families where the majority of children lacked antibody to EBV at the age of 10 years, evidence of new infection could only be found in about one-third of family groups; transmission from parents to their children was an irregular event. Also, spread among siblings was infrequent. A smaller study of four households, in which the children ranged in age from 6 to 17 years and which was conducted over an interval of one year, did not demonstrate a single seroconversion event (63). Three children in two different families failed to acquire infection despite sharing a bedroom with persistent excretors of the virus. In an extensive study of 67 seronegative members of 75 Canadian families conducted over a period of approximately two years, only about one-tenth of the susceptibles seroconverted; all infections were unaccompanied by symptoms (64).

In the most primitive societies, such as among the tribesmen of the New Guinea Highlands and among the New Hebridean and Solomon Islanders, it has been suggested that the exceedingly high prevalence of infection, even among the youngest age groups, can be accounted for by the "intensity and promiscuity of interpersonal contact, together with the prevalence of spreaders" (65). In some of these societies, saliva and nasal mucus on the hands are rarely washed off, and direct mouth-to-mouth sharing of premasticated food, especially with infants, is a common practice among a wide circle of individuals who care for the youngsters. Finally, in all these communities, babies are seldom out of the arms of child or adult caregivers during the day and many relatives (up to a dozen adults) hold, carry, and kiss the infant and engage in mouth-to-mouth contact. This intense level of interpersonal contact with many individuals each day easily increases the opportunity for transmission of virus, when compared to the rather meager number of such interactions that take place in nuclear Western families. Modern daycare centers obviously afford a greater opportunity for such interactions to occur, as do cultures or families in which many adults and children share the care of infants and toddlers.

Comprehensive investigations of military and college populations have also confirmed the low risk of transmission to susceptible, exposed roommates of index cases of IM (6–8,66). In a study of Yale University undergraduates, 18 antibody-negative roommates or close contacts of 17 patients with IM were followed for nine months; only one contact developed clinical illness and a heterophile antibody response 41 days after exposure (67). This secondary attack rate, 5.5%, was lower than the overall university seroconversion rate of 13.1%, suggesting the presence of routes and of persons responsible for transmission that exist outside the traditional domiciliary units common to colleges and military institutions.

Clues to the low rates of acquisition of infection among close contacts of acutely infected persons and the great difficulty in tracing the routes of transmission of disease (i.e., IM) on a case-to-case basis were forthcoming only after techniques became available for culturing the etiologic agent from saliva and throat wash material (68,69). Such techniques, all based on the capacity of EBV to transform human leukocytes into continuously dividing cell lines, made it possible to conduct studies which ultimately revealed why the transmission patterns of EBV were different from those of highly contagious diseases, such as measles and influenza, infections for which case-to-case tracing is easily accomplished. Early studies using the transformation assay revealed that approximately 20% of adults attending an outpatient clinic excreted the virus from time to time, with no significant differences in prevalence among age groups, between sexes, by season, or among broad medical categories of patients (68). In contrast, the rates of excretion of the virus were much higher among cancer patients, especially those on intensive chemotherapy regimens. Furthermore, cross-sectional studies of healthy adults have also revealed excretion in approximately 20% of patients; once again the excretion rates were discovered to be higher among persons receiving immunosuppressive drugs (70). Excretion rates were found to be just as high among those whose primary infection was unaccompanied by symptoms as among those who had experienced IM in the past. Because shedders of virus are so prevalent in the general population and because so much shedding occurs asymptomatically, the source of new infections can rarely be traced.

In studies of patterns of shedding of EBV in the saliva and oropharynx of patients with IM, the majority of infected individuals demonstrate intermittent excretion over a period of three months, whereas a smaller number shed virus more regularly; in a few individuals, no virus can be detected (71). Quantitative analyses of oral secretions have revealed that the amounts of biologically active virus that can be detected in patients with IM are very small: on the 12th day following the onset of disease, some patients have as few as 3 to 10 "50% transforming units" in saliva or throat washings; in some cases, no herpesvirus particles were seen, even in concentrated specimens by electron microscopy (71). These patterns of oropharyngeal excretion of virus help to define the epidemiologic features of this disease. Low titers of infectious virus account for the low-to-moderate contagiousness of the disease and the apparent requirement of intimate contact for disease transmission. Intermittent excretion of EBV, even in those who are currently or recently infected, also accounts for the relatively low risk of secondary spread. Lastly, prolonged excretion of EBV in some patients with IM and the relatively high rates of excretion among normal persons and, most particularly, among those who are immunocompromised help to explain the wide, but "low grade," continuous spread of virus from shedders to seronegatives. Thus, in age groups and societies where salivary exchange and contact with saliva are high, transmissibility of the disease is high and, conversely, in age groups and social groups in which this type of contact is uncommon, rates of contagion are low.

Transmission by Way of Blood and Other Body Fluids

In early attempts to trace the various means by which IM might be spread from person to person, nearly 100 human volunteers received inocula, including blood, serum, throat and nasal washings, and lymph node and stool suspensions from acutely ill patients; none of these was successful in transmitting the disease. However, in 1942, Wising was able to produce the disease in a 23-year-old female volunteer who received 250 mL of whole blood from a donor during the first week of IM; the recipient developed full-blown clinical disease three weeks following the inoculation and, concurrently, a heterophile antibody response (72). Additional attempts of this sort performed by Evans (73,74) and, later still, by Niederman and Scott (75), using whole blood, serum, or throat washings, produced inconclusive results. (Using stored serum specimens, it was later shown that all the recipients had antibody to EBV in their blood prior to the inoculations and were, therefore, almost certainly immune.)

A few cases in the literature provide strong evidence that transmission of infection may occur by the parenteral route. In one instance, transmission occurred after plasma from a healthy male in the incubation period of IM was transfused into his leukemic brother (76). The recipient, on the development of signs of the disease 30 days later, mounted a heterophile antibody response and seroconverted to EBV. In another report, four of five patients undergoing open-heart surgery and cardiopulmonary bypass seroconverted: two remained symptom free, one had a nonspecific febrile episode, and one developed a mononucleosis-like illness characterized by fever, splenomegaly, lymphadenopathy, atypical lymphocytosis, and heterophile antibody response (77). IM has also been reported to occur after transfusion of packed red blood cells (78) and following accidental subcutaneous injection of tissue materials derived from cultured Burkitt lymphoma cells (79).

EBV shedding from the female genital tract has been documented using newer molecular assays (80–84). The overall rate of detection among these studies is 33%, this rate must be interpreted cautiously because these studies were among patients with sexually transmitted infections. Intermittent genital tract EBV carriage was detected in 5 of 36 (14%) girls followed from 16 to 18 years of age (85). Genital tract shedding suggests that sexual transmission is a possible, though minor, mode of EBV transmission. There is no recognized disease associated with genital tract shedding of EBV.

REFERENCES

1. Evans AS. Infectious mononucleosis: observations from a public health laboratory. Yale J Biol Med 1961; 34:261–276.
2. Evans AS. Complications of infectious mononucleosis. Recognition and management. Hospital Med 1967; 3:24–25, 28–33.
3. Evans AS. New discoveries in infectious mononucleosis. Mod Med 1974; 1:18–24.
4. Chang RS, Rosen L, Kapikian AZ. Epstein–Barr virus infections in a nursery. Am J Epidemiol 1981; 113(1):22–29.
5. Tischendorf P, Shramek GJ, Balagtas RC, et al. Development and persistence of immunity to Epstein–Barr virus in man. J Infect Dis 1970; 122(5):401–409.
6. Niederman JC, Evans AS, Subramahnyan L, McCollum RW. Prevalence, incidence and persistence of EBV antibody in young adults. N Engl J Med 1970; 282(7):361–365.
7. Hallee TJ, Evans AS, Niederman JC, Brooks CM, Voegtly H. Infectious mononucleosis at the United States Military Academy. A prospective study of a single class over four years. Yale J Biol Med 1974; 47(3):182–195.
8. Laboratories, J.I.b.U.H.P.a.P.H.L.S. Infectious mononucleosis and its relationship to EBV antibody. Br Med J 1971; 4:643–646.
9. McKinnon GT, Pringle RC. A serological study of antibody to Epstein–Barr virus in an Australian population. Med J Aust 1974; 2(7):243–246.
10. Demissie A, Svmyr A. Age distribution of antibodies to EBV in Swedish females as studied by indirect immunofluorescence on Burkitt cells. Acta Pathol Microbiol Scand 1969; 75(3):457–465.
11. Pereira MS, Blake JM, Macrae AD. EBV antibody at different ages. BMJ 1969; 4(682): 526–527.
12. Centers for Disease Control: Annual summary 1983. MMWR Morb Mortal Wkly Rep 1984; 32(54):v–121.
13. Christine B. Infectious mononucleosis. Connecticut Health Bull 1968; 82:115–119.
14. Rosdahl N, Larsen SO, Thamdrup AB. Infectious mononucleosis in Denmark. Epidemiological observations based on positive Paul–Bunnell reactions from 1940–1969. Scand J Infect Dis 1973; 5(3):163–170.
15. Heath CW Jr, Brodsky AL, Potolsky AI. Infectious mononucleosis in a general population. Am J Epidemiol 1972; 95(1):46–52.
16. Henke CE, Kurland LT, Elveback LR. Infectious mononucleosis in Rochester, Minnesota, 1950 through 1969. Am J Epidemiol 1973; 98(6):483–490.
17. Centers for Disease Control: Infectious Mononucleosis Surveillance, 1972.
18. Evans AS. Infectious mononucleosis in University of Wisconsin students: report of a five-year investigation. Am J Hyg 1960; 71:342–362.
19. Brodsky AL, Heath CW Jr. Infectious mononucleosis: epidemiologic patterns at United States colleges and Universities. Am J Epidemiol 1972; 96(2):87–93.

20. Hoagland R. The transmission of infectious mononucleosis. Am J Med Sci 1955; 229: 262–272.
21. Evans AS. Infectious mononucleosis in the Armed Forces. Mil Med 1970; 135(4): 300–304.
22. Black FL, Hierholzer WJ, Pinheiro F, et al. Evidence for persistence of infectious agents in isolated human populations. Am J Epidemiol 1974; 100(3):230–250.
23. Strom J. Infectious mononucleosis—Is the incidence increasing? ACTA Med Scand 1960; 168:35–39.
24. Hoagland RJ. Infectious Mononucleosis. Grune and Stratton. New York and London, 1967.
25. Jennings E. Prevalence of EBV Antibody in Hawaii. New Haven: Yale University School of Medicine, 1973.
26. Biggar RJ, Henle W, Fleisher G, Bocker J, Lennette ET, Henle G. Primary Epstein–Barr virus infections in African infants. I. Decline of maternal antibodies and time of infection. Int J Cancer 1978; 22(3):239–243.
27. Biggar RJ, Henle G, Bocker J, Lennette ET, Fleisher G, Henle, W. Primary Epstein–Barr virus infections in African infants. II. Clinical and serological observations during seroconversion. Int J Cancer 1978; 22(3):244–250.
28. Sohier R. La Mononucleose Infectieuse. Paris: Masson, 1943.
29. Gardner H, Paul J. Infectious mononucleosis at the New Haven Hospital 1921–1946. Yale J Biol Med 1947; 19:839–853.
30. Davidson RJ. A survey of infectious mononucleosis in the North-East Regional Hospital Board area of Scotland, 1960–1969. J Hyg (Lond) 1970; 68(3):393–400.
31. Munoz N, Davidson RJ, Witthoff B, Ericsson JE, de The G. Infectious mononucleosis and Hodgkin's disease. Int J Cancer 1978; 22(1):10–13.
32. Pannuti CS, Carvalho RP, Evans AS, Cenabre LC, et al. A prospective clinical study of the mononucleosis syndrome in a developing country. Int J Epidemiol 1980; 9(4): 349–353.
33. Henle G, Henle W. Observations on childhood infections with the Epstein–Barr virus. J Infect Dis 1970; 121(3):303–310.
34. Sumaya CV. Primary Epstein–Barr virus infections in children. Pediatrics 1977; 59(1): 16–21.
35. Shapiro LR, Hirshaut Y, Kanef DM, Glade P. Epstein–Barr virus in infancy. J Pediat 1972; 80(6):1025–1026.
36. Joncas J, Boucher J, Granger-Julien M, Filion C. Epstein–Barr virus infection in the neonatal period and in childhood. Can Med Assoc J 1974; 110(1):33–37.
37. Visintine AM, Gerber P, Nahmias AJ. Leukocyte transforming agent (Epstein–Barr virus) in newborn infants and older individuals. J Pediat 1976; 89(4):571–575.
38. Tamir D, Benderly A, Levy J, Ben-Porath E, Vonsover A. Infectious mononucleosis and Epstein–Barr virus in childhood. Pediatrics 1974; 53(3):330–335.
39. Ginsburg CM, Henle W, Henle G, Horwitz CA. Infectious mononucleosis in children. Evaluation of Epstein–Barr virus-specific serological data. JAMA 1977; 237(8):781–785.
40. Hornsleth A, Siggaard-Andersen J, Hjort L. Epidemiology of herpesvirus and respiratory virus infections. Part 1. Serologic findings. Geriatrics 1975; 30(8):61–68.
41. Sumaya CV, Henle W, Henle G, Smith MH, Leblanc D. Seroepidemiologic study of Epstein–Barr virus infections in a rural community. J Infect Dis 1975; 131(4):403–408.
42. Gurtsevich V, Le Riverend E, Ruiz R. Sero-epidemiologic study of the Epstein–Barr virus infectivity in a healthy Cuban population. Neoplasma 1979; 26(6):677–683.
43. Henle W, Henle G. Seroepidemiology of the virus. In: Epstein M, Achong B, eds. Epstein–Barr Virus. Berlin: Springer-Verlag, 1979:63.
44. Glaser R, Strain EC, Tarr KL, Holliday JE, Donnerberg RL, Kiecolt-Glaser JK. Changes in Epstein–Barr virus antibody titers associated with aging. Proc Soc Exp Biol Med 1985; 179(3):352–355.

45. Schmader KE, van der Horst CM, Klotman ME. Epstein–Barr virus and the elderly host. Rev Infect Dis 1989; 11(1):64–73.
46. Hehlmann R, Walther B, Zollner N, Wolf H, Deinhardt F, Schmid M. Fatal lymphoproliferation and acute monocytic leukemia-like disease following infectious mononucleosis in the elderly. Klinische Wochenschrift 1981; 59(10):477–483.
47. Talamo TS, Borochovitz D, Atchison RW. Fatal Epstein–Barr virus infection in a 63-year-old man. An autopsy report. Arch Pathol Lab Med 1981; 105(9):465–469.
48. Axelrod P, Finestone AJ. Infectious mononucleosis in older adults. Am Fam Physician 1990; 42(6):1599–1606.
49. Horwitz CA, Henle W, Henle G, et al. Heterophil-negative infectious mononucleosis and mononucleosis-like illnesses. Laboratory confirmation of 43 cases. Am J Med 1977; 63(6): 947–957.
50. Horwitz CA, Henle W, Henle G, et al. Infectious mononucleosis in patients aged 40 to 72 years: report of 27 cases, including 3 without heterophil-antibody responses. Medicine 1983; 62(4):256–262.
51. Corr WP. Infectious mononucleosis in the elderly. JAMA 1966; 195(13):1158.
52. Acikalin T, Akdamar K. Infectious mononucleosis in the elderly. J Louisiana State Med Soc 1980; 132(1):1–3.
53. Jones J, Gardner W, Newman T. Severe optic neuritis in infectious mononucleosis. Ann Emergency Med 1988; 17(4):361–364.
54. West J. An epidemic of glandular fever. Arch Pediat 1986; 13:889–900.
55. Carlson G, Brooks EH, Marshall VG. Acute glandular fever: recent epidemic, report of cases. Wisconsin Med J 1926; 25:176–178.
56. Moir JI. Glandular fever in the Falkland Islands. Br Med J 1930; 2:822–823.
57. Halchrow JPA, Owen LM, Roger NO. Infectious mononucleosis with an account of an epidemic in E.M.S. Hospital. Br Med J 1943; 2:443–447.
58. Hobson FG, Lawson B, Wigfield M. Glandular fever, a field study. Br Med J 1958; 1: 845–852.
59. Ginsburg CM, Henle G, Henle W. An outbreak of infectious mononucleosis among the personnel of an outpatient clinic. Am J Epidemiol 1976; 104(5):571–575.
60. Armstrong CW, Hackler RL, Miller GB Jr. Two pseudo-outbreaks of infectious mononucleosis. Pediat Infect Dis 1986; 5(3):325–327.
61. Centers for Disease Control: Pseudo-outbreak of Infectious Mononucleosis—Puerto Rico, 1990. MMWR Morb Mortal Wkly Rep 1991; 40(32):552–555.
62. Wechsler H, Rosenblum A, Sills C. Infectious mononucleosis: report of an epidemic in an Army Post. Ann Int Med 1945; 25:113–133.
63. Chang RS. Letter: interpersonal transmission of EB-virus infection. N Engl J Med 1975; 293(9):454–455.
64. Joncas J, Mitnyan C. Serological response of the EBV antibodies in pediatric cases of infectious mononucleosis and in their contacts. CMAJ 1970; 102(12):1260–1263.
65. Lang DJ, Garruto RM, Gajdusek DC. Early acquisition of cytomegalovirus and Epstein–Barr virus antibody in several isolated Melanesian populations. Am J Epidemiol 1977; 105(5):480–487.
66. Evans AS, Niederman JC, McCollum R. Seroepidemiologic studies of infectious mononucleosis with EBV. N Engl J Med 1968; 279(21):1121–1127.
67. Sawyer RN, Evans AS, Niederman JC, McCollum RW. Prospective studies of a group of Yale University freshmen. I. Occurrence of infectious mononucleosis. J Infect Dis 1971; 123(3):263–270.
68. Chang RS, Lewis JP, Abildgaard CF. Prevalence of oropharyngeal excretors of leukocyte-transforming agents among a human population. N Engl J Med 1973; 289(25): 1325–1329.
69. Miller G, Niederman JC, Andrews LL. Prolonged oropharyngeal excretion of Epstein–Barr virus after infectious mononucleosis. N Engl J Med 1973; 288(5):229–232.

70. Gerber P, Lucas S, Nonoyama M, Perlin E, Goldstein LI. Oral excretion of Epstein–Barr virus by healthy subjects and patients with infectious mononucleosis. Lancet 1972; 2(7785):988–989.

71. Niederman JC, Miller G, Pearson HA, Pagano JS, Dowaliby JM. Infectious mononucleosis. Epstein–Barr virus shedding in saliva and the oropharynx. N Engl J Med 1976; 294(25):1355–1359.

72. Wising P. A study of infectious mononucleosis (Pfeiffer's disease) from the etiological point of view. ACTA Med Scand 1942; 133:1–102.

73. Evans AS. Experimental attempts to transmit infectious mononucleosis to man. Yale J Biol Med 1947; 20:19–26.

74. Evans AS. Further experimental attempts to transmit infectious mononucleosis to man. J Clin Invest 1950; 29:508–512.

75. Niederman JC, Scott RB. Studies on infectious mononucleosis: attempts to transmit the disease to human volunteers. Yale J Biol Med 1965; 38(1):1–10.

76. Turner AR, MacDonald RN, Cooper BA. Transmission of infectious mononucleosis by transfusion of pre-illness plasma. Ann Intern Med 1972; 77(5):751–753.

77. Gerber P, Walsh JH, Rosenblum EN, Purcell RH. Association of EB-virus infection with the post-perfusion syndrome. Lancet 1969; 1(7595):593–595.

78. Blacklow NR, Watson BK, Miller G, Jacobson BM. Mononucleosis with heterophil antibodies and EBV infection. Acquisition by an elderly patient in hospital. Am J Med 1971; 51(4):549–552.

79. Grace JT, Blakeslee J, Jones R. Induction of infectious mononucleosis in man by the herpes-type virus (HTV) in Burkitt lymphoma cells in tissue culture. Proc Am Assoc Cancer Res 1969; 10:31.

80. Sixbey JW, Lemon SM, Pagano JS. A second site for Epstein–Barr virus shedding: the uterine cervix. Lancet 1986; 2:1122–1124.

81. Näher H, Gissmann L, Freese UK, Petzoldt D, Helfrich S. Subclinical Epstein–Barr virus infection of both the male and female genital tract—indication for sexual transmission. J Invest Dermatol 1992; 98:791–793.

82. Taylor Y, Melvin WT, Sewell HF, Flannelly G, Walker F. Prevalence of Epstein–Barr virus in the cervix. J Clin Pathol 1994; 47:92–93.

83. Voog E, Ricksten A, Löwhagen GB. Prevalence of Epstein–Barr virus and human papillomavirus in cervical samples from women attending an STD-clinic. Int J STD AIDS 1995; 6:208–210.

84. Gradilone A, Vercillo R, Napolitano M, et al. Prevalence of human papillomavirus, cytomegalovirus, and Epstein-Barr virus in the cervix of healthy women. J Med Virol 1996; 50:1–4.

85. Andersson-Ellstrom A, Bergstrom T, Svennerholm B, Milsom I. Epstein–Barr virus DNA in the uterine cervix of teenage girls. Acta Obstet Gynaecol Scand 1997; 76(8): 779–783.

4
Pathology of Primary and Persistent Epstein–Barr Virus Infection

Gerald Niedobitek
Institut für Pathologie, Friedrich-Alexander-Universität, Erlangen, Germany

Hermann Herbst
Gerhard-Domagk-Institut für Pathologie, Westfälische Wilhelms-Universität, Münster, Germany

INTRODUCTION

The Epstein–Barr virus (EBV) is a B-lymphotropic human herpesvirus that infects over 90% of adults worldwide, including tribal populations in remote areas (1). Primary infection is usually asymptomatic when it occurs during childhood. Primary infection during adolescence or early adulthood is associated with a clinical syndrome, designated infectious mononucleosis (IM) or glandular fever, which develops in approximately 50% of individuals (2,3). In either circumstance, primary EBV infection is followed by lifelong persistence of the infection that is asymptomatic in the vast majority of individuals.

IM is a self-limiting lymphoproliferative disease usually running a benign course. However, it can be associated with a number of complications other than those affecting the lymphoreticular tissues, e.g., hepatitis, interstitial nephritis, hematological abnormalities, and neurological symptoms. Rarely, IM may take a fulminant and rapidly fatal course (fatal IM). This may either occur as a sporadic disease or associated with the inherited condition, X-linked lymphoproliferative disease (XLPD) (see Chapter 16). Another rare complication of primary EBV infection is EBV-associated hemophagocytic syndrome (EBV-AHS). Finally, in some individuals, IM may not resolve but may evolve into a remitting or chronic disorder, sometimes known as chronic active EBV (CAEBV) infection.

This chapter discusses the histopathological changes seen in lymphoreticular and other tissues in IM, fatal IM, EBV-AHS, and CAEBV, and considers possible pathogenic mechanisms contributing to organ manifestations of these disorders.

INFECTIOUS MONONUCLEOSIS

Typical symptoms of acute IM include fever, fatigue, sore throat, tonsillitis with ulceration, cervical lymphadenopathy, and splenomegaly (3–6). Patients commonly show an absolute lymphocytosis with atypical mononuclear cells (5–7). Not uncommonly, there is also evidence of liver involvement as shown by elevated transaminase levels, while other organ manifestations are comparatively rare (5).

Tonsils and Other Lymphoreticular Tissues

Histopathology and Immunophenotype

Cervical lymphadenopathy and tonsillar hyperplasia are common features of acute IM while splenomegaly is relatively uncommon (5). In cases of clinically established IM, lymph node biopsy or tonsillectomy are only rarely performed, the latter usually because of severe upper airways obstruction. Occasionally, IM may be suspected in cases without clinically established diagnosis, but presenting typical histopathological changes. The tonsils of IM show a striking expansion of the interfollicular areas that may lead to the impression of a destroyed architecture (Fig. 1A) (8,9). This is largely due to a massive proliferation of polymorphic lymphoid cells including large immunoblasts and cells showing plasmacytoid differentiation (8,9). Not uncommonly, atypical cells are seen resembling Hodgkin and Reed–Sternberg (HRS) cells—HRS-like cells (Fig. 1A) (8–10). Histiocytes are regularly present, frequently forming clusters or microgranulomas (9). Follicular hyperplasia is usually not a prominent feature, but may develop later in the disease (8,11). In addition, tonsillar sinuses may contain numerous monocytoid B-cells, the so-called "immature sinus histiocytosis" (8,11). Necrosis with ulceration may also be present (8). None of these features is diagnostic of the disease, but in combination they should suggest the possibility of EBV infection and IM. The diagnosis of lymphoma is generally excluded by the lack of monoclonal immunoglobulin gene rearrangements (12). EBV studies may also help in the differential diagnosis. Changes seen in other lymphoreticular tissues, such as the lymph nodes and appendix, are similar to those seen in tonsils (13). In lymph nodes, capsular and extranodal infiltration may be observed (9). The spleen usually shows less dramatic alterations consisting mainly of an expansion of the red pulp by lymphoid blasts and plasma cells (9,10).

The proliferating extrafollicular lymphoid blasts seen in IM tissues display mostly a B-cell phenotype (Fig. 1B) (10,14). The larger cells, particularly the HRS-like cells, also express the CD30 antigen (Fig. 1D) (14). However, in contrast to HRS cells of Hodgkin's disease (HD), these cells are CD15 negative (10). Variable numbers of T-cells are admixed with the proliferating B-cells, including large activated cells (Fig. 1C) (10,14). Notably, the atypical mononuclear cells characteristically found in the peripheral blood of IM patients have been shown to be largely of T-cell phenotype (7).

EBV Studies and Phenotype of EBV-Infected Cells

By in situ hybridization, EBV DNA and expression of the small EBV-encoded nuclear RNAs (EBER1 and EBER2) are detected in extrafollicular cells (Fig. 1D) (9,14–16). In IM, these EBV-infected cells are usually quite numerous, exceeding 1000 cells per 0.5 cm^2 (16). These cells typically accumulate in the extrafollicular areas of lymphoreticular tissues, sparing germinal centers (14,16,17). By reverse

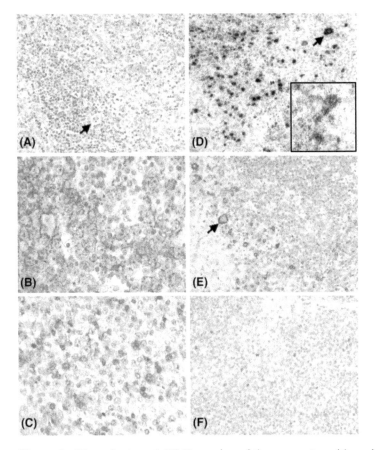

Figure 1 (*See color insert.*) (**A**) Expansion of the paracortex with proliferation of lymphoid blasts is seen in an infectious mononucleosis tonsil (H and E). Note occasional Reed-Sternberg–like cells (*arrow*). (**B**) Immunohistochemistry reveals expression of the CD20 B-cell antigen in most lymphoid blasts (red membrane staining). (**C**) There are also numerous admixed CD3-positive T-cells, including larger, activated cells (red membrane staining, *arrows*). (**D**) In situ hybridization with radiolabeled EBER-specific probes reveals numerous EBV-positive cells in the paracortex (black labeling), including multinucleated Reed-Sternberg–like cells (*arrow*). (**D**, inset) A proportion of these cells express the CD30 activation antigen as shown by double labeling (inset red staining). (**E**) Variable proportions of lymphoid cells express LMP1 (red membrane staining). Note a LMP1-positive Reed-Sternberg–like cell (*arrow*). (**F**) Variable proportions of lymphoid cells express EBNA2 [red nuclear labeling (*arrows*)]. *Abbreviations*: EBNA, Epstein–Barr nuclear antigen; EBER, EBV encoded RNA; EBV, Epstein–Barr virus; LMP, latent membrane protein.

transcriptase polymerase chain reaction and immunohistochemistry, a pattern of EBV latent gene expression that corresponds to latency III has been identified in IM (see Chapter 2) (18). Immunohistochemical double-labeling studies, however, have shown a heterogeneous picture (19). Thus, only a minority of the cells show simultaneous expression of Epstein–Barr nuclear antigen (EBNA)-2 and latent membrane protein (LMP)-1 consistent with type III latency (19). A small proportion of cells express LMP1 but not EBNA2 (latency II), and these cells tend to be larger cells, including HRS-like cells (Fig. 1E) (19). EBNA2-positive cells are also detected and can be more numerous than LMP1-expressing cells (Fig. 1F) (19). Double-staining studies have identified a population of cells positive for EBNA2 but negative for LMP1 (19). This pattern of viral latent gene expression is observed early in EBV infection when EBNA2 is expressed before LMP1 and, thus, these cells may represent newly infected cells (20). Finally, there is a variable proportion of cells expressing the EBERs but not EBNA2 or LMP1, suggesting type I latency (19). In addition, expression of LMP2A has been demonstrated in IM (21).

The nature of the lineage of EBV-infected cells in IM has been a matter of controversy. Double-labeling studies have demonstrated that the vast majority of EBV-infected cells display a B-cell phenotype (16,19,22). The detection of EBV-infected T-cells in IM has also been reported; however, these results have been controversial and EBV-infected T-cells are at best rare in acute IM (17,19,23). Conflicting results regarding the possibility of EBV infection in epithelial cells have also been published. Studies conducted in the late 1970s and early 1980s have reported the detection of EBV replication in desquamated oropharyngeal epithelial cells from IM patients (24,25). These results, however, could not be reproduced in two independent recent studies (22,26). Studies of tissue sections from IM tonsils have also consistently failed to detect EBV-infected epithelial cells (15,16,27). Thus, the combined evidence of these studies suggests that B-cells are the primary target of EBV infection in IM.

Involvement of Other Tissues

Heart

Up to 6% of patients with acute IM may display electrocardiographic abnormalities suggesting involvement of the heart (28). However, there are only a few reports of fatal myocarditis associated with primary EBV infection (29). Hebert et al. reported a single case of a young girl who had recurrent episodes of myocarditis associated with chicken pox (30). The ultimately fatal episode of myocarditis in this case was associated with primary EBV infection. Immunohistochemistry revealed a T-cell infiltration of the myocardium, and EBV DNA was detected by polymerase chain reaction (PCR) in myocardial tissue suggesting EBV infection of T-cells (30).

Bone Marrow

Anemia may develop in the course of acute IM. It may occur as autoimmune hemolytic anemia (31). Severe aplastic anemia with pancytopenia has also been reported (32–34). While this may be fatal, most patients appear to recover and may benefit from treatment with corticosteroids (34). In a case report, Shadduck et al. describe a 17-year-old girl who developed severe aplastic anemia in the course of IM. The patient's bone marrow was shown to suppress colony formation when mixed with normal marrow. The patient recovered after therapy with antithymocyte globulin suggesting that the EBV-induced immune response was responsible for bone marrow damage (33). In support of this notion, bone marrow infiltration by atypical lymphocytes, immunoblasts, and plasma cells has been observed in patients with fatal IM (see below) (35).

Liver

Biochemical evidence of hepatic dysfunction is not uncommon in patients with acute IM, with over 50% of individuals showing elevated transaminase levels (5,36). Thus, minor histological changes in the liver are also common, although there is no indication to perform liver biopsy in the majority of IM cases. Literature descriptions of hepatitis associated with IM are rare (37,38). In the cases reported, a polymorphous lymphoid cell infiltrate has been observed expanding the portal tracts but not breaching the limiting plate (36,39). The lobular architecture is preserved and there are only small and discrete foci of necrosis (36,39). Typically, there is also sinusoidal leukostasis with an "Indian file" pattern of lymphoid cells (36,39). Cirrhosis does not develop (36). The mechanism causing liver damage in IM is uncertain. It is generally agreed that EBV infection of hepatocytes does not occur or is at best a rare event (38,40). Thus, EBV hepatitis differs from classical viral hepatitis in this respect. EBV appears to be detectable in infiltrating lymphocytes, but the phenotype of these cells is uncertain. Feranchak et al. reported the case of a young girl who developed fulminant hepatic failure in association with primary EBV infection. In this case, the infiltrate consisted mainly of T-cells with a minor component of EBV-positive B-cells (40). In another case, Kimura et al. reported that the inflammatory infiltrate consisted mainly of CD8-positive T-cells and that the majority of these cells were EBV positive (38). Thus, the question remains unresolved. Nevertheless, the absence of EBV from hepatocytes suggests that liver injury is caused in a nonspecific manner either by the host T-cell response to EBV-infected B-cells or by an abnormal EBV-positive T-cell population.

Respiratory Tract

Involvement of the lungs in patients with acute IM has rarely been described. Andersson et al. reported the case of a 26-year-old woman with primary EBV infection who developed pulmonary interstitial infiltrates with epithelioid granulomas and admixed LMP1-positive lymphoid blasts (41). The patient recovered upon therapy with interferon (IFN)-γ (41). In another case, development of marked pulmonary edema that improved with corticosteroids was reported (32). A case of interstitial pneumonia occurring in association with IM has also been reported (42). In this case, numerous EBV-infected lymphoid cells were detected in a lung biopsy (42). However, it has not been determined whether these were B or T-cells (42). Most complications of IM affecting the lungs and the upper respiratory tract, including pneumonia, pleural empyema, pharyngeal abscess, and mediastinitis appear to be caused by bacterial superinfection (43,44).

Kidneys

Renal failure may develop as a rare complication of IM. In such cases, histological examination usually shows an interstitial nephritis with an infiltration by CD8-positive T-cells (45,46). Using in situ hybridization, only rare EBV-infected lymphocytes have been detected in such cases (45,46). Again, it appears likely that the kidney is an innocent bystander damaged in the course of the host immune response to EBV infection (45).

Genital Mucosa

The occurrence of genital ulcers associated with IM has been reported in women, but not in men (41,47,48). Such ulcers may be the presenting symptom of IM (48). In one of these cases, shedding of EBV in the lesion was demonstrated using the lymphocyte transformation assay (47). This would seem to indicate virus replication in the lesion.

In another case, detection of LMP1- and EBNA2-positive cells by immunohisto-chemistry was reported (41). However, it is not known which cell type is infected in these ulcers, and it has not been established to what extent the infection is latent or replicative. Thus, the pathogenesis of genital ulcers in IM remains unknown.

Nervous System

Some degree of neurological involvement is quite common in acute IM with up to 50% of patients complaining of headache at presentation (49,50). However, serious neurological complications are rare (49). Domachowske et al. have noted headache, seizures, and electroencephalographic abnormalities in children with acute IM lead-ing to the diagnosis of EBV encephalitis (51). In some of these children, long-term sequelae remained (51). Moreover, meningitis, cranial nerve palsies, and demyelinat-ing disease have been reported in IM (49,52). Guillain–Barre syndrome can also occur as a complication of IM (43). A single case of recurrent laryngeal nerve palsy associated with IM has been reported (53). The pathological basis of these varied complications remains uncertain. Detection of EBV genomes and anti-EBV anti-bodies in cerebrospinal fluids from IM patients with neurological complications has been reported, suggesting a direct involvement of the central nervous system (CNS) (54,55). However, whether this is due to direct infection of the CNS or through infiltration of the CNS by EBV-infected lymphocytes remains uncertain. The occasional detection of mainly perivascular infiltration of EBV-infected lym-phoid cells of brain and spinal cord in patients with fatal IM and CAEBV infection would suggest the latter (56,57).

Placenta

Ornoy et al. studied five cases of pregnancy interruption associated with IM (58). They noted perivascular inflammatory infiltrates in the decidua. The chorionic mem-branes and placental villi showed stromal infiltration with lymphocytes and plasma cells, and vascular inflammatory changes. In three cases, the fetuses were studied and two displayed myocarditis (58). This supports the suggestion that placental transmis-sion of EBV is possible (59). In further support of this notion, development of an EBV-associated placental lymphoma of fetal origin in a 20-week stillborn fetus has been described (60).

PERSISTENT EBV INFECTION

Following primary infection, EBV establishes a lifelong persistent infection that is usually asymptomatic. It is now generally accepted that persistent EBV infection is mostly, if not exclusively, mediated by B-cells, and the available evidence points to memory B-cells as the most likely site of virus persistence (61,62). EBV-infected memory B-cells are resting and express a very limited set of viral latent genes (63,64). At the messenger ribonucleic acid level, expression of LMP2A has been detected regularly, and there is also possibly some EBNA1 expression (18,65,66). How EBV enters the memory B-cell pool is uncertain. Based on a single cell analysis of EBV-infected cells, Kurth et al. have concluded that EBV can infect naive and memory B-cells in acute IM, but that only EBV-infected memory B-cells show evi-dence of clonal expansion (67). By contrast, Thorley-Lawson et al. have provided evidence to suggest that EBV may utilize physiological B-cell pathways to gain access to the memory B-cell pool (62,68). It has been proposed that two EBV-encoded LMPs, LMP1 and LMP2A, may substitute for CD40 and B-cell receptor signaling, respectively; this facilitates the differentiation of EBV-infected cells into memory B-cells (62,69–71). This notion has been supported by the occasional detection of an expansion of EBV-positive B-cells in germinal center reactions (16). Whether this process occurs in an antigen-dependent or -independent fashion remains uncertain.

The number of EBV-infected B-cells varies among individuals; however, it has been shown to be remarkably constant in any one individual, suggesting that a level of homeostasis is maintained (72). Immunosuppressed persons generally show higher levels of EBV-infected cells in the peripheral blood and tonsils (73,74). However, these cells are again resting memory B-cells (73). The mechanism contributing to the elevated numbers of EBV-infected cells in these patients is unknown. In addition to peripheral blood, EBV-infected cells are detectable in various lymphoid and non-lymphoid tissues in chronic virus carriers. In general, the number of EBV-infected cells appears to be higher in tonsils than in lymph nodes and other lymphoid tissues (75). In addition, EBV-infected cells have been detected in solid organs, e.g., liver, and at other mucosal sites, e.g., stomach and intestines (76–78). To some extent, these cells probably belong to the pool of circulating EBV-positive memory B-cells. There is some evidence, however, that the numbers of EBV-infected cells may be influenced by certain disease conditions. Thus, elevated numbers of EBV-infected cells have been detected in intestinal mucosa samples from patients with chronic inflammatory bowel disease, notably ulcerative colitis (77). By contrast, only rare EBV-positive cells are detectable in chronic gastritis (78). Different patterns of cytokine expression may, in part, account for this difference. Thus, it is held that ulcerative colitis is characterized by a Th2 milieu (79–81). Some Th2 cytokines have been shown to be growth factors for EBV-positive B-cells (82–84); this may at least partly explain the increased number of EBV-infected B-cells at these sites.

EBV REPLICATION IN PRIMARY AND PERSISTENT INFECTION

The site of EBV replication is an unresolved issue. It is well documented that infectious virus is shed into the saliva in primary as well as persistent EBV infection (85). The source of this virus, however, is uncertain. Several studies have suggested that EBV may replicate in oropharyngeal epithelial cells, and there is clear evidence that this is indeed the case in epithelial cells of oral hairy leukoplakia, an AIDS-associated lesion of the tongue (24,25,86,87). However, the significance of this model has been questioned. Recent studies have failed to detect evidence of EBV replication in desquamated oropharyngeal epithelial cells from IM patients as well as from chronic carriers (22,26). In a large study of autopsy cases, evidence of EBV replication was detected in tongue epithelial cells in 4 of 168 samples (88). Although there was no evidence of human immunodeficiency virus infection, all individuals with evidence of EBV replication were either on immunosuppressive therapy for autoimmune disease or were terminally ill cancer patients, raising the possibility that an impairment of the immune system may have allowed EBV replication to occur at this site (88). Thus, the combined evidence of these studies would appear to suggest that EBV replication in oropharyngeal epithelial cells is at best a rare event of uncertain significance for EBV biology. In IM tonsils, a small number of EBV-positive lymphocytes with evidence of plasmacytoid differentiation has been shown to enter the lytic cycle (19,89,90). Whether this is followed by full-scale virus production or remains abortive is uncertain. Nevertheless, these results support the notion that terminal differentiation of EBV-infected B-cells may trigger entry into the EBV lytic cycle (91). In addition, a small number of EBV-infected cells showing lytic cycle antigen expression has been detected in mucosal samples from patients with ulcerative colitis (77). This observation raises the possibility that fecal transmission may occur in addition to transmission through the established salivary route. Similarly, patients with EBV-positive Hodgkin lymphoma (HL) displayed viremia and high titers of *Bam*HI Z EBV replication activator (ZEBRA/BZLF1) protein–specific antibodies (92). Because BZLF1 is only infrequently expressed in HL tissues (93), viral replication in tissues outside the Hodgkin's lymphoma lesions is suggested. Thus, EBV replication may be favored in conditions of decreased efficacy of the immune system. The occurrence of genital ulcers in patients with IM and the recovery of EBV from such lesions suggest yet another route for EBV spread, although this requires further investigation (47).

FATAL IM, CAEBV INFECTION, AND EBV-AHS

Fatal IM

IM may run a fatal course in approximately 1 in 3000 IM cases as a sporadic disease (94). In addition, fatal IM may occur as a familial disease affecting males in association with XLPD (94,95). Patients with XLPD are unable to establish T-cell control of EBV infection; approximately 65% of patients with XLPD develop fatal IM following primary EBV infection (94,96). Recently, defects in the *SAP* [signaling lymphocytic activation molecule (SLAM)–associated protein] gene have been identified in XLPD patients (97). It has been proposed that signaling through SLAM may induce a Th1 immune response, contribute to the activation of natural killer (NK) cells, and sensitize B-cells to Fas-induced apoptosis (97). Thus, defects in SLAM signaling through *SAP* mutations could inhibit T and NK cell–mediated clearance of EBV-infected B-cells (97). Two surface molecules, 2B4 (CD244) and NTB-A, have been shown to contribute to NK cell activation through interaction with *SAP* (98,99). One of these, 2B4 (CD244), is a receptor for the B-cell antigen, CD48, expression of which is upregulated by EBV infection (98,100). In NK cells from XLPD patients, both 2B4 and NTB-A inhibit rather than activate NK cell function (98,99). It has also been suggested that *SAP* mutations may make B-cells resistant to Fas-induced apoptosis, thus further increasing the pool of EBV-infected B-cells (97). However, the B-cells in XLPD patients have been shown to be susceptible to lysis by EBV-specific T-cells suggesting that B-cell defects do not contribute significantly to the disease (101).

Histopathology and Immunophenotype

The pathological features of sporadic and XLPD-related fatal IM are similar and result from an excessive proliferation of B-cells accompanied by variable numbers of T-cells. Immunophenotypic studies of affected tissues have shown a predominance of B-cells over T-cells. The infiltrating B-cells are usually polyclonal, but transition into a monoclonal proliferation is possible (94,102,103). Patients typically present with lymphadenopathy and splenomegaly. In initial stages, the lymphoreticular tissues show an expansion of the paracortex with proliferation of immunoblasts, small and medium-sized lymphocytes, and plasma cells. Germinal centers are usually small and prominent necrosis may be present (35). In later stages, lymphoid tissues may be depleted of lymphocytes with plasma cells and histiocytes remaining (35). The splenic white pulp is infiltrated by numerous immunoblasts and plasma cells (35). Again, necrosis may be present, but splenic rupture appears to be rare (35). The thymus may show extensive lymphocytic infiltration with effacement of the architecture (104). There is also usually a reduction or even a complete loss of Hassal bodies (104). The major causes of death in fatal IM relate to liver damage and EBV-AHS (35,105). The bone marrow changes are initially nonspecific consisting of granulocytic hyperplasia and only minimal lymphoid cell infiltration. With progression of the disease, the bone marrow shows a polymorphic lymphoid infiltrate and necrosis (35). There is also an increase in histiocytes with prominent hemophagocytosis. During the course of the disease, the marrow becomes depleted with only histiocytes and plasma cells remaining (35). Histiocytes showing evidence of hemophagocytosis may also be seen in the sinusoids of lymph nodes (94). The liver is also usually affected and displays periportal and sinusoidal infiltration (94). Parenchymal necrosis may occur in severe cases and hepatic failure is a major cause of death (94,106). In some cases, bile duct damage has also been observed (106,107). Notably, in situ studies have detected EBV in infiltrating lymphocytes but not in hepatocytes (106). The precise mechanism of liver damage in such cases is uncertain, but is believed to be caused by the infiltrating T and NK cells rather than by the EBV-infected B-cells (106). Other tissues including the heart, lungs, CNS, kidneys, and gastrointestinal tract may show perivascular infiltration (94,103,107).

EBV Studies and Phenotype of EBV-Infected Cells

There are only limited studies regarding the phenotype of EBV infected cells and the pattern of viral latent gene expression in fatal IM. The available evidence suggests that B-cells represent the major cell population carrying the virus in this condition (102). Notably, EBV infection has been shown to be absent from hepatocytes in fatal IM (106). In most cases, the infiltrating B-cells display a phenotype reminiscent of EBV-transformed lymphoblastoid cell lines with expression of activation markers in the absence of antigens typically expressed in Burkitt lymphoma (CD10, CD77) (102). In agreement with this, most cases displayed the full spectrum of EBV latent gene expression, including EBNA1, EBNA2, and LMP1 (latency III) (102). However, in some instances, expression of EBNA1 alone was observed, as seen in Burkitt lymphoma (102). Notably, this pattern was observed mainly in cases with a monoclonal B-cell proliferation suggesting transition to malignant lymphoma (102).

EBV-AHS and CAEBV Infection

IM commonly is a self-limiting disease. However, there are occasional reports of a fulminant and usually rapidly fatal illness developing in primary EBV infection, mainly in children (108,109). This illness is characterized by fever, hepatosplenomegaly, pancytopenia, and CNS involvement (108,109). The presence of hemophagocytic histiocytes in bone marrow samples is a defining feature of this disease which has been termed EBV-AHS. Mutations of the *perforin* gene have been suggested as a possible contributory factor (110). Occasionally, a chronic disease termed CAEBV infection or chronic IM may develop subsequent to primary EBV infection (111,112). This disease is characterized by symptoms such as fever, lymphadenopathy, splenomegaly, hematological abnormalities, and elevated antibody titers against lytic EBV antigens persisting for more than six months (111,112). Mutations of the *SAP* gene have not been identified in patients with CAEBV (113).

Histopathology

Patients having EBV-AHS present with fever, hepatosplenomegaly, liver dysfunc-tion, and pancytopenia (108,109). Even though the disease is usually fatal, there are only limited autopsy studies on these patients. A histiocytic hyperplasia of bone marrow with hemophagocytosis and infiltration by small lymphocytes has been reported (108,109). The liver may also show periportal and sinusoidal lymphocytes (109). Lymph nodes have been described as showing lymphocyte depletion and sinu-soidal histiocytes with evidence of hemophagocytosis (109). Organ manifestations of CAEBV include persistent hepatitis, interstitial pneumonitis, interstitial nephritis, and uveitis. However, histopathological studies of involved tissues are rare. Several authors have reported the occurrence of vasculitis with aneurysms involving the cor-onary arteries and the aortic arch in patients with CAEBV (108,114–116). Myocar-dial infarction may develop as a complication (115). Recently, a case of CAEBV and massive myocarditis in a Caucasian patient has been reported (56). This patient also displayed involvement of other organs showing perivascular T-cell infiltration in the gastrointestinal tract and the CNS (56). Chronic pericarditis with detection of EBV in pericardial tissue samples was also reported (117). Kikuchi et al. reported a case of CAEBV with vanishing bile duct syndrome (118). Interstitial nephritis and even immune complex–mediated glomerulonephritis have also been reported in CAEBV patients (115,119). Evidence of hemophagocytosis has also been reported in patients with CAEBV, and thus distinction from EBV-AHS may not always be clear (113).

EBV Studies and Phenotype of EBV-Infected Cells

Several studies have demonstrated that, unlike in acute IM, T-cells and NK cells are the major EBV-infected cell population in EBV-AHS and in CAEBV (56,109, 113,114,116). Kasahara et al. have reported the detection of EBV in CD8+ T-cells in patients with EBV-AHS, while patients with CAEBV showed EBV infection mainly of CD4+ T-cells and in CD16 NK cells (120). In agreement with this, Kimura et al. identified subsets of CAEBV patients with EBV infection predominantly of CD3-positive T-cells and CD16-positive NK cells, respectively (113). In that study, patients with NK cell type CAEBV were reported to have a better prognosis than those with T-cell type (113). Tissue damage in patients with EBV-AHS or CAEBV likely results from tissue infiltration by EBV-infected T or NK cells and abnormal patterns of cytokine expression (111). EBV-infected T-cells were detected in bone marrow and liver samples from patients with EBV-AHS and around bile ducts in a case of vanishing bile duct syndrome associated with CAEBV (109,118). EBV-infected T-cells have been reported to infiltrate vascular walls in CAEBV patients showing vasculitis and coronary artery aneurysms, and in myocardium and spinal cord samples of a CAEBV patient with myocarditis and neurological symptoms (56,116). The detection of EBV in isolated hepatocytes has also been reported in EBV-AHS (108). Similarly, Joh et al. (119) demonstrated the presence of EBV-posi-tive renal tubular epithelial cells in interstitial nephritis associated with CAEBV while there were only rare EBV-infected interstitial lymphocytes detectable. These observations raise the possibility that, in addition to T-cells, aberrant EBV infection of parenchymal cells may contribute to the disease process. However, this notion requires confirmation. Interestingly, Schwarzmann et al. described the isolation of an EBV strain with an impaired ability to transform B-cells and an inclination for lytic replication from a CAEBV patient, suggesting that viral factors may have contributed to the disease (121). However, the significance of this finding currently remains uncertain. Peripheral blood EBV load has been shown to correlate with disease severity in CAEBV (113). Viral episomes as well as T-cell receptor gene rearrangements have been shown to be polyclonal or monoclonal in CAEBV, and there is a clear possibility of transition to malignant T–cell lymphoma (see Chapter 13) (56,108,109,122,123).

EXPRESSION OF CYTOKINE AND CHEMOKINE GENES IN IM AND CAEBV INFECTION

The expression patterns of cytokine genes in EBV-associated lymphoproliferative disorders are only incompletely understood. This is important because some cytokines and chemokines are likely to stimulate the development of T-cell immunity in response to proliferating EBV-infected B-cells. On the other hand, other cytokines may serve to inhibit EBV-specific immunity, or even serve as (autocrine) growth factors for EBV-infected B-cells. The issue is further complicated by the heterogeneity of the cell populations present, e.g., in IM. Thus, high levels of interleukin (IL)-6 expression have been demonstrated in IM tissues, but this cytokine appears to be expressed mainly in EBV-negative cells (124). The expression of IL-6 may contribute to the disease owing to its known immune-modulating functions and its possible role as a growth factor in EBV-infected B-cells (82). In contrast, lymphotoxin and tumor necrosis factor-α (TNF-α) are mainly produced by EBV-positive cells in IM (124). In comparison to reactive lymphoid tissues, elevated expression of monokine induced by interferon (IFN)-γ (Mig), interferon-inducible protein-10 (IP-10), IL-18, as well as human and viral IL-10 has been observed in IM (125). Expression of IL-10 in IM tissues and abnormally high levels of circulating IL-10 in IM patients have been reported (126,127). IL-10 is a known autocrine growth factor for EBV-transformed B-cells (84). IL-10 may inhibit EBV-specific cytotoxic T-cells, thus contributing to immune escape of EBV-infected cells (128). However, IL-10 has also been shown to inhibit apoptotic death of T-cells in IM, suggesting that it may contribute to the development of T-cell memory (129). Mig and IP-10 are CXC chemokines induced by IFN-γ in monocytes (130). Both Mig and IP-10 are chemoattractant for activated T-cells through a joint receptor, CXCR3, and both have been suggested to contribute to tissue damage in EBV-associated lymphoproliferation (130,131). Together with IL-12, IL-18 is known to promote expression of IFN-γ, and thus may promote the development of a Th1 immune response (132). Recently, expression of Epstein–Barr virus induced gene 3 (EBI3) has also been reported in IM (133). EBI3 is an EBV-induced cytokine homologous to the IL-12 p40 subunit (134). EBI3 can be secreted as a monomer or can heterodimerize with IL-12 p35 (135). It has been speculated that EBI3 may act as an IL-12 antagonist (136). However, EBI3 is also able to heterodimerize with p28 to form IL-27 (137). IL-27 has been shown to stimulate proliferation of naive CD4 T-cells and, in conjunction with IL-12, to promote Th1 reactions (137). Thus, the function of EBI3 may depend on the context of its expression. High levels of human and viral IL-10 have also been reported in patients with CAEBV (138). Higher expression levels of IFN-γ, IL-2, IL-10, and transforming growth factor (TGF) β have been reported in activated T-cells in CAEBV than in IM suggesting that expression of both Th1 and Th2 cytokines may be deregulated in CAEBV (139). Particularly, human and viral IL-10 may contribute to the disease by inhibiting host immunity (138). Patients with CAEBV and EBV-AHS show elevated blood and tissue levels of Th1 and Th2 cytokines capable of macrophage activation, e.g., TNF-α, IL-1, and IFN-γ (111). It is possible that these are produced by EBV-infected T-cells (111). However, the full significance of these observations is currently uncertain, and thorough studies at the single cell level will be required to define cytokine patterns and the contribution of EBV-infected cells more clearly.

CONCLUSIONS

Primary EBV infection in children usually is asymptomatic. However, IM may develop in up to 50% of individuals when primary infection is delayed into adolescence or early adulthood (2,3). What is known about primary EBV infection largely stems from studies of IM cases and is based on the implicit assumption that what is seen in IM is also found in asymptomatic primary infection albeit at a lower level. This, however, is by no means certain. Indeed, fundamental immunological differences between IM patients and individuals with asymptomatic primary infection have recently been identified (140). Thus, lymphocytosis with an increase of CD8 T-cells and selective expansions of Vβ-expressing T-cells was observed in IM while these changes were undetectable in asymptomatic primary infection (140–142). The hallmark of acute IM is the proliferation of EBV-infected B-cells, which in turn triggers a vigorous EBV-specific T-cell response. This is reflected in the histopathological changes in lymphoid tissues. EBV infection of other cell types in IM, notably T-cells, has not been well documented and if at all occurring, is at best a rare event. Damage in nonlymphoid tissues such as the liver is probably the result of excessive T-cell infiltration that may or may not be EBV specific. In any case, this is likely to be a nonspecific side effect of the EBV-specific immune response and not a specific reaction against EBV-infected non–B-cells. Imbalances in the cytokine milieu in IM may contribute to this effect. The end result of IM as well as of asymptomatic primary EBV infection is a lifelong carrier state in which the virus is present in a small number of resting B-cells (62). A contribution of other cell types, notably T-cells and epithelial cells, to virus persistence remains doubtful. Virus replication in IM as well as in persistent infection may occur in plasma cells and/or in oropharyngeal epithelial cells, resulting in shedding of virus into saliva and renewed infection of the B-cell compartment. The inter-relationship between epithelial and B-cell–derived EBV is uncertain. Recently, it has been suggested that B-cell–derived virus may preferentially infect epithelial cells while epithelial-derived EBV has an increased ability to infect B-cells (143); whether this mechanism is relevant for EBV infection in vivo remains to be established. Fatal IM represents an exaggerated form of IM precipitated by an inherited or sporadic failure to mount a sufficient EBV-specific immunity. In most tissues, a slight predominance of EBV-positive B-cells over T-cells is observed. Tissue damage is thought to be a nonspecific result of T-cell proliferation, although an effect of EBV-positive B-cells cannot be excluded (94).

In typical as well as fatal IM, EBV infection of T-cells occurs only rarely if at all. In contrast, EBV infection of T-cells is a characteristic feature of EBV-AHS and CAEBV. Interestingly, it appears that different T-cell subsets are infected in EBV-AHS and CAEBV. Thus, in EBV-AHS, infection of CD8+ T-cells has been observed, while in CAEBV, EBV has been detected in CD4+ T-cells and NK cells (120). Moreover, subsets of CAEBV patients showing predominant infection of either T-cells or NK cells have been identified, and it appears that patients with NK cell type CAEBV have a better prognosis than those with a T-cell type (113). Thus, these findings raise the intriguing possibility that the infected cell type may influence clinical symptomatology and outcome of EBV infection. The tissue damage observed in EBV-AHS and CAEBV is likely to be the result of tissue infiltration by EBV-infected T or NK cells. EBV infection of T or NK cells may induce an abnormal cytokine expression pattern that may contribute to the disease, e.g., by activating macrophages in EBV-AHS. When and how EBV infection of T-cells occurs remains uncertain. It has been speculated that this may occur as an accident during the cytotoxic T lymphocyte (CTL)-mediated killing of EBV-infected B-cells (144). In any case, it remains unclear at present if accidental EBV infection of T-cells is the primary event in EBV-AHS and CAEBV, or if it is merely an epiphenomenon reflecting an underlying immune defect.

REFERENCES

1. International Agency for Research on Cancer. Epstein–Barr Virus and Kaposi's Sarcoma Herpesvirus/Human Herpesvirus 8. Lyon, France: WHO, 1997.
2. Infectious mononucleosis and its relationship to EB virus antibody. A joint investigation by university health physicians and P.H.L.S. laboratories. Br Med J 1971; 4:643–646.
3. Evans AS. Clinical syndromes associated with EB virus infection. Ann Intern Med 1972; 18:77–93.
4. Pfeiffer E. Drüsenfieber. Jahrb Kinderheilkd 1889; 29:257–264.
5. Rea TD, Russo JE, Katon W, Ashley RL, Buchwald DS. Prospective study of the natural history of infectious mononucleosis caused by Epstein–Barr virus. J Am Board Fam Pract 2001; 14:234–242.
6. Svedmyr E, Ernberg I, Seeley J, et al. Virologic, immunologic, and clinical observations on a patient during the incubation, acute, and convalescent phases of infectious moononucleosis. Clin Immunol Immunopathol 1984; 30:437–450.
7. Pattengale PK, Smith RW, Perlin E. Atypical lymphocytes in acute infectious mononucleosis. Identification by multiple T and B lymphocyte markers. N Engl J Med 1974; 291:1145–1148.
8. Lennert K, Schwarze E-W, Krüger G. Lymph node lesions caused by viral infections. Verh Dtsch Ges Pathol 1981; 65:151–171.
9. Strickler JG, Fedeli F, Horwitz CA, Copenhaver CM, Frizzera G. Infectious mononucleosis in lymphoid tissue. Histopathology, in situ hybridization, and differential diagnosis. Arch Pathol Lab Med 1993; 117:269–278.
10. Isaacson PG, Schmid C, Pan L, Wotherspoon AC, Wright DH. Epstein–Barr virus latent membrane protein expression by Hodgkin and Reed–Sternberg-like cells in acute infectious mononucleosis. J Pathol 1992; 167:267–271.
11. Frizzera G. The clinico-pathological expressions of Epstein–Barr virus infection in lymphoid tissues. Virchows Arch B Cell Pathol Incl Mol Pathol 1987; 53:1–12.
12. Plumbley JA, Fan H, Eagan PA, Schnitzer B, Gulley ML. Lymphoid tissues from patients with infectious mononucleosis lack monoclonal B and T cells. J Mol Diagn 2002; 4:37–43.
13. O'Brien A, O'Briain DS. Infectious mononucleosis. Appendiceal lymphoid tissue involvement parallels characteristic lymph node changes. Arch Pathol Lab Med 1985; 109:680–682.
14. Niedobitek G, Hamilton-Dutoit S, Herbst H, et al. Identification of Epstein–Barr virus-infected cells in tonsils of acute infectious mononucleosis by in situ hybridization. Hum Pathol 1989; 20:796–799.

15. Weiss LM, Movahed LA. In situ demonstration of Epstein–Barr viral genomes in viral-associated B cell lymphoproliferations. Am J Pathol 1989; 134:651–659.

16. Niedobitek G, Herbst H, Young LS, et al. Patterns of Epstein–Barr virus infection in non-neoplastic lymphoid tissue. Blood 1992; 79:2520–2526.

17. Reynolds DJ, Banks PM, Gulley ML. New characterisation of infectious mononucleosis and a phenotypic comparison with Hodgkin's disease. Am J Pathol 1995; 146:379–388.

18. Tierney RJ, Steven N, Young LS, Rickinson AB. Epstein–Barr virus latency in blood mononuclear cells: analysis of viral gene transcription during primary infection and in the carrier state. J Virol 1994; 68:7374–7385.

19. Niedobitek G, Agathanggelou A, Herbst H, Whitehead L, Wright DH, Young LS. Epstein–Barr virus (EBV) infection in infectious mononucleosis: virus latency, replication and phenotype of EBV-infected cells. J Pathol 1997; 182:151–159.

20. Alfieri C, Birkenbach M, Kieff E. Early events in Epstein–Barr virus infection of human lymphocytes-B. Virology 1991; 181:595–608.

21. Niedobitek G, Kremmer E, Herbst H, et al. Immunohistochemical detection of the Epstein–Barr virus-encoded latent membrane protein 2A (LMP2A) in Hodgkin's disease and infectious mononucleosis. Blood 1997; 90:1664–1672.

22. Karajannis MA, Hummel M, Anagnostopoulos I, Stein H. Strict lymphotropism of Epstein–Barr virus during acute infectious mononucleosis in nonimmunocompromised individuals. Blood 1997; 89:2856–2862.

23. Deamant FD, Albujar PF, Chen YY, Weiss LM. Epstein–Barr virus distribution in nonneoplastic lymph nodes. Mod Pathol 1993; 6:729–732.

24. Lemon SM, Hutt LM, Shaw JE, Li JL, Pagano JS. Replication of EBV in epithelial cells during infectious mononucleosis. Nature 1977; 70:268–270.

25. Sixbey JW, Nedrud JG, Raab-Traub N, Hanes RA, Pagano JS. Epstein–Barr virus replication in oropharyngeal epithelial cells. N Engl J Med 1984; 310:1225–1230.

26. Niedobitek G, Agathanggelou A, Steven N, Young LS. Epstein–Barr virus (EBV) in infectious mononucleosis: detection of the virus in tonsillar B lymphocytes but not in desquamated oropharyngeal epithelial cells. J Clin Pathol: Mol Pathol 2000; 53:37–42.

27. Niedobitek G, Finn T, Herbst H, Stein H. Detection of viral genomes in the liver by in situ hybridisation using 35S-, bromodeoxyuridine-, and biotin-labeled probes. Am J Pathol 1989; 134:633–639.

28. Hoagland RJ. Mononucleosis and heart disease. Am J Med Sci 1964; 248:35–40.

29. Frishman W, Kraus ME, Zabkar J, Brooks V, Alonso D, Dixon LM. Infectious mononucleosis and fatal myocarditis. Chest 1977; 72:535–538.

30. Hebert MM, Yu C, Towbin JA, Rogers BB. Fatal Epstein–Barr virus myocarditis in a child with repetitive myocarditis. Pediatr Pathol Lab Med 1995; 15:805–812.

31. Brncic N, Sever-Prebilic M, Crnic-Martinovic M, Prebilic I. Severe autoimmune hemolytic anemia as a potentially fatal complication of EBV infectious mononucleosis. Int J Hematol 2001; 74:352–353.

32. Koppes GM, Ratkin GA, Coltman CA. Pancytopenia and "capillary leak syndrome" with infectious mononucleosis. South Med J 1976; 69:145–148.

33. Shadduck RK, Winkelstein A, Zeigler Z, et al. Aplastic anemia following infectious mononucleosis: possible immune etiology. Exp Hematol 1979; 7:264–271.

34. Lazarus KH, Baehner RL. Aplastic anemia complicating infectious mononucleosis: a case report and review of the literature. Pediatrics 1981; 67:907–910.

35. Mroczek EC, Weisenburger DD, Lipscomb Grierson H, Markin R, Purtilo DT. Fatal infectious mononucleosis and virus-associated hemophagocytic syndrome. Arch Pathol Lab Med 1987; 111:530–535.

36. White NJ, Juel-Jensen BE. Infectious mononucleosis hepatitis. Semin Liver Dis 1984; 4:301–306.

37. Jacobson IM, Gang DL, Schapiro RH. Epstein–Barr viral hepatitis: an unusual case and review of the literature. Am J Gastroenterol 1984; 79:628–632.

38. Kimura H, Nagasaka T, Hoshino Y, et al. Severe hepatitis caused by Epstein–Barr virus without infection of hepatocytes. Hum Pathol 2001; 32:757–762.

39. Markin RS. Manifestations of Epstein–Barr virus-associated disorders in the liver. Liver 1994; 14:1–13.

40. Feranchak AP, Tyson RW, Narkewicz MR, Karrer FM, Sokol RJ. Fulminant Epstein–Barr virus hepatitis: orthotopic liver transplantation and review of the literature. Liver Transpl Surg 1998; 4:469–476.

41. Andersson J, Isberg B, Christensson B, Veress, Linde A, Bratel T. Interferon γ (IFN-γ) deficiency in generalized Epstein–Barr virus infection with interstitial lymphoid and granulomatous pneumonia, focal cerebral lesions, and genital ulcers: remission following IFN-γ substitution therapy. Clin Infect Dis 1999; 28:1036–1042.

42. Sriskandan S, Labreque LG, Schofield J. Diffuse pneumonia associated with infectious mononucleosis: detection of Epstein–Barr virus in lung tissue by in situ hybridization. Clin Infect Dis 1996; 22:578–579.

43. Alpert G, Fleisher GR. Complications of infection with Epstein–Barr virus during childhood: a study of children admitted to the hospital. Pediat Infect Dis 1984; 3: 304–307.

44. Andrianakis IA, Kotanidou AN, Pitraridis MT, et al. Life-threatening bilateral empyema and mediastinits complicating infectious mononucleosis. Intensive Care Med 2002; 28:663–664.

45. Mayer HB, Wanke CA, Williams M, Crosson AW, Federman M, Hammer SM. Epstein–Barr virus-induced infectious mononucleosis complicated by acute renal failure: case report and review. Clin Infect Dis 1995; 22:1009–1018.

46. Lei PS, Lowichik A, Allen W, Mauch TJ. Acute renal failure: unusual complication of Epstein–Barr virus-induced infectious mononucleosis. Clin Exp Immunol 2000; 31:1519–1524.

47. Portnoy J, Ahronheim GA, Ghibu F, Clecner B, Joncas JH. Recovery of Epstein–Barr virus from genital ulcers. N Engl J Med 1984; 311:966–968.

48. Hudson LB, Perlman SE. Necrotizing genital ulcerations in a premenarcheal female with mononucleosis. Obstet Gynecol 1998; 92:642–644.

49. Connelly KP, DeWitt LD. Neurologic complications of infectious mononucleosis. Pediat Neurol 1994; 10:181–184.

50. Corssmit EP, Leverstein van Hall MA, Portegies P, Bakker P. Severe neurological complications in association with Epstein–Barr virus infection. J Neurovirol 1997; 3: 460–464.

51. Domachowske JB, Cunningham CK, Cummings DL, Crosley CJ, Hannan WP, Weiner LB. Acute manifestations and neurologic sequelae of Epstein–Barr virus encephalitis in children. Pediat Infect Dis 1996; 15:871–875.

52. Bray PF, Culp KW, McFarlin DE, Panitch HS, Torkelson RD, Schlight JP. Demyelinating disease after neurologically complicated primary Epstein–Barr virus infection. Neurology 1992; 42:278–282.

53. Parano E, Pavone L, Musumeci S, Giambusso F, Trifiletti RR. Acute palsy of the recurrent laryngeal nerve complicating Epstein–Barr virus infection. Neuropediatrics 1996; 27:164–166.

54. Imai S, Usui N, Sugiura M, et al. Epstein–Barr virus genomic sequences and specific antibodies in cerebrospinal fluid in children with neurological complications of acute and reactivated EBV infections. J Med Virol 1993; 40:278–284.

55. Schiff JA, Schaefer JA, Robinson JE. Epstein–Barr virus in cerebrospinal fluid during infectious mononucleosis encephalitis. Yale J Biol Med 1982; 55:59–63.

56. Hauptmann S, Meru N, Schewe C, et al. Fatal atypical T-cell proliferation associated with Epstein–Barr virus infection. Br J Haematol 2001; 112:377–380.

57. Talamo TS, Borochovitz D, Atchison RW. Fatal Epstein–Barr virus infection in a 63-year-old man. Arch Pathol Lab Med 1981; 105:465–469.

58. Ornoy A, Dudai M, Sadovsky E. Placental and fetal pathology in infectious mononu-
    cleosis. Diagn Gynecol Obstetr 1982; 4:11–16.
59. Meyohas M-C, Marechal V, Desire N, Bouillie J, Frottier J, Nicolas J-C. Study of
    mother-to-child Epstein–Barr virus transmission by means of nested PCRs. J Virol
    1996; 70:6816–6819.
60. Fritsch M, Jaffe ES, Griffin C, Camacho J, Raffeld M, Kingma DW. Lymphoprolifera-
    tive disorder of fetal origin presenting as oligohydramnios. Am J Surg Pathol 1999;
    23:595–601.
61. Niedobitek G, Young LS. Epstein–Barr virus persistence and virus-associated tumours.
    Lancet 1994; 343:333–335.
62. Thorley-Lawson DA, Babcock GJ. A model for persistent infection with Epstein–Barr
    virus: the stealth virus of human B cells. Life Sci 1999; 14:1433–1453.
63. Miyashita EM, Yang B, Lam KMC, Crawford DH, Thorley-Lawson DA. A novel form
    of Epstein–Barr virus latency in normal B cells in vivo. Cell 1995; 80:593–601.
64. Babcock GJ, Decker LL, Volk M, Thorley-Lawson DA. EBV persistence in memory B
    cells in vivo. Immunity 1998; 9:395–404.
65. Qu L, Rowe DT. Epstein–Barr virus latent gene expression in uncultured peripheral
    blood lymphocytes. J Virol 1992; 66:3715–3724.
66. Babcock G, Thorley-Lawson DA. Tonsillar memory B cells, latently infeced with
    Epstein–Barr virus, express the restricted pattern of latent genes previously found only
    in Epstein–Barr virus-associated tumors. Proc Natl Acad Sci USA 2000; 97:12,250–
    12,255.
67. Kurth J, Spieker T, Wustrow J, et al. EBV-infected B cells in infectious mononucleosis:
    viral strategies for spreading in the B cell compartment and establishing latency. Immu-
    nity 2000; 13:485–495.
68. Babcock GJ, Hochberg D, Thorley-Lawson DA. The expression pattern of Epstein–
    Barr virus latent genes in vivo is dependent upon the differentiation stage of the infected
    B cell. Immunity 2000; 13:497–506.
69. Kilger E, Kieser A, Baumann M, Hammerschmidt W. Epstein–Barr virus-mediated B-
    cell proliferation is dependent upon latent membrane protein 1, which simulates an acti-
    vated CD40 receptor. EMBO J 1998; 17:1700–1709.
70. Floettmann JE, Eliopoulos AG, Jones M, Young LS, Rowe M. Epstein–Barr virus
    latent membrane protein-1 (LMP1) signalling is distinct from CD40 and involves phy-
    sical cooperation of its two C-terminus functional regions. Oncogene 1998; 17:2383–
    2392.
71. Caldwell RG, Wilson JB, Anderson SJ, Longnecker R. Epstein–Barr virus LMP2A
    drives B cell development and survival in the absence of normal B cell receptor signals.
    Immunity 1998; 9:405–411.
72. Khan G, Miyashita EM, Yang B, Babcock GJ, Thorley-Lawson DA. Is EBV persis-
    tence in vivo a model for B cell homeostasis? Immunity 1996; 5:173–179.
73. Babcock GJ, Decker LL, Freeman RB, Thorley-Lawson DA. Epstein–Barr virus-
    infected resting memory B cells, not proliferating lymphoblasts, accumulate in the per-
    ipheral blood of immunosuppressed patients. J Exp Med 1999; 190:567–576.
74. Meru N, Davison S, Whitehead L, et al. Epstein–Barr virus infection in paediatric liver
    transplant recipients: detection of the virus in posttransplant tonsilectomy specimens. J
    Clin Pathol: Mol Pathol 2001; 54:264–269.
75. Laichalk LL, Hochberg D, Babcock GJ, Freeman RB, Thorley-Lawson DA. The dis-
    persal of mucosal memory B cells: evidence from persistent EBV infection. Immunity
    2002; 16:745–754.
76. Hubscher SG, Williams A, Davison SM, Young LS, Niedobitek G. Epstein–Barr virus
    in inflammatory diseases of the liver and liver allografts: an in situ hybridization study.
    Hepatology 1994; 20:899–907.
77. Spieker T, Herbst H. Distribution and phenotype of Epstein–Barr virus-infected cells in
    inflammatory bowel disease. Am J Pathol 2000; 157:51–57.

78. Hungermann D, Müller S, Spieker T, Lisner R, Niedobitek G, Herbst H. Low prevalence of latently Epstein–Barr virus infected cells in chronic gastritis. Microsc Res Tech 2001; 53:409–413.

79. Mullin GE, Lazenby AJ, Harris ML, Bayless TM, James SP. Increased interleukin-2 messenger RNA in the intestinal mucosal lesions of Crohn's disease but not ulcerative colitis. Gastroenterology 1992; 102:1620–1627.

80. Fuss IJ, Neurath M, Boirivant M, et al. Disparate CD4+ lamina propria (LP) lymphokine secretion profiles in inflammatory bowel disease. Crohn's disease LP cells manifest increased secretion of IFN-gamma, whereas ulcerative colitis LP cells manifest increased secretion of IL-5. J Immunol 1996; 157:1261–1270.

81. Christ AD, Stevens AC, Koeppen H, et al. An interleukin 12-related cytokine is up-regulated in ulcerative colitis but not in Crohn's disease. Gastroenterology 1998; 115:307–313.

82. Tosato G, Tanner J, Jones KD, Revel M, Pike SE. Identification of interleukin-6 as an autocrine growth factor for Epstein–Barr virus-immortalized B cells. J Virol 1990; 64:3033–3041.

83. Baumann MA, Paul CC. Interleukin-5 is an autocrine growth factor for Epstein–Barr virus-transformed B lymphocytes. Blood 1992; 79:1763–1767.

84. Beatty PR, Krams SM, Martinez OM. Involvement of IL-10 in the autonomouos growth of EBV-transformed B cell lines. J Immunol 1997; 158:4045–4051.

85. Niederman JC. Infectious mononucleosis: observations on transmission. Yale J Biol Med 1982; 55:259–264.

86. Greenspan JS, Greenspan D, Lennette ET, et al. Replication of Epstein–Barr virus within the epithelial cells of oral hairy leukoplakia, an AIDS-associated lesion. N Engl J Med 1985; 313:1564–1571.

87. Niedobitek G, Young LS, Lau R, et al. Epstein–Barr virus infection in oral hairy leukoplakia: virus replication in the absence of a detectable latent phase. J Gen Virol 1991; 72:3035–3046.

88. Herrmann K, Frangou P, Middeldorp J, Niedobitek G. Epstein–Barr virus replication in tongue epithelial cells. J Gen Virol 2002; 83:2995–2998.

89. Robinson JE, Smith D, Niederman J. Plasmacytic differentiation of circulating Epstein–Barr virus-infected B lymphocytes during acute infectious mononucleosis. J Exp Med 1981; 153:235–244.

90. Anagnostopoulos I, Hummel M, Kreschel C, Stein H. Morphology, immunophenotype, and distribution of latently and/or productively Epstein–Barr virus-infected cells in acute infectious mononucleosis: implications for the interindividual infection route of Epstein–Barr virus. Blood 1995; 85:744–750.

91. Crawford DH, Ando I. Epstein–Barr virus induction is associated with B-cell maturation. Immunology 1986; 59:405–409.

92. Drouet E, Brousset P, Fares F, et al. High Epstein–Barr virus serum load and elevated titers of anti-ZEBRA antibodies in patients with EBV-harboring tumor cells of Hodgkin's disease. J Med Virol 1999; 57:383–389.

93. Pallesen G, Sandvej K, Hamilton-Dutoit SJ, Rowe M, Young LS. Activation of Epstein–Barr virus replication in Hodgkin and Reed–Sternberg cells. Blood 1991; 78:1162–1165.

94. Purtilo DT, Strobach RS, Okano M, Davis JR. Epstein–Barr virus-associated lymphoproliferative disorders. Lab Invest 1992; 67:5–23.

95. Bar RS, DeLor J, Clausen KP, Hurtubise P, Henle W, Hewetson JF. Fatal infectious mononucleosis in a family. N Engl J Med 1974; 290:363–367.

96. Yasuda N, Lai PK, Rogers J, Purtilo DT. Defective control of Epstein–Barr virus-infected B cell growth in patients with X-linked lymphoproliferative disease. Clin Exp Immunol 1991; 83:10–16.

97. Howie D, Sayos J, Terhorst C, Morra M. The gene defective in X-linked lymphoproliferative disease controls T cell dependent immune surveillance against Epstein–Barr virus. Curr Opin Immunol 2000; 12:474–478.

98. Parolini S, Bottino C, Falco M, et al. X-linked lymphoproliferative disease: 2B4 mole-
    cules displaying inhibitory rather than activating function are responsible for the inabil-
    ity of natural killer cells to kill Epstein–Barr virus infected cells. J Exp Med 2000;
    192:337–346.

99. Bottino C, Falco M, Parolini S, et al. NTB-A, a novel SH2D1A-associated surface
    molecule contributing to the inability of natural killer cells to kill Epstein–Barr virus-
    infected B cells in X-linked lymphoproliferative disease. J Exp 2001; 194:235–246.

100. Thorley-Lawson DA, Schooley RT, Bhan AK, Nadler LM. Epstein–Barr virus super-
     induces a new human B cell differentiation antigen (B-LAST 1) expressed in trans-
     formed lymphocytes. Cell 1982; 30:415–425.

101. Jäger M, Benninger-Döring G, Prang N, et al. Epstein–Barr virus-infected B cells of
     males with the X-linked lymphoproliferative syndrome stimulate and are susceptible
     to T-cell-mediated lysis. Int J Cancer 1998; 76:694–701.

102. Falk K, Ernberg I, Sakthivel R, et al. Expression of Epstein–Barr virus-encoded proteins
     and B-cell markers in fatal infectious mononucleosis. Int J Cancer 1990; 46:976–984.

103. Yatabe Y, Mori N, Oka K, et al. Fatal Epstein–Barr virus-associated lymphoprolifera-
     tive disease in children. Arch Pathol Lab Med 1995; 119:409–417.

104. Mroczek EC, Seemayer TA, Grierson HL, et al. Thymic lesions in fatal infectious
     mononucleosis. Clin Immunol Immunopathol 1987; 43:243–255.

105. Okano M, Gross TG. From Burkitt's lymphoma to chronic active Epstein–Barr virus
     (EBV) infection: an expanding spectrum of EBV-associated diseases. Pediat Hematol
     Oncol 2001; 18:427–442.

106. Markin RS, Linder J, Zuerlein K, et al. Hepatitis in fatal infectious mononucleosis.
     Gastroenterology 1987; 93:1210–1217.

107. Iijima T, Sumazaki R, Mori N, et al. A pathological and immunological case report of
     fatal infectious mononucleosis, Epstein–Barr virus infection, demonstrated by in situ
     and Southern blot hybridization. Virchows Archiv A Pathol Anat Histopathol 1992;
     421:73–78.

108. Kikuta H, Sakiyama Y, Matsumoto S, et al. Fatal Epstein–Barr virus-associated hemo-
     phagocytic syndrome. Blood 1993; 82:3259–3264.

109. Kawaguchi H, Miyashita T, Herbst H, et al. Epstein–Barr virus-infected T lymphocytes
     in Epstein–Barr virus-associated hemophagocytic syndrome. J Clin Invest 1993; 92:
     1444–1450.

110. Stepp SE, Dufourcq-Lagelouse R, Le Deist F, et al. Perforin gene defects in familial
     hemophagocytic lymphohistiocytosis. Science 1999; 286:1957–1959.

111. Maia DM, Peace-Brewer AL. Chronic active Epstein–Barr virus infection. Curr Opin
     Hematol 2000; 7:59–63.

112. Straus SE. The chronic mononucleosis syndrome. J Infect Dis 1988; 157:405–412.

113. Kimura H, Hoshino Y, Kanegane H, et al. Clinical and virologic characteristics of
     chronic active Epstein–Barr virus infection. Blood 2001; 98:280–286.

114. Kikuta H, Taguchi Y, Tomizawa K, et al. Epstein–Barr virus genome-positive T lym-
     phocytes in a boy with chronic active EBV infection associated with Kawasaki-like dis-
     ease. Nature 1988; 333:455–457.

115. Muso E, Fujiwara H, Yoshida H, et al. Epstein–Barr virus genome-positive tubulo-
     interstitial nephritis associated with Kawasaki disease-like coronary aneurysms. Clin
     Nephrol 1993; 1:7–15.

116. Nakagawa A, Ito M, Iwaki T, Yatabe Y, Asai J, Hayashi K. Chronic active Epstein–Barr
     virus infection with giant coronary aneurysms. Am J Clin Pathol 1996; 105:733–736.

117. Satoh T, Kojima M, Ohshima K. Demonstration of the Epstein–Barr genome by poly-
     merase chain reaction and in situ hybridisation in a patient with viral pericarditis. Br
     Heart J 1993; 69:563–564.

118. Kikuchi K, Miyakawa H, Abe K, et al. Vanishing bile duct syndrome associated with
     chronic EBV infection. Digest Dis Sci 2000; 45:160–165.

119. Joh K, Kanetsuna Y, Ishikawa Y, et al. Epstein–Barr virus genome-positive tubulointerstitial nephritis associated with immune complex-mediated glomerulonephritis in chronic active EB virus infection. Virchows Archiv 1998; 432:567–573.

120. Kasahara Y, Yachie A, Takei K, et al. Differential cellular targets of Epstein–Barr virus (EBV) infection between acute EBV-associated hemophagocytic lymphohistiocytosis and chronic active EBV infection. Blood 2001; 98:1882–1888.

121. Schwarzmann F, von Baehr R, Jager M, et al. A case of severe chronic active infection with Epstein–Barr virus: immunologic deficiencies associated with a lytic virus strain. Clin Infect Dis 1999; 29:626–631.

122. Kanegane H, Bhatia K, Gutierrez M, et al. A syndrome of peripheral blood T-cell infection with Epstein–Barr virus (EBV) followed by EBV-positive T-cell lymphoma. Blood 1998; 91:2085–2091.

123. Quintanilla-Martinez L, Kumar S, Fend F, et al. Fulminant EBV+ T-cell lymphoproliferative disorder following acute/chronic EBV infection: a distinct clinicopathologic syndrome. Blood 2000; 96:443–451.

124. Foss HD, Herbst H, Hummel M, et al. Patterns of cytokine gene expression in infectious mononucleosis. Blood 1994; 83:707–712.

125. Setsuda J, Teruya-Feldstein J, Harris NL, et al. Interleukin-18, interferon-, IP-10, and Mig expression in Epstein–Barr virus-induced infectious mononucleosis and posttransplant lymphorpoliferative disease. Am J Pathol 1999; 155:257–265.

126. Herbst H, Foss H-D, Samol J, et al. Frequent expression of interleukin-10 by Epstein–Barr virus-harboring tumor cells of Hodgkin's disease. Blood 1996; 87:2918–2929.

127. Taga H, Taga K, Wang F, Chretien J, Tosato G. Human and viral interleukin-10 in acute Epstein–Barr virus-induced infectious mononucleosis. J Infect Dis 1995; 171:1347–1350.

128. Bejarano MT, Masucci MG. Interleukin-10 abrogates the inhibition of Epstein–Barr virus-induced B-cell transformation by memory T-cell reponses. Blood 1998; 92:4256–4262.

129. Taga K, Chretien J, Cherney B, Diaz L, Brown M, Tosato G. Interleukin-10 inhibits apoptotis cell death in infectious mononucleosis T cells. J Clin Invest 1994; 94:251–260.

130. Farber JM. Mig and IP-10: CXC chemokines that target lymphocytes. J Leukoc Biol 1997; 61:246–257.

131. Teruya-Feldstein J, Jaffe ES, Burd PR, et al. The role of Mig, the monokine induced by interferon-γ, and IP-10, the interferon-γ-induced protein-10, in tissue necrosis and vascular damage associated with Epstein–Barr virus-positive lymphoproliferative disease. Blood 1997; 90:4099–4105.

132. Okamura H, Kashiwamura S-i, Tsutsui H, Yoshimoto T, Nakanishi K. Regulation of interferon-γ production by IL-12 and IL-18. Curr Opin Immunol 1998; 10:259–264.

133. Niedobitek G, Päzolt D, Teichmann M, Devergne O. Expression of the Epstein–Barr virus (EBV)-induced gene, EBI3, an IL-12 p40 related cytokine, in EBV-associated tumors: frequent detection in Hodgkin and Reed–Sternberg cells. J Pathol 2002; 198:310–316.

134. Devergne O, Hummel M, Koeppen H, et al. A novel interleukin-12 p40-related protein induced by latent Epstein–Barr virus infection in B lymphocytes. J Virol 1996; 70:1143–1153.

135. Devergne O, Birkenbach M, Kieff E. Epstein–Barr virus-induced gene 3 and the p35 subunit of interleukin 12 form a novel heterodimeric hematopoietin. Proc Natl Acad Sci USA 1997; 94:12,041–12,046.

136. Devergne O, Coulomb-L'Hermine A, Capel F, Moussa M, Capron F. Expression of EBI3, an IL-12 p40 related molecule, throughout human pregnancy: involvement of syncytiotrophoblasts and extravillous trophoblast. Am J Pathol 2001; 159:1763–1776.

137. Pflanz S, Timans JC, Cheung J, et al. IL-27, a heterodimeric cytokine composed of EBI3 and p28 protein, induces proliferation of naive CD4+ T cells. Immunity 2002; 16:779–790.

138. Kanegane H, Wakiguchi H, Kanegane C, Kurashige T, Tosato G. Viral interleukin-10 in chronic active Epstein–Barr virus infection. J Infect Dis 1997; 176:254–257.

139. Ohga S, Nomura A, Takada H, et al. Epstein–Barr virus (EBV) load and cytokine gene expression in activated T cells of chronic active EBV infection. J Infect Dis 2001; 183:1–7.

140. Sillins SL, Sherritt MA, Silleri JM, et al. Asymptomatic primary Epstein–Barr virus infection occurs in the absence of blood T-cell repertoire perturbations despite high levels of systemic viral load. Blood 2001; 98:3739–3744.

141. Silins SL, Cross SM, Elliott SL, et al. Development of Epstein–Barr virus-specific memory T-cell receptor clonotypes in acute infectious mononucleosis. J Exp Med 1996; 184:1815–1824.

142. Steven NM, Annels NE, Kumar A, Leese AM, Kurilla MG, Rickinson AB. Immediate early and early lytic cycle proteins are frequent targets of the Epstein–Barr virus-induced cytotoxic T-cell response. J Exp Med 1997; 185:1605–1617.

143. Borza CM, Hutt-Fletcher LM. Alternate replication in B cells and epithelial cells switches tropism of Epstein–Barr virus. Nat Med 2002; 8:594–599.

144. Meijer CJLM, Jiwa NM, Dukers DF, et al. Epstein–Barr virus and human T-cell lymphomas. Semin Cancer Biol 1996; 7:191–196.

5

The Immune Response to Epstein–Barr Virus

Scott R. Burrows
Cellular Immunology Laboratory, Queensland Institute of Medical Research, Herston, Brisbane, Australia

Andrew D. Hislop
Cancer Research U.K., Institute for Cancer Studies, University of Birmingham, Edgbaston, Birmingham, U.K.

INTRODUCTION

Epstein–Barr virus (EBV) is the best known and most widely studied herpesvirus because of its clinical and oncogenic importance. It is also widely utilized as an important general model for investigating the antiviral immune response in humans because of its ubiquity in human populations, the ease with which virus-infected cells can be maintained in vitro, and the strength of the T-cell response during primary as well as persistent infection. Early interest in the immune response to EBV revolved primarily around the seroepidemiology of the virus, particularly in relation to the EBV-associated diseases. These studies exploited immunofluorescence assays that quantitatively assessed the antibody responses to various serologically defined viral antigens including viral capsid antigen (VCA), membrane antigen (MA), and Epstein–Barr nuclear antigen (EBNA).

The observation that atypical lymphocytes expressed during acute infectious mononucleosis (IM) are not virus-infected B-cells but lymphoblasts of thymic origin led to an early suspicion that a cellular response might be important in controlling EBV infection. The huge increase in CD8 T-cell numbers during primary infection provided further evidence of a critical role for the cellular immune response. More direct evidence for a strong T-cell response to EBV was provided in the late 1970s by Moss et al. (1) with their observation that virus-induced transformation of B-cells from healthy virus carriers was inhibited by T-cells in vitro. This T-cell response is generally a classic virus-specific response [CD8 human leukocyte antigen (HLA) class I-restricted] (2), although EBV-specific CD4 class II–restricted cytotoxic T lymphocytes (CTLs) have also been described (3,4). Following these observations, considerable interest was directed toward defining the EBV antigens that are the targets for this potent T-cell response. Although the MAs were initially considered the most likely candidates for CTL recognition, attention soon focused on the EBNA proteins after work with the influenza model demonstrated that nuclear antigens are frequently the sites of CTL epitopes. Further evidence indicating that the EBNA proteins are recognized by T-cells was provided by the key observation that EBV-reactive CTL clones are often specific for autologous B-cells transformed with type 1 but not type 2 EBV strains (3). As outlined in earlier chapters, the EBNA proteins display EBV–type-specific sequence polymorphism (see Chapter 2). The direct mapping of CTL epitopes within the EBNA proteins later supported this indirect evidence (5–7). More recent work has shown that a wide array of EBV antigens are targeted by CD8 T-cells during primary and persistent infection, including the latent membrane proteins (LMPs) (8,9) and several early and immediate early proteins of the lytic cycle (10,11). This basic knowledge of the anti-EBV immune response is now being directed toward the development of vaccine formulations that might have broad application in the control of acute infection and EBV-associated malignancies (see Chapter 19).

HUMORAL RESPONSE

The humoral response during acute IM is characterized by a pronounced immuno-globulin (Ig) antibody response to autoantigens and heterophile antigens presumably associated with the well-documented role of the virus as a polyclonal B-cell activator (12). This feature has been exploited as a diagnostic marker for the disease whereby heterophile antibodies agglutinate sheep and horse erythrocytes in the Paul–Bunnell–Davidsohn test (see Chapter 7). The EBV-specific antibody response has traditionally been studied with reference to serologically defined "antigens" that have been found to be a composite of several distinct viral proteins. These include (i) EBNA, which is a complex of six distinct nuclear proteins; (ii) MA, which is expressed on the surface of cells late in the lytic cycle and consists predominantly of the glycoprotein (gp350); (iii) VCA, which is expressed within cells late in the lytic cycle and consists of the BFRF3, BLRF2, BcLF1, and glycoprotein gp110; and (iv) early antigen (EA), which is expressed within cells early in the lytic cycle and consists of many viral proteins including BZLF1, BHRF1, BMLF1, BMRF1, and BALF2.

The combination of antibody reactivities associated with primary EBV infection is characterized by detectable IgM and IgG antibodies to VCA and EA, a detectable IgM but relatively weak IgG response to MA, and the absence of a detectable IgG response in the EBNA immunofluorescence test. The IgM anti-VCA response subsequently disappears either during convalescence or over the next few months. Notably, the anti-MA response is directed primarily toward gp85 rather than gp350 (13). Because antibody to gp350 is the most potent source of neutralization of the virus, this result appears to bring into question the role of the neutralizing response in the recovery from acute infection. Most patients with acute IM also show a transient IgG response to the EBNA2 protein, whereas the IgG response to EBNA1 is not usually detectable until the convalescence phase (14). During convalescence, the IgM response falls while the IgG response to VCA and EBNA1 plateaus without any obvious protective role. It has been suggested that antibody to gp350 does play an important role in controlling primary infection by binding to productively infected cells rendering them susceptible to antibody-dependent cellular cytotoxicity–mediated lysis (15).

There has been considerable interest in using the humoral response to various EBV proteins in the diagnosis and prognosis of nasopharyngeal carcinoma (NPC).

Although technical differences among laboratories have prevented a universal agreement on the most accurate serological marker for active NPC, an early observation that NPC patients frequently present with an IgA response to VCA and EA is widely accepted (16). Other reports have suggested the possible diagnostic value of antibody responses to the immediate early proteins of the lytic cycle, BRLF1 and BZLF1 (17,18), to LMP1 (19), and to EBNA2 (20).

T-CELL RESPONSE DURING IM AND AFTER RESOLUTION OF DISEASE

The cell-mediated immune response to EBV during IM represents one of the most dramatic examples of a cellular response to an infectious agent. IM is observed in some primary infections of adolescents and is a self-limiting febrile illness associated with splenomegaly, lymphadenopathy, and tonsillitis (see Chapter 6).

During the symptomatic phase of the disease, large expansions of CD8 T-cells occur in the peripheral circulation, such that there is an inversion of the CD4 to CD8 ratio and significant disruptions to the T-cell repertoire (21–23). Initially this expansion was thought to be due to stimulation by a virus-encoded or -induced superantigen. However, later studies indicated that a spectrum of Vβ T-cell receptors (TCRs) was used by these expanded cells, suggestive of an antigen-specific response (24).

Further studies on the peripheral blood mononuclear cells (PBMCs) of IM patients suggested that at least some of these expanded cells were specific for EBV-encoded antigens. Cytotoxicity assays of IM patients' PBMCs, where the cells were used directly in ex vivo assays against targets sensitized with EBV-derived CD8 epitopes, indicated that EBV-specific cytotoxic effectors were present in this population of cells (25). Furthermore, in vitro clonal outgrowth and limiting dilution analysis of IM patients' PBMCs, where the cells are serially diluted and cultured at limiting numbers with antigen-specific stimulator cells and subsequently tested for cytotoxicity against targets sensitized with EBV epitopes allowing quantitation of the EBV-specific CD8 T-cells in the PBMC population, indicated that a substantial proportion of these cells were specific for EBV-encoded antigens (10,25).

Recently, innovative techniques for analyzing T-cell populations at the single-cell level have indicated that the majority of the cells that expanded during acute IM are indeed EBV specific (26–29). The study of CTL responses has been revolutionized by the development of novel methods to quantitatively analyze effector and memory CD8 T-cell populations by flow cytometry. These approaches include functional assays in which T-cells are stimulated ex vivo with antigen and recognition of the antigen is assayed by cytokine secretion (30). Alternatively, direct TCR binding assays using major histocompatibility complex (MHC)–peptide multimers (tetramers) (31) have demonstrated far larger primary CD8 T-cell responses to a variety of pathogens than that which was generally realized previously. In these assays, PBMCs are incubated with complexes of four synthetic class I MHC molecules containing EBV epitopes, which are tethered by a fluorescent linker. This allows a sufficiently avid interaction of the MHCs with epitope-specific TCRs to permit stable binding of the fluorescent complex to the T-cell, making it suitable for flow cytometry analysis. Using such reagents, acute infection with EBV, for instance, has been shown to have a dramatic impact on the composition of the host's T-cell pool with epitope-specific T-cell frequencies of up to 44% of the CD8 subset within peripheral blood being reported (26). The MHC class I–peptide tetrameric complex is arguably the most important of these technological advances because of its potential additional application in sorting live antigen-specific T-cells for adoptive transfer in the clinic.

The surprisingly high magnitude of individual epitope-specific CD8 T-cell responses within the PBMC populations in acute IM have been shown to be dominated by a limited range of epitope specificities. Of these specificities, immediate early gene products have been shown to generate potent responses visualized on HLA class I tetramer staining of PBMCs from IM patients. CD8 T-cells specific for the BZLF1-derived HLA-B8–presented RAKFKQLL epitope can account for up to 44% of the CD8 response, while the response to the BRLF1-derived A2-presented YVLDHLIVV epitope can represent 33% of the CD8 population (26,29). Responses to epitopes from the early gene products, such as the BMLF1-derived HLA-A2-GLCTLVAML response or the BMRF1-derived HLA-A2-TLDYKPLSV response are generally smaller than responses to the immediate EA, but can still represent up to 12% of the CD8 population (26,28,29). Responses to BALF2 and BHLF1 have also been observed by cloning PBMCs from IM patients; however, the epitope identity and size of these responses remain to be determined (Steven, Annels, and Hislop, unpublished observations). The magnitude of responses to epitopes derived from late lytic cycle proteins has not been as well defined, but preliminary EliSpot analysis of PBMCs from IM patients suggests that these responses are substantially weaker than those made to epitopes derived from the early lytic cycle proteins (32). Responses to epitopes from the latent cycle proteins are generally much smaller than the immediate early and EA-specific responses, but can contribute up to 3% of the CD8 response during acute IM (25,26,29).

Circulating EBV-specific CD8 cells examined during IM express cell-surface markers characteristic of highly activated cells such as CD38, HLA-DR, and CD69 (26,32). Markers expressed on CTLs that have been associated with a memory or effector phenotype are also observed; namely, perforin, CD27, CD45RO, and lack of expression of CCR7 (a homing receptor proposed to discriminate between a "central memory" and "effector memory" population) (27,29,33). Furthermore, these cells are in cycle, expressing the proliferation marker Ki-67; they also express low levels of bcl-2 and high levels of annexin V, and as such are highly susceptible to apoptosis (27,34–37).

With the resolution of symptomatic infection, viral loads decrease and marked changes occur in the numbers and relative representation of EBV-specific CTL within the PBMC population. Dramatic reductions in the representation of highly expanded immediate early and EA-specific CD8 cells are observed in the aftermath of IM (26–29,38). Interestingly, the size of some of these responses to lytic cycle antigens following IM is not reflective of their peak sizes during IM; i.e., the burst size of the response is not necessarily the primary determinant of the long-term response. Such examples are seen in the response to the two HLA-A2–presented epitopes, YVLDHLIVV and GLCTLVAML, whereby the response during IM to YVLDH-LIVV is generally greater than that to GLCTLVAML, and yet after resolution of the primary infection these responses are codominant (29). Similarly, other examples are now emerging that support the idea that the CD8 repertoire present during persistent infection is not reflective of the initial pool of CD8 responses (38). The longitudinal dynamics of latent-epitope–specific responses are not as clear. Latent-antigen specificities that have been substantially expanded during IM tend to be moderately decreased in their representation after IM. However, in cases where the representation of latent-antigen–specific responses is modest during IM, they may increase their representation after resolution of the disease (26). Indeed, some latent-antigen–specific responses may not be detected during IM but may be subsequently found after resolution of acute infection (29,38).

The phenotype of the EBV-specific CTL post-IM can be quite different to that seen during acute infection. The EBV-specific CD8 T-cells no longer express activation markers such as CD38, MHC class II, or CD69 but contain intermediate levels of perforin (26,27,32). These cells are mostly no longer cycling as evidenced by no or low levels of cells expressing Ki-67, but express bcl-2 and as such are much more resistant to apoptosis (39). These cells still retain their CD27 expression and show variable expression of CC chemokine receptor 7 (CCR7), thus suggesting that some of these antigen-experienced cells now constitute part of the "central memory" population. Interestingly, a dramatic proportion of CD8 T-cells that are specific for EBV lytic epitopes may downregulate CD45RO expression and upregulate CD45RA, a marker whose expression has been previously associated with naive lymphocytes or possibly "terminally differentiated" CTL effectors. The reason why these cells re-express CD45RA is unclear. This re-expression does not correlate with the degree of antigen-specific expansion as proposed in other herpesvirus infections [e.g., human cytomegalovirus (HCMV)] but rather with the source from which the epitope is derived, namely lytic versus latent cycle proteins (29).

The reason for such differences in the magnitude of responses to the immediate early lytic epitopes and latent cycle epitopes is not clear. Certainly, at symptomatic presentation, both lytic and latent replications are well established (40). It is possible that the antigenic load of lytic replicating virus is much higher than that of latently infected cells or that latent-antigen–specific CTL is sequestered in secondary lymphoid tissue presumably where latent replication is occurring. The relationship between virus load and the strength of the immune response remains largely unexplored at present, but quantitation of virus levels by real time polymerase chain reaction analysis, as a surrogate marker for antigen load, and analysis of epitope-specific responses within donors may clarify this issue.

T-cell responses in IM patients are almost always directed to the immunodominant epitopes derived from immediate early lytic, early lytic, and latent cycle antigens (26,29,38). A preliminary analysis of a range of subdominant responses has suggested a link between the breadth of the response to EBV during IM and the clinical outcome, such that donors who make a broad response targeting multiple epitopes have a shorter duration of illness (32). This raises the interesting possibility that a successful immune response to EBV may be broadly based, similar to that seen in other viral infections such as hepatitis C (41).

During IM, expansions of activated CD4 T-cells are observed; however, relatively little is known about the specificity of these cells and their importance in containing EBV replication at this stage of infection. Direct ex vivo cytolytic assays from IM patients have demonstrated CD4 T-cell–mediated EBV-specific cytotoxicity, and in one case, this response has been mapped to an epitope in BHRF1 (42). Given the importance of CD4 T-cells in maintaining CD8 T-cell responses, it will be of great value to further characterize these cells and their target epitopes to define their role in IM.

T-CELL RESPONSE IN ASYMPTOMATIC PRIMARY INFECTION

In contrast to the substantial amount of information known about the immune response to EBV during IM, relatively little is known about the EBV-specific response that occurs during asymptomatic primary infection. This is primarily because of the difficulty in identifying donors undergoing asymptomatic primary infection, with studies that have been performed mostly relying on retrospective serological analysis of samples. Early studies on infants undergoing asymptomatic seroconversion indicated that no lymphocytosis was apparent in these individuals and that they had a delayed development of EBV-specific antibodies (43).

A recent study of an adolescent EBV-seronegative cohort in which several individuals were identified as having an asymptomatic primary infection has indeed confirmed that such individuals do not have an overt lymphocytosis like that seen during IM. Furthermore, these individuals did not develop significant disruptions to their T-cell repertoire, despite having viral genome loads at levels similar to those seen in IM patients (23). This raises the interesting possibility that the high viral loads, and thus presumably high antigen loads seen in IM patients, may not be directly responsible for the profound expansion of EBV-specific CD8 T-cells. Similarly it is possible that the CD8 T-cell expansions seen in IM may not be entirely responsible for the control of the infection but represent an overreaction to the virus, given that these asymptomatic individuals appear to control primary EBV infection successfully without a dramatic expansion of lymphocytes. Further analysis of these asymptomatic donors is required to clarify how their immune response copes so successfully with EBV infection.

T-CELL RESPONSE IN HEALTHY VIRUS CARRIERS

The size and specificity of EBV-induced CTL responses in healthy immunocompetent individuals have been analyzed in detail. The pioneering experiments of Moss et al. (1) first demonstrated the existence of a cellular response to EBV with their observation that PBMCs from EBV-exposed individuals prevent the outgrowth of EBV-transformed B lymphoblastoid cell lines (LCLs), or cause the "regression" of growth of LCL cultures. Further analysis of LCL regression assays demonstrated that CD8 T-cells are primarily responsible for these effects, with a smaller contribution from CD4 T-cells.

EBV-transformed LCLs have been subsequently used either to stimulate PBMCs from EBV-infected donors in an effort to expand these EBV-specific T-cells and identify their target antigens or to stimulate cells for quantitation of latent-antigen–specific responses using limiting dilution analysis. Initially, such studies used clones derived from individuals infected with a type 1 strain of EBV and these clones were screened against peptide-sensitized LCLs transformed with a distinct type 2 strain of EBV to which the clones did not react (3). Such T-cell lines and clones are predominantly CD8 T-cells and have been characterized by assaying first against target cells infected with recombinant vaccinia viruses that express individual EBV genes, or target cells sensitized with synthetic peptides (5,44–46). Because LCLs predominantly express EBV-latent proteins as opposed to lytic proteins, numerous epitopes have been identified within the EBV-latent gene products (Fig. 1) and a hierarchy of immunodominance is observed to these products. The EBNA3 family of proteins appears to be the frequent target of CD8 T-cell response, while LMP2 is less frequently recognized. Responses to EBNA2 and LMP1 are rarely detected and EBNA1-specific responses are exceptionally rare (45,46). This pattern of immunodominance appears to be conserved across at least several different HLA types, possibly suggesting that the EBNA3 family proteins may have preferential access to the class I antigen–processing pathway.

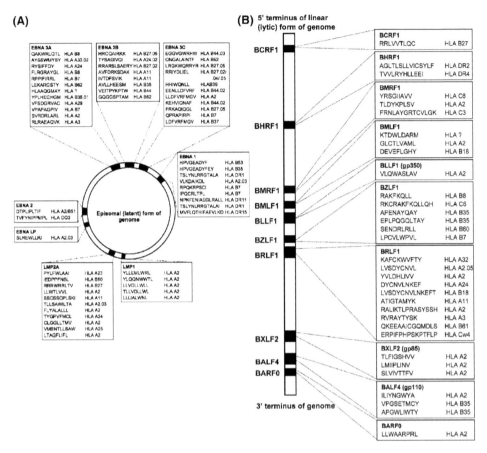

Figure 1 Diagrammatic representation of (**A**) the episomal form of the Epstein–Barr virus genome found in latently infected cells and (**B**) the linear form of the EBV genome found in cells supporting lytic replication of the virus. Black regions represent open reading frames that encode the highlighted proteins with the tables indicating the defined epitopes derived from these proteins and their restriction elements. *Source*: From Refs. 5, 7–11, 25, 29, 42, 51, 57–59.

The use of LCLs to stimulate EBV-specific T-cells has biased the spectrum of responses identified toward latent cycle epitopes, as only a low proportion of LCLs contain cells with virus lytic replication occurring in them. Sources of productively infected cells that express lytic cycle epitopes for use as antigen-presenting cells have not been found and so identifying and quantifying EBV lytic epitope responses remain a challenging proposition. LCL stimulation has, however, been used to restimulate some relatively strong lytic cycle responses from healthy donors, and these are at least codominant with responses to epitopes derived from the latent antigens (47,48).

Analysis of EBV-specific CD8 T-cells from healthy donors using single-cell analytical techniques such as tetramer staining and cytokine production has allowed a more direct examination of these responses without excessive ex vivo manipulation. These assays have demonstrated several important details with respect to the immune response to EBV, most notably that in healthy carriers the global CD8 T-cell response to EBV is much greater than had been previously estimated (49–51). These techniques also represent a more convenient way of analyzing responses to lytic cycle antigens. Using tetramer-staining analysis, up to 5.5% of the total CD8 T-cell population has been described as being specific for the HLA-B8–presented RAKFKQLL epitope derived from the immediate early BZLF1-encoded protein. Responses to the latent cycle EBNA3A-derived HLA-B8–presented FLRGRAYGL epitope can range up to 2% of the CD8 cells and responses to the EBNA3B-derived IVTDFSVIK epitope presented by HLA-A11 can range up to 3.8% of the CD8 cells (50). CTL responses made to EBV appear to be relatively stable over time (38). Interestingly, there are differences between the patterns of responses made by healthy donors and recovered IM donors with respect to the ultimate size of the response to some epitopes. As noted above, the responses to the HLA-A2–presented YVLDHLIVV and GLCTLVAML epitopes in recovered IM patients are in general codominant. In healthy donors who have not been affected by IM, however, the responses made to YVLDHLIVV are significantly smaller than the responses detected in recovered IM donors. Furthermore, the YVLDHLIVV-specific responses made by such donors are significantly smaller than the coresident GLCTLVAML-specific responses (29).

The pattern of phenotypic marker expression observed on EBV-specific CD8 T-cells is similar to that seen long-term in recovered IM patients. CD8 T-cells specific for latent cycle antigens express CD45RO, CD27, and CD28, with variable levels of CD62-L and CCR7 expression. Although most lytic cycle epitope–specific CD8 T-cells express CD45RO, substantial numbers may express CD45RA although not at the dramatic levels observed in some post-IM patients. These EBV-specific cells are predominantly CD27 and express variable levels of CD28, CD62-L, and CCR7, usually at lower levels than that observed on latent cycle antigen–specific CD8 T-cells (50,52,53). Neither the latent nor lytic cycle antigen–specific CD8 T-cells express activation markers such as CD38, CD69, or HLA-DR, yet in direct ex vivo cytotoxicity assays these cells are potent effectors (54).

Single-cell analytical techniques have further highlighted an interesting point with respect to immune evasion by EBV in that responses to the latent cycle protein EBNA1 that are very rarely detected after LCL stimulation of PBMCs can be relatively frequent in vivo. The EBNA1 protein includes a glycine–alanine repeat sequence which interferes with proteosomal degradation and abrogates presentation of its epitopes on class I MHC molecules, thus rendering endogenously synthesized EBNA1 immunologically silent to CD8 T-cell detection (55,56). Identification of epitopes using overlapping peptide mapping techniques has demonstrated the existence of CD8 T-cells specific for EBNA1, and the target epitopes have been used to quantify epitope-specific responses to EBNA1. These responses can be as frequent as those made to EBNA3-derived epitopes (57,58). Presumably, these responses have been generated by cross-presentation of EBNA1, whereby protein released by EBV-infected cells is taken up, reprocessed, and presented by dendritic cells to T-cells. This raises the question of the relevance of these EBNA1-specific CD8 T-cells in vivo, given that endogenously processed EBNA1 will not be presented to them.

The CD4 T-cell–mediated response to EBV is much less characterized. Responses to epitopes from BHRF1, EBNA1, and EBNA3C have been described, and cells specific for epitopes derived from these proteins have been found to be cytotoxic effectors and to produce cytokines (42,59). Currently CD4 T-cell responses to EBV are being characterized more closely, not just for their capacity to provide help to CD8 T-cell responses, but as effectors that may be useful for targeting MHC class II positive tumors associated with EBV infection such as Burkitt lymphoma (BL).

T-CELL–MEDIATED CONTROL OF EBV-ASSOCIATED TUMORS

Polyclonal Lymphomas

Most of the EBV-associated malignancies arise in individuals whose immune system is intact. The exceptions to this are the polyclonal lymphomas that emerge from the uncontrolled expansion of EBV-infected B-cells in patients whose T-cell function has been impaired. Polyclonal lymphomas frequently present as multifocal lesions within lymphoid tissue and/or in the central nervous system, and are often seen in organ transplant patients and individuals infected with HIV. The discovery that these immunoblastic lymphomas are composed of EBV-transformed LCL-like cells expressing the full spectrum of virus latent proteins (60–62) suggested the important role of the immune surveillance in limiting the proliferation of EBV-infected B-cells in vivo. It also implied that the outgrowth of these EBV-transformed cells would be reversed by a restoration of CTL control. Indeed, a planned reduction of immuno-suppression is now the first treatment option in many cases of posttransplant lymphoproliferative disease (PTLD) (63). The critical role of CTLs in controlling the outgrowth of EBV-infected B-cells has now been dramatically demonstrated in both bone marrow and solid organ transplant patients. Thus in bone marrow transplant (BMT) patients in whom the lymphomas that arise are of donor origin, the adoptive transfer of in vitro reactivated EBV-specific CTL preparations from the donor can rapidly reverse tumor growth (64). Similarly, adoptive transfer of autologous CTLs into solid organ transplant patients with active PTLD can lead to a very significant regression of the tumor mass (see Chapter 18) (65).

Burkitt Lymphoma

BL provides a most amenable model for experimental analysis of mechanisms of immune evasion by tumor cells. The model draws strength from the availability of BL cell lines carrying the relevant translocation plus LCLs derived from normal circulating B-cells from the same patient by infection with EBV in vitro. Thus, it is possible to compare the sensitivity to immune lysis of tumor-derived and non–tumor-derived tissue from the same patient. Cell lines established in vitro from BL biopsies at first display the original biopsy cell phenotype and grow as a single-cell suspension with no intercellular adhesions. On serial passage, some BL cell lines retain this biopsy cell phenotype (referred to as group I lines), whereas other lines show a marked phenotypic shift with expression of the full spectrum of B-cell activation antigens and adhesion molecules (referred to as group II or III lines).

    Although only a limited number of BL patients have been studied thus far, no detectable EBV-specific CTL dysfunction is evident (66). However, it is well established that EBV-positive group I BL cell lines are highly resistant to virus-specific CTL lysis and are poorly immunogenic in their ability to stimulate an alloresponse (67). Thus, when matched sets of LCL and BL cell lines from the same patient are compared, it is found that the group I cell lines are not lysed in vitro by polyclonal EBV-specific T-cell lines or CTL clones (68,69). As EBV-positive BL cell lines switch from a group I to group III phenotype, they show increased susceptibility to EBV-specific CTL recognition (69).

    There are several mechanisms by which BL cells resist virus-specific CTL lysis in vitro. One of the first to be highlighted was a selective downregulated expression of certain HLA class I alleles (70,71). Another suggestion was that the very low expression of adhesion molecules, especially lymphocyte function associated 3 (LFA3) and intra cellular adhesion molecule 1 (ICAM1), plays a major role (72). However, this factor now appears to be of little importance since BL cells consistently express high levels of ICAM2. Furthermore, BL cells and normal lymphocytes from the same patient show equal sensitivity to lysis by EBV-specific CTLs when EBV-peptide epitopes are added exogenously to the cells (68).

The viral phenotype of BL cells is likely to be a very important factor in reducing tumor susceptibility to EBV-specific CTL surveillance. Viral antigen expression in EBV-positive BL cells in vivo is restricted to a single protein, EBNA1, with all other EBNAs and LMPs downregulated (73). As discussed in an earlier section, the EBNA1 protein is shielded from CD8 T-cell recognition because of a glycine–alanine (Gly-Ala) repeat domain that protects endogenously expressed EBNA1 from proteosomal processing and presentation (55). Thus it is not hard to realize the advantage that this highly restricted form of EBV latency offers BL cells in terms of immune evasion, because EBNA2, EBNA3A–C, and the LMPs, which constitute important targets of virus-specific CTL recognition (45,46), are not expressed. It seems unlikely that restricted EBV gene expression in BL cells is a result of immune pressure in vivo, that is, downregulation of latent protein expression is a key selective step in the pathogenesis of BL. Indeed, the latency program in BL may reflect that of its progenitor B lymphocyte, rather than a unique feature of a malignant cell clone selected for its ability to evade EBV-specific CTL recognition.

Another possible mechanism by which BL cells escape CTL recognition involves a defect in the endogenous antigen-processing function in these cells. It is now clear that the class I antigen–processing pathway that delivers peptide from endogenously synthesized proteins for presentation on the cell surface in association with HLA class I molecules is much less active in BL cells than in LCLs (74). This is reflected in very low expression of the transporter proteins transporter associated with antigen processing 1 (TAP1) and TAP2 in a number of BL cell lines. These proteins are involved in peptide transport from the cytosol to the endoplasmic reticulum (ER) (75). Deficiencies in this antigen-processing pathway are generally associated with reduced stability and surface expression of MHC class I molecules in laboratory-generated antigen-processing mutant cell lines (such as RMA-S and T2) (76). This reduction is apparently due to a deficient supply of peptide epitopes into the ER for MHC stabilization. Indeed, BL cells show a similar phenomenon, with a very low proportion of the MHC class I molecules expressed in the cytoplasm being transported onto the cell surface. Furthermore, the endogenous presentation of CTL epitopes on BL cells can be restored by transfection with an expression vector encoding a CTL epitope fused to an ER translocation signal sequence (74). In contrast to the RMA-S and T2 cell lines, in which the TAP genes are deleted, BL cell lines show a transcriptional deficiency with significantly reduced levels of TAP1 and TAP2 mRNA protein expression (77). Thus, downregulated expression of both viral antigens and the TAP proteins may contribute to evasion from the normal EBV-specific CTL response in BL patients.

NPC and Hodgkin's Disease

Like BL, NPC and Hodgkin's disease (HD) are seen in relatively immunocompetent individuals. Very limited information is available on the role of specific T-cells in controlling these tumors, although IgA-positive NPC patients show a significantly depressed EBV-specific CTL response (78). However, it is unlikely that this diminished T-cell response is the sole basis for tumor outgrowth, because a proportion of the IgA-positive NPC patients showed a normal response. An immunohistochemical analysis of fresh biopsies and laboratory-established tumor lines indicates that malignant cells in both NPC and HD express normal levels of HLA class I, TAP1, and TAP2 (79,80).

The effectiveness of the T-cell response is presumably limited by the pattern of viral gene expression, which is restricted to EBNA1 and in some cases to LMP1 and LMP2 as well. Thus, the EBV proteins that are a rich source of immunodominant CTL epitopes are not expressed. Indeed, the frequency of CTLs reactive to epitopes within the LMP1 protein is generally much lower than that of CTLs reactive to the immunodominant EBNA3A, EBNA3B, and EBNA3C proteins. Furthermore, evidence is emerging that sequence variation within the LMP1 gene can lead to a loss of immunogenicity. A murine model used by Trivedi et al. showed that the LMP1 gene from NPC cells when expressed in mouse carcinoma cells was completely nonimmunogenic, while the LMP1 gene from the B95.8 cell line was highly immunogenic (81). Interestingly, LMP1 encoded by NPC isolates shows numerous amino acid changes compared with the B95.8 sequence (82). Similar amino acid changes in the LMP1 gene have been found in EBV isolates from HD (83). It is therefore possible that mutations in the LMP1 sequence will render tumor cells nonimmunogenic for CTLs.

LMP2 is a latent antigen that is generally conserved among EBV isolates worldwide, and is also a common target for the CTL response in healthy Chinese and Caucasian virus carriers (9). The inability of the CTL response to reject LMP2-expressing tumors may reflect some local cytokine-mediated suppression of CTL activation in the vicinity of the tumor itself. This possibility is consistent with the observation that EBV-specific CTLs could be reactivated from the blood of patients with EBV-positive HD, but not from the tumor-infiltrating lymphocyte population (84). Indeed, interleukin-10 is made by EBV-positive HD cells (85), and this cytokine clearly has the capacity to alter tumor immunogenicity (86).

TCR SELECTION

In common with other acute viral infections in murine and simian models and with acute HIV infection in man, a dramatic perturbation of the peripheral TCR repertoire occurs during the primary T-cell response to EBV infection that subsequently resolves during convalescence (24). Recent studies of TCR usage have investigated the clonal composition and dynamic regulation of the EBV-specific CTL response. These TCR analyses have concentrated on the selection events during IM and on the repertoire composition in the healthy virus carrier state. Prospective studies on IM patients have provided an important opportunity to track the developmental process that T-cells undergo from the primary to memory state, by TCR typing of CTL clones generated at different stages of the infection (22,87,88). Importantly, these studies have demonstrated the potential for different levels of TCR diversity selection depending on the viral epitope that is the target of the response. For example, the TCR repertoire utilized in the response to two HLA-B8–restricted epitopes from the latent antigen EBNA3A (FLRGRAYGL and QAKWRLQTL) was found to be oligoclonal in one IM patient, with preservation of distinct clonotypes in the memory T-cell pool (22). In contrast, T-cell populations that rose against an HLA-B8–binding epitope from the lytic antigen BZLF1 (RAKFKQLL) were highly diverse in several IM patients, with no dramatic signs of repertoire focusing over time (87). Overall, the developing picture in IM is that a broad range of TCRs are selected and maintained within the composite CTL response against natural EBV infection. This multiclonotypic T-cell population may be especially important in the establishment and maintenance of an effective lifelong CTL control.

In the persistent virus carrier state, EBV-specific CD8 CTL responses also appear to cover a wide spectrum of TCR usage. At one extreme, a single expansion of a TCR BV6/BJ2S7 clonotype can dominate the response to the HLA-B8–binding latent-antigen epitope FLRGRAYGL (89), while at the other extreme, a high degree of clonotype diversity can exist to two different epitopes within the lytic antigen BZLF1 (87,90). Indeed, the strength and monoclonal nature of the CTL response to the FLRGRAYGL epitope is such that it dramatically skews the entire memory repertoire to near oligoclonality leaving a permanent immunological footprint of previous EBV infection in the T-cell pool of healthy adults (91). This effect was observed in a number of HLA-B8+ virus carriers because the clonotype response is remarkably conserved among different individuals at both the TCR-alpha and -beta chain loci (89).

Detailed analysis of this highly conserved TCR structure that is commonly utilized in response to the B8-binding FLRGRAYGL epitope revealed that it can mediate cross-reactive lysis of EBV-positive and EBV-negative target cells expressing the HLA-B*4402 alloantigen (92). Such is the strength of this EBV epitope–specific memory response in HLA-B8+ virus carriers that their alloreactive response to HLA-B*4402 in conventional mixed lymphocyte culture is dominated by CTLs from virus-specific memory with the relevant cross-reactive TCR. This illustrates how a prior history of infection with an immunogenic virus such as EBV can influence an individual's level of responsiveness to an alloantigen. Such mechanisms may underlie the observed clinical association between herpesvirus exposure and graft-versus-host disease in BMT patients (92). Not surprisingly, T-cells with this particular TCR are not detected within the EBV-induced memory CTL population in individuals who coexpress HLA-B8 and B*4402 because of their potential for self-reactivity (93). Interestingly, however, such individuals do still make a response to the FLRGRAYGL-B8 complex through a variety of TCRs, thereby illustrating the flexibility and reserve strength of the TCR repertoire in the response to a target epitope.

CONCLUDING REMARKS AND FUTURE DIRECTIONS

The immune response to EBV represents one of the most intensely studied responses to a viral pathogen. The high frequency of infected individuals, genetic stability of the virus, and the immunogenicity of at least some of the viral proteins make it not only a convenient host–pathogen model to study, but also an attractive model to address fundamental immunological questions.

Detailed information of the immune response to EBV in healthy infected individuals is available, and the response that IM patients make is being further characterized. However, basic questions remain relating to the immune response made to EBV by individuals who undergo asymptomatic primary infection. As these individuals mount what may be considered a successful immune response in that they are able to control the virus infection without developing symptoms or dramatic CD8 T-cell expansions like those seen in IM patients, characterization of such responses is likely to be highly informative. Analysis of the spectrum of epitope-specific responses made by these individuals and whether it is different from those made by IM patients may reveal that a broadly based response is more beneficial, as suggested for some

IM patients with less severe symptoms (32) and in cases of other persistent viral infections (e.g., hepatitis C infection). It will also be of interest to correlate the T-cell response with virus or antigenic load at different anatomical sites (such as peripheral B-cells as a measure of latent virus load and oropharynx as a measure of lytic viral load) in IM and primary asymptomatic donors. Evidence is now emerging that subtle differences in the patterns of CD8 T-cell responses occur many years following primary infection and are influenced by the severity of disease during the primary infection. For example, asymptomatic donors have a weak, if any, response to the BRLF1-encoded YVLDHLIVV epitope, while IM donors can have a relatively strong response to this epitope during and many years after IM. Whether this represents a reaction to high levels of lytic virus replication is unknown.

More fundamental immunological questions remain as to how the distinct hierarchies of CD8 T-cell responses to EBNA3 are generated. Such analysis may address how accessible these proteins are to the antigen-processing pathway, whether the concentration of the antigen has an effect, or whether the order in which the immune response is exposed to the antigens affects the preferential response to these proteins. In a similar vein, responses made to lytic cycle epitopes also appear to be highly focused, with only a few epitopes apparently constituting most of the lytic cycle response. So far, a relatively small proportion of the 80 lytic cycle proteins have been examined as potential targets for T-cells and so it remains possible that other proteins are also targeted by the immune response.

Further analysis of factors controlling the maintenance of these responses is worthy, especially in the context of CTL responses to the immediate early gene products, and may offer some insight into the maintenance of immunological memory. IM patients usually make very strong responses to the BZLF1-derived HLA-B8–presented RAKFKQLL epitope and maintain this response at relatively high levels after resolution of symptoms (26,29). Interestingly, when responses have been quantified to epitopes derived from this protein and presented by other HLAs, albeit in different individuals, these responses are extinguished or rarely detected (38). The reason why the anti-RAKFKQLL response is maintained at higher levels is not clear; however, self and bacterial antigens that are cross-reactive with this viral epitope have been identified and may have a role in the maintenance of this response (48). A similar theme of results is now emerging for responses to CTL epitopes derived from the BRLF1 gene product. IM donors who are HLA-A2+ maintain sizeable responses to the YVLDHLIVV epitope after IM, while other donors who initially respond to an HLA-A3–presented epitope appear to poorly maintain this response (38). Dissection of these responses for cross-reactivity remains to be performed, yet may cast some light on the fundamental concept of maintenance of immunological cellular memory.

An understanding of whether all components of the immune response to EBV are truly effective would help clarify the role of certain epitope specificities. For example, some doubt exists as to what role EBNA1-specific CD8 CTL play in immune control of EBV, given that in general, these CTL cannot respond to endogenously synthesized EBNA1. Because these CTL are presumably generated by cross-priming, it is not clear what other epitope specificities are also generated in this manner and thus whether the immunodominant responses observed are a genuine reflection of classical antigen stimulation and perhaps represent effective responses.

A much neglected facet of the immune response to EBV alluded to in earlier sections is the role that CD4 T-cells play in the response to EBV infection. The paucity of defined HLA class II–binding EBV epitopes is hampering this analysis;

however, concerted efforts are now under way to define epitopes by the use of peptide epitope mapping with EliSpot technology. These cells are likely to be critical, not only for the provision of T-cell help and maintenance of CD8 T-cell responses, but possibly also as effectors. This is of particular interest because some EBV-associated malignancies express class II molecules and may be targets for such cells. Furthermore, such malignancies express the EBNA1 protein which has evolved strategies to avoid CD8 CTL recognition but may be processed and presented in a class II context. Further studies are required to determine whether such cells are capable of endogenous presentation of epitopes to CD4 effectors and whether these effectors will kill tumor cell targets.

Finally, our understanding of the immune response to EBV allows for the development of effective immunotherapeutic interventions to combat EBV-associated diseases as well as the rational development of prophylactic vaccination strategies (see Chapters 18 and 19). Established immunotherapy regimes that range from a reduction of immune suppression to allow host cellular immunity to control the lymphoma, to the adoptive transfer of polyclonal cytotoxic T-cell lines now exist for treating immunoblastic lymphoma in BMT and solid organ transplant recipients. Currently EBV vaccination strategies are being pursued for the prevention of IM in adolescents and for boosting responses in pretransplant patients prior to immune suppression. However, the challenge remains to understand how the immune response to EBV can be used to target EBV-associated malignancies that are associated with a more restricted pattern of EBV gene expression such as BL, HD, and NPC.

REFERENCES

1. Moss DJ, Rickinson AB, Pope JH. Long-term T-cell-mediated immunity to Epstein–Barr virus in man. I. Complete regression of virus-induced transformation in cultures of seropositive donor leukocytes. Int J Cancer 1978; 22:662–668.
2. Misko IS, Moss DJ, Pope JH. HLA antigen-related restriction of T lymphocyte cytotoxicity to Epstein–Barr virus. Proc Natl Acad Sci USA 1980; 77:4247–4250.
3. Moss DJ, Misko IS, Burrows SR, Burman K, McCarthy R, Sculley TB. Cytotoxic T-cell clones discriminate between A and B type Epstein–Barr virus transformants. Nature 1988; 331:719–721.
4. Misko IS, Schmidt C, Moss DJ, Burrows SR, Sculley TB. Cytotoxic T lymphocyte discrimination between type A Epstein–Barr virus transformants is mapped to an immunodominant epitope in EBNA 3. J Gen Virol 1991; 72:405–409.
5. Burrows SR, Sculley TB, Misko IS, Schmidt C, Moss DJ. An Epstein–Barr virus-specific cytotoxic T-cell epitope in EBNA3. J Exp Med 1990; 171:345–350.
6. Burrows SR, Misko IS, Sculley TB, Schmidt D, Moss DJ. An Epstein–Barr virus-specific cytotoxic T-cell epitope present on A- and B- type transformants. J Virol 1990; 64:3974–3976.
7. Burrows SR, Gardner J, Khanna R, et al. Five new cytotoxic T-cell epitopes identified within Epstein–Barr virus nuclear antigen 3. J Gen Virol 1994; 75:2489–2493.
8. Khanna R, Burrows SR, Nicholls J, Poulsen LM. Identification of cytotoxic T cell epitopes within Epstein–Barr virus (EBV) oncogene latent membrane protein 1 (LMP1): evidence for HLA-A2 supertype-restricted immune recognition of EBV-infected cells by LMP1-specific cytotoxic T lymphocytes. Eur J Immunol 1998; 28:451–458.
9. Lee SP, Tierney RJ, Thomas WA, Brooks JM, Rickinson AB. Conserved cytotoxic T lymphocyte (CTL) epitopes within Epstein- Barr virus (EBV) latent membrane protein 2, a potential target for CTL-based tumour therapy. J Immunol 1997; 158:3325–3334.

10. Steven NM, Annels N, Kumar A, Leese A, Kurilla MG, Rickinson AB. Immediate early and early lytic cycle proteins are frequent targets of the Epstein–Barr virus-induced cytotoxic T-cell response. J Exp Med 1997; 185:1605–1617.

11. Bogedain C, Wolf H, Modrow S, Stuber G, Jilg W. Specific cytotoxic T-lymphocytes recognize the immediate-early transactivator ZTA of Epstein–Barr virus. J Virol 1995; 69:4872–4879.

12. Garzelli C, Taub FE, Scharff JE, et al. Epstein–Barr virus-transformed lymphocytes produce monoclonal autoantibodies that react with antigens in multiple organs. J Virol 1984; 52:722–725.

13. Henle G, Lennette ET, Alspaugh MA, Henle W. Rheumatoid factor as a cause of positive reactions in tests for Epstein–Barr virus-specific IgM antibodies. Clin Exp Immunol 1979; 36:415–422.

14. Henle W, Henle G, Andersson J, et al. Antibody responses to Epstein–Barr virus-determined nuclear antigen (EBNA)-1 and EBNA 2 in acute and chronic Epstein–Barr virus infection. Proc Natl Acad Sci USA 1987; 84:570–574.

15. Patarroyo M, Blazar B, Pearson G, Klein E, Klein G. Induction of the EBV cycle in B-lymphocyte-derived lines is accompanied by increased natural killer (NK) sensitivity and the expression of EBV-related antigen(s) detected by the ADCC reaction. Int J Cancer 1980; 26:365–375.

16. Henle W, Henle G. Epstein–Barr virus-specific IgA serum antibodies as an outstanding feature of nasopharyngeal carcinoma. Int J Cancer 1976; 17:1–7.

17. Dardari R, Khyatti M, Benider A, et al. Antibodies to the Epstein–Barr virus transactivator protein (ZEBRA) as a valuable biomarker in young patients with nasopharyngeal carcinoma. Int J Cancer 2000; 86:71–75.

18. Yoshizaki T, Miwa H, Takeshita H, Sato H, Furukawa M. Elevation of antibody against Epstein–Barr virus genes BRLF1 and BZLF1 in nasopharyngeal carcinoma. J Cancer Res Clin Oncol 2000; 126:69–73.

19. Xu JW, Ahmad A, D'Addario M, et al. Analysis and significance of anti-latent membrane protein-1 antibodies in the sera of patients with EBV-associated diseases. J Immunol 2000; 164:2815–2822.

20. Shimakage M, Dezawa T, Chatani M. Proper use of serum antibody titres against Epstein–Barr virus in nasopharyngeal carcinoma: IgA/virus capsid antigen for diagnosis and EBV-related nuclear antigen-2 for follow-up. Acta Otolaryngol 2000; 120:100–104.

21. Tomkinson BE, Wagner DK, Nelson DL, Sullivan JL. Activated lymphocytes during acute Epstein–Barr virus infection. J Immunol 1987; 139:3802–3807.

22. Silins SL, Cross SM, Elliott SL, et al. Development of Epstein–Barr virus-specific memory T-cell receptor clonotypes in acute infectious mononucleosis. J Exp Med 1996; 184:1815–1824.

23. Silins SL, Sherritt MA, Silleri JM, et al. Symptomatic primary Epstein–Barr virus infection occurs in the absence of blood T-cell repertoire perturbations despite high levels of systemic viral load. Blood 2001; 98:3739–3744.

24. Callan MFC, Steven N, Krausa P, et al. Large clonal expansions of CD8+ T-cells in acute infectious mononucleosis. Nat Med 1996; 2:906–911.

25. Steven NM, Leese AM, Annels N, Lee S, Rickinson AB. Epitope focusing in the primary cytotoxic T-cell response to Epstein–Barr virus and its relationship to T-cell memory. J Exp Med 1996; 184:1801–1813.

26. Callan MFC, Tan L, Annels N, et al. Direct visualization of antigen-specific CD8(+) T-cells during the primary immune response to Epstein–Barr virus in vivo. J Exp Med 1998; 187:1395–1402.

27. Callan MFC, Fazou C, Yang HB, et al. CD8+ T-cell selection, function, and death in the primary immune response in vivo. J Clin Invest 2000; 106:1251–1261.

28. Annels NE, Callan MFC, Tan L, Rickinson AB. Changing patterns of dominant TCR usage with maturation of an EBV-specific cytotoxic T-cell response. J Immunol 2000; 165:4831–4841.

29. Hislop AD, Annels N, Gudgeon N, Leese A, Rickinson A. Epitope-specific evolution of human CD8+ T-cell responses from primary to persistent phases of Epstein–Barr virus infection. J Exp Med 2002; 195:893–905.

30. Butz EA, Bevan MJ. Massive expansion of antigen-specific CD8+ T-cells during an acute virus infection. Immunity 1998; 8:167–175.

31. Doherty PC. The new numerology of immunity mediated by virus-specific CD8(+) T-cells. Curr Opin Microbiol 1998; 1:419–422.

32. Bharadwaj M, Burrows SR, Burrows JM, Moss DJ, Catalina M, Khanna R. Longitudinal dynamics of antigen-specific CD8+ cytotoxic T lymphocytes following primary Epstein–Barr virus infection. Blood 2001; 98:2588–2589.

33. Sallusto F, Lenig D, Forster R, Lipp M, Lanzavecchi A. Two subsets of memory T lymphocytes with distinct homing potentials and effector functions. Nature 1999; 401:708–712.

34. Uehara T, Miyawaki T, Okta K, et al. Apoptotic cell death of primed CD45RO+ T lymphocytes in Epstein–Barr virus-induced infectious mononucleosis. Blood 1992; 80:452–458.

35. Akbar AN, Borthwick N, Salmon M, et al. The significance of low Bcl-2 expression by CD45RO-T-cells in normal individuals and patients with acute viral infections—The role of apoptosis in T-cell memory. J Exp Med 1993; 178:427–438.

36. Borthwick NJ, Bofill M, Hassan I, et al. Factors that influence activated CD8+ T-cell apoptosis in patients with acute herpes virus infections: loss of costimulatory molecules CD28, CD5 and CD6 but relative maintenance of Bax and Bcl-x expression. Immunology 1996; 88:508–515.

37. Roos MTL, van Lier RAW, Hamann D, et al. Changes in the composition of circulating CD8+ T-cell subsets during acute Epstein–Barr and human immunodeficiency virus infections in humans. J Infect Dis 2000; 182:451–458.

38. Catalina M, Sullivan JL, Bak KR, Luzuriaga K. Differential evolution of epitope-specific CD8+ T-cell responses in EBV infection. J Immunol 2001; 167:4450–4457.

39. Dunne PJ, Faint JM, Gudgeon NH, et al. Epstein–Barr virus-specific CD8(+) T cells that re-express CD45RA are apoptosis-resistant memory cells that retain replicative potential. Blood 2002; 100:933–940.

40. Rickinson AB, Kieff E. Epstein–Barr Virus. In: Fields BN, Knipe DM, Howley PM, Chanock RM, Melnick JL, Monath TP, Roizman B, Strauss SE, eds. Fields Virology. 4th ed. Philadelphia: Lippincott Williams & Wilkins, 2001:2575–2627.

41. Lechner F, Wong DKH, Dunbar PR, et al. Analysis of successful immune responses in persons infected with hepatitis C virus. J Exp Med 2000; 191:1499–1512.

42. Schmidt CW, Misko IS. The ecology and pathology of Epstein–Barr virus. Immunol Cell Biol 1995; 73:489–504.

43. Biggar RJ, Henle W, Fleisher G, Bocker J, Lennette ET, Henle G. Primary Epstein–Barr virus infections in African infants. I. Decline of maternal antibodies and time of infection. Int J Cancer 1978; 22:239–243.

44. Murray RJ, Kurilla MG, Griffin HM, et al. Human cytotoxic T-cell responses against Epstein–Barr virus nuclear antigens demonstrated using recombinant vaccinia viruses. Proc Natl Acad Sci USA 1990; 87:2906–2910.

45. Murray RJ, Kurilla MG, Brooks JM, et al. Identification of target antigens for the human cytotoxic T-cell response to Epstein–Barr virus (EBV): implications for the immune control of EBV-positive malignancies. J Exp Med 1992; 176:157–168.

46. Khanna R, Burrows SR, Kurilla MG, et al. Localisation of Epstein–Barr virus cytotoxic T-cell epitopes using recombinant vaccinia: implications for vaccine development. J Exp Med 1992; 176:169–178.

47. Elliott SL, Pye SJ, Schmidt C, Cross SM, Silins SL, Misko IS. Dominant cytotoxic T lymphocyte response to the immediate-early trans-activator protein, BZLF1, in persistent type A or B Epstein–Barr virus infection. J Infect Dis 1997; 176:1069–1072.

48. Misko IS, Cross SM, Khanna R, et al. Cross-reactive recognition of viral, self, and bacterial peptide ligands by human class I-restricted cytotoxic T lymphocyte clonotypes: implications for molecular mimicry in autoimmune disease. Proc Natl Acad Sci USA 1999; 96:2279–2284.

49. Kuzushima K, Hoshino Y, Fujii K, et al. Rapid determination of Epstein–Barr virus-specific CD8+ T-cell frequencies by flow cytometry. Blood 1999; 94:3094–3100.

50. Tan LC, Gudgeon N, Annels NE, et al. A re-evaluation of the frequency of CD8(+) T-cells specific for EBV in healthy virus carriers. J Immunol 1999; 162:1827–1835.

51. Saulquin X, Ibisch C, Peyrat A, et al. A global appraisal of immunodominant CD8 T-cell responses to Epstein–Barr virus and cytomegalovirus by bulk screening. Eur J Immunol 2000; 30:2531–2539.

52. Faint JM, Annels NE, Curnow SJ, et al. Memory T-cells constitute a subset of the human CD8+CD45RA+ pool with distinct phenotypic and migratory characteristics. J Immunol 2001; 167:212–220.

53. Tussey L, Speller S, Gallimore A, Vessey R. Functionally distinct CD8+ memory T-cell subsets in persistent EBV infection are differentiated by migratory receptor expression. Eur J Immunol 2000; 30:1823–1829.

54. Hislop AD, Gudgeon NH, Callan MFC, et al. EBV-specific CD8+ T-cell memory: relationships between epitope specificity, cell phenotype, and immediate effector function. J Immunol 2001; 167:2019–2029.

55. Levitskaya J, Coram M, Levitsky V, et al. Inhibition of antigen processing by the internal repeat region of the Epstein–Barr virus nuclear antigen 1. Nature 1995; 375:685–688.

56. Levitskaya J, Sharipo A, Leonchiks A, Ciechanover A, Masucci MG. Inhibition of ubiquitin/proteasome-dependent protein degradation by the Gly-Ala repeat domain of the Epstein–Barr virus nuclear antigen 1. Proc Natl Acad Sci USA 1997; 94:12616–12621.

57. Blake N, Lee SP, Redchenko I, et al. Human CD8(+) T-cell responses to EBV EBNA1: HLA class I presentation of the (Gly-Ala)-containing protein requires exogenous processing. Immunity 1997; 7:791–802.

58. Blake N, Haigh T, Shaka'a G, Croom-Carter D, Rickinson A. The importance of exogenous antigen in priming the human CD8+ T-cell response: lessons from the EBV nuclear antigen EBNA1. J Immunol 2000; 165(12):7078–7087.

59. Leen A, Meji P, Redchenko I, et al. Differential immunogenicity of Epstein–Barr virus latent-cycle proteins for human CD4(+) T-helper 1 responses. J Virol 2001; 75:8649–8659.

60. Young LS, Finerty S, Brooks L, Scullion F, Rickinson AB, Morgan AJ. Epstein–Barr virus gene expression in malignant lymphomas induced by experimental virus infection of cottontop tamarins. J Virol 1989; 63:1967–1974.

61. Thomas JA, Hotchin N, Allday MJ, Yacoub M, Crawford DH. Immunohistology of Epstein–Barr virus associated antigens in B-cell disorders from immunocompromised individuals. Transplant 1990; 49:944–953.

62. Gratama JW, Zutter MM, Minarovits J, et al. Expression of Epstein–Barr virus growth-transformation-associated proteins in lymphoproliferations of bone-marrow transplant recipients. Int J Cancer 1991; 47:188–192.

63. Paya CV, Fung JJ, Nalesnik MA, et al. Epstein–Barr virus-induced, post-transplant lymphoproliferative disorders. Transplant 1999; 68:1517–1525.

64. Rooney CM, Smith CA, Ng CYC, et al. Use of gene-modified virus-specific T lymphocytes to control Epstein–Barr virus-related lymphoproliferation. Lancet 1995; 345:9–13.

65. Khanna R, Bell S, Sherritt M, et al. Activation and adoptive transfer of Epstein–Barr virus-specific cytotoxic T-cells in solid organ transplant patients with post-transplant lymphoproliferative disease. Proc Natl Acad Sci USA 1999; 96:10391–10396.

66. Rooney CM, Rickinson AB, Moss DJ, Lenoir GM, Epstein MA. Cell-mediated immunosurveillance mechanisms and the pathogenesis of Burkitt's lymphoma. In: Lenoir GM, O'Conor GT, Olweny CLM, eds. Burkitt's Lymphoma: A Human Cancer Model. Lyon: IARC, 1985:249–264.

67. Rooney CM, Edwards CF, Lenoir GM, Rupani H, Rickinson AB. Differential activation of cytotoxic responses by Burkitt's lymphoma (BL)-cell lines: relationship to the BL-cell surface phenotype. Cell Immunol 1986; 102:99–112.

68. Khanna R, Burrows SR, Suhrbier A, et al. EBV peptide epitope sensitisation restores human cytotoxic T-cell recognition of Burkitt's lymphoma cells. Evidence for a critical role for ICAM2. J Immunol 1993; 150:5154–5162.

69. Rooney CM, Rowe M, Wallace LE, Rickinson AB. Epstein–Barr virus-positive Burkitt's lymphoma cells not recognised by virus-specific T-cell surveillance. Nature 1985; 317:629–631.

70. Masucci MG, Torsteindottir S, Colombani BJ, Brautbar C, Klein E, Klein G. Down-regulation of class I HLA antigens and of the Epstein–Barr virus (EBV)-encoded latent membrane protein (LMP) in Burkitt lymphoma lines. Proc Natl Acad Sci USA 1987; 84:4567–4571.

71. Torsteinsdottir S, Brautbar C, Klein E, Klein G, Masucci MG. Differential expression of HLA antigens on human B-cell lines of normal and malignant origin: a consequence of immune surveillance of a phenotypic vestige of the progenitor cells? Int J Cancer 1988; 41:913–919.

72. Gregory CD, Murray RJ, Edwards CF, Rickinson AB. Down regulation of cell adhesion molecules LFA-3 and ICAM-1 in Epstein–Barr virus-positive Burkitt's lymphoma under-lies tumour cell escape from virus-specific T-cell surveillance. J Exp Med 1988; 167:1811–1824.

73. Rowe M, Rowe DT, Gregory CD, et al. Differences in B-cell growth phenotype reflect novel patterns of Epstein–Barr virus latent gene expression in Burkitt's lymphoma cells. EMBO J 1987; 6:2743–2751.

74. Khanna R, Burrows SR, Argaet V, Moss DJ. Endoplasmic reticulum signal sequence facilitated transport of peptide epitopes restores immunogenicity of an antigen processing defective tumour cell line. Int Immunol 1994; 6:639–645.

75. Spies T, Bresnahan M, Bahram S, et al. A gene in the human major histocompatibility complex class II region controlling the class I antigen presentation pathway. Nature 1990; 348:744–747.

76. Ljunggren HG, Stam NJ, Ohlen C, et al. Empty MHC class I molecules come out in the cold. Nature 1990; 346:476–480.

77. Rowe M, Khanna R, Jacob CA, et al. Restoration of endogenous antigen processing in Burkitt's lymphoma cells by Epstein–Barr virus latent membrane protein-1: co-ordinate up-regulation of peptide transporters and HLA class I antigen expression. Eur J Immunol 1995; 25:1374–1384.

78. Moss DJ, Chan SH, Burrows SR, et al. Epstein–Barr virus T-cell response in nasopharyngeal carcinoma patients. Int J Cancer 1983; 32:301–305.

79. Khanna R, Busson P, Burrows SR, et al. Molecular characterisation of antigen-processing function in nasopharyngeal carcinoma (NPC): evidence for efficient presentation of Epstein–Barr virus cytotoxic T-cell epitopes by NPC cells. Cancer Res 1998; 58:310–314.

80. Lee SP, Constandinou CM, Thomas WA, et al. Antigen presenting phenotype of Hodgkin Reed-Sternberg cells: analysis of the HLA class I processing pathway and the effects of interleukin-10 on Epstein–Barr virus-specific cytotoxic T-cell recognition. Blood 1998; 92:1020–1030.

81. Trivedi P, Hu LF, Chen F, et al. Epstein–Barr virus (EBV)-encoded membrane protein LMP1 from a nasopharyngeal carcinoma is non-immunogenic in a murine model system, in contrast to a B-cell-derived homologue. Eur J Cancer 1994; 30:84–88.

82. Hu LF, Zabarovsky ER, Chen F, et al. Isolation and sequencing of the Epstein–Barr virus BNLF-1 gene (LMP1) from a Chinese nasopharynx carcinoma. J Gen Virol 1991; 72:2399–2409.

83. Knecht H, Bachmann E, Brousset P, et al. Deletions within the LMP1 oncogene of Epstein–Barr virus are clustered in Hodgkin's Disease and identical to those observed in nasopharyngeal carcinoma. Blood 1993; 82:2937–2942.

84. Frisan T, Sjoberg J, Dolcetti R, et al. Local suppression of Epstein–Barr virus (EBV)-specific cytotoxicity in biopsies of EBV-positive Hodgkin's disease. Blood 1995; 86: 1493–1501.

85. Herbst H, Foss HD, Samol J, et al. Frequent expression of interleukin-10 by Epstein–Barr virus harboring tumor cells of Hodgkin's disease. Blood 1996; 87:2918–2929.

86. Matsuda M, Salazar F, Petersson M, et al. Interleukin 10 pretreatment protects target cells from tumor- and allo-specific cytotoxic T-cells and down-regulates HLA class I expression. J Exp Med 1994; 180:2371–2376.

87. Silins SL, Cross SM, Elliott SL, et al. Selection of a diverse TCR repertoire in response to an Epstein–Barr virus-encoded transactivator protein BZLF1 by CD8+ cytotoxic T lymphocytes during primary and persistent infection. Int Immunol 1997; 9:1745–1755.

88. Callan MFC, Annels N, Steven N, et al. T-cell selection during the evolution of CD8+ T-cell memory in vivo. Eur J Immunol 1998; 28:4382–4390.

89. Argaet VP, Schmidt CW, Burrows SR, et al. Dominant selection of an invariant T-cell antigen receptor in response to persistent infection by Epstein–Barr virus. J Exp Med 1994; 180:2335–2340.

90. Couedel E, Bodinier M, Peyrat MA, et al. Selection and long-term persistence of reactive CTL clones during an EBV chronic response are determined by avidity, CD8 variable contribution compensating for differences in TCR affinities. J Immunol 1999; 162: 6351–6358.

91. Silins SL, Cross SM, Krauer KG, Moss DJ, Schmidt CW, Misko IS. A functional link for major TCR expansions in healthy adults caused by persistent Epstein–Barr virus infection. J Clin Invest 1998; 102:1551–1558.

92. Burrows SR, Khanna R, Burrows JM, Moss DJ. An alloresponse in humans is dominated by cytotoxic T lymphocytes (CTL) cross-reactive with a single Epstein–Barr virus CTL epitope: implications for graft versus host disease. J Exp Med 1994; 179:1155–1161.

93. Burrows SR, Silins SL, Moss DJ, Khanna R, Misko IS, Argaet VP. T-cell receptor repertoire for a viral epitope in humans is diversified by tolerance to a background major histocompatibility complex antigen. J Exp Med 1995; 182:1703–1715.

6

Clinical Features of Infectious Mononucleosis

Jan Andersson
Division of Infectious Diseases, Karolinska University Hospital, Huddinge, Stockholm, Sweden

CLINICAL CHARACTERIZATION OF ACUTE INFECTIOUS MONONUCLEOSIS

The clinical syndrome of infectious mononucleosis (IM) is most frequently manifested during adolescence and young adulthood. After the age of 15, primary infection with Epstein–Barr virus (EBV) leads to the clinical syndrome of IM in approximately 30% to 40% cases (1). Filatov and Pfeiffer initially described the IM syndrome at the end of the 19th century (2,3). However, the association between primary EBV infection and IM was first established in 1968 when a laboratory technician in Dr. Werner Henle's laboratory seroconverted to EBV during the course of classical IM (4). The mononucleosis syndrome includes a clinical triad of pharyngitis, lymphadenopathy, and fever (5). Patients may experience several days of prodromal symptoms including malaise, fatigue, arthralgia, fever, chills, dysphagia, and anorexia (6). As symptoms of sore throat and fever worsen, patients typically seek medical attention. However, the classic symptoms of IM may be mistaken for those of other common infections including streptococcal pharyngitis. IM is a benign lymphoproliferative disorder caused by a disseminating EBV infection in B-lymphocytes and mucosal epithelial cells that may lead to abnormal clinical signs and symptoms involving almost any organ (7). During the acute phase of IM, roughly one in 10^3 to 10^4 circulating B-cells are infected with EBV (8,9). They are proliferating, lymphoblastic plasmacytoid cells, are highly immunogenic, and can trigger potent cellular immune activation (10). In fact, EBV replication is predominantly mediated via cellular DNA polymerase in B-cells, resulting in the transformation of B-lymphocytes (11). In contrast, epithelial mucosal cells become lytically infected and release infectious viral particles (12). This results in oropharyngeal EBV shedding as well as presence of infectious EBV particles in genital secretions (13).

EBV infection is ubiquitous and predominantly occurs during childhood (14). Thus, most children in underdeveloped countries have had asymptomatic EBV infection by the age of five and more than 90% of all infants are seropositive by the age of four (15). However, in developed countries, primary EBV infection and the subsequent manifestations vary with socioeconomic class. Epidemiological studies have revealed that more than 15% of individuals in higher socioeconomic class remain EBV seronegative at the age of 20 (9). Thus, IM is more prevalent in areas with higher standards of hygiene. The incidence of IM in these countries has been estimated at 45 per 100,000 overall. However, a much higher incidence is reported among adolescents, 15 to 19 years (320–370 per 100,000) (16). The infection is contracted through saliva or genital secretions but may occasionally be acquired through blood transfusion or via organ transplantation. The incubation period is estimated to be around 30 to 50 days (6). Vertical transmission of the virus probably occurs but has not been definitely associated with any single malformation or pattern of congenital abnormality. This is in sharp contrast to infection with cytomegalovirus (CMV), herpes simplex virus, and varicella. There are, however, rare cases of virologically verified intrauterine EBV infection with apparent sequelae (17).

Clinical Course of IM

The clinical course of IM is exceedingly variable (Table 1). In one prospective study, the time to full clinical recovery varied from 6 to 174 days (18). The dominating clinical picture includes sore throat, generalized lymphadenopathy, tonsillitis, and fever. The clinical illness normally has a duration of one to four weeks, occasionally

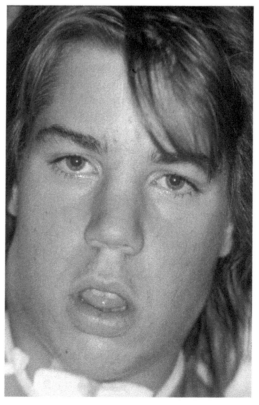

Figure 1 A fulminant case of infectious mononucleosis with periorbital edema and cervical lymphadenopathy. A tracheotomy was performed because of upper respiratory obstruction.

Table 1 Clinical Manifestations of Infectious Mononucleosis

Signs	Prevalence (%)
Pharyngitis	>90
Lymphadenopathy	>90
Fever	60–90
Pharyngotonsillitis	50–90
Splenomegaly	50
Periorbital edema	20–50
Skin rash	5–10
Hepatomegaly	≤10
Jaundice	≤5
Interstitial pneumonia	≤2
CNS involvement	1–5
Myocarditis	≤1
Genital ulcerations	≤1

Abbreviation: CNS, central nervous system.

lasting for up to six weeks. During the first week of illness, the patient may develop a generalized rash, which may be morbilliform and transient or occasionally of urticarial phenotype (1,19). Arthralgia, gastrointestinal symptoms, and headache are not uncommon. Jaundice may develop in a minority of patients in the second or third week of illness, and splenomegaly may develop during the same period in more than 50% of the patients (20). The pharyngotonsillitis may generate difficulties in swallowing as well as respiration. This is due to a generalized pharyngotonsillar edema as well as generation of fibrinous membranes not only in the tonsillary region, but also in the nasopharynx in patients with severe disease (21). Malaise and exhaustion are the most persistent symptoms (6).

Hematological Findings

The clinical entity of IM reflects symptoms generated via extensive activation of both the humoral and the cellular immune system. Lymphocytosis is a hallmark of IM and is considered to be a prerequisite for the diagnosis (Table 2). Lymphocytosis, both relative (>50%) and absolute (>4500 cells/μL), is generally noted between the 5th and 20th day of illness (22). Many (>5%) of the lymphocytes are atypical

Table 2 Hematological Abnormalities in Infectious Mononucleosis

Signs	Prevalence (%)
Lymphocytosis (>4.5 × 10^3 cells/μL)	>80
Atypical lymphocytes (>5%)	>80
Granulocytopenia (<3.0 × 10^3 cells/μL)	60–80
Thrombocytopenia (<80 × 10^3 cells/μL)	4–7
Hemolytic anemia (Hb <90 g/L)	≤5
Lymphopenia (<1.5 × 10^3 cells/μL)	≤5
Aplastic anemia	Rare

in appearance, characterized by large mononuclear cells with irregular contour of the cytoplasm and nucleus and the presence of cytoplasmic vacuoles (22). These cells are significantly increased in size compared to normal cells and have been called Downey–McKinlay cells after their discoverers in 1923 (23). However, these cells also can be present in acute infections with CMV, HIV-1, hepatitis B, rubella, and measles (Table 3).

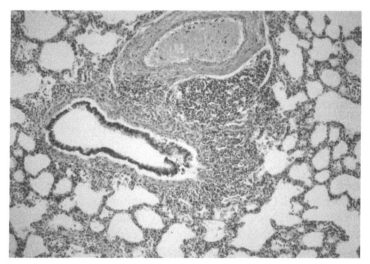

Figure 2   A transbronchial biopsy performed in an infectious mononucleosis case with interstitial pneumonia. The pathological anatomical description shows peribronchial lymphoid infiltrates, which is a common finding and may cause obliteration of the bronchioles.

Lymphopenia in the early onset of IM is a poor prognostic sign and is often associated with protracted and more extensively disseminated disease (24). Neutropenia (neutrophilic granulocyte counts $<3000/\mu L$) is common among IM patients.

Table 3   Etiologies Demonstrating Signs and Symptoms Similar to Infectious Mononucleosis

---

Infectious etiological agents
  Group A streptococcus
  CMV
  Adenovirus
  Herpes simplex type I
  Acute primary HIV-1
  Toxoplasma gondii
  Chlamydophila pneumoniae
  Corynebacterium diphtheriae
Non-infectious etiological agents
  Diphenylhydantoin hypersensitivity
  Hodgkin lymphoma
  Non-Hodgkin lymphoma
  Histiocytosis

Abbreviations: CMV, cytomegalovirus; HIV, human immunodeficiency virus.

Formations of autoantibodies against granulocytes are believed to be the pathogenic mechanism for this condition. Anemia in IM is usually due to autohemolysis (25). Although excessive autohemolysis is not uncommon, anemia is a rare manifestation in IM patients. Autoantibodies are also believed to be the pathogenic mechanism (26). Mild thrombocytopenia (platelet counts <140,000 cells/μL) is a common occurrence. However, severe thrombocytopenia with bleeding is rare but does occur in IM, in particular in patients with disseminated intravascular coagulopathy (7). In most cases, thrombocytopenia is transient and the platelet levels return to normal during convalescence ≤3 weeks from clinical onset. While it is tempting to explain thrombocytopenia on the basis of the production of the abnormal antibodies against autologous platelets, not all IM patients with a severe thrombocytopenia have demonstrable platelet antibodies (7). Abnormal platelet function may reflect a defect that predisposes to premature platelet destruction.

Diagnosis

Diagnosis of IM is usually based on a combination of clinical, hematological, and serological findings. The great majority of IM patients (>80%) have absolute lymphocytosis that peaks during the first and second week of illness. This is often concomitant with greater than 5% atypical lymphocytes, which can be detectable for weeks after onset of disease (8,27).

Serologic Diagnosis

Serology testing is the gold standard for confirmation of acute IM in immunocompetent persons. Serologic diagnosis is based on the presence of heterophile antibodies combined with EBV-specific antibodies. The classic EBV-induced heterophile antibodies were first reported by Paul, Bunnell, and Davidsohn in 1932, who observed erythrocyte agglutinins directed against sheep erythrocytes during acute IM illness (28). These immunoglobulin M (IgM) antibodies bind to antigens on heterologous erythrocytes but have no affinity against any EBV-associated antigens. Traditionally, the Paul-Bunnell-Davidsohn test detects production of heterophile antibodies that generate an agglutination reaction in sheep erythrocytes. More modern commercially available tests use a latex agglutination assay or enzyme-linked immunosorbant assay for detection of IgM heterophile antibodies against horse red blood cells. Heterophile antibodies are present in the first week after onset of disease but peak during two to five weeks of illness. However, 10% to 20% of the patients may remain heterophile antibody negative (28). This occurs particularly in children younger than 10 years as well as in adults older than 40 years. The use of EBV-specific serology is unnecessary in patients with typical clinical symptoms, lymphocytosis, and positive heterophile antibody response.

EBV-Specific Antibody Response

EBV-specific serology should be performed in IM patients with severe symptoms or in those with a negative heterophile test result (Table 4). EBV antigens most commonly used for serologic diagnosis include viral capsid antigen (VCA), early antigen (EA) of the anti-D subset (EA-D), and EBV nuclear antigen (EBNA) 1–6 (29). VCA and EA-D proteins are expressed during the lytic phase of viral infection, and EBNA is expressed in transformed or latently infected B-cells (29). The development of EBV-specific antibodies throughout the course of IM is illustrated in Figure 3.

Table 4 Diagnosis of Primary Epstein–Barr Virus Infection

	Acute IM	Convalescence
Serology		
Heterophil antibodies IgM	+	−
Anti-EBV capsid antigens		
Immunoglobulin M	+	−
Immunoglobulin G	+	+
Anti-EBV early antigens	+	−
Anti-EBNA	−	+
Virus detection		
Virus isolation oropharynx[a]	+	+(−)
EBV-DNA by PCR[b]		
Blood	+	+
Plasma (>50 EBV-DNA c/mL)	+	−
In situ hybridization[c]	+	−
EBV-antigens[d]	+	−

[a]EBV isolated from mouthwash samples.
[b]EBV-DNA detection by PCR from peripheral blood mononuclear cells or plasma.
[c]Detection of the EBV-gene EBER in tissue biopsies.
[d]EBV-antigen, LMP-1, EBNA-1 by the use of immunohistochemical technique in tissue biopsy or blood.
Abbreviations: EBER, EBV-encoded RNA; EBNA, EBV nuclear antigen; EBV, Epstein–Barr virus; LMP, latent membrane protein; PCR, polymerase chain reaction; IM, infectious mononucleosis.

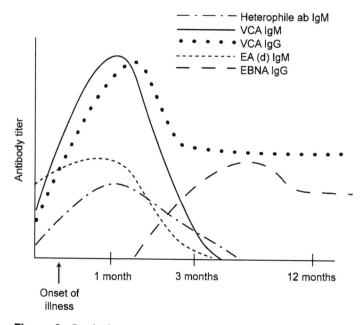

Figure 3 Serologic response determined on 160 patients with infectious mononucleosis. *Source*: From Ref. 18.

VCA IgM antibodies are almost universally present at onset of disease and may be detected up to three months after contracting the illness (29). False VCA-positive cross-reacting IgM occurs during primary CMV and in patients with rheumatoid arthritis (30). The generation of VCA IgG antibodies is almost parallel with the IgM response (31). However, these latter antibodies persist throughout life in immunocompetent individuals (29). In contrast to anti-VCA, EBNA antibodies tend to appear later in the course of infection, from 6 to 12 weeks after clinical onset (29). Thus, the assessment of these antibodies should be combined with VCA-IgG and VCA-IgM in the diagnosis of primary EBV infection. The presence of anti-EBNA antibodies early in the course of illness excludes primary EBV infection, while the presence of anti–VCA IgM combined with lack of EBNA antibodies is consistent with acute IM. Two subsets of anti-EA antibodies, diffuse (cytoplasmatic anti-D) and perinuclear restricted (anti-R), are identified based on cellular distribution of the antigens. The anti-D subset is associated with primary infection. However, more than 30% of patients never develop antibodies to this antigen. Thus, absence does not exclude acute infection. Patients rarely have anti-R antibodies in primary EBV and therefore these antibodies have no clinical significance. In general, it is difficult to demonstrate a VCA or EA antibody seroconversion or a significant rise in the antibody titers in patients with a suspected diagnosis of IM, because EBV-specific antibodies, with the exception of anti-EBNA antibodies, are usually at their peak around onset of the disease.

Diagnosis in Immunocompromised Persons

Viral DNA Detection

In patients with a selective immunodeficiency against EBV, some or many of the EBV-specific antibodies may be absent. These patients usually do not develop anti-EBNA antibodies that normally occur once the affected patient generates a significant EBV-specific cellular immune response. Diagnosis in these patients

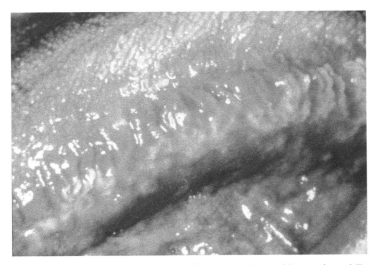

Figure 4   Oral hairy leukoplakia in an HIV-1 infected patient with reactivated Epstein–Barr virus infection. The lesions are characterized by whitish hyperplastic epithelial ridges a few millimeters in size on the lateral margin of the tongue.

may be based on direct isolation of the virus or detection of viral genes (Table 4). Virus isolation of EBV from mouthwash samples or blood usually has limited clinical value because EBV shedding in the oropharynx as well as EBV latency persists in circulating B-cells and continues throughout life following infection. EBV-DNA detection by the polymerase chain reaction (PCR) may be positive in peripheral blood samples because of the presence of latent EBV-infected B-cells throughout life (at the frequency of 1–50 DNA copies/10^6 cells) (32). In contrast, EBV-DNA positivity in serum or plasma predominantly occurs in primary infection and in immunocompromised individuals with reactivated EBV, which may be associated with lytic replication in B-cells (33,34). Recently, it has been observed that there is a relation between the EBV-DNA load in plasma and the infected peripheral blood lymphocytes with severity of IM as well as with risk for development of EBV-related posttransplant lymphoproliferative disorder (PTLD) (35). Assessment of plasma viral load by real-time PCR quantitative assay for detection of EBV-DNA has demonstrated that healthy immunocompetent EBV seropositive individuals lack detectable EBV-DNA in plasma while patients with IM had a mean of 64,000 copies/mL (26). There is a rapid decline in EBV-DNA after onset of clinical symptoms, and thus the timing of plasma EBV-DNA analysis is critical; positivity is dramatically reduced after more than 10 days of illness. Use of quantitative EBV-DNA measurement by real-time PCR or competitive PCR assay is also of value for the determination of clinical effect of antiviral therapy as well as effects of immune reconstitution in cases with life-threatening EBV disorders (26). EBV-DNA detection methods should also be used in cerebrospinal fluid in individuals with suspected EBV-associated central nervous system (CNS) infection in particular, because assays based on detection of intrathecal antibody production have failed in these conditions.

In Situ Hybridization

In situ hybridization for detection of the EBV gene EBV-encoded RNA (EBER) is considered the gold standard for detection and localization of latent EBV in tissue samples (36). This assay is universally positive in lymphoid tissue biopsies obtained from patients with IM while it is rarely positive in samples obtained from EBV seropositive healthy carriers. Because EBER transcripts are naturally amplified, they represent a more reliable target for detecting and localizing EBV in tissue sections by in situ hybridization. In situ hybridization for detection of the EBV gene Z Epstein–Barr replication activator (ZEBRA), also known as BZLF1, is a valuable tool for detection of the lytic EBV replication that occurs predominantly in epithelial cells (36). ZEBRA complexes with viral proteins that are collectively referred to as EAs and VCA. These antigens elicit a humoral immune response resulting in abnormal elevated antibody titers that are thus associated with lytic virus production in the diseased patient (Table 4).

In Situ Viral Antigen Detection

Detection of viral proteins can be achieved by immunohistochemical staining in tissue sections. In fact, latent membrane protein (LMP)-1 immunostaining is nearly as sensitive and specific as EBER in situ hybridization for identifying EBV in IM and PTLD cases, as well as in Hodgkin's disease. LMP-1 is reliably expressed in lymph nodes from IM patients, with some EBER-positive small lymphocytes failing to coexpress LMP-1, and immunoblasts coexpressing both markers (36). Therefore, EBER and LMP-1 stains appear to be equally informative in confirming the diagnosis of IM (Table 4).

Differential Diagnosis

Primary HIV-1 infection is a self-limited viral syndrome characterized by fever, rash, pharyngitis, and lymphadenopathy, thus resembling the clinical presentation of IM. Out of 600 patients testing negative for heterophile antibodies, but with clinical suspicion of IM, 1.2% turned out to be positive for primary HIV-1 infection (37). Furthermore, false-positive heterophile antibody tests have also been reported in primary HIV-1 infection (even though reactivation of EBV was not excluded) (38).

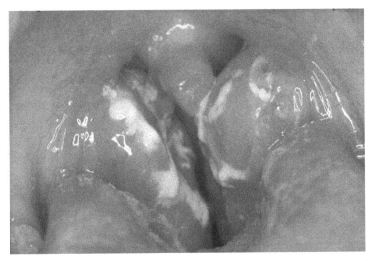

Figure 5 Classic tonsillar enlargement with membranous exudates and edema of the uvula during the acute phase of infectious mononucleosis.

Therefore, clinicians considering a diagnosis of IM should review the patient's HIV-1 risk behavior and consider the diagnosis of acute primary HIV-1 syndrome (39). Symptomatic primary CMV and adenovirus infection may resemble the clinical picture of acute IM (Table 3) (40). False-positive IgM VCA responses have been noticed in primary CMV infection (40). The latter though has only rarely been associated with pharyngotonsillitis, which is a much more common phenomenon in adenovirus and primary herpes simplex type 1 infection in the adolescent population. In addition, groupA streptococcal pharyngotonsillitis may present with identical symptoms of acute IM. Nasopharyngeal endoscopy shows reliable differences in mucosal pathology between IM and streptococcal pharyngitis—patients with IM normally present with generalized enlarged lymphoid tissue and fibrinous membranes in the nasopharynx, which do not occur in streptococcal group A-induced pharyngotonsillitis or peritonsillitis (21). Furthermore, toxoplasmosis and chlamydia infection as well as diphtheria may generate symptoms and orpharyngeal signs that are difficult to distinguish from those of acute IM. In addition, fulminant IM cases often show extensive T-cell lymphoproliferative disorders that may present histological pictures of histocytic hyperplasia and erythrophagocytosis, events which may also be found in histiocytosis, virus-associated hemophagocytic syndrome (VAHS), and Hodgkin's and non-Hodgkin's lymphoma (41–43). Studies on lymphoid tissue have also demonstrated the presence of large binucleated cells indistinguishable from the Reed–Sternberg cells in multiple IM cases. Occasionally, drug-induced toxicity or hypersensitivity may generate symptoms associated with acute IM (43). Detection of EBV-DNA (PCR), EBV genes (hybridization), and EBV antigens (immunohistological stains) in affected tissue is of clinical importance in these settings (Table 4) (36).

ATYPICAL PRESENTATIONS OF ACUTE IM

Clinical signs and symptoms of primary EBV infection can be extremely variable. In particular, children younger than five years and adults older than 40 years may have unusual presentations of primary EBV infection (44).

Primary EBV Infection in Infants Younger Than Five Years

Primary EBV infection in infants is predominantly an asymptomatic infection (45). Occasionally, these children develop pharyngitis (45). There are scattered reports of hepatitis combined with intrahepatic cholestasis. Liver histology shows extensive lymphoid infiltration and, in a few cases, extensive liver necrosis also.

Primary EBV Infection in Adults Older Than 40 Years

Symptomatic primary EBV infection in this cohort is often associated with fever of unknown origin (46). Sore throat and generalized lymphadenopathy may be absent. Heterophile antibodies are not a reliable diagnostic tool in this cohort (47). Fever of unknown origin is sometimes combined with cholestatic liver involvement and jaundice. Focal lymphadenopathy may be present (46). The diagnosis should be based on complete EBV serology and/or quantitative assessments of EBV-DNA in serum, plasma, or peripheral blood mononuclear cells.

Atypical Primary EBV Infection

In spite of the fact that primary EBV infection is a systemic disorder, patients may present with symptoms emanating from only one organ. Atypical cases may have isolated meningitis, encephalitis, focal lymphadenopathy, interstitial pneumonia, myocarditis, or hematological abnormalities including thrombocytopenia, hemolytic anemia, or granulocytopenia (44). Painful, multiple, superficial genital ulcerations may occur with severe infection (48). A common finding in these cases is lack of heterophile antibodies, with only marginal elevation of atypical lymphocytes and variable degree of lymphocytosis. Therefore, these patients can normally only be diagnosed after complete EBV serology and/or assessment of EBV genes or antigens. Alternatively, EBV-DNA should be detected by PCR in blood, serum, plasma, or cerebrospinal fluid. Biopsies obtained from affected organs may be assessed for the EBV gene expression by in situ hybridization of EBER or EBNA and LMP-1, utilizing immunohistochemical staining.

Fulminant EBV Lymphoproliferative Disorder

Fatal IM (FIM) is an uncommon presentation of primary EBV infection (42). It predominately occurs in children younger than seven years, but has also been reported in adolescents as well as in adults. This entity can be subdivided into several subgroups of patients who reflect different mechanisms of an underlying impairment of the immune system (41,42). There is a high incidence of FIM in patients with the X-linked lymphoproliferative (XLP) disease (Duncan's disease) (49), which recently has been linked to mutation in the src-homology 2 (SH-2) domain-encoding gene (see Chapter 16) (50). However, FIM also occurs sporadically in female children with a similar clinical presentation, suggesting additional immunodeficiencies yet to be identified. One subgroup of patients with FIM is characterized by an uncontrolled B-cell lymphoproliferation (50). This is due to a defect in the T-cell–mediated EBV-specific immune control (50). Recently, a fulminant EBV-associated T-cell lymphoproliferative disorder has also been described by several groups (42).

Virus-Associated Hemophagocytic Syndrome

The clinical characteristics of patients with FIM may be acute or insidious in onset. Most of the cases demonstrate a spiking fever, generalized lymphadenopathy, extensive hepatosplenomegaly, liver failure, and interstitial bilateral pneumonitis (51,52).

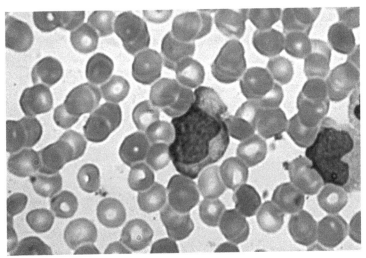

Figure 6 An acute blood sample from a case with infectious mononucleosis with large atypical lymphocytes, characterized by irregular nucleus, and large granular cytoplasm. These cells are three times larger than normal nonactivated lymphocytes.

CNS involvement with disseminated encephalitis is not uncommon. Death is usually caused by liver failure or extensive interstitial pneumonia. Chronic cases may develop lymphoma, agammaglobulinemia, or aplastic anemia (49). These categories of patients have hematological abnormalities. Lymphocytopenia and histiocytic infiltration are common, and thrombocytopenia is often a consequence of a long-lasting extensive inflammation and is also common (53). Almost all cases show evidence of erythrophagocytosis (53). A full-blown VAHS develops in more than 80% of the cases of FIM (42). EBV is the virus most frequently found in VAHS. However, multiple other viral etiologies including adenovirus, CMV, and hepatitis virus have also been described.

T-cell–associated lymphoproliferative disorders may develop shortly after primary, acute EBV infection. These cases are more frequent among Asian children, and similar cases have also been described on the American continent. Histologically, two subgroups can be identified. The clinical syndrome of FIM could be the end result of either uncontrolled polyclonal B-cell lymphoproliferative disorder (classical form) or a monoclonal proliferation of activated predominantly cytotoxic T-cells of either CD4 or CD8 T-cell phenotype (53–56). Histiocytic hyperplasia occurs in both cases. Liver biopsies show a prominent lymphoid infiltration and a striking hemophagocytosis. There is often intracellular and intracanalicular cholestatis, steatosis, and focal necrosis (57). Lymphoid tissue may show extensive hyperplasia and proliferation of B-cells and/or T-cells combined with sinus histiocytosis and erythrophagocytosis. Pulmonary tissue typically shows extensive peribronchial lymphoid infiltration combined with extensive edema in the matrix (53–56). These patients often lack EBV-specific antibodies to one or several of the commonly expressed antigens, including VCA and EA. They universally lack expression of anti-EBNA antibodies. Heterophile antibodies are also lacking. The diagnosis should be based on the detection of EBV-DNA in blood, often demonstrating excessively high viral load, in addition to identification of EBV gene expression in B-cells and/or T-cells by in situ hybridization (36). Detection of EBER-1 or other EBV antigens (LMP-1 and EBNA) utilizing an immunohistochemical technique may be an alternative. There are scattered cases presenting only with fatal myocarditis, interstitial pneumonia, or acute liver failure in a subgroup of these patients. The development of these clinical conditions may be due to selective impairment of EBV-specific immunity, and patients may, therefore, have contracted a number of infections in the past without demonstrating abnormal symptoms or disease patterns. Underlying genetic disorders responsible for this broad entity of VAHS need to be further characterized (53–56).

ACUTE COMPLICATIONS OF EBV IM

The vast majority of patients with IM recover uneventfully without any complications. However, due to the disseminated nature of the disease with generalized spread of infected B-cells combined with reactive infiltrating lymphocytes and histiocytes, virtually all organs in the body may be affected (Table 5). Therefore, IM may be associated with a vast number of symptoms and complications (58). Because of lack of systematic prospective studies, a direct cause of association of IM with unusual symptoms or complications is sometimes weak. In addition, many studies were performed during the 1960s and 1970s when molecular-based detection techniques of the virus were unavailable, which limits the interpretations of these data. There is, however, a vast cumulative clinical experience and, in some cases, also experimental data that supports the causal association of many complications described in the literature with EBV-induced IM, which is summarized in Table 5.

Skin Complications

Approximately 10% of patients with clinical signs of IM develop skin rash that resembles mild rubella but is more morbilliform and transient. Urticaria, erythema multiforme, and even erythema nodosum have also been reported. A great majority of patients treated with ampicillin develop skin rash. The rash first appears on the trunk

Table 5 Acute Complications in Primary Epstein–Barr Virus Infection

Complication	Frequency (%)
Skin	
Rash	~10
Ampicillin rash	90
β-Lactam antibiotics	30–40
Hepatitis	
Elevated transaminases	50–80
Jaundice	5–7
Fulminant hepatitis	Rare
Splenomegaly	50–80
Splenic rupture	Rare (<0.1–0.5%)
Upper respiratory tract	
Airway obstruction	1–3,5
Lower respiratory tract	
Interstitial pneumoniae	Rare
Pleuritis	Rare
Cardiologic	
ECG abnormalities	5–8
Myocarditis	Rare
Pericarditis	Rare
Neurologic	
CNS pleocytosis	25
Meningoencephalitis	Rare
Encephalitis	Rare
Transverse myelitis	Rare
Cranial neuritis	
Bell palsy	Rare
Opticus neuritis	Rare
Mono- or polyneuritis	Rare
Guillian Barré syndrome	<1
Hematologic	
Hemolytic anemia	3–5
Aplastic anemia	Rare
Thrombocytopenia (early)	30–50
Severe ($<$20,000 cells/μL)	Rare
Neutropenia (early)	50–80
Severe ($<$1000 cells/μL)	<2
Agranulocytosis	Rare
Pancytopenia	Rare
Agammaglobulinemia	Rare
Lymphoproliferative disorders	Rare
Psychological	
Fatigue (≥6 months)	5–8
Depression	Rare
Psychosis	Rare
Fatal IM (historical data)	Rare ($<1/3000$ cases)

Abbreviations: CNS, central nervous system; ECG, electrocardiogram; FIM, fatal infectious mononucleosis.

5 to 14 days after intake of ampicillin and becomes generalized, involving the face and palm, within the next few days (59,60). It is a pruritic, florid maculopapular rash sometimes accompanied by fever. Use of other β-lactam antibiotics has also been associated with a similar type of rash (Table 5).

Liver Complications

Abnormal liver function characterized by elevation of hepatic transaminases is a common phenomenon occurring in 50% to 80% of patients. A much lower proportion of the patients develop jaundice from cholestatic hepatitis. This type of hepatitis is a benign condition with complete recovery as a general rule. However, there are rare cases of fulminant hepatitis, in children younger than 10 years and in patients older than 40 years (61,62). A few of these patients also develop ascites (62). Severe life-threatening hepatitis is particularly prevalent in IM cases associated with impairment of cellular EBV-specific immune responses (Table 5).

Splenic Complications

Splenomegaly is common, occurring in 50% to 80% of patients with IM. However, due to the roundish enlargement of the organ it may be missed on simple palpation but can be verified by ultrasound (63). King first reported spontaneous splenic rupture in 1941. In a large series of proven cases of IM, the incidence of spontaneous splenic rupture was between 0.1% and 0.5% (63). Estimates for mortality have varied between 30% and 60%. Splenic rupture in children is much less common than in adolescents and young adults (64,65). The peak incidence is during the second and third week of illness. Abrupt or insidious onset of acute left upper quadrant abdominal pain, which may radiate to the left shoulder, suggests the possibility of splenic hemorrhage. This may be accompanied by development of circulatory shock. The mechanism of spontaneous rupture of the spleen in IM remains unclear (65). Grossly, the spleen appears edematous and often shows signs of subcapsular hematoma. Histologically, there are extensive lymphoid infiltrates characterized by excessive numbers of atypical lymphocytes extending through the trabeculae, capsule, and blood vessel walls. Laboratory findings include leucocytosis with a large number of atypical lymphocytes and anemia (63). However, anemia may not be detectable within the initial 6 to 12 hours following hemorrhage. Potential splenic rupture can be investigated by computed tomography, magnetic resonance imaging, or ultrasonography. However, direct transfer to the operating room may be indicated in the presence of hemodynamic compromise. There is a debate on surgical versus conservative treatment for splenic rupture. A diseased spleen may remain susceptible to delayed rupture for several weeks. Therefore, a patient considered for conservative treatment should be advised to avoid physical contact activities for a considerable time (Table 5).

Upper Respiratory Tract Complications

Patients with extensive pharyngotonsillitis have an increased risk of developing secondary bacterial tonsillitis for several months after the acute disease. Upper airway obstruction may result from palatal and nasopharyngeal tonsil hypertrophy and inflammatory edema of surrounding soft tissue (64). This can result in odynophagia, dysphagia, dehydration, and toxicity associated with secondary bacterial infection. The incidence of upper airway obstruction complicating acute IM has been reported to be between 1% and 3.5% (64–66). It is difficult to identify a standard clinical definition of upper airway obstruction or consensus guidelines with respect to monitoring, management, and decision-making for potential acute tonsillectomy, endotracheal intubation, or acute tracheotomy. The cardinal signs of severe upper airway obstruction include stridor predominantly in inspiration, dyspnea, intercostal and substernal retraction, tachypnea, and cyanosis (67). However, it is clear that most of these symptoms can be absent until late in the disease process. Continuous pulse oximetry and nasopharyngeal endoscopy add to reliability as adjunctive measurements. An electrocardiogram is recommended to evaluate for concomitant myocarditis because even mild hypoxemia secondary to upper airway obstruction may lead to arrhythmia and secondary progressive hypoxemia in these patients. Pharyngeal complications are the most common indications for hospitalization in IM, and younger children appear to be at a greater risk (64–66). Conservative treatment includes elevation of the head of the bed, intravenous hydration, ventilation with humidified air, and potential addition of systemic corticosteroids. Temporary nasopharyngeal stenting to bypass the lymphoid hyperplasia and soft tissue edema may be warranted.

Lower Respiratory Tract Complications

Pulmonary infiltrates are not an uncommon finding in routinely performed radiographs in IM patients. However, most of these cases are completely asymptomatic. Symptomatic lower respiratory tract infection is uncommon and occurs predominantly in FIM and in persons with impairment of EBV-specific cellular immunity (68). Bilateral interstitial infiltrates are frequently associated with unilateral or bilateral pleural effusions (42). Histologically, the pulmonary tissue is infiltrated with lymphocytes and histiocytes predominantly generating peribronchial infiltrates. The secondary edema may lead to occlusion of bronchioles with increased risk for secondary bacterial infections (Table 5).

Cardiac Complications

Asymptomatic electrocardiogram abnormalities are the most frequent cardiac complications occurring approximately in 5% of cases within the first two weeks of illness (58). It normally resolves without any sequelae. Symptomatic myocarditis or pericarditis is a rare complication. It predominantly occurs in fatal and fulminant IM cases (69). Histologically, histiocytes and lymphoid infiltration of the myocardium may affect the conductivity and generate arrhythmia (69). Chest pain is a warning sign that should prompt urgent medical attention (Table 5).

Neurological Complications

More than 25% of patients with EBV-associated IM have cerebrospinal fluid abnormalities, in particular, pleocytosis (70). The great majority of these patients have asymptomatic or nonspecific CNS symptoms. The nervous system is, however, clinically involved in IM patients in 0.5% to 5% of all cases (70). There is a vast spectrum of neurological manifestations that includes meningitis, encephalitis, cranial nerve palsies (especially Bell's palsy), optic neuritis, transverse myelitis, polyradiculitis, and Guillain–Barré syndrome (70–72). The prognosis is good in more than 85% of the cases. However, encephalitis cases with severe polyradiculitis may be fatal due to autonomic dysfunction with cardiac arrhythmias as complications.

Seizures are not an uncommon complication in encephalitis. The acute neurological manifestations include combative behavior in 50%, seizures in 35%, headache in 35%, and focal involvement in 25%. Approximately 15% of all patients develop persistent neurological abnormalities including global impairment, perseverative autistic-like behavior, or persistent pareses (73,74). Lumbar puncture and magnetic resonance imaging combined with electroencephalography are valuable methods in addition to single photon emission computed tomography, which detects the abnormal perfusion more precisely in a substantial number of patients with CNS involvement. Pathology is generated most likely via both infectious and immunological mechanisms. EBV-DNA can normally be detected by PCR of cerebrospinal fluid, while evidence of intrathecal antibody production is absent in most of the cases. Encephalitis is sometimes accompanied by myelitis, which may present as paraplegia or quadriplegia. The prognosis of spinal cord involvement is normally good. Cranial nerve involvement in patients with IM has been reported frequently (70). Facial nerve involvement has been reported most often, but neuropathies of cranial nerve I, II, III, IV, V, VI, VIII, and XII have also been described (Table 5).

Hematological Abnormalities

Anemia

Excessive autoimmune hemolytic anemia is relatively rare in IM (71–74). It normally occurs during the first weeks of illness and lasts for another four weeks. Aplastic anemia and agranulocytosis are much less common and occur three weeks after the onset of illness with usual recovery within 4 to 10 days (75,76). Both conditions are believed to be due to autoantibody formation (Table 5).

Thrombocytopenia

Mild thrombocytopenia is a common occurrence among IM. In contrast, severe thrombocytopenia with bleeding manifestations is rare. In most cases, thrombocytopenia is transient with platelet levels returning to normal during convalescence (77). Both hypersplenism and antiplatelet antibodies may contribute to this condition. Purpura, epistaxis, gingival bleeding, hematuria, splenic hemorrhage with rupture, and cerebral hemorrhage are warning signs (Table 5).

Neutropenia

Neutropenia, defined as an absolute neutrophil count less than 3000 cells/μL, is common among IM patients. This is particularly found in the early onset of illness but may occasionally persist for several weeks. Severe neutropenia at less than 1000 cells/μL typically lasts only a few days even if it has been reported two weeks after onset and is probably caused by antineutrophil antibodies and leucoagglutinins (78–80). In addition, these antibodies may arrest promyelocyte or myelocyte differentiation. Toxic changes in neutrophils are common findings in these cases. Agranulocytosis has been described in a few cases (Table 5).

Lymphocytes

Even if lymphocytosis is a cardinal sign of IM, lymphophenia may be present at the onset of disease. This is a prognostic bad sign and these patients often develop protracted IM (24). Lymphoproliferative disorders of either B-lymphocyte or T-lymphocyte origin may occur in fulminant IM (42). These cases may sometimes be difficult to distinguish from Hodgkin lymphoma, T-cell lymphoma, or malignant histiocytosis (Table 5).

Psychological Complications

Fatigue occurs initially in the great majority of IM patients. The duration of this condition is extremely variable, ranging from 5 to 180 days (81). Several studies have reported a prevalence of up to 25% of postinfectious fatigue lasting for up to six months after acute IM. A longitudinal study observed persistent fatigue after six months in 9% of the patients, and is thus much more common than after viral upper respiratory tract infections (82). One additional report confirmed failure to recover at two months in one-third of the patients, while 12% had not completely recovered at six months (83). Predictors of psychological stress included severity of symptoms during the first two weeks of illness, excessive elevation of hepatic transaminases, as well as poor social functioning in the month prior to diagnosis (83). The long-term prognosis, however, is good with few reported chronic disabilities. Depression or psychosis is exceedingly rare in the convalescence period of the illness (Table 5).

Fatal Infectious Mononucleosis

Death is exceedingly rare in IM and historically is estimated to occur in less than 1 per 3000 cases (84). However, more recent improvements in diagnosis have resulted in a number of case reports of fulminant atypical primary EBV infection associated with a fatal outcome (42). These patients often present with a persistent or intermittent fever, a generalized lymphadenopathy, excessive hepatosplenomegaly, initial lymphopenia, and extremely high antibody production of anti-VCA, anti-EA with lack of EBNA antibodies, and a high viral burden (41,42,50). Most of these cases have VAHS and a generalized histiocytic proliferation combined with infiltration of abnormal activated lymphocytes, resulting in pulmonary infiltrates, rash, liver dysfunction, and myocarditis (41,42,50).

THERAPY OF ACUTE INFECTION

Antiviral Treatment

A total of five placebo-control trials of treatment of IM with acyclovir have been performed in 340 patients between 1990 and 1999. These studies show no statistically significant clinical benefit or effectiveness of acyclovir treatment (Table 6). Acyclovir has been administered via peroral or intravenous routes. The studies have shown a significant reduction in the rate of oropharyngeal EBV shedding during therapy (18,85–88). However, within two weeks after cessation of treatment, no difference in shedding was apparent. Thus, there is no evidence that antiviral therapy with acyclovir leads to resolution of symptoms or prevents development of complications of IM. These results suggest that IM symptoms are predominantly caused by the immune response to EBV-infected activated B-lymphocytes, rather than as a direct result of virus replication. However, another plausible explanation might be that EBV replicates through cellular DNA polymerases in the great majority of infected B-lymphocytes (89). This is a process that would be resistant to current antiviral drugs. Furthermore, in vitro studies have shown that nucleoside analogues and DNA polymerase inhibitors do not prohibit EBV-induced transformation of B-lymphocytes, again an action mediated via cell-specific DNA

Table 6 Suggested Treatment Strategies in Primary Epstein–Barr Virus Infection

Clinical condition	Recommended treatment
Uncomplicated infectious mononucleosis	None
Generalized meningo-encephalitis	Acyclovir 10 mg/kg × q8 hr/tid i.v. + prednisolone 0.6 mg/kg × 1 p.o. for 7–10 days
Post-infectious asthenia[a]	Serotonin blockade, escitalopram 10–20 mg/day p.o.
Obstructive pharyngotonsillitis	Acyclovir 5 mg/kg × q8 hr/tid i.v. + prednisolone 0.6 mg/kg × 1 p.o. for 7–10 days
Hypoxic pneumonia (interstitial)	Acyclovir 5 mg/kg × q8 hr/tid i.v. + prednisolone 0.6 mg/kg × 1 p.o for 7–10 days + IFN-γ 2 × 10⁶ U/m² three times/wk s.c.
Cholestatic hepatitis	Plasmapheresis, IVIG 0.5 g/kg every two days until clinical improvement
Hematological abnormalities	
Thrombocytopenia	Prednisolone 1 mg/kg × 1 p.o. or IVIG 0.5 g/kg × 1 for 2–4 days
Hemolytic anemia	Prednisolone 0.6 mg/kg × 1 p.o. for 2–4 days
Disseminated coagulopathy	Plasmapheresis + IVIG 0.5 g/kg every two days until clinical recovery
Immunosuppressed persons	Adoptive transfer by LAK cells (in vitro, IL-2 treated HLA-matched EBV-specific T cells) until clinical recovery or IFN-γ 2.0 MU/m² s.c. three times/wk + acyclovir 10 mg/kg × q6 hr/tid p.o. daily
XLP disease	Prophylaxis; IVIG 0.5 g/kg i.v. every four wks + valacyclovir 10 mg/kg × q8 hr/tid p.o. until BMT procedure. Therapeutic; bone marrow transplantation

[a]Sustained post-infectious asthenia is defined as mental asthenia persisting more than six months from onset of IM.
Abbreviations: BMT, bone marrow transplant; HLA, human leukocyte antigen; i.v., intravenous; IFN-γ, interferon gamma; IM, infectious mononucleosis; IVIG, intravenous immunoglobulin; LAK, lymphokine-activated killer cells; p.o., peroral; s.c., subcutaneous; tid, three times daily; XLP, X-linked lympho-proliferative.

enzymatic activity (90). There are, however, specific IM-associated subsets of life-threatening events, which may be considered for treatment as outlined in Table 6. More recently, in the mid-1990s, a placebo-controlled study of combined predniso-lone and acyclovir therapy in the early onset of IM showed no significant reduction in duration of symptoms or signs of IM (87). This therapeutic approach may be of some clinical value in patients with autoantibody-induced cytopenia including leu-copenia, thrombocytopenia, and hemolytic anemia. Potentially, it may also be worth considering combination treatment to reduce swelling in patients with severe upper respiratory tract obstruction. However, no such prospective study has been performed as yet.

Corticosteroids

Corticosteroids are unnecessary in uncomplicated cases and should not be routinely administrated to IM patients. Throughout the 1970s and 1980s, several studies, including prospective placebo-control trials, evaluated the use of oral prednisolone in uncomplicated IM (64,65,71,72,91). It did not significantly shorten the time to complete resolution of symptoms. The benefit of corticosteroids in complications of IM has been advocated based on anecdotal experience, without well-conducted prospective studies. Conditions requiring potential treatment include incipient upper respiratory tract obstruction, autoimmune hemolytic anemia or neutropenia, thrombocytopenia with hemorrhage, and meningoencephalitis plus other neurological complications. Intravenous dexamethasone 0.25 mg/kg every six hours, methylprednisolone 1 mg/kg every six hours, or oral prednisolone 40 mg/day given for one to three days have each been used with similar results. Dramatic subjective improvements within one to two days and objective improvements within three days have been reported (64,65,71,72,91). Care should be exercised in using corticosteroids because of the unknown long-term effects of using an immunosuppressive drug for a virus that invariably establishes intracellular latency. It has clearly been shown that normal immune responses are of vital importance for effectively preventing disease progression. Furthermore, EBV-specific cellular immune responses have clearly been associated with the control of the long-lasting EBV infection. Thus, use of corticosteroids in the initial setting of IM may possibly affect the risk for subsequent development of later EBV-associated malignancies (Table 6).

Alternative Treatment Strategies

Severe isolated thrombocytopenia with hemorrhage may be treated with intravenous immunoglobulin or prednisolone (92). Polyspecific intravenous IgG has been shown to have significantly more rapid effect compared to steroids and also may be effective in steroid-resistant conditions (92). Plasmapheresis, combined with pooled human intravenous immunoglobulins, has also been shown to be effective in some patients with severe cholestatic hepatitis and disseminated intravascular coagulation (Table 6) (93,94).

When IM is complicated by interstitial, symptomatic pneumonitis, potential selective immunodeficiencies contributing to this complication should be considered (95). Anecdotal reports exist of EBV-specific downregulation of interferon (IFN) -γ in T-cells affecting development of EBV-specific cytotoxic T-lymphocyte (CTL). Combination therapy of subcutaneous recombinant IFN-γ 2×10^6 U/m^2, three times per week in combination with oral steroids (prednisolone 0.6 mg/kg) and acyclovir (800 mg, five times daily) may be an alternative, although it has never been carefully evaluated (95). In patients with severe encephalitis, meningoencephalitis, or transverse myelitis, intravenous acyclovir (10 mg/kg, three times daily) may be combined with prednisolone (0.6 mg/kg, once daily) for 10 days (96). Steroids have been shown to have a positive effect on some EBV-associated neurological disorders. However, in other studies, prednisolone has been associated with increased risk for neurological complications in IM (96,97). Low dose serotonin-blockade (citalopram) has been shown to result in response rates of 50% in an open label study of patients with sustained postinfectious asthenia (Table 6) (7).

Treatment of Acute EBV Infection in Individuals with Cellular Immune Deficiency Disorders

XLP syndrome, polyclonal lymphoproliferative disorders, and fulminant acute IM have anecdotally been treated with acyclovir, IFN-α, IFN-γ, or intravenous immunoglobulins (98). Although these treatment strategies have reported positive effects in scattered cases, there are no published prospective studies demonstrating 100% significant effect on EBV-induced symptoms. Some patients with VAHS have been treated with intravenous podophyllin derivatives, such as etoposide (53,99). There are no conclusive results as to whether this should be the treatment of choice (Table 6).

Future Directions

Adoptive transfer of EBV-specific immunity via infusion of unmodified lymphocytes from human leukocyte antigen (HLA)-matched healthy EBV-seropositive donors or of in vitro expanded HLA-matched reactivated EBV-specific CTLs are the future treatments of choice (100). Exposing T-cells to autologous EBV-infected B-cells in the presence of interleukin (IL)-2 may generate CTLs (101). This approach has shown clinical efficacy, not only in the treatment of PTLD, but also prophylactically in T-cell–depleted allogeneic bone marrow–transplanted patients (102,103). In addition, adoptive transfer of EBV immunity has been used for treatment of EBV-associated malignancies (102). Use of adoptive therapy, however, requires strategic planning, either by generating cell lines prospectively from individuals with risk of severe EBV infection, or from HLA-matched donors (104) (Table 6).

Monoclonal Antibody Therapy in EBV-Induced Lymphoproliferative Disorders

The monoclonal antibody (mAb) therapy approach has mainly been used for treatment of monoclonal PTLD in allogeneic B and T-cells and in solid organ–transplanted

Table 7 Treatment and Prevention of Polyclonal and Monoclonal Lymphoproliferative Diseases

Diagnosis	Treatment
Prophylaxis for primary EBV	Acyclovir 10 mg/kg, maximum 4 times/day p.o. or ganciclovir 5 mg/kg × once/day i.v.
Polyclonal PTLD	Reduce the immunosuppression to a minimal level + acyclovir 10 mg/kg maximum 4 times/day p.o. or ganciclovir 5 mg × 2 times/day i.v.
Monoclonal PTLD	Adoptive T-cell immunotherapy: MHC-matched donor lymphocyte infusions $2–10 \times 10^5$ cells/kg every wk Or in vitro stimulated MHC-matched PBMC stimulated with IL-2 + EBV-infected B-lymphocytes to induce EBV-specific T-cells. Give 10^7 to 5×10^7 cells/m^2 every other wk
Monoclonal PTLD	Anti-CD20 mAb. Rituximab i.v. every wk or anti-CD21 + anti-CD24 mAb 0.2 mg/kg i.v. every wk

Abbreviations: EBV, Epstein–Barr virus; i.v., intravenous; mAb, monoclonal antibody; MHC, major histocompatibility complex; p.o., peroral; PBMC, peripheral blood mononuclear cells; PTLD, post-transplant lymphoproliferative disorder.

patients (30,105). A recent multicenter study using anti-B-cell mAb treatment by combining anti-CD21 and anti-CD24 reported a remission rate of 61% (106). Similar results have also previously been shown for the use of anti-CD20 mAb (Rituximab®) therapy. However, currently there are no reports of use of mAb therapy in acute EBV or in IM-associated polyclonal proliferative disorders. Furthermore, one may consider a combined approach of adoptive therapy of EBV-specific CTL and anti–B-lympho-cyte monoclonal treatment (Table 7).

Vaccines Against EBV Disease

There is currently no licensed vaccine against EBV infection. However, vaccine trials aiming to control IM, PTLD, nasopharyngeal carcinoma, and Hodgkin's disease are warranted. Multicenter trials are now evaluating the potential prophylactic efficacy of an EBV vaccine candidate designed around the structure of the EBV antigen glycoprotein 350 (gp350) (see Chapter 19) (107).

CONCLUSIONS

The prognosis for IM is very favorable. There is, however, a variety of acute com-plications. Therapy in these patients must be individualized, depending on the type of complication. Fatal cases of IM result from uncontrolled lymphoproliferative disorders. Immune EBV-specific reconstitution is a potential, future therapeutic option in this setting. There is no evidence for the benefit of antiviral therapy in uncomplicated cases. Even though corticosteroids may reduce duration of upper air-way obstruction and appear to improve resolution of immune-mediated anemia and thrombocytopenia, they should be used with caution in IM.

REFERENCES

1. Fleisher G, Henle W, Henle G, Lennette ET, Biggar RJ. Primary infection with Epstein–Barr virus in infants in the United States: clinical and serologic observations. J Infect Dis 1979; 139:553–558.
2. Filatov N. In: Lolleznyak N, ed. Lectures on Acute Infectious Diseases of Children. Moscow: U. Deitel, 1885.
3. Pfeiffer L. Jahrbuch für Kinderheilkunde. 1889; 29:257–266.
4. Henle G, Henle W, Diehl V. Relation of Burkitt's tumor-associated herpes-type virus to infectious mononucleosis. Proc Natl Acad Sci USA 1968; 59:94–101.
5. Hoagland R. The clinical manifestations of infectious mononucleosis: a report of two hundred cases. Am J Med Sci 1960; 240:55–62.
6. Straus SE, Cohen JI, Tosato G, Meier J. Epstein–Barr virus infections: biology, patho-genesis, and management. Ann Intern Med 1993; 118:45–58.
7. Andersson J. Clinical and immunological considerations in Epstein–Barr virus-associated diseases. Scand J Infect Dis Suppl 1996; 100:72–82.
8. Cohen JI. Epstein–Barr virus infection. N Engl J Med 2000; 343:481–492.
9. Niederman JC, Evans AS, Subrahmanyan L, McCollum RW. Prevalence, incidence and persistence of EB virus antibody in young adults. N Engl J Med 1970; 282:361–365.
10. Cohen JI. Epstein–Barr virus and the immune system. Hide and seek. JAMA 1997; 278:510–513.
11. Anagnostopoulos I, Hummel M, Kreschel C, Stein H. Morphology, immunophenotype, and distribution of latently and/or productively Epstein–Barr virus-infected cells in

acute infectious mononucleosis: implications for the interindividual infection route of Epstein–Barr virus. Blood 1995; 85:744–750.

12. Gerber P, Lucas S, Nonoyama M, Perlin E, Goldstein LI. Oral excretion of Epstein–Barr virus by healthy subjects and patients with infectious mononucleosis. Lancet 1972; 2:988–989.

13. Sixbey JW, Lemon SM, Pagano JS. A second site for Epstein–Barr virus shedding: the uterine cervix. Lancet 1986; 2:1122–1124.

14. Biggar RJ, Henle G, Bocker J, Lennette ET, Fleisher G, Henle W. Primary Epstein–Barr virus infections in African infants II. Clinical and serological observations during seroconversion. Int J Cancer 1978; 22:244–250.

15. de-The G, Geser A, Day NE, et al. Epidemiological evidence for causal relationship between Epstein–Barr virus and Burkitt's lymphoma from Ugandan prospective study. Nature 1978; 274:756–761.

16. Chetham MM, Roberts KB. Infectious mononucleosis in adolescents. Pediatr Ann 1991; 20:206–213.

17. Meyohas MC, Marechal V, Desire N, Bouillie J, Frottier J, Nicolas JC. Study of mother-to-child Epstein–Barr virus transmission by means of nested PCRs. J Virol 1996; 70:6816–6819.

18. Andersson J, Britton S, Ernberg I, et al. Effect of acyclovir on infectious mononucleosis: a double-blind, placebo-controlled study. J Infect Dis 1986; 153:283–290.

19. Moffat LE. Infectious mononucleosis. Prim Care Update Ob Gyns 2001; 8:73–77.

20. Papesch M, Watkins R. Epstein–Barr virus infectious mononucleosis. Clin Otolaryngol 2001; 26:3–8.

21. Weber R, Hegenbarth V, Kaftan H, Krupe H, Jaspersen D, Keerl R. Nasopharyngeal endoscopy adds to reliability of clinical diagnosis of infectious mononucleosis. J Laryngol Otol 2001; 115:792–795.

22. Pattengale PK, Smith RW, Perlin E. Atypical lymphocytes in acute infectious mononucleosis. Identification by multiple T and B lymphocyte markers. N Engl J Med 1974; 291:1145–1148.

23. Downey H, McKinlay C. Acute lymphadenosis compared with acute lymphatic leukemia. Part I. Clinical Study. Arch Intern Med 1923; 32:82–112.

24. Bar RS, Adlard J, Thomas FB. Lymphopenic infectious mononucleosis. Arch Intern Med 1975; 135:334–337.

25. Chapman CJ, Spellerberg MB, Smith GA, Carter SJ, Hamblin TJ, Stevenson FK. Autoanti-red cell antibodies synthesized by patients with infectious mononucleosis utilize the VH4-21 gene segment. J Immunol 1993; 151:1051–1061.

26. Niesters HG, van Esser J, Fries E, Wolthers KC, Cornelissen J, Osterhaus AD. Development of a real-time quantitative assay for detection of Epstein–Barr virus. J Clin Microbiol 2000; 38:712–715.

27. Lahat E, Berkovitch M, Barr J, Paret G, Barzilai A. Abnormal visual evoked potentials in children with "Alice in Wonderland" syndrome due to infectious mononucleosis. J Child Neurol 1999; 14:732–735.

28. Davidsohn I, Lee C. Serologic diagnosis of infectious mononucleosis. A cooperative study of five tests. Am J Clin Pathol 1964; 41:115–125.

29. Henle W, Henle G, Andersson J, et al. Antibody responses to Epstein–Barr virus-determined nuclear antigen (EBNA)-1 and EBNA-2 in acute and chronic Epstein–Barr virus infection. Proc Natl Acad Sci USA 1987; 84:570–574.

30. Lang D, Vornhagen R, Rothe M, Hinderer W, Sonneborn HH, Plachter B. Cross-reactivity of Epstein–Barr virus-specific immunoglobulin M antibodies with cytomegalovirus antigens containing glycine homopolymers. Clin Diagn Lab Immunol 2001; 8:747–756.

31. Farber I, Hinderer W, Rothe M, Lang D, Sonneborn HH, Wutzler P. Serological diagnosis of Epstein–Barr virus infection by novel ELISAs based on recombinant capsid antigens p23 and p18. J Med Virol 2001; 63:271–276.

32. Meerbach A, Gruhn B, Egerer R, Reischl U, Zintl F, Wutzler P. Semiquantitative PCR analysis of Epstein–Barr virus DNA in clinical samples of patients with EBV-associated diseases. J Med Virol 2001; 65:348–357.
33. Berger C, Day P, Meier G, Zingg W, Bossart W, Nadal D. Dynamics of Epstein–Barr virus DNA levels in serum during EBV-associated disease. J Med Virol 2001; 64:505–512.
34. Kimura H, Nishikawa K, Hoshino Y, Sofue A, Nishiyama Y, Morishima T. Monitoring of cell-free viral DNA in primary Epstein–Barr virus infection. Med Microbiol Immunol (Berl) 2000; 188:197–202.
35. Kanegane H, Wakiguchi H, Kanegane C, Kurashige T, Miyawaki T, Tosato G. Increased cell-free viral DNA in fatal cases of chronic active Epstein–Barr virus infection. Clin Infect Dis 1999; 28:906–909.
36. Gulley ML. Molecular diagnosis of Epstein–Barr virus-related diseases. J Mol Diagn 2001; 3:1–10.
37. Rosenberg ES, Caliendo AM, Walker BD. Acute HIV infection among patients tested for mononucleosis. N Engl J Med 1999; 340:969.
38. Vidrih JA, Walensky RP, Sax PE, Freedberg KA. Positive Epstein–Barr virus heterophile antibody tests in patients with primary human immunodeficiency virus infection. Am J Med 2001; 111:192–194.
39. Walensky RP, Rosenberg ES, Ferraro MJ, Losina E, Walker BD, Freedberg KA. Investigation of primary human immunodeficiency virus infection in patients who test positive for heterophile antibody. Clin Infect Dis 2001; 33:570–572.
40. Lajo A, Borque C, Del Castillo F, Martin-Ancel A. Mononucleosis caused by Epstein–Barr virus and cytomegalovirus in children: a comparative study of 124 cases. Pediatr Infect Dis J 1994; 13:56–60.
41. Kojima M, Nakamura S, Itoh H, Yoshida K, Suchi T, Masawa N. Acute viral lymphadenitis mimicking low-grade peripheral T-cell lymphoma. A clinicopathological study of nine cases. Apmis 2001; 109:419–427.
42. Quintanilla-Martinez L, Kumar S, Fend F, et al. Fulminant EBV(+) T-cell lymphoproliferative disorder following acute/chronic EBV infection: a distinct clinicopathologic syndrome. Blood 2000; 96:443–451.
43. Greiner T, Armitage JO, Gross TG. Atypical lymphoproliferative diseases. Hematology (Am Soc Hematol Educ Program) 2000:133–146.
44. Taga K, Taga H, Tosato G. Diagnosis of atypical cases of infectious mononucleosis. Clin Infect Dis 2001; 33:83–88.
45. Chan KH, Tam JS, Peiris JS, Seto WH, Ng MH. Epstein–Barr virus (EBV) infection in infancy. J Clin Virol 2001; 21:57–62.
46. Horwitz CA, Henle W, Henle G, Schapiro R, Borken S, Bundtzen R. Infectious mononucleosis in patients aged 40 to 72 years: report of 27 cases, including 3 without heterophil-antibody responses. Medicine (Baltimore) 1983; 62:256–262.
47. Kirov SM, Marsden KA, Wongwanich S. Seroepidemiological study of infectious mononucleosis in older patients. J Clin Microbiol 1989; 27:356–358.
48. Portnoy J, Ahronheim GA, Ghibu F, Clecner B, Joncas JH. Recovery of Epstein–Barr virus from genital ulcers. N Engl J Med 1984; 311:966–968.
49. Seemayer TA, Gross TG, Egeler RM, et al. X-linked lymphoproliferative disease: twenty-five years after the discovery. Pediatr Res 1995; 38:471–478.
50. Sayos J, Wu C, Morra M, et al. The X-linked lymphoproliferative-disease gene product SAP regulates signals induced through the co-receptor SLAM. Nature 1998; 395:462–469.
51. Imashuku S, Teramura T, Morimoto A, Hibi S. Recent developments in the management of haemophagocytic lymphohistiocytosis. Expert Opin Pharmacother 2001; 2:1437–1448.
52. Hiraki A, Fujii N, Masuda K, Ikeda K, Tanimoto M. Genetics of Epstein–Barr virus infection. Biomed Pharmacother 2001; 55:369–372.

53. Okano M, Gross TG. Epstein–Barr virus-associated hemophagocytic syndrome and fatal infectious mononucleosis. Am J Hematol 1996; 53:111–115.

54. Ohshima K, Shimazaki K, Sugihara M, et al. Clinicopathological findings of virus-associated hemophagocytic syndrome in bone marrow: association with Epstein–Barr virus and apoptosis. Pathol Int 1999; 49:533–540.

55. Kikuta H, Sakiyama Y, Matsumoto S, et al. Fatal Epstein–Barr virus-associated hemophagocytic syndrome. Blood 1993; 82:3259–3264.

56. Ross CW, Schnitzer B, Weston BW, Hanson CA. Chronic active Epstein–Barr virus infection and virus-associated hemophagocytic syndrome. Arch Pathol Lab Med 1991; 115:470–474.

57. Cohen JI. Epstein–Barr virus lymphoproliferative disease associated with acquired immunodeficiency. Medicine (Baltimore) 1991; 70:137–160.

58. Jenson HB. Acute complications of Epstein–Barr virus infectious mononucleosis. Curr Opin Pediatr 2000; 12:263–268.

59. Pullen H, Wright N, Murdoch JM. Hypersensitivity reactions to antibacterial drugs in infectious mononucleosis. Lancet 1967; 2:1176–1178.

60. Patel BM. Skin rash with infectious mononucleosis and ampicillin. Pediatrics 1967; 40:910–911.

61. Fuhrman SA, Gill R, Horwitz CA, et al. Marked hyperbilirubinemia in infectious mononucleosis. Analysis of laboratory data in seven patients. Arch Intern Med 1987; 147:850–853.

62. Devereaux CE, Bemiller T, Brann O. Ascites and severe hepatitis complicating Epstein–Barr infection. Am J Gastroenterol 1999; 94:236–240.

63. Rothwell S, McAuley D. Spontaneous splenic rupture in infectious mononucleosis. Emerg Med (Fremantle) 2001; 13:364–366.

64. Wohl DL, Isaacson JE. Airway obstruction in children with infectious mononucleosis. Ear Nose Throat J 1995; 74:630–638.

65. Farley DR, Zietlow SP, Bannon MP, Farnell MB. Spontaneous rupture of the spleen due to infectious mononucleosis. Mayo Clin Proc 1992; 67:846–853.

66. Ganzel TM, Goldman JL, Padhya TA. Otolaryngologic clinical patterns in pediatric infectious mononucleosis. Am J Otolaryngol 1996; 17:397–400.

67. Chan SC, Dawes PJ. The management of severe infectious mononucleosis tonsillitis and upper airway obstruction. J Laryngol Otol 2001; 115:973–977.

68. Haller A, von Segesser L, Baumann PC, Krause M. Severe respiratory insufficiency complicating Epstein–Barr virus infection: case report and review. Clin Infect Dis 1995; 21:206–209.

69. Frishman W, Kraus ME, Zabkar J, Brooks V, Alonso D, Dixon LM. Infectious mononucleosis and fatal myocarditis. Chest 1977; 72:535–538.

70. Portegies P, Corssmit N. Epstein–Barr virus and the nervous system. Curr Opin Neurol 2000; 13:301–304.

71. Grose C, Henle W, Henle G, Feorino PM. Primary Epstein–Barr-virus infections in acute neurologic diseases. N Engl J Med 1975; 292:392–395.

72. Whitelaw F, Brook MG, Kennedy N, Weir WR. Haemolytic anaemia complicating Epstein–Barr virus infection. Br J Clin Pract 1995; 49:212–213.

73. Gelati G, Verucchi G, Chiodo F, Romeo M. Hemolytic anemia as a complication of Epstein–Barr virus infection: a report of two cases. J Exp Pathol 1987; 3:485–489.

74. Domachowske JB, Cunningham CK, Cummings DL, Crosley CJ, Hannan WP, Weiner LB. Acute manifestations and neurologic sequelae of Epstein–Barr virus encephalitis in children. Pediatr Infect Dis J 1996; 15:871–875.

75. Levy M, Kelly JP, Kaufman DW, Shapiro S. Risk of agranulocytosis and aplastic anemia in relation to history of infectious mononucleosis: a report from the international agranulocytosis and aplastic anemia study. Ann Hematol 1993; 67:187–190.

76. Lazarus KH, Baehner RL. Aplastic anemia complicating infectious mononucleosis: a case report and review of the literature. Pediatrics 1981; 67:907–910.

77. Carter RL. The mitotic activity of circulating atypical mononuclear cells in infectious mononucleosis. Blood 1965; 26:579–586.
78. Cantow EF, Kostinas JE. Studies on infectious mononucleosis IV. Changes in the granulocytic series. Am J Clin Pathol 1966; 46:43–47.
79. Hammond WP, Harlan JM, Steinberg SE. Severe neutropenia in infectious mononucleosis. West J Med 1979; 131:92–97.
80. Schooley RT, Densen P, Harmon D, et al. Antineutrophil antibodies in infectious mononucleosis. Am J Med 1984; 76:85–90.
81. Rea TD, Russo JE, Katon W, Ashley RL, Buchwald DS. Prospective study of the natural history of infectious mononucleosis caused by Epstein–Barr virus. J Am Board Fam Pract 2001; 14:234–242.
82. Katon W, Russo J, Ashley RL, Buchwald D. Infectious mononucleosis: psychological symptoms during acute and subacute phases of illness. Gen Hosp Psychiat 1999; 21:21–29.
83. White PD, Thomas JM, Amess J, et al. Incidence, risk and prognosis of acute and chronic fatigue syndromes and psychiatric disorders after glandular fever. Br J Psychiat 1998; 173:475–481.
84. Penman HG. Fatal infectious mononucleosis: a critical review. J Clin Pathol 1970; 23:765–771.
85. Andersson J, Skoldenberg B, Henle W, et al. Acyclovir treatment in infectious mononucleosis: a clinical and virological study. Infection 1987; 15(suppl 1):S14–S20.
86. van der Horst C, Joncas J, Ahronheim G, et al. Lack of effect of peroral acyclovir for the treatment of acute infectious mononucleosis. J Infect Dis 1991; 164:788–792.
87. Tynell E, Aurelius E, Brandell A, et al. Acyclovir and prednisolone treatment of acute infectious mononucleosis: a multicenter, double-blind, placebo-controlled study. J Infect Dis 1996; 174:324–331.
88. Torre D, Tambini R. Acyclovir for treatment of infectious mononucleosis: a meta-analysis. Scand J Infect Dis 1999; 31:543–547.
89. Norio P, Schildkraut CL. Visualization of DNA replication on individual Epstein–Barr virus episomes. Science 2001; 294:2361–2364.
90. Pagano JS, Sixbey JW, Lin JC. Acyclovir and Epstein–Barr virus infection. J Antimicrob Chemother 1983; 12(suppl B):113–121.
91. Steeper TA, Horwitz CA, Moore SB, et al. Severe thrombocytopenia in Epstein-Barr virus-induced mononucleosis. West J Med 1989; 150:170–173.
92. Cyran EM, Rowe JM, Bloom RE. Intravenous gammaglobulin treatment for immune thrombocytopenia associated with infectious mononucleosis. Am J Hematol 1991; 38:124–129.
93. Geurs F, Ritter K, Mast A, Van Maele V. Successful plasmapheresis in corticosteroid-resistant hemolysis in infectious mononucleosis: role of autoantibodies against triosephosphate isomerase. Acta Haematol 1992; 88:142–146.
94. Levi M, Ten Cate H. Disseminated intravascular coagulation. N Engl J Med 1999; 341:586–592.
95. Andersson J, Isberg B, Christensson B, Veress B, Linde A, Bratel T. Interferon gamma (IFN-gamma) deficiency in generalized Epstein–Barr virus infection with interstitial lymphoid and granulomatous pneumonia, focal cerebral lesions, and genital ulcers: remission following IFN-gamma substitution therapy. Clin Infect Dis 1999; 28:1036–1042.
96. Corssmit EP, Leverstein-van Hall MA, Portegies P, Bakker P. Severe neurological complications in association with Epstein–Barr virus infection. J Neurovirol 1997; 3:460–464.
97. McGowan JE Jr, Chesney PJ, Crossley KB, LaForce FM. Guidelines for the use of systemic glucocorticosteroids in the management of selected infections Working Group on Steroid Use, Antimicrobial Agents Committee, Infectious Diseases Society of America. J Infect Dis 1992; 165:1–13.

98. Purtilo DT. X-linked lymphoproliferative disease (XLP) as a model of Epstein–Barr virus-induced immunopathology. Springer Semin Immunopathol 1991; 13:181–197.

99. Maia DM, Peace-Brewer AL. Chronic, active Epstein–Barr virus infection. Curr Opin Hematol 2000; 7:59–63.

100. Heslop HE, Rooney CM. Adoptive cellular immunotherapy for EBV lymphoproliferative disease. Immunol Rev 1997; 157:217–222.

101. Smith CA, Ng CY, Heslop HE, et al. Production of genetically modified Epstein–Barr virus-specific cytotoxic T-cells for adoptive transfer to patients at high risk of EBV-associated lymphoproliferative disease. J Hematother 1995; 4:73–79.

102. Rooney CM, Roskrow MA, Smith CA, Brenner MK, Heslop HE. Immunotherapy for Epstein–Barr virus-associated cancers. J Natl Cancer Inst Monogr 1998; 23:89–93.

103. Roskrow MA, Suzuki N, Gan Y, et al. Epstein–Barr virus (EBV)-specific cytotoxic T lymphocytes for the treatment of patients with EBV-positive relapsed Hodgkin's disease. Blood 1998; 91:2925–2934.

104. Regn S, Raffegerst S, Chen X, Schendel D, Kolb HJ, Roskrow M. Ex vivo generation of cytotoxic T lymphocytes specific for one or two distinct viruses for the prophylaxis of patients receiving an allogeneic bone marrow transplant. Bone Marrow Transplant 2001; 27:53–64.

105. Verschuuren EA, Stevens SJ, van Imhoff GW, et al. Treatment of posttransplant lymphoproliferative disease with rituximab: the remission, the relapse, and the complication. Transplantation 2002; 73:100–104.

106. Benkerrou M, Jais JP, Leblond V, et al. Anti-B-cell monoclonal antibody treatment of severe posttransplant B-lymphoproliferative disorder: prognostic factors and long-term outcome. Blood 1998; 92:3137–3147.

107. Jung S, Chung YK, Chang SH, et al. DNA-mediated immunization of glycoprotein 350 of Epstein-Barr virus induces the effective humoral and cellular immune responses against the antigen. Mol Cells 2001; 12:41–49.

7

Epstein–Barr Virus Disease—Serologic and Virologic Diagnosis

Alex Tselis
Department of Neurology, Wayne State University, Detroit, Michigan, U.S.A.

Joseph R. Merline
DMC University Laboratories and Department of Pathology, Wayne State University, Detroit, Michigan, U.S.A.

Gregory A. Storch
Department of Pediatrics, Washington University School of Medicine, St. Louis Children's Hospital, St. Louis, Missouri, U.S.A.

INTRODUCTION

The Epstein–Barr virus (EBV) is a member of the herpesvirus family that infects more than 90% of the world's population. The consequences of infection with this virus depend on age and degree of immunocompetence and can lead to a broad spectrum of disease manifestations, from a subacute febrile illness with pharyngitis and lymphadenopathy to viral encephalitis, to posttransplant lymphoproliferative diseases (PTLDs).

To confirm if EBV infection is the cause of specific symptoms, a careful choice among a variety of laboratory tests is required. The choice, in turn, is based on the manifestations that require the identification of an etiological diagnosis.

HETEROPHILE ANTIBODIES

Early History

The syndrome of fatigue, malaise, fever, sore throat, and cervical lymphadenopathy with splenomegaly was first described in the late 1800s. While the syndrome was etiologically heterogeneous, as experience accumulated, a distinct clinical entity with characteristic clinical and laboratory findings gradually emerged. The first formal descriptions of infectious mononucleosis (IM) were given by Filatov in 1885 and by Pfeiffer in 1889 (1). In 1920, Sprunt and Evans introduced the term "infectious mononucleosis" and described the characteristic hematological finding of "atypical lymphocytes" (2).

It has been known since the work of Forssman in 1911 that normal human serum contains antibodies that agglutinate sheep red blood cells (3). The antigen on sheep red cells to which these antibodies are directed is the Forssman antigen. The Forssman antigen is a pentahexosyl ceramide and is widely distributed in sheep and horse erythrocytes and in some human cancer cells, as well as in the guinea pig kidney. Most human sera contain antibodies to the Forssman antigen. Hanganutziu in 1924 and Deicher in 1926 observed that patients with serum sickness also had antibodies that agglutinated sheep red cells (4,5). The antigen in the sheep erythrocytes to which these antibodies react is called the Hanganutziu–Deicher (H-D) antigen, which is associated with sialic acid groups in gangliosides and glycoproteins. The H-D antigen is different from the Forssman antigen.

The observation that IM also gave rise to antibodies that coincidentally agglutinated sheep red blood cells (heterophile antibodies) was reported by Paul and Bunnell in 1932 (6). These authors investigated the specificity of the observation that sheep cell–agglutinins occurred in serum sickness, and tested a number of control sera. One serum sample taken from a patient with IM gave extremely high titers of activity. The authors followed this up by comparing the sheep cell–agglutinating-ability of IM sera with that of healthy persons as well as patients with various other infectious and neoplastic illnesses. The titers were consistently greater in the IM patients, although there was some overlap with serum sickness patients. These antibodies also agglutinate horse and goat erythrocytes and cause lysis of bovine red cells in the presence of a complement (7). Because these antibodies agglutinate antigens of different origins, they are known as heterophile antibodies. These so-called Paul–Bunnell (PB) antigens found on sheep, horse, goat, and beef cells are not necessarily identical.

Formally, heterophile antibodies were defined as those that were elicited by one type of infectious antigen and reacted to a different, completely unrelated antigen. Probably the most famous example is that of the rapid plasma reagin test, which detects infection by *Treponema pallidum* by the measurement of antibodies against cardiolipin. Other examples include antibodies ("cold agglutinins"), elicited by *Mycoplasma pneumoniae*, that react with certain human red cell antigens (I antigens) and antibodies induced by the scrub typhus rickettsia, which agglutinate the OX-K strain of the bacillus *Proteus* (Weil-Felix test) (8).

Acute EBV infection is usually accompanied by heterophile (or PB) antibodies that agglutinate sheep erythrocytes, as well as horse and goat erythrocytes. The PB antigens on these erythrocytes have been isolated (from red cell membranes by a hot ethanol extraction procedure) and purified by various methods, including ion exchange chromatography and immunoabsorption chromatography. The PB antigens on erythrocytes from different species are only partially cross-reactive, as shown by Ouchterlony precipitin arcs and cross-absorption of IM sera, and therefore not identical. The precise nature of the PB antigen is unknown, although purified fractions contain a sialoglycopeptide with cross-reactivity to erythrocyte glycophorin (Fig. 1). The PB antigen is not an EBV-encoded antigen. Indeed, if sheep red cells are used to absorb heterophile-positive serum, there is no change in antibody titers to the usual EBV antigen complexes [viral capsid antigen (VCA) and early antigens (EAs)] or in neutralizing antibody titers (9). In a study of nine volunteers who were inoculated with sheep red cells, one had negative previous serology for EBV infection. The serum from this subject was used to test for antibodies to EBV-specific antigens (VCA and EA) by the method of immunofluorescence. No such antibodies could be found despite the presence of very high titers of antibodies that bound to

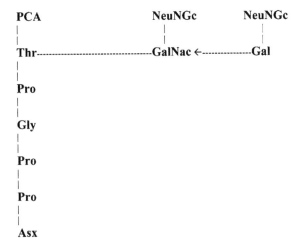

```
PCA                      NeuNGc          NeuNGc
 |                          |               |
 |                          |               |
Thr---------------------------GalNac ←---------------Gal
 |
 |
Pro
 |
 |
Gly
 |
 |
Pro
 |
 |
Pro
 |
 |
Asx
```

Figure 1 Model of Bovine Paul–Bunnell determinant. *Abbreviation*: PCA, 2-pyrridolinone-5-carboxylic acid (a cyclized glutamine residue). *Source*: From Ref. 7.

sheep erythrocytes. This suggests that the heterophile antibody is not directed to the usual EBV antigens elicited during primary infection (9). Indeed, acute EBV infection is known to lead to the production of a number of antibodies, some of which are autoantibodies, probably resulting from the generalized nonspecific activation of B-cells that occurs with this infection.

PB heterophile antibodies are mainly of the immunoglobulin M (IgM) class, but most patients will have heterophile antibodies of the IgG, IgA, and IgE classes, although the titers are much lower than those of the IgM class (10,11).

PB Test

The PB test was historically performed using sheep erythrocytes. In this test, serial twofold dilutions of the patient's serum are tested against a standard amount of sheep red cells that is added to each dilution of serum. The highest dilution of serum that agglutinates the sheep red cells is the reported titer. While high titers strongly imply the diagnosis of IM, lower titers can be nonspecific because there are nonspecific antibodies to sheep red cells in normal serum (antibodies to Forssman antigen, as mentioned above) and in the serum of those persons with serum sickness (H-D antibodies, more common historically than now) (Fig. 2). A more specific test is the Davidsohn differential absorption test.

Davidsohn Differential Absorption Test

This test is more specific than the PB test for the IM or PB heterophile antibody (12). The test is based on the fact that sheep cells have the Forssman antigen as well as the PB antigen. Guinea pig kidney contains the Forssman antigen as well as the H-D antigen, while beef cells express PB and H-D antigens, and horse cells express Forssman and PB antigens. These different types of cells are used to test the specificity of the sheep cell agglutinins in the patient's serum (Fig. 2).

Serial dilutions of the test serum are made as for the PB test. Standard amounts of guinea pig kidney are added to each aliquot of serum and incubated, which

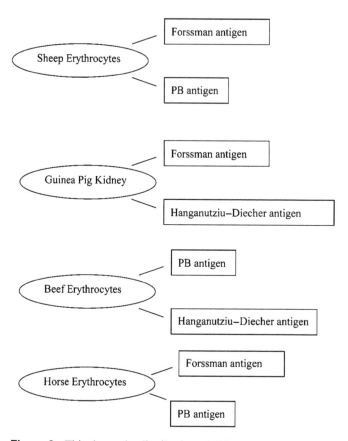

Figure 2 This shows the distribution of different antigens among different types of cells used in detection of red cell agglutinating heterophile antibodies.

absorbs Forssman and H-D antibodies. The serum samples are centrifuged and the supernatants are tested with sheep red cells. If the sheep cells agglutinate, then PB heterophile antibodies are present. Duplicate aliquots are treated with beef erythrocytes. Because beef erythrocytes absorb PB heterophile antibodies, the ability of the heterophile-positive sera to agglutinate sheep red cells is abolished, thus confirming the specificity of the finding.

Current Tests for Heterophile Antibodies

Current tests with high sensitivity for IM-specific heterophile antibodies include latex agglutination slide tests, in which the IM-specific heterophile antigen (PB antigen) is obtained from bovine red cell membranes. This antigen is coated onto latex particles, which are mixed with the patient's serum (or plasma) that is to be tested. A positive test is indicated by agglutination of the latex particles. Bovine-based material used for screening tests is more sensitive than that obtained from horse, which in turn is more sensitive than that from sheep. Indeed, testing for heterophile antibody (by the Davidsohn differential absorption test) in the sera of children with acute EBV infection (confirmed by specific EBV antibody testing) showed that the use of horse cells gave greater sensitivity than sheep cells. Interestingly, these tests were relatively insensitive in younger children: 83.6% of sera from children aged over four years were positive while for children aged less than four years only 31.8% of the sera were heterophile positive. A rapid slide test was even less sensitive (13).

Tests that use purified or selected sialoglycopeptide with PB activity are more sensitive and specific than whole red cell or stroma-based assays (14). Furthermore, preabsorption with guinea pig kidney to remove nonspecific Forssman and H-D antibodies is not necessary. These tests can be used to semiquantitate the titer of heterophile antibodies by using serial dilutions of the serum that is to be tested (15).

CONVENTIONAL EBV SEROLOGIC TESTS

After an infection by EBV, an immune reaction, both cellular and humoral, develops against EBV antigens. Historically, EBV-specific antibodies have been extensively studied in this disease because detection of antibodies against viral antigens is simpler than lymphocyte proliferation tests. The spectrum of antibodies expressed during particular clinical situations has been defined (9). Specifically, antibodies to several antigens (or antigen complexes) are measured: antibodies to the proteins expressed during lytic viral infection that develop acutely during infection—VCA and EA—and antibodies to proteins expressed during latent viral infection that develop later—Epstein–Barr nuclear antigen (EBNA).

In the original work of Werner and Gertrude Henle (16), total anti-EBV antibodies were detected by indirect immunofluorescence. EB-3 cells (an EBV producer cell line) were smeared onto a glass slide and fixed. Serial dilutions of the serum to be tested were overlaid on the slide, incubated, and then washed off. The slides were then overlaid with fluorescent dye–conjugated antihuman IgG. This would detect any IgG molecules in the test sera that specifically bind to the EBV antigens expressed in the EB-3 cells. After washing, the slides were examined under a fluorescent microscope. The highest dilution of the test serum showing fluorescence was defined as the EBV antibody titer. Defined this way, anti-EBV antibody titers varied from 1:40 to 1:640 during the acute illness, and decayed slowly over months to years.

Different groups of antibodies were subsequently characterized based on their immunofluorescent detection in different cell lines. These different antibodies were noted to occur at different times of infection (with blood samples obtained serially from patients recruited in the original studies of IM), as defined by immunostaining of particular cell lines in vitro. Thus, three types of antigen were defined using indirect immunofluorescence assays (IFAs) (Fig. 3). The antigens are VCA, EA, and EBNA.

EBV VCA IgM and IgG

The VCA consists of several proteins that constitute the structural capsomers of the virus. These are expressed late, after viral DNA replication, in cells undergoing lytic infection. Both IgG- and IgM-specific tests are commonly used for VCA detection. VCA IgG increases rapidly in the acute stage, peaks, and then declines to a steady state level. VCA IgM is present only transiently in the acute stage and disappears within weeks.

Early literature descriptions of VCA reactivity were based on IFAs that measured antigen complexes using producer cell lines such as EB-3 or HR-1, which undergo lytic infection (and therefore express VCA, a lytic antigen complex). Unfortunately, the fluorescence-based tests are technically demanding and require highly trained personnel for interpretation, not easily standardized, and not amenable to large volume testing.

Indirect Immunofluorescence Assay—VCA, EA antibody Assay

—Starts with standard cell line expressing the appropriate
 EBV antigen = △

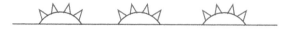

—Add serial dilutions of test (patient) serum, containing the
 appropriate antibodies. ⤙

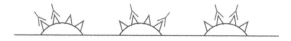

—Incubate and wash off.

—Add antihuman IgG conjugated globulin ⤙ to fluorescent
 dye ○∗ (usually obtained from appropriately prepared animal)

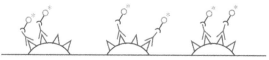

—View under fluorescent microscope.

Figure 3 Steps in the procedure for an indirect immunofluorescence assay for the detection of EBV-specific antibodies to VCA and EA in test serum. The antigen can be VCA or EA. See text. *Abbreviations*: EBV, Epstein–Barr virus; EA, early antigen; VCA, viral capsid antigen.

Newer enzyme-linked immunosorbent assays (ELISAs) that use viral lysate proteins, recombinant proteins, or synthetic peptides are now available, but are not directly comparable with fluorescent antigen complexes. The major antigens in the VCA complex are p150 (BcLF1), p18 (BFRF3), p23 (BLRF2), and the glycoprotein gp110, also known as gp125 (BALF4). In ELISA tests, diluted serum is added to microwells containing antigen (the Wampole Laboratories kit uses BALF4) fixed to a plastic substrate. The wells are washed, and goat antihuman IgM globulin conjugated with horseradish peroxidase is added. This will bind to any test serum IgM that is bound to the antigen in the wells. The wells are washed and a chromogen is added (e.g., tetramethylbenzidine), which turns blue in the presence of horseradish peroxidase. The reaction is allowed to continue for a standard period and is then stopped. The change in optical density of the wells is measured by a spectrophotometer and compared with the positive controls.

Three recombinant proteins are currently available to represent VCA in ELISA: p18, p23, and gp125. Studies of assays using the synthetic peptide VCA p18 have shown 95% correlation with fluorescent IgG tests and 95% correlation with VCA IgM presence in confirmed IM cases. The lack of p18 sequence homologues with other human herpesviruses should limit cross-reactivity.

Serum samples tested using VCA p23 in an immunoblot showed a delay in p23 detection during the early phase of infection (17). An enzyme immunoassay developed using a fusion protein of p18 and p23 has been shown to closely match results of the VCA IFA antigen that are still considered the gold standard by many experts (18). gp125, another capsid antigen, is similar to other herpesvirus proteins and may be more problematic for use in diagnosis because of decreased specificity (19). Tests using smaller fragments of gp125 were found to be insensitive in diagnostic use (18). The development of a VCA IgG p150 commercial assay is unlikely because studies have shown a low sensitivity to the assay in patients with recent or acute EBV infection (20).

The presence of VCA IgM antibodies is used as a marker of recent EBV infection. VCA IgM antibody is usually positive at the time of presentation with IM and persists for only a few weeks. Because most EBV infections occur in childhood and are not associated with IM, it is difficult to determine if the antibody patterns are similar in inapparent versus symptomatic disease. Some studies have shown that testing for antibodies to p18 may be insensitive in early IM, and therefore, may be less suitable for use in an IgM test (19,21). Tranchand-Bunel reports the opposite using a p18-based VCA IgM test that has increased reactivity than the traditional ELISA IgM tests. False positive EBV IgM tests can occur as a heterologous response due to cytomegalovirus infection (22). IgA assays for VCA have utility in nasopharyngeal carcinoma (NPC) where they are used along with EA IgA tests as markers of elevated tumor risk and treatment effectiveness (23,24).

Another approach used to distinguish recent seroconversion from longstanding antibodies is avidity of the antibody. The early antibody response consists of antibodies with low avidity binding to EBV. Over time, the avidity of the antibodies increases. Low avidity antibodies can be determined in both IFA and ELISA tests by the decrease in the strength of the reaction following treatment with a reducing agent such as urea. Along with ELISA, a 50% decrease in optical density post-treatment is an indicator of recent infection (25). On comparing supplementary immunoblot and avidity assays in the testing of problematic sera that could not be classified by the commonly used EBV markers, IgG avidity assays differentiated between acute and past infections, whereas the use of immunoblots alone left some specimens unresolved (26).

EBV EA IgG

EAs are expressed prior to viral DNA replication. These antigens are expressed in nonproducer cell lines (e.g., Raji cells) that have been superinfected with EBV. The infection is abortive and only EAs are synthesized, but not EBV VCA and virions. Originally, anti-EA antibodies were detected by indirect immunofluorescence in which Raji cells were superinfected with EBV several days before titration, smeared onto a glass slide, and fixed. Serial dilutions of the serum to be tested were overlaid on the slides, incubated, and washed off. The slides were then overlaid with fluorescein isothiocyanate–conjugated antihuman globulin, incubated, washed, and examined under fluorescent microscope. The highest dilution yielding fluorescence was read as the titer (Fig. 3) (27). In that study, anti-EA titers were compared with anti-VCA titers that were measured in the same way, except that a producer cell line EB-3 was used. There was no correlation between the titers to VCA and those to EA. The EA titers were generally transitory, with 75% being at levels of 1:5 to 1:320 during the acute illness, and then decreasing from their peak at three to four weeks after illness onset, although they could persist for years. Indeed, 12% of patients had titers of level greater than 1:40 when measured at 40 to 104 months after the initial infection (28).

The EAs that were originally described using fluorescent antibody methodologies were labeled as: diffuse (EA-D), with a nuclear and cytoplasmic distribution, and restricted (EA-R), presenting as cytoplasmic aggregates. In addition, EA-R was methanol sensitive. Anticomplement fluorescent methods and EBV lysate–derived ELISA commonly use the Raji cell line, which is an active producer of EA following exposure to DNA inhibitors.

The active components of EA-D are p54 (BMRF1), p44 (BSMLF1), and p138 (BALF2), which function as DNAase polymerase processivity factor, DNA binding protein homolog, and promiscuous transactivator, respectively. In IM infection, IgG antibodies are produced mostly to EA-D. Antibody to EA-D arises at the onset of IM symptoms and peaks within a few weeks. The p54 recombinant antigen is commonly used in ELISA EA-D IgG kits (29). EA-R IgG is seen in only a small number of patients (10–15%) with acute IM and has been associated with severe disease (30). Using p90 (BORF2) as the recombinant protein representing EA-R, Ginsburg found a good correlation with NPC (20 of 33 serum samples positive), and no correlation with Burkitt lymphoma (BL) (0 of 15) (31). This contrasts with early data from immunofluorescent studies showing high levels of EA-R with BL (32). In an evaluation of 11 EBV kits for IgM, Weber et al. found little clinical relevance for EA IgM (33).

The presence of EA has often been used as an indicator of active infection because it is usually a short-lived antibody. However, EAs are found in low levels in 10% to 20% of the healthy population. In addition, long-term follow-up of patients has shown that EAs may persist for 30 to 104 months, which lessens their use as a sole active infection indicator (28).

Another EA that has diagnostic significance is Z Epstein–Barr replication activator (ZEBRA) (BZLF1), which is also termed as "immediate EA" because it is produced very early in viral replication. ZEBRA is a transactivator that is involved in the activation of EBV from its latent to productive cycle. Recent studies have demonstrated that antibodies to ZEBRA and EA IgA in NPC patients may be more valuable biomarkers than the commonly used VCA IgG and EA IgG assays (34).

EBNA IgG

EBNA was discovered when there was an attempt to localize EBV-associated antigens that induced complement-fixing (CF) antibodies (35). Briefly, indicator cells were smeared and fixed on a glass slide. Serial dilutions of the test serum were applied to the slide, incubated, and washed off. Serum from EBV-negative subjects was obtained and layered on the slide; this served as a source of complement. After incubation, this was washed. Any CF antibody would have bound to the relevant antigen in the indicator cells (Raji cells), and the complement in the EBV-negative serum would have bound to the CF antibody from the test serum. The slides were then overlaid with fluorescent-conjugated antihuman complement antibody, incubated, washed, and examined under a fluorescent microscope (Fig. 4). The antibodies to EBNA were found to occur late in IM; most of them became positive between two and three months after onset, and persisted indefinitely (36).

Multiple EBNAs exist (EBNA-1, EBNA-2, EBNA-3A, EBNA-3B, EBNA-3C, and EBNA-LP). EBNA-1 is the major protein in this group and functionally appears to tether EBV DNA to the host chromosome, as well as plays a vital role in cell transformation. Most antibody response to EBNA in humans is toward EBNA-1 and EBNA-2 (36,37). Antibodies to EBNA-1 increase slowly. Following acute IM,

Indirect Immunofluorescence Assay—EBNA Antibody Assay

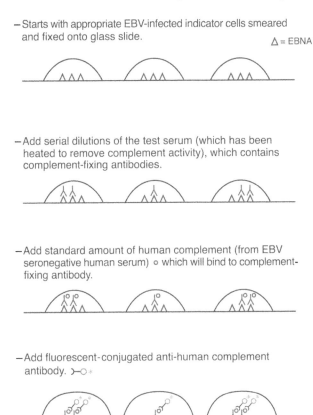

— Starts with appropriate EBV-infected indicator cells smeared
  and fixed onto glass slide.

Δ = EBNA

— Add serial dilutions of the test serum (which has been
  heated to remove complement activity), which contains
  complement-fixing antibodies.

— Add standard amount of human complement (from EBV
  seronegative human serum) ○ which will bind to complement-
  fixing antibody.

— Add fluorescent-conjugated anti-human complement
  antibody. >—○ *

— View under fluorescent microsope.

Figure 4 Steps in the procedure for an indirect immunofluorescence assay for the detection of EBV-specific antibodies to EBNA in test serum. The antigen is EBNA, and is detected by using its property of fixing complement. See text. *Abbreviations*: EBV, Epstein–Barr virus; EBNA, Epstein-Barr nuclear antigen.

most patients do not respond serologically to EBNA until one to two months after acute infection (36). EBNA antibody is long lasting in most individuals. A subpopulation of EBV-infected individuals (5%) do not make EBNA-1 antibody (38). Because the presence of EBNA-1 antibody is commonly used as a marker of past infection, this subpopulation can be misclassified as recently infected. EBNA-2 can be present early in the primary infection in 30% of those studied, thus leading to misclassification when tests that do not discriminate between EBNA-1 and EBNA-2 are used (39). To avoid this problem, EBNA-1 recombinant protein and synthetic peptide ELISA using p72 (BKRF1 corresponds to EBNA-1) are used.

Membrane-Associated Antibodies

Membrane-associated antibodies are formed in response to antigens found in the envelope of the virion. Their location on the surface makes them targets for neutralizing antibodies. The EBV glycoprotein gp350 is the predominant membrane antigen, as well as the attachment protein that binds to CD21. Antibody to gp350 has neutralizing activity and has been used as the antigen in experimental vaccines (40,41). Two other membrane antibodies have been described, gp250 and gp85. Fluorescent tests use unfixed cells that limited antibody reaction to surface components. Diagnostic use of EBV membrane antibodies has little utility at this time.

DETERMINING EBV STATUS BASED ON SEROLOGICAL PANELS

A number of different antibody patterns have been used to determine the stage of EBV infection. For determining acute disease, the factors that are commonly taken into account are the presence of EBV VCA IgM and the absence of antibodies to EBNA-1. Additional markers such as VCA IgA have also proved useful. Reactivation of virus is not clearly defined clinically and is more difficult to establish serologically, and definite criteria have not been established. Newer molecular methods, such as viral load, may be more appropriate. Reactivation may cause significant rises from the VCA IgG steady state level, with higher antibody titers suggestive of increased levels of replication. Because individuals vary in the level of their immune response and baseline levels are rarely available, it has been proposed that geometric mean titers be used as the norm with values 8 to 10 times normal indicating significantly higher titers (32). Very strong reactions on immunoblotting were seen with VCA p23 and/or EA p54 IgG with serological reactivations, which were not seen during primary infections (17). Other early studies have shown that VCA and EA titers at the upper limit of normal do not always correlate with virus levels from throat washing measured by culture transformation (42). High titers may have some role in the determination of reactivation in immunocompetent individuals, but they are probably insensitive in immunocompromised individuals. Polymerase chain reaction (PCR) viral loads, which will be discussed below, may offer the best solution once lower limits of normal are established in various patient populations.

Limitations

Conventional EBV serology has its limitations, the most serious of which may be the unreliability of measurements in immunocompromised patients. Fluorescence-based methods are labor intensive, involve serum titration, and are subjective in reading of the results. Enzyme immunoassays can be automated, objectively read, and standardized with the use of recombinant proteins or synthetic peptides. The available number of EBV proteins that can be selected as antigens is enormous. Commercial products continue to undergo modification and are used widely in clinical diagnostic laboratories.

DETECTION OF EBV BY VIRAL CULTURE

The seminal discovery in 1964 by Epstein et al. of a herpes group virus in BL cells using electron microscopy was the first indication of the cell types favored for growth by EBV (43). By 1967 Pope and associates had shown that lymphoblastoid cell lines (LCL) from the peripheral leukocytes of IM patients could be readily established (44). Similar LCL were shown in the same year to harbor EBV-specific antigens (45).

At about the same time Glade described continuous cell culture suspensions for EBV and bone marrow methods were also developed (46,47). In 1971, Nillson et al. (48) found EBV in the peripheral cells of normal adults without recent IM. In the same paper they described their inability to establish EBV-infected cell lines from fetal tissue unless they were exposed to cell-free extracts from EBV-carrying cell lines. By this time it was clear that EBV transformed lymphocytes and permitted their continuous culture in perpetuity. Because this transformation is not to malignancy, it is termed immortalization.

Cell culture of EBV is performed using the original procedures with minor variations for establishing LCL. The method involves collecting peripheral blood using heparin as an anticoagulant. Leukocytes are separated by dextran solution or other column materials. After washing in buffer, the cells are suspended in Roswell Park Memorial Institute (RPMI) 1640 medium with 20% fetal calf serum at a concentration of 10^6 cells/mL, and placed in cell culture. The cell cultures are examined twice weekly for change. EBV-transformed cells will show clumped cells at the periphery due to loss of cell contact inhibition. Over time, the transformed cells will increase in number, and the mass of cells will increase. These changes occur gradually over a period of two to eight weeks. Cells must have the medium changed at least twice weekly, which is best accomplished by removing half the depleted medium and adding an equal volume of fresh medium. Once a rapid increase in the size of the cell pellet is observed, the cells can be stained with EBV fluorescence to identify EBNA antigen, which predominates in this type of EBV-infected cells (35).

The use of culture methods for diagnosis is compromised by the ability to grow the virus from many seropositive individuals if a large enough inoculum of cells is used. Dilution studies using 10^3 to 10^6 lymphocytes/mL per tube may be used to sort those patients with a higher proportion of infected cells, but viral load studies using PCR are more useful (49).

EBV has been shown to be periodically present in throat washings of a proportion of healthy individuals at any given time (50). Successful culture of EBV from saliva or throat washings requires cord blood lymphocytes as the cell substrate. The addition of fibroblasts or placental cells has been shown to enhance the isolation rate (51). Tissue such as lymph nodes can also be examined for the presence of EBV. The tissue is supported on a moist matrix, such as sterile tea paper on an elevated stainless steel screen, and placed in a petri dish containing RPMI 1640 with 20% fetal calf serum. Within days, the lymphocytes fall to the bottom of the dish. After sufficient cells have accumulated they are transferred to a tube and the culture proceeds in the same manner as with LCL. The long time required to confirm the presence of EBV and the low specificity render these methods impractical for most diagnostic situations.

DETECTION OF EBV GENOME

Viral Load Determination

The most sensitive way of detecting EBV DNA is by PCR; studies of EBV by PCR were initiated soon after its description (52). In these studies, primers from the EBNA-1 gene were used to detect EBV DNA from a variety of specimens including blood from acute IM patients and seropositive controls and from cell lines established from Hodgkin's lymphoma (HL), lymphomas from transplant and AIDS patients, and lymphomas from immunocompetent persons; EBV was not detected in the latter group. Controls consisting of other viruses were negative. No EBV DNA could be amplified from other negative controls. DNA obtained from formalin-fixed specimens of HL (known to contain EBV by Southern blot) embedded in paraffin was also amplified, showing that archival tissues could be successfully tested for EBV.

In another early study, DNA extracted from clotted blood from five patients with IM, 25 transplant patients, 13 healthy controls (11 of whom were seropositive for EBV), and 29 patients with various lymphoproliferative disorders was tested for EBV DNA by amplification using primers to the genes for EBV capsid protein gp220 (*Bam*HI L region) and to EBNA-1 (*Bam*HI K region). The PCR products were detected by two methods: agarose gel electrophoresis with ethidium staining and by Southern blot. EBV was detected in all five IM patients, in no healthy controls, in 11 of the 25 (44%) transplant patients, and in 11 of the 29 (38%) patients with lymphoproliferative disease (LPD). Of the patients with LPD, those with an immunodeficiency-related lymphoproliferation had EBV DNA in the blood, along with one patient with B-cell lymphoma (out of seven), but EBV DNA was found in none of the six other patients with B-cell lymphoma, the seven patients with Hodgkin's disease, or the four patients with T-cell lymphocytic leukemia. It was found that EBV DNA was detected more sensitively with the gp220 primers and with Southern blotting than with gel electrophoresis and ethidium bromide staining (53). In another early study, EBV was detected in mononuclear cells of 17 healthy EBV-seropositive donors by PCR using primers generated from the *Bam*HI W region of the EBV genome. This consists of the repeating unit of the long direct internal repeat IR-1 (see Chapter 2) and is repeated up to 11 times, thus conferring sensitivity to the probe (54). The finding that EBV DNA can be detected in the blood of some EBV-seropositive normal and many EBV-seropositive immunocompromised individuals who are not ill emphasizes the need for quantitative tests to distinguish those individuals with significant EBV disease.

Viral load is determined by quantitative polymerase chain amplification of EBV genomes. The optimal blood component for determining EBV viral load is controversial. Testing may be performed on DNA extracted from either whole blood or from plasma, and the outcome is expressed as genome copies per milliliter of whichever component is being tested. Testing may also be performed on DNA extracted from isolated leukocytes, and the outcome is expressed as genome copies per microgram of leukocyte DNA or as genome copies per 100,000 leukocytes. While differences in specimen type and preparation make it difficult to easily summarize the literature, viral load generally appears to be proportional to the severity of disease regardless of which component is tested. Elevated EBV viral loads may predict EBV-related complications in immunosuppressed patients, especially transplant patients, who are at risk of posttransplant LP. Using primers to the *Bam*HI W region, Yamamoto et al. were able to determine viral loads in plasma of patients with acute IM, EBV-related acute hemophagocytic syndrome, fatal IM, and chronic active EBV (CAEBV) disease (see section "Chronic Active EBV") (55). The sensitivity of their assay was 1000 copies/mL. In acute IM, serial determinations showed mean loads of 6×10^4 copies/mL in the acute phase (less than seven days after onset), 10^4 copies/mL in the second week of illness (8–14 days after onset), and less than 10^3 copies/mL in early convalescence (greater than 15 days after onset of illness in the 6 of the 12 subjects for which data were available). Mean viral loads in other clinical situations were as shown in Table 1.

Different PCR methods have been used and these methods vary in sensitivity. There are no standard primers for detection of EBV DNA and various genes, such as

Table 1 Plasma EBV viral load in various EBV-related diseases

PTS	EBV-related illness	Plasma load (copies/mL)
20	Acute IM	6×10^4
4	Acute EBV-AHS	5×10^5
4	Convalescent EBV AHS	2×10^4
2	Fatal IM	3×10^7
4	CAEBV disease	6×10^4
	Deteriorating CAEBV	10^6

Abbreviations: AHS, associated hemophagocytic syndrome; CAEBV, chronic active Epstein–Barr virus; EBV, Epstein–Barr virus; IM, infectious mononucleosis.

EBNA, VCA-p23 region, the *Bam*HI W segment and BZLF1, and the BNRF1 membrane protein has been targeted with specifically designed primers.

EBV Clonality Assay by Southern Blot Analysis

The detection of EBV in a tissue, particularly a neoplasm, does not necessarily imply that the virus has an important pathogenetic role in the disease. However, if the virus population in the tumor is shown to be monoclonal, the inference is that EBV infection preceded the onset of the neoplastic process. An assay to establish the clonality of the virus in such circumstances was devised by Raab-Traub and Flynn in 1986 (56).

The clonality assay is based on the presence of variable numbers of terminal repeat sequences at the end of each EBV DNA molecule. Assuming that each cell is initially infected with a single EBV genome, a population of cells arising from a single EBV-positive progenitor will each have an exact copy of the original EBV DNA molecule, with the same number of terminal repeats as the original. If the cells in the population have been infected with different strains of EBV, then it is likely that several viral populations, with different numbers of terminal repeats, will be present in the tissue sample. The assay can also detect whether the EBV DNA is present in circular form (latent infection) or linear form (lytic infection).

The procedure is as follows. DNA is extracted from the lesion and digested with *Bam*HI restriction enzyme. This cuts the genome at sequences right next to the terminal repeats. The DNA fragments are separated by electrophoresis through a gel and then transferred to a nylon membrane (or other such solid support). A labeled internal DNA probe is applied to the blot, and the result is visualized by standard means (Fig. 5). Internal DNA probes include the restriction fragments *Xho*I and *Eco*RI I, which label the EBV genome near the right and left termini, respectively. The molecular weights of the fragments can be obtained as follows. The distance between the *Bam*HI restriction site at the right side of the EBV genome and the first terminal repeat is 4.0 kb. Supposing that the number of terminal repeats at the right end of the genome is TR, each of which has a length of 0.5 kb, then the total length of the fragment generated from the right side of the genome is 4.0 + 0.5 (TR) kb. On the left side of the genome, the distance between the *Bam*HI cut site and the beginning of the terminal repeats is 3.5 kb and if the number of terminal repeats (each of length 0.5 kb) is TR, then the total length of the fragment generated from the right side is 3.5 + 0.5 (TR) kb (Fig. 6). The number of terminal repeats can be

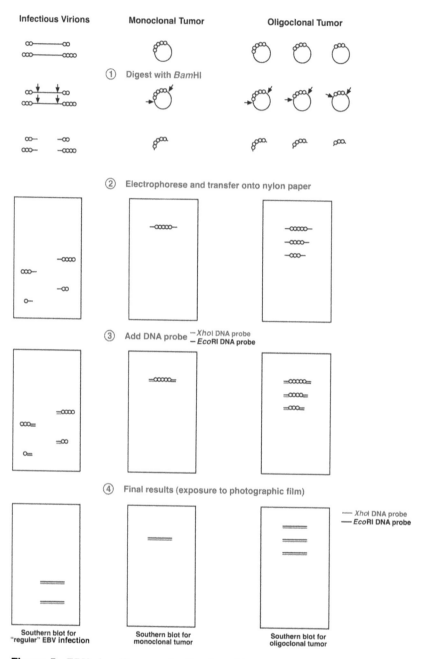

Figure 5 EBV clonality assay by Southern blot. This shows the steps in this procedure in which the clonality of EBV is tested by detecting the number of terminal repeats in the viral DNA. The viral DNA is digested with a restriction enzyme and electrophoresed through a gel. It is then transferred to nylon paper and a DNA probe which anneals to the nucleotide sequences of choice is added. This results in a pattern which can give information about the clonality of the virus in the sample as well as its configuration (linear vs. circular). *Abbreviation*: EBV, Epstein–Barr virus. *Source*: From Ref. 57.

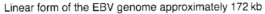

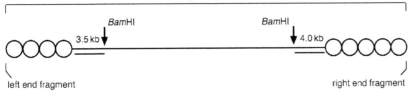

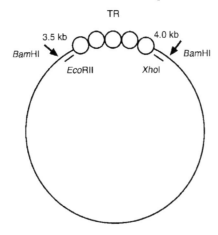

Figure 6 This shows the EBV genome in linear and circular configurations, explicitly showing the terminal repeats and binding sites for the EcoRII and XhoI restriction fragment probes. *Abbreviation*: EBV, Epstein–Barr virus. *Source*: From Ref. 58.

estimated from the results and depending on the number of bands detected, monoclonality can be differentiated from oligoclonality. This assay has been used to demonstrate the monoclonality of EBV in some cases of primary gastric carcinoma in Japanese patients (59).

DIRECT DETECTION OF LATENT EBV INFECTION

Latent EBV infection forms the pathogenetic basis of a number of lymphoproliferative disorders and epithelial neoplasms. Demonstration of EBV presence in neoplastic cells is useful because this confirms EBV involvement in lymphoproliferation and has important diagnostic and therapeutic implications. An example of this cited by Gulley is that the finding of latency-associated EBV antigens in a metastatic carcinoma of unknown primary would direct the search for primary tumor in the nasopharynx, because 75% of NPCs in North America are associated with EBV (57). Furthermore, PTLD involving the liver can resemble recurrent viral hepatitis or acute rejection pathologically, and the demonstration of EBV infection in the infiltrating lymphocytes differentiates between these possibilities. This is an important point because the usual treatment for PTLD is *decreased* immunosuppression (at least initially) while rejection requires *increased* immunosuppression. Stereotactic biopsy of a possible brain lymphoma in an AIDS patient can yield a specimen which is too small to show specific histopathology (lymphoma vs. reactive inflammation), but positive staining for certain EBV nucleic acids would support the diagnosis.

EBV Latency–Associated Antigens by Immunostaining

The latency-associated proteins of EBV include the six members of the EBNA complex, latent membrane protein LMP-1, LMP-2A, and LMP-2B. These are expressed in latently EBV infected cells, which are prevented from proliferating by an intact immune system. Conversely, in EBV-driven LP, many of the cells will stain for these antigens, and this staining can be used to differentiate EBV-driven neoplastic disease from viral-induced inflammation and transplant rejection.

There are three basic patterns of latency that are found in EBV-infected lymphoid cells in different milieux. These patterns (Patterns I, II, and III: see Table 2 of Chapter 2) are found in hosts presenting with decreasing immunocompetence. Thus, Pattern I is found in the infected B-cells in a normal healthy carrier or in BL patients, who are relatively immunocompetent. EBNA-1 is a relatively poorly immunogenic protein (for cell-mediated immunity), and thus is expressed in infected lymphocytes in those patients with intact immune systems. The other patterns are not seen in such patients because cells expressing Patterns II and III are quickly eliminated by competent immune systems. Pattern II is found in those who are moderately immunosuppressed, such as patients with Hodgkin's disease. Finally, Pattern III is found in the most immunosuppressed patients, particularly transplant patients, although it can be found in peripheral blood lymphocytes in acute IM, before the host develops immunity.

It may be noted that all EBV-driven LP lymphocytes express EBNA-1, and at first glance, this would be a reasonable marker to look for. However, EBNA-1 is expressed at a low level, the protein is sensitive to the effects of common fixatives, and reagents to detect it after fixation are not easily available (60). The next most commonly expressed latency protein is LMP-1. While immunostaining for LMP-1 tends to be sparse, if enough microscopic sections are carefully examined, it can be found that most EBV-driven lymphomas stain positive for it and nonlymphomatous inflammatory infiltrates do not (61). However, methods such as in situ hybridization (ISH) and PCR are more sensitive, though technically more demanding. In one study, all methods of EBV detection (EBV RNA, EBV-encoded RNA (EBER) ISH, and LMP immunostaining) were sensitive (all were positive in four cases of PTLD) and specific (all were negative in control sections from patients with acute cellular rejection) (62). Both staining for LMP-1 and EBER ISH are used for detection of latent EBV in lymphoid neoplasms and lymphoproliferations (see Chapter 1).

EBV-Encoded RNA by ISH

In all latent EBV infections, two different EBER species are transcribed but not translated (EBER-1 and EBER-2, together known as "EBERs"). These are short transcripts of unknown function and limited homology to cellular RNA species, and are expressed at very high levels (10^6–10^7 copies per cell) in latently EBV-infected cells making them attractive targets for in situ detection (60). ISH is used to detect EBERs in latently infected cells. Labeled antisense riboprobes can easily be made in vitro, and signal-recorded according to the label that is used (^{3}H, ^{35}S, digoxigenin, biotin, and fluorescein). The hybridization target is robust to various treatments and can be detected in fixed archival tissues and autopsy specimens. EBER ISH has been used to detect latent EBV in samples from PTLD and in gastric carcinomas (59,62).

USE OF EBV DIAGNOSTIC TESTS IN SELECTED CLINICAL CIRCUMSTANCES

Infectious Mononucleosis

A diagnosis of acute IM requires only lymphocytosis with atypical lymphocytes and a positive heterophile test in a patient with a subacute malaise, fever, cervical lymphadenopathy, and sore throat. For a clinical illness compatible with acute IM, but with a negative heterophile test, EBV-specific serologic testing can be used. The most useful test is an assay for EBV VCA IgM, because the presence of these antibodies indicates current or very recent infection. Likewise, for an illness that has prominent atypical lymphocytosis, but unusual clinical features (see Chapter 6), an EBV panel (EBV VCA IgM and IgG, EBV EA IgG, and EBNA IgG titers) may be helpful in documenting an acute simultaneous EBV infection to which the illness may be attributable. EBV-specific serology, especially EBV VCA IgM, is useful in young children in whom heterophile antibody testing may yield false negatives (13).

Posttransplant Lymphoproliferative Disease

EBV viral load testing of blood is useful in predicting PTLD. Liver transplant patients at risk for PTLD were followed with serial determinations of EBV in whole blood by quantitative PCR using primers detecting EBNA-1 gene sequences (63). With this assay, levels were considered significant only when they exceeded 2000 copies/mL, because levels below that could be detected in healthy EBV-seropositive individuals. Patients who developed PTLD had significantly higher viral loads than those who did not. The blood EBV loads overall (from 141 blood samples tested) in six PTLD patients were in the range 2000 to 308,000 copies/mL, while in patients without PTLD the maximum level was 6600 copies/mL. In the PTLD patients, viral loads before PTLD developed were above the cutoff value (2000 copies/mL) in 50 of the 64 (78%) samples, while in the non-PTLD group only 4 of the 117 (3.4%) samples had viral loads above the cutoff value. Similar results have been found by other investigators who performed tests on plasma or on leukocytes. This information has been used in deciding on preemptive therapy with a B-cell depleting monoclonal antibody, rituximab (64).

Burkitt Lymphoma

BL (see Chapters 1 and 10) is a lymphoid neoplasm existing in endemic and sporadic forms. The pathogenesis of the tumor involves one of several chromosomal translocations which dysregulated the c-myc proto-oncogene. The endemic cases of BL occur in Africa and are strongly (and monoclonally) associated with EBV while only about 20% of sporadic BL, in the rest of the world, contain EBV (65).

Patients with endemic BL were found to have higher titers of total anti-EBV antibody than controls matched for age, gender, and geography (32). A large epidemiologic prospective study of a pediatric African population in an endemic area identified high titers of antibodies to VCA, but not EA or EBNA, as risk factors for the development of BL (66). The data on the relation between antibody titers and disease burden is very meager. Titers have been noted to increase just before clinical relapse of BL (32).

Nasopharyngeal Carcinoma

EBV-associated NPC is endemic in Southeast Asia, but uncommon in North America and Europe. The epithelial tumor cells contain EBV in episomal form, and occasionally the EBV DNA is integrated into cellular DNA. Infiltrating lymphocytes do not contain EBV (67).

Serology can be used to help define NPC tumor burden and response to therapy. In patients with EBV-related NPC, serum titers of both IgG and IgA antibodies directed against VCA and EA are considerably increased compared to controls (23,68). In normal subjects, serum IgA antibodies to EBV antigens are rare and present only in low titer (23). The high levels of IgA antibody to VCA and EA that are seen in NPC patients are not seen in patients with other cancers of the head and neck (68). The antibody titers are proportional to the tumor burden, and decrease with successful therapy of the tumor (29). Persistent high titers indicate residual or relapsing tumor.

Serological methods can be predictive for the development of NPC in populations at risk of the disease. Recently, it was shown that the presence of EBV VCA IgA antibodies and neutralizing antibodies to EBV DNAase are highly predictive for the development of NPC in Taiwanese men, with a relative risk of four in those subjects positive for one marker and 33 in those with both markers (69).

Detection of cell-free EBV DNA by PCR in serum has also been used to define the extent of NPC and its response to therapy (70,71). In a recent study, a 35-cycle PCR technique was used to detect cell-free EBV DNA, and compared with a 50-cycle method (71). While EBV DNA can be detected in normal controls (positive in 10.7% of subjects with 50 cycles), the probability of detection in NPC is much higher (positive in 75% of patients with 50 cycles). Reduction of tumor burden is accompanied by a decrease in the detection rate of EBV DNA (36.5% of patients with 50 cycles), while local recurrence of NPC and distant metastases were associated with the detection of EBV in 88.9% and 100% of patients, respectively.

Tissue diagnosis is dependent on detection of EBV (most easily and sensitively by PCR) in tumor samples obtained at biopsy of a nasopharyngeal tumor or of cervical lymph nodes in the case of an unknown primary (72,73).

Thus, serologic methods can be used to define those at risk of NPC and to follow the response of the disease to therapy, and may possibly be useful for detection of relapsed disease and distant metastases. The use of PCR methods for EBV detection remains to be validated.

Chronic Active EBV

CAEBV is characterized by a severe, unremitting, IM-like illness possibly encompassing two (and possibly more) pathogenetic entities; in one, T-cells are infected and proliferate, and in the other, natural killer cells are involved (74). This illness can resemble autoimmune diseases such as lupus erythematosus and rheumatoid arthritis, and neoplastic diseases such as leukemia, Hodgkin's disease, or other lymphoid neoplasms (75). This illness can become life threatening, with a mortality rate of 50% in 14 years (74). Some cases evolve into a lymphoproliferative disorder.

Diagnostic criteria have recently been proposed by Okano et al., and are listed in the Table 2 of Chapter 2 (75). EBV viral load in the blood is high in CAEBV patients (55).

EBV Reactivation

EBV reactivation is a term used to describe ill-defined clinical scenarios in which there is an increase in antibody titers to EBV antigens, an increase in viral shedding in saliva or other secretions, or an increase in EBV viral load.

In immunocompetent-seropositive adults, serologic reactivation as defined by an increase in anti-EA antibodies appears to be asymptomatic. In a community survey, Sumaya studied EBV antibody panels in adults (76). In this group of 462 adults, 95% were VCA IgG seropositive, indicating recent or remote infection with EBV. The sera from some of the patients were further tested for VCA IgM (to detect recent infection), EA IgG (to detect serologic response to active lytic infection), EBNA IgG (which is positive in patients infected with EBV in the remote past), and heterophile antibody (to test for acute infection). Twenty patients were seropositive for EA antibodies, which were compared to a matched group of EA-seronegative persons. All of the EA-seropositive subjects had anti-EBNA antibodies, indicating that their primary EBV infection had occurred in the remote past. Most of these subjects had high titers of VCA IgG and were VCA IgM positive. In contrast, the EA-seronegative subjects had lower titers of VCA IgG and none were VCA IgM positive. None of the subjects had heterophile antibodies. Two months before the antibody testing, the EA-seropositive and EA-seronegative subjects had similar rates of mild, nonspecific illnesses. Thus purely serologic reactivation does not necessarily appear to correlate with disease, although it is possible that it may be associated with a minor illness. Thus, in a small series of cases of recurrent tonsillitis, EA reactivation with no other evident microbial etiology was noted (76).

Reactivation can also be defined by the detection of EBV DNA in the blood by PCR, as discussed above (see Chapter 12) in the context of PTLD. Serial monitoring of viral load in the blood in such patients appears to be useful in detecting those at risk for PTLD.

REFERENCES

1. Evans AS. The history of infectious mononucleosis. Am J Med Sci 1974; 267:198–194.
2. Sprunt T, Evans F. Mononuclear leucocytosis in reaction to acute infections ("infectious mononucleosis"). Bull Johns Hopkins Hosp 1920:410–416.
3. Forssman J. Die Herstellung hochwertiger spezifischer Schafhamolysine ohne Verwendung von Schafblut. Biochem Ztschr 1911; 37:78.
4. Hanganutziu M. Hemagglutinines heterogenetiques apres injection de serum de cheval. C R Soc Biol 1924; 91:1457–1459.
5. Deicher H. Uber die Erzeugung heterospezifischer Hamagglutinine durch Injektion artfremden Serums. I. Mitteilung. Ztschr Hyg Infektionskr 1926; 106:561–579.
6. Paul JR, Bunnell WW. The presence of heterophile antibodies in infectious mononucleosis. Am J Med Sci 1932; 183:191–194.
7. Patarca R, Fletcher MA. Structure and pathophysiology of the erythrocyte membrane-associated Paul–Bunnell heterophile antibody determinant in Epstein–Barr virus-associated disease. Crit Rev Oncog 1995; 6:305–326.
8. Smadel J. Scrub typhus. In: Rivers T, Horsfall FJ, eds. Viral and Rickettsial Infections of Man. PhiladelphiaJB Lippincott, 1959:869–879.
9. Henle W, Henle GE, Horwitz CA. Epstein–Barr virus specific diagnostic tests in infectious mononucleosis. Hum Pathol 1974; 5(5):551–565.

10. Tamura T, Kano K, Milgrom F. Studies on Paul–Bunnell (PB) antigen-antibody system. V. Immunoglobulin classes of P-B antibodies. Diagn Immunol 1984; 2:191–196.
11. Duverlie G, Driencourt M, Rouseel C, Orfila J. Heterophile IgM, IgA, and IgE antibodies in infectious mononucleosis. J Med Virol 1989; 28:38–41.
12. Davidsohn I. Serologic diagnosis of infectious mononucleosis. J Am Med Assoc 1937; 108:289–295.
13. Sumaya CV, Ench Y. Epstein–Barr virus infectious mononucleosis in children. II. Heterophil antibody and viral-specific responses. Pediatrics 1985; 75:1011–1019.
14. Farhat SE, Finn S, Chua R, et al. Rapid detection of infectious mononucleosis-associated heterophile antibodies by a novel immunochromatographic assay and latex agglutination test. J Clin Microbiol 1993; 31:1597–1600.
15. Elgh F, Linderholm M. Evaluation of six commercially available kits using purified heterophile antigen for the rapid diagnosis of infectious mononucleosis compared with Epstein–Barr virus-specific serology. Clin Diagn Virol 1996; 7:17–21.
16. Niederman J, McCollum RW, Henle G, Henle W. Infectious mononucleosis. Clinical manifestations in relation to EB virus antibodies. JAMA 1968; 203:139–142.
17. Buisson M, Fleurent B, Mak M, et al. Novel immunoblot assay using four recombinant antigens for diagnosis of Epstein–Barr virus primary infection and reactivation. J Clin Microbiol 1999; 37:2709–2714.
18. Hinderer W, Lang D, Rothe M, Vornhagen R, Sonneborn HH, Wolf H. Serodiagnosis of Epstein–Barr virus infection by using recombinant viral capsid antigen fragments and autologous gene fusion. J Clin Microbiol 1999; 37:3239–3244.
19. van Grunsven WM, Spaan WJ, Middeldorp JM. Localization and diagnostic application of immunodominant domains of the BFRF3-encoded Epstein–Barr virus capsid protein. J Infect Dis 1994; 170:13–19.
20. Gorgievski-Hrisoho M, Hinderer W, Nebel-Schickel H, et al. Serodiagnosis of infectious mononucleosis by using recombinant Epstein–Barr virus antigens and enzyme-linked immunosorbent assay technology. J Clin Microbiol 1990; 28:2305–2311.
21. Shedd D, Angeloni A, Niederman J, Miller G. Detection of human serum antibodies to the BFRF3 Epstein–Barr virus capsid component by means of a DNA-binding assay. J Infect Dis 1995; 172:1367–1370.
22. Aalto SM, Linnavuori K, Peltola H, et al. Immunoreactivation of Epstein–Barr virus due to cytomegalovirus primary infection. J Med Virol 1998; 56:186–191.
23. Henle G, Henle W. Epstein–Barr virus-specific IgA serum antibodies as an outstanding feature of nasopharyngeal carcinoma. Int J Cancer 1976; 17:1–7.
24. Zeng Y. Seroepidemiological studies on nasopharyngeal carcinoma in China. Adv Cancer Res 1985; 44:121–138.
25. Gray JJ. Avidity of EBV VCA-specific IgG antibodies: distinction between recent primary infection, past infection and reactivation. J Virol Meth 1995; 52:95–104.
26. Schubert J, Zens W, Weissbrich B. Comparative evaluation of the use of immunoblots and of IgG avidity assays as confirmatory tests for the diagnosis of acute EBV infections. J Clin Virol 1998; 11:161–172.
27. Henle W, Henle G, Niederman JC, Klemola E, Haltia K. Antibodies to early antigens induced by Epstein–Barr virus in infectious mononucleosis. J Infect Dis 1971; 124:58–67.
28. Horwitz C, Henle W, Henle G, Rudnick H, Latts E. Long term serologic follow-up of patients for Epstein–Barr virus after recovery from infectious mononucleosis. J Infect Dis 1985; 151:1150–1153.
29. Halprin J, Scott AL, Jacobson L, et al. Enzyme-linked immunosorbent assays of antibodies to Epstein–Barr virus nuclear and early antigens in patients with infectious mononucleosis and nasopharyngeal carcinoma. Ann Intern Med 1986; 104:331–337.
30. Ophoven J. Infectious mononucleosis: Part 2. Serological aspects. Lab Med 1979; 10:203–206.
31. Ginsburg M. Antibodies against the large subunit of the EBV-encoded ribonucleotide reductase in patients with nasopharyngeal carcinoma. Int J Cancer 1990; 45:1048–1053.
32. Henle G, Henle W, Clifford P, et al. Antibodies to Epstein–Barr virus in Burkitt's lymphoma and control groups. J Nat Cancer Inst 1969; 43:1147–1157.

33. Weber B, Brunner M, Preiser W, Doerr HW. Evaluation of 11 enzyme immunoassays for the detection of immunoglobulin M antibodies to Epstein–Barr virus. J Virol Methods 1996; 57:87–93.

34. Dardari R, Hinderer W, Lang D, et al. Antibody response to recombinant Epstein–Barr virus antigens in nasopharyngeal carcinoma patients: complementary test of ZEBRA protein and early antigens p54 and p138. J Clin Microbiol 2001; 39:3164–3170.

35. Reedman B, Klein G. Cellular localization of an Epstein–Barr virus-associated complement-fixing antigen in producer and non-producer lymphoblastoid cell lines. Int J Cancer 1973; 11:499–520.

36. Henle G, Henle W, Horwitz C. Antibodies to Epstein–Barr virus-associated nuclear antigen in infectious mononucleosis. J Infect Dis 1974; 130:231–239.

37. Henle W, Henle G, Andersson J, et al. Antibody responses to Epstein–Barr virus-determined nuclear antigen (EBNA)-1 and EBNA-2 in acute and chronic Epstein–Barr virus infection. Proc Natl Acad Sci USA 1987; 84:570–574.

38. Bauer G. Simplicity through complexity: immunoblot with recombinant antigens as the new gold standard in Epstein–Barr virus serology. Clin Lab 2001; 47:223–230.

39. Schillinger M, Kampmann M, Henninger K, Murray G, Hanselmann I, Bauer G. Variability of humoral immune response to acute Epstein–Barr virus (EBV) infection: evaluation of the significance of serological markers. Med Microbiol Lett 1993; 2:296–303.

40. Jackman WT, Mann KA, Hoffman HJ, Spaete RR. Expression of Epstein–Barr virus gp350 as a single chain glycoprotein for an EBV subunit vaccine. Vaccine 1999; 17:660–668.

41. Jung S, Chung YK, Chang SH, et al. DNA-Mediated immunization of glycoprotein 350 of Epstein–Barr virus induces the effective humoral and cellular immune response against the antigen. Mol Cells 2001; 12:41–49.

42. Yao QY, Rickinson AB, Epstein MA. A re-examination of the Epstein–Barr virus carrier state in healthy seropositive individuals. Int J Cancer 1985; 35:35–42.

43. Epstein MA, Achong BG, Barr YM. Virus particles in cultured lymphoblasts from Burkitt's lymphoma. Lancet 1964:702–703.

44. Pope JH. Establishment of cell lines from peripheral leucocytes in infectious mononucleosis. Nature 1967; 216:810–811.

45. Diehl V, Henle G, Henle W, Kohn G. Demonstration of a herpes group virus in cultures of peripheral blood leucocytes from patients with infectious mononucleosis. J Virol 1968; 2:663–669.

46. Glade PR, Kasel JA, Moses HL, et al. Infectious mononucleosis: continuous suspension culture of peripheral blood leucocytes. Nature 1968; 217:564–565.

47. Benyesh-Melnick M, Phillips CF, Lewis RT, Seidel EH. Studies on acute leukemia and infectious mononucleosis of childhood IV. Continuos propagation of lymphoblastoid cells from spontaneously transformed bone marrow cultures. J Natl Cancer Inst 1968; 40:123–134.

48. Nillson K, Klein G, Henle W, Henle G. The establishment of lymphoblastoid lines from adult and fetal human lymphoid tissue and its dependence on EBV. Int J Cancer 1971; 8:443–450.

49. Fan H, Gulley ML. Molecular methods for detecting Epstein–Barr virus. In: T.N. Killeen AA, ed. Molecular Pathology Protocols. New Jersey: Humana Press, 2001:869–879.

50. Chang R, Golden H. Transformation of human lymphocytes by throat washings from infectious mononucleosis patients. Nature 1971; 234:359–360.

51. Grogan EA, Enders JF, Miller G. Trypsinized placental cell cultures for the propagation of viruses and as "feeder layers." J Virol 1970; 5:406–409.

52. Ambinder R, Lambe BC, Mann RB, et al. Oligonucleotides for polymerase chain reaction amplification and hybridization detection of Epstein–Barr virus DNA in clinical specimens. Mol Cell Probes 1990; 4:397–407.

53. Telenti A, Marshall W, Smith T. Detection of EBV by polymerase chain reaction. J Clin Microbiol 1990; 28:2187–2190.

54. Wagner H, Bein G, Bitsch A, Kirchner H. Detection and quantification of latently infected B lymphocytes in Epstein–Barr virus-seropositive, healthy individuals by polymerase chain reaction. J Clin Microbiol 1992; 30:2826–2829.

55. Yamamoto M, Kimura H, Hironaka T, et al. Detection and quantification of virus DNA in plasma of patients with Epstein–Barr virus-associated diseases. J Clin Microbiol 1995; 33:1765–1768.

56. Raab-Traub N, Flynn K. The structure of the termini of the Epstein–Barr virus as a marker of clonal cell proliferation. Cell 1986; 47:883–889.

57. Gulley ML. Molecular diagnosis of Epstein–Barr virus-related diseases. J Mol Diagn 2001; 3:1–10.

58. Tsuchiya S. Cirt Rev Hematol Oncol 2002; 44:227–238.

59. Imai S, Koizumi S, Sugiura M, et al. Gastric carcinoma: monoclonal epithelial malignant cells expressing Epstein–Barr virus latent infection protein. Proc Natl Acad Sci 1994; 91:9131–9135.

60. Ambinder R, Mann R. Epstein–Barr-encoded RNA in situ hybridization: diagnostic applications. Hum Pathol 1994; 25:602–605.

61. Lones M, Shintaku P, Weiss LM, Thung SN, Nichols WS, Geller SA. Posttransplant lymphoproliferative disorder in liverallograft biopsies: a comparison of three methods for the demonstration of Epstein–Barr virus. Hum Pathol 1997; 28:533–539.

62. Niedobitek G, Mutimer DJ, Williams, N, et al. Epstein–Barr virus infection and malignant lymphomas in liver transplant recipients. Int J Cancer 1997; 73:514–520.

63. Verschuuren EA, Stevens S, Pronk I, et al. Frequent monitoring of Epstein–Barr virus DNA load in unfractionated whole blood is essential for early detection of post-transplant lymphoproliferative disease in high risk patients. Blood 2001; 97:1165–1171.

64. van Esser J, Niesters HG, van der Holt B, et al. Prevention of Epstein–Barr virus lymphoproliferative disease by molecular monitoring and preemptive rituximab in high-risk patients after allogeneic stem cell transplantation. Blood 2002; 99:4364–4369.

65. Magrath I. African Burkitt's lymphoma. History, biology, clinical features and treatment. Amer J Pediat Hematol Oncol 1991; 13:222–246.

66. de-The G, Geser A, Day NE, et al. Epidemiological evidence for causal relationship between Epstein–Barr virus and Burkitt's lymphoma from Ugandan prospective study. Nature 1978; 274:756–761.

67. Spano J, Busson P, Atlan D, et al. Nasopharyngeal carcinomas: an update. Eur J Cancer 2003; 39:2121–2135.

68. Ringborg U, Henle W, Henle G, Ingimarsson S, Silfversward C, Strander H. Epstein–Barr virus-specific serodiagnostic tests in carcinomas of the head and neck. Cancer 1983; 52:1237–1243.

69. Chien Y, Chen JY, Liu MY, et al. Serologic markers of Epstein–Barr virus infection and nasopharyngeal carcinoma in Taiwanese men. N Engl J Med 2001; 345:1877–1882.

70. Lo YM. Prognostic implications of pretreatment plasma/serum concentration of Epstein–Barr virus DNA in nasopharyngeal carcinoma. Biomed Pharmacother 2001; 55:362–365.

71. Hsiao JR, Jin YT, Tsai ST. Detection of cell free Epstein–Barr virus DNA in sera from patients with nasopharyngeal carcinoma. Cancer 2002; 94:723–729.

72. Feinmesser R, Miyazaki I, Cheung R, Freeman JL, Noyek AM, Dosch HM. Diagnosis of nasopharyngeal carcinoma by DNA amplification of tissue obtained by fine needle aspiration. N Engl J Med 1992; 326:17–21.

73. Walter MA, Menarguez-Palanca J, Peiper SC. Epstein–Barr virus detection in neck metastases by polymerase chain reaction. Laryngoscope 1992; 102:481–485.

74. Kimura H, Morishima T, Kanegane H, et al. Prognostic factors for chronic active Epstein–Barr virus infection. J Infect Dis 2003; 187:527–533.

75. Okano M, Matsumoto S, Osato T, Sakiyama Y, Thiele GM, Purtilo DT. Severe chronic active Epstein–Barr virus infection syndrome. Clin Microbiol Rev 1991; 4:129–135.

76. Sumaya CV. Endogenous reactivation of Epstein–Barr virus infections. J Infect Dis 1977; 135:374–379.

77. Veltri RW, Sprinkle PM, McClung JE. Epstein–Barr virus associated with episodes of recurrent tonsillitis. Arch Otolaryngol 1975; 101:552–556.

8

Epstein–Barr Virus and the Nervous System

Alex Tselis and Kumar Rajamani
Department of Neurology, Wayne State University, Detroit, Michigan, U.S.A.

EBV-RELATED NEUROLOGICAL DISEASES

The clinical manifestations of Epstein–Barr virus (EBV) infection depend on factors such as age and state of immunocompetence, and include an astonishing array of multisystemic involvements (see Chapter 6). The neurological manifestations of EBV infection were first noted by Epstein and Dameshek (1), who reported a case of encephalitis, and then by Johansen (2), who reported aseptic meningitis, in patients with acute infectious mononucleosis (IM). Since then, a large number of neurological manifestations of EBV infection that affect both the central nervous system (CNS) and the peripheral nervous system have been documented.

Neurological complications of IM are not rare, and are occasionally the basis for hospitalization of patients with EBV infection. In a series of 109 cases with IM admitted to a London hospital between May 1957 and May 1964, neurological manifestations were seen in eight (7.3%) (3). Of these, five patients had encephalitis, one had meningitis, and two had polyneuropathy and mononeuropathy. In another series of 144 hospitalized IM patients, 5.5% had neurological problems as the prominent or major presentation (4). In a Mayo Clinic series of 1285 cases of IM, 12 had confirmed neurological problems directly attributed to EBV infection (5). In a series of 10 children hospitalized with EBV infection collected from among all infection-related neurologic admissions to the University Hospital Rhine-Westphalia Institute of Technology (RWTH), Aachen, Germany during 1999–2000, two had acute EBV infection with cerebellitis and cranial neuropathies, and one had chronic active EBV infection with lymphomatous cranial neuropathy (6). Seven were described as having "reactivated infections," including three with "Alice-in-Wonderland" syndrome, one with facial nerve palsy, one with progressive macrocephaly, and two with a prolonged encephalitic illness that resulted in prolonged seizures and cognitive deficit. Some of these seven patients had baseline neurologic deficits, with unclear relationship to EBV (6).

Aseptic Meningitis

Aseptic meningitis is a common complication of acute EBV infection, and is probably underappreciated in IM. Headaches are not uncommon in the acute illness, and it is likely that some of these are due to mild aseptic meningitis. One of the first mentions of a neurological complication of EBV infection was the report by Johansen (2) of a case of aseptic meningitis. In a review of the neurological complications of IM, 14 of 34 cases (41%) reported in the literature as of 1950 had associated aseptic meningitis (7). The presentation is similar to that of other causes of aseptic meningitis with headache, fever, and stiff neck, and usually, but not always, occurs in the context of the other common manifestations of IM. The meningitis associated with acute EBV infection is self-limited.

EBV Encephalitis

EBV-associated encephalitis is characterized by fever, headache, confusion, seizures, and paresis, as in the other forms of viral encephalitis. The encephalitis often occurs with other manifestations of clinical IM, but it also has been reported without systemic signs (4,5,8–10). Focal features are often seen, and occasionally EBV encephalitis resembles herpes encephalitis (11). Of the three cases of brainstem encephalitis that have been reported, one recovered completely, another was left with mild residual gait ataxia and nystagmus, and the third died. However, all these cases were diagnosed by serology (12–14). Occasionally, the onset of EBV encephalitis is slow and insidious, and can consist of behavioral and focal neurological deficits (15). A few rare cases of relapsing–remitting disease, satisfying the criteria of multiple sclerosis (MS), following acute EBV infection with neurological manifestations have been described (16). The relation between acute EBV disease and the subsequent MS-like illness is not clear, but recent serological studies have suggested a contributory role of EBV in MS (17).

A broad spectrum of CNS disorders is associated with acute EBV infection. One reported patient developed opsoclonus, myoclonus, and unsteadiness 10 days after a febrile rash and sore throat. The patient had EBV in the cerebrospinal fluid (CSF), which was detected by polymerase chain reaction (PCR), and a serology appropriate for acute EBV infection [high viral capsid antigen (VCA)-immunoglobulin M (IgM) as well as a positive early antigen (EA)]. However, the EBV nuclear antigen (EBNA) antibody titers were not listed, and a negative EBNA antibody would have clinched the issue of it being a primary case of EBV infection. The patient was treated with intravenous methylprednisolone followed by intravenous immunoglobulin for five days. The patient improved gradually, and was able to return to work as a barber five months later and was completely normal at one year (18). Four other cases of EBV-associated opsoclonus–myoclonus were reviewed and the prognosis was generally benign, unlike paraneoplastic opsoclonus–myoclonus syndrome (18).

Reports of pathological findings are scarce because death from EBV encephalitis is rare. Variable findings obtained on pathological examination of the brain have been described, which point to several possible pathogenetic processes including typical viral encephalitis and postinfectious acute disseminated encephalomyelitis. Perivascular infiltrates of lymphocytes as well as diffuse parenchymal infiltrates consisting of both lymphocytes and microglia have been found in the cortex, as is typical with viral encephalitis (19). In one patient, both meningeal and diffuse parenchymal white matter perivascular infiltrates of lymphocytes and lymphoblastoid cells were found, some of which showed mitotic figures reminiscent of neoplasm. Most of these cells were EBV-infected B-cells, but a few T-cells and microglia or macrophages were also found (10). Some patients have had typical histopathological findings of acute disseminated encephalomyelitis with perivenular infiltrates of lymphocytes in the white matter, with lipid-laden macrophages and demyelination (20,21).

The pathologic data suggest several possible pathogeneses, although there appears to be no direct effect of the virus on neural cells. Indeed, as far as is known, EBV does not infect neurons or other specifically neural cells, so that the damage to neural tissue is probably of a "bystander" type, similar to that in HIV dementia. As is known to happen with IM (see Chapter 4), there is systemic infiltration of B-cells in multiple organs, and the brain is likely no exception. A particularly heavy infiltration of infected B-cells and reactive T-cells in the brain might therefore give rise to encephalitis associated with EBV mononucleosis. Indeed, activated CD8 cells [expressing CD45RO and the activation antigens CD29 and human leukocyte antigen (HLA)-DR] were found in the CSF of a patient with EBV-associated meningoencephalitis (22). Similarly an infiltration of the meninges may cause aseptic meningitis (which is seen in EBV mononucleosis) or cranial nerve palsies coinciding with or following the acute febrile illness. It is tempting to speculate that the timing of the insult to neural tissues from the local immune activation resulting from B-cell–T-cell interaction may be variable and so the same basic immunopathologic mechanisms may underlie an acute EBV neurologic manifestation as well as a postinfectious neurologic disease. Furthermore, there are possibilities of molecular mimicry between EBV antigens and myelin that can initiate and possibly sustain an attack on CNS myelin, in the midst of an acute EBV infection (see the discussion of the possible relation of EBV to MS that follows). Thus, "infectious" and "postinfectious" may not be completely distinct from each other, and "parainfectious" may be the best description.

A peculiar case of a fatal EBV-associated acute encephalopathy in an adult was described with pathological findings of scattered neuronal pyknosis, diffuse cortical edema, and visual cortical perivascular edema, but no perivascular infiltrates or microglial nodules (23). These findings are reminiscent of what has been called a "toxic encephalopathy," which is a poorly understood parainfectious process mostly seen in children (24).

Radiographic and Electroencephalographic Findings

The imaging findings reported with EBV encephalitis are nonspecific. In one case, the brain magnetic resonance image (MRI) showed normal parenchyma, but there was leptomeningeal enhancement, particularly in the basal cisterns (9). Abnormal signal in the basal ganglia has also been described (15).

Electroencephalography (EEG) of EBV-associated encephalitis usually shows nonspecific abnormalities, such as focal and diffuse slowing (5). Periodic EEG complexes have been described, reminiscent of those seen in herpes encephalitis (25,26).

CSF Findings

The CSF in EBV encephalitis typically shows variable pleocytosis and normal to mildly increased protein. Occasionally, the atypical lymphocytes characteristic of IM are also seen in the CSF (9,27). The CSF glucose is normal. Oligoclonal bands (OCBs) in the CSF have been reported, and in one case, these appeared about three weeks after the onset of IM (9). Specific antibodies against EBV VCA have been detected in the CSF in a case of EBV encephalitis (28). Similar CSF abnormalities can be seen in other EBV-associated neurologic disease.

EBV has been cultured from CSF of patients with EBV encephalitis, but this is a tedious process with unknown sensitivity for EBV encephalitis (29,30). PCR methods have also been used to identify EBV in CSF. EBV PCR is often positive in primary CNS lymphoma patients with AIDS. PCR of CSF has also been used for patients with EBV encephalitis, although this has not yet been validated as a diagnostic test. EBV detected in the CSF may reflect contamination with EBV-infected lymphocytes rather than reflecting a causal role. However, several cases in which EBV was detected by PCR in the CSF of patients with CNS disease and serologic evidence of acute EBV infection have been reported, including two patients, one with encephalopathic illness (9), and the other with myelitis (31). These cases suggest that the best means to diagnose EBV-associated encephalitis is with an EBV serologic profile that shows acute EBV infection and also EBV PCR–positive in the CSF, supporting CNS involvement. Indeed, in a very informative study of 528 CSF samples from patients with an acute neurologic disease, 39 (7.4%) had EBV DNA in the CSF detectable by PCR (32). The patients were divided into three groups: acute EBV encephalitis, primary CNS lymphoma, which is frequently EBV-driven, especially in immunocompromised patients, and postinfectious complications of acute systemic EBV, which include Guillain–Barré syndrome (GBS), acute transverse myelitis, polyradiculomyelitis, and acute disseminated encephalomyelitis (Table 1). In the patients diagnosed with EBV encephalitis, the viral burden and leukocyte count were both high, while in those with primary CNS lymphoma the viral burden was high but the leukocyte count was low. In the patients with postinfectious complications, the viral load was low, but the CSF leukocyte count was high. This makes sense because EBV encephalitis is an acute infection of the brain with significant viral presence and an inflammatory reaction, while primary CNS lymphoma is a neoplasm without significant inflammation. Postinfectious complications are primarily inflammatory and not particularly driven by EBV. It would not be unreasonable to do a simultaneous PCR for other viruses, such as herpes simplex virus (HSV), to help exclude the possibility of nonspecific viral reactivation.

Cranial Nerve Palsy

The classical cranial nerve palsy associated with EBV infection is facial nerve palsy, or Bell's palsy. In three cases of young adults with IM who were diagnosed serologically, unilateral peripheral facial palsy was noted (33). Bell's palsy in very young children has also been reported in association with IM (34). In several of these patients, facial nerve palsy was the presenting and sole symptom of IM, and the findings of lymphadenopathy and splenomegaly led to blood studies that confirmed the diagnosis. Bell's palsy can be bilateral. In one case, a facial diplegia occurred two weeks after clinical IM with fever, malaise, and cervical lymphadenopathy (35). Bell's palsy can occur with involvement of other cranial nerves. In one patient, clinical IM was followed by left-sided deafness, and then by left-sided Bell's palsy. Examination revealed left

Table 1 Comparison of Relative CSF Pleocytosis and EBV Viral Burden in EBV-Related CNS Diseases

	CSF white cell count	CSF EBV viral load
Acute EBV encephalitis	High	High
Primary CNS lymphoma	Low	High
EBV postinfectious complications	High	Low

Abbreviations: CNS, central nervous system; CSF, cerebrospinal fluid; EBV, Epstein–Barr virus.

facial numbness as well, confirming involvement of the left cranial nerves V, VII, and VIII. Nine months later, the patient had recovered completely (36). Hypoglossal nerve palsy was reported in one patient six days after the onset of a febrile pharyngitis and malaise, with IM diagnosed by a positive heterophile antibody test (37). Other cranial palsies occasionally have been reported to occur with IM.

Optic neuritis has also been reported to occur with EBV infection, with several cases of bilateral optic nerve involvement (38–40). Several of these cases occurred before IM was diagnosed.

Transverse Myelitis

Transverse myelitis is a rare complication of EBV infection. The myelitis may be very rapid in onset. In one case, a young woman had a two-week history of fever, sore throat, and malaise, followed by dysesthesias in the legs thus making them weak (41). Three days later she was unable to walk. Examination showed a spinal sensory level, and upgoing toes. The patient's CSF had a protein of 100 mg/dL and a cell count of 2/μL. CSF viral culture was negative. The heterophile screen was positive, and a blood film showed atypical lymphocytes. She was treated with adrenocorticotropic hormone (ACTH) and prednisone and had a slow, almost complete recovery over six months. In another case, a young woman noted difficulty in voiding, which was followed by paresthesias and weakness in the legs within 24 hours, leading to flaccid paraplegia two days later with a thoracic sensory level. There was no systemic illness. The CSF had an increased protein of 106 mg/dL and pleocytosis of 249 cells/μL. Recent EBV infection was diagnosed by the presence of very high anti-EBV antibody titers in the blood. A slow recovery over several months ensued (42).

Recently, EBV DNA has been detected in the CSF of a patient with EBV-associated myelitis (43). In another case, a young man was diagnosed with IM 10 days before developing a transient tetraparesis. Examination showed a spinal sensory level, a bilateral Babinski sign, and normal gait. Serology was consistent with an acute EBV infection. The CSF showed a minor pleocytosis of 27 cells/μL and a normal protein. EBV was detected in the CSF by PCR, in a higher concentration than in blood or saliva. A month later, there were only mild residua.

Cerebellar Ataxia

Cerebellar ataxia has been reported to occur with EBV infection, although acute varicella-zoster virus infection is the most common cause of acute cerebellar ataxia in children. While cerebellar ataxia has typically been thought to involve children (44,45), it has been reported in both young and older adults (46–48). In most cases, the patients had a systemic illness, which was often mild, before developing gait ataxia and dysarthria. All those patients were found to have atypical lymphocytes in the blood and a positive heterophile screen. Pleocytosis was absent or mild, up to 15 cells/μL, and CSF protein was at most modestly elevated. Recovery was complete within a few weeks. One of the patients who was treated with ACTH improved. Usually remission is permanent, but relapses have been reported. One patient developed scanning speech, ataxic gait, and dysmetria coincident with a positive EBV VCA-IgM that resolved after a course of oral prednisone (49). A year later, these symptoms recurred and then resolved spontaneously after two months. Given the uniformly good prognosis of the neurological complications of EBV infection, it is likely that these patients with cerebellar ataxia would have improved without treatment.

No pathological findings are available to explain the pathogenesis of EBV-associated cerebellar ataxia. It is unknown whether this is a manifestation of a direct viral cerebellitis or a postinfectious demyelination, or whether there is even a clear distinction between the two. Indeed, two cases of documented EBV infection followed by cerebellar ataxia responded to plasmapheresis therapy (50).

Psychiatric Manifestations and the Alice-in-Wonderland Syndrome

Occasionally, EBV infection is complicated by prominent psychiatric symptoms that occur in the course of the illness. One such patient, a 25-year-old married college student, developed aggressive, impulsive, unpredictable, and sexually inappropriate behavior, delusional thinking, and auditory and visual hallucinations during the course of clinical IM, which was diagnosed by a positive heterophile test. Atypical lymphocytes were found in the blood. The patient was fully oriented, and the CSF examination was normal. His clinical picture was thought to resemble an acute schizophrenic episode (51). Two other patients, both teenagers, developed severe depression during acute IM (52). Neither of these patients had any premorbid psychiatric history and both were well adjusted and doing well in school. The depression persisted after the clinical illness resolved but led to suicidal ideation in both. The neurological examination was remarkable for normal cognition in both patients. One of them had minimal left-sided clumsiness and hyperreflexia, and trace bilateral intention tremor. The EEG showed diffuse slowing during the depression in both patients. The depressions resolved in a few months in one case, and in several years in the other. Two other patients with acute depression coincident with IM that required electroconvulsive therapy have been reported (53). The pathogenesis of this depression is unknown.

A very interesting and characteristic neuropsychiatric syndrome has been reported to occur with IM, the so-called Alice-in-Wonderland syndrome in which metamorphopsia (bizarre distortions of spatial sense) occurs, similar to that of migraine. This was first reported in three patients, two teenagers and one nine-year-old boy (54). The syndrome consisted of several anxiety-provoking episodes a day, each lasting up to half an hour, with distortions in the size, shape, and orientation of objects in the environment. These episodes were coincident with or shortly followed acute IM. One of the patients reported bumping into objects while she walked. EEG was normal in one case, and only minor abnormalities were reported in another. Neurologic examination was usually normal. One patient was given a single dose of corticosteroids that caused improvement in the IM but did not affect the metamorphopsia. Another patient who was put on phenytoin did not show any improvement. The metamorphopsia resolved after several weeks in all the patients. In another case, a six-year-old boy had similar intermittent episodes of metamorphopsia beginning several days after the onset of a fever accompanied by sore throat (55). He was noted to have fever, a reddened throat, lymphadenopathy, and hepatosplenomegaly. Neurologic examination was normal. Liver function tests were mildly abnormal and atypical lymphocytes were found in the blood. EBV serology showed acute EBV infection. The metamorphopsia gradually resolved over the next three weeks.

The resemblance of the Alice-in-Wonderland syndrome to hemiplegic migraine is noteworthy. A study of the visual evoked responses in five children with Alice-in-Wonderland syndrome showed high amplitude of the P100-N145 wave complex, when compared to normal controls (56). Another study of children with Alice-in-Wonderland syndrome (in some of whom it was associated with EBV infection), using hexamethylpropylene amine oxime single-photon emission computed tomo-graphy (which measures cerebral perfusion), showed decreased perfusion near the visual tract and visual cortex (57).

Acute Hemiplegia

Acute hemiplegia resembling an acute vascular event has been reported in EBV infection. Hemiplegia of childhood, a recognized clinical entity, often does not have a clear etiology. A few such cases have been associated with acute EBV infection. In one case, a 14-year-old girl had a left-sided hemiplegia that developed over several hours accompanied by right-sided headache, photophobia, and emesis (58). Exami-nation showed left hemiplegia, left-sided numbness, and left hyperreflexia. These resolved over several hours, but recurred later on the same day, and then resolved again. Two days later, she had two seizures accompanied by fever and cervical lym-phadenopathy. CSF examination showed a moderate pleocytosis of 103 cells/μL. Several days later, the patient became confused and ataxic, with diffuse slowing in the EEG. EBV serology was consistent with acute primary EBV infection. She recov-ered completely after three months. In another case, a nine-year-old girl with fever and sore throat developed a right-sided headache, fever, vomiting, and left-sided hemiparesis with left hyperreflexia and left homonymous hemianopsia (59). CSF examination showed 63 cells/μL and brain computed tomography (CT) was normal. EEG showed diffuse slowing. EBV serology was consistent with acute primary EBV infection. The hemiplegia resolved completely over the next few days. A similar case has been reported in an adult (60). A 32-year-old man had fever, sore throat, and headache, and developed left-sided weakness several days later. Examination showed mild left hemiparesis with hyperreflexia as well as fever, lymphadenopathy, and sple-nomegaly. A slide test for heterophile antibodies was positive. A CT scan of the brain was normal. He was given oral dexamethasone, and the hemiparesis resolved over the next 24 hours.

GBS and Other Peripheral Neuropathies

EBV infection can be associated with the GBS, which was first described by Zohman and Silverman (61). Grose and Feorino (62) compared EBV antibody titers of five patients with GBS to those of age-matched controls, and found that the GBS patients had considerably higher titers, which are usually seen with acute IM. Two of the patients had positive heterophile antibodies that indicated acute EBV infec-tion. Both patients had generalized lymphadenopathy, and one had a pleocytosis of 8 cells/μL. While EBV-associated GBS is well documented, it is not a common complication of IM. In a series of 109 hospitalized patients with IM, only one had GBS coincident with fever, headache, lymphadenopathy, and appropriate serology (3). However, GBS as a complication of EBV infection can be fatal. In one fatal case, the patient's illness was characterized by cranial nerve palsies progressing to areflexia and complete flaccid paralysis necessitating intubation after three days. Autopsy showed inflammatory demyelination of both dorsal and ventral roots, as well as the cranial nerves and cauda equina (63).

Several other forms of peripheral nerve involvement have been reported in con-junction with EBV infection. Lumbosacral radiculoplexopathy, with pain and lower extremity weakness, has been reported in five patients (64). In all cases, pain in the gluteal area and the thigh was an early complaint, followed by leg weakness that was severe enough for the patients to require ambulatory assistance, and two patients were wheelchair bound. Electromyography (EMG) showed acute denervation and mild slowing of motor nerve conduction. Serology showed acute EBV infection in all patients. CSF was examined in the five patients and showed mild elevation in protein in three patients and a very mild pleocytosis in two. Two patients received oral prednisone and seemed to improve. All patients recovered completely or nearly completely, and were independently ambulatory several months after onset.

IM has also preceded brachial radiculoplexopathy. In one case, a 19-year-old man developed acute pain in the shoulders about two weeks after developing IM, which was diagnosed by a positive heterophile test (65). Several days later, he was unable to lift his arms above his head, developing atrophy of the shoulder girdle muscles. Electromyography showed bilateral brachial plexopathy. Complete recovery occurred over the next four months. Another patient developed a bilateral brachial plexopathy with pain and weakness of the arms along with unilateral facial nerve palsy, about a week after a febrile pharyngitis with IM diagnosed by a positive heterophile test (66). Two siblings who had an acute EBV infection within weeks of one another developed acute shoulder pain and weakness within 10 days of onset of symptoms (67). One had bilateral shoulder weakness. EMG showed severe axonal loss in both patients. Because of the rapidly progressive weakness, one was treated with intravenous methylprednisolone, without apparent benefit, followed by intravenous immunoglobulin, which appeared to improve both pain and weakness significantly. The other was treated with intravenous acyclovir, which had no effect. She was then treated with intravenous immunoglobulin, which had little immediate effect, but considerable improvement was noted a year later.

Mixed central and peripheral nervous system disease has also been reported with acute EBV infection. Majid et al. (68) described four patients with various combinations of myeloradiculitis, encephalomyeloradiculitis, and meningoencephalomyeloradiculitis showing involvement of multiple parts of the neuraxis simultaneously. The CSF was abnormal in all four patients with elevated protein and mononuclear pleocytosis but normal glucose. Serum and CSF antibodies to EBV were detected, with the diagnosis confirmed in all four patients by the presence of EBV DNA in the CSF and the demonstration of intrathecal synthesis of EBV antibodies, based on serum-to-CSF ratios. None of the patients died, although they were all left with residual leg weakness and two patients with additional sensory changes.

Acute autonomic neuropathy with blurred vision, orthostatic hypotension, constipation, and burning dysesthesias has also been reported in IM (69). Besnard et al. (70) reported a case of a boy with acute pandysautonomia resulting in intestinal pseudo-obstruction. The 13-year-old presented with pharyngitis and acute ileus. Histological examination of the appendix and rectum showed destruction of ganglion cells, and a mononuclear cell infiltrate in the myenteric neural plexus. EBV PCR was positive in the blood as well as the CSF. The virus was demonstrated in the inflammatory cells in the gut, but not in enteric neurons, by in situ hybridization. The authors proposed that the pathogenesis is immune mediated rather than due to direct infection of intestinal cells by EBV.

A very rare form of T-cell lymphoproliferative disease (LPD) has been reported to affect peripheral nerves causing paresthesias and motor weakness of the arms and legs, as well as progressive dilated cardiomyopathy in a young man without any previous history of immune disease (71). He was treated with acyclovir, methylprednisolone, cyclophosphamide, and immunoglobulin, which resulted in improvement of the neuropathy and ejection fraction. At autopsy, multiple organs were found to be infiltrated by monoclonal and polyclonal atypical T-cell populations that were shown to contain EBV. The relationship between this disorder and systemic EBV-driven T-cell lymphomas (see Chapter 13) is unclear. A precedent for such a disease may be the Marek's disease of chickens in which a herpesvirus infects B-cells acutely followed by infection of T-cells, and results in neoplastic transformation and T-cell lymphoma. The neoplastic T-cells characteristically invade and proliferate in peripheral nerves, causing a neurolymphomatosis that may resemble GBS (72).

Neurologic Manifestations of EBV-Driven LPDs

There is a broad distinction to be made between neurological disease associated with or shortly following acute EBV infection, and neurological disease caused by lymphoproliferation that is driven by EBV. In LPD, the neuropathology is related to the lymphoproliferation per se, rather than the EBV infection underlying it. For example, endemic or African Burkitt lymphoma (BL) is well known to affect the nervous system, and is always driven by EBV. However, sporadic BL may also affect the nervous system, though it is not EBV driven. This is also true of posttransplant lymphoproliferations. Although a lymphoma may manifest independent of whether it is EBV driven or not, the presence or absence of EBV may have prognostic and therapeutic implications.

Primary CNS Lymphoma

Primary CNS lymphoma (PCNSL) is a neoplasm of the brain usually seen in the elderly and in immunocompromised persons. With the emergence of HIV and the AIDS epidemic, PCNSL has become much more common, especially in patients with advanced HIV disease. In a series of 20 cases of PCNSL reported in 1986, all but one patient had one or more opportunistic infections or neoplasms such as Kaposi's sarcoma (73). The known oncogenic effects of EBV and its association with systemic lymphomas suggest that the virus may play an important role in this tumor. In fact, the virus is found in all AIDS-associated PCNSLs (74,75), but only in about 50% of systemic lymphomas in HIV patients. In situ hybridization studies have shown that all the neoplastic cells express the latency molecules, EBV encoded RNA (EBER) and latent membrane protein (LMP) which are associated with immortalization of infected lymphocytes. Control tissues from brains of both HIV positive and negative patients with other diagnoses showed no such expression (74). In another study, PCNSL samples from 26 patients with AIDS and 22 HIV-negative patients were tested for EBV by in situ hybridization for EBER and immunostaining for LMP-1. All the cases with AIDS-associated PCNSL were positive for EBV infection, but none from the HIV-negative patients (75). Rare instances of EBV positive PCNSL in HIV-negative patients have been reported (76).

Clinically, PCNSL presents with subacute, progressive mental status changes such as apathy and confusion with a variable combination of focal weakness, seizures, and headaches. The MRI typically shows a deeply situated ring-enhancing lesion (Fig. 1) with a thick rim of enhancement (Fig. 2) and a nodularity of the rim (Fig. 3). Often the lesion is periventricular, and occasionally there is periventricular spread with a lumpy-bumpy appearance (77). In HIV-infected persons, the lesions can strongly resemble those seen in toxoplasmic encephalitis caused by the protozoan *Toxoplasma gondii*. Points of possible differentiation include the presence of multiple, contrast-enhancing lesions in toxoplasmosis, while a single lesion is more suggestive of lymphoma. HIV-infected persons with toxoplasmic encephalitis

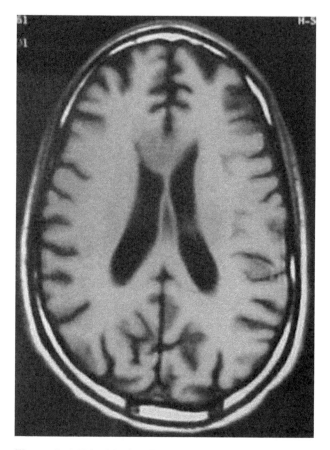

Figure 1 MRI of brain of AIDS patient with primary CNS lymphoma, T1 weighted, non contrast. Note area of decreased intensity in the anterior corpus callosum, medial to the right frontal horn, with perilesional edema. The CSF was positive for EBV DNA by PCR. *Abbreviations*: MRI, magnetic resonance image; EBV DNA, Epstein–Barr virus DNA; PCR, polymerase chain reaction. *Source*: Courtesy of Dr. I. Zak, Division of Neuroradiology, Department of Radiology, Harper University Hospital, Detroit, Michigan, U.S.A.

are usually seropositive for antitoxoplasma IgG antibodies. Seronegative status for antitoxoplasma antibodies makes toxoplasmosis extremely unlikely. Clinical or radiologic deterioration during the first week of therapy, or lack of clinical improvement within weeks to *Toxoplasma* therapy, usually a combination of pyrimethamine plus sulfadiazine plus leucovorin, strongly suggests another diagnosis, with lymphoma becoming more likely. In these circumstances, a biopsy of the lesion is necessary to confirm the diagnosis.

The detection of EBV DNA in the CSF by PCR is very strongly suggestive of PCNSL in HIV-infected patients (78). Recently, thallium-201 single-photon emission CT scans have been used to differentiate between PCNSL and toxoplasmosis (or other ring-enhancing mass lesions). Thallium is a potassium analog that is taken up by tumor, but not inflammatory, cells. Typically, PCNSL "lights up" on thallium scans, but toxoplasmosis or other types of brain abscesses do not (Fig. 4) (77). Biopsy of the lesions typically shows an angiocentric distribution of neoplastic cells (Fig. 5), which stain positively for B-cell markers (Fig. 6) and for latency-associated proteins such as LMP-1 (Fig. 7).

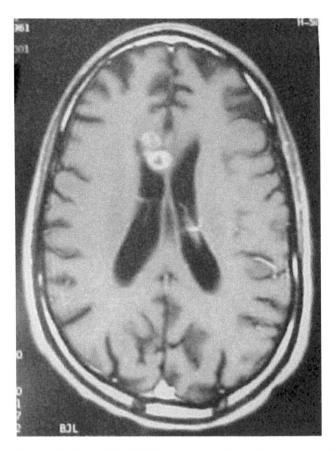

Figure 2 T1 weighted MRI showing contrast enhancement of the lesions shown in Figure 1. Note that two dintinct lesions, one anterolateral and the other posteromedial, are resolved on this image. *Abbreviation*: MRI, mechanical resonance image. *Source*: Courtesy of Dr. I. Zak, Division of Neuroradiology, Department of Radiology, Harper University Hospital, Detroit, Michigan, U.S.A.

The prognosis of PCNSL is poor. In the days before highly active antiretroviral therapy (HAART), the average survival reported for 20 patients with AIDS PCNSL was less than two months (73). Whole brain radiation therapy may increase survival; 10 patients with AIDS who underwent whole brain radiation had a median survival of 5.5 months. Deaths were due to progression of disease and to development of other AIDS-associated complications (79). Cases of significant improvement after treatment with hydroxyurea (80) and HAART (81) have also been reported. One small study demonstrated that decrease in the burden of EBV in the CSF, as measured by quantitative EBV PCR, correlated with clinical improvement (82).

Burkitt Lymphoma

African BL (see Chapter 10) was first described as a "sarcoma" involving the four quadrants of the jaw, but further pathologic studies showed this to be a systemic lymphoma involving multiple viscera, including the nervous system. In early autopsy series, 21 of 25 patients had tumors involving the CNS or the meninges (83). Clinically, paraplegia was the most common manifestation of nervous system involvement,

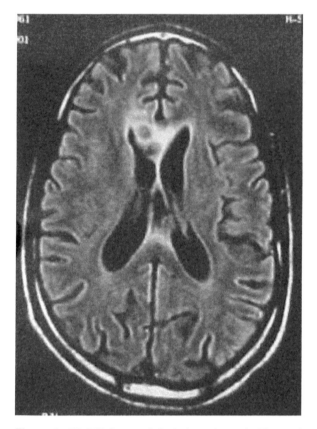

Figure 3 FLAIR image of the lesions shown in Figures 1 and 2. *Abbreviation*: FLAIR, fluid attenuated inversion recovery. *Source*: Courtesy of Dr. I. Zak, Division of Neuroradiology, Department of Radiology, Harper University Hospital, Detroit, Michigan, U.S.A.

affecting 10% to 18% of patients. Intracranial involvement was usually the result of direct extension of maxillary or orbital tumors. Extension usually causes facial or ocular motor palsies, but occasionally visual loss, hearing loss, and dysphagia may result (Fig. 8).

Approximately 25% of patients were found to have neoplastic cells in the CSF on admission (83). Mass lesions forming in the brain manifest, as would be expected, with increased intracranial pressure and altered consciousness (Fig. 9) (83). In a more recent report of BL in 1005 Kenyans, 39% of cases had CNS involvement (84).

X-Linked LPD

X-linked LPDs (XLPDs) (see Chapter 16) occur in males in affected families. Most XLPDs manifest as a systemic illness such as fatal IM and systemic lymphoprolifera-tion, as well as aplastic anemia. Neurologic disease in the context of severe systemic illness is not unknown. In one of the first cases reported, a 16-year-old boy died of ful-minant IM. Autopsy showed extensive lymphoproliferation, with extensive perivascu-lar infiltration of mitotic immature cells with plasmacytoid differentiation in the brain, as well as systemically (85). In one of the original papers describing this disease, autop-sies of several patients who had died of severe systemic illness showed lymphoid

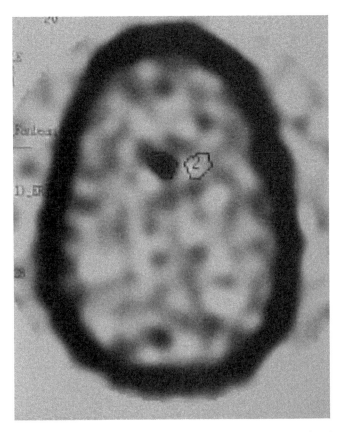

Figure 4 Thallium-201 SPECT image of the lesions seen in Figure 2. There is an increased uptake of the tracer in the locations coinciding with the lesions seen in Figures 1–3. The lesion-to-background ratio of tracer uptake in the posteromedial lesion is 4.9 while that in the anterolateral lesions is 2.1. Any ratio greater than 2.0 suggests malignancy. *Abbreviation*: SPECT, single photon emission computed tomography. *Source*: Courtesy of Dr. Larry Davis, Division of Nuclear Medicine, Department of Radiology, Harper University Hospital, Detroit, Michigan, U.S.A.

proliferation in the brain identical to that present systemically (86). One of the patients had presented with facial twitching and convulsions in the context of a progressive febrile illness with pharyngitis and lymphadenopathy, and occasionally neurologic symptoms occurred during life. There appeared to be no specific neurologic manifestations of XLPD, but these were part of a severe systemic illness affecting all the viscera.

Posttransplant Lymphoproliferative Disease

Posttransplant lymphoproliferative disease (PTLD) is an EBV-driven polyclonal B-cell proliferation seen in patients who were immunosuppressed after solid organ transplants (see Chapter 12). The early form of the disease, beginning between 6 and 12 months posttransplant, presents as a rapidly progressive severe form of IM that can evolve into a sepsis-like syndrome. CNS involvement appears to be uncommon, and is present primarily among patients with very advanced disease (87). However, in a series of 1332 transplant patients examined at the University of Cincinnati

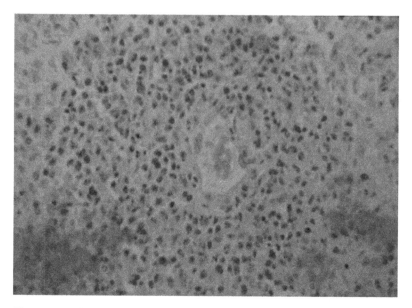

Figure 5 Primary central nervous system lymphoma is an AIDS patient. Biopsy specimen. Note the angiocentric distribution of the neoplastic cells. Hematoxylin and eosin stain. 100×. *Source*: Courtesy of Dr. William Kupsky, Division of Neuropathology, Harper University Hospital, Detroit, Michigan, U.S.A.

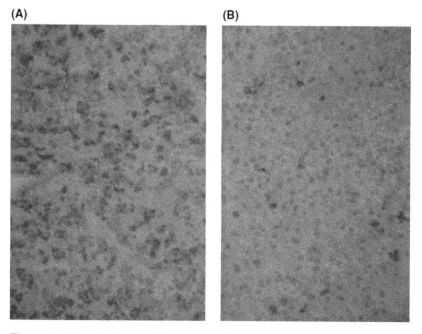

Figure 6 (*See color insert.*) Primary central nervous system lymphoma in an AIDS patient. Same patient as in Figure 5. (**A**) Stained for L26, a B lymphocyte marker. (**B**) Stained for CD3, a T lymphocyte marker. This shows that the neoplastic cells are B lymphocytes, in accord with the known tropism of Epstein–Barr virus. *Source*: Courtesy of Dr. William Kupsky, Division of Neuropathology, Harper University Hospital, Detroit, Michigan, U.S.A.

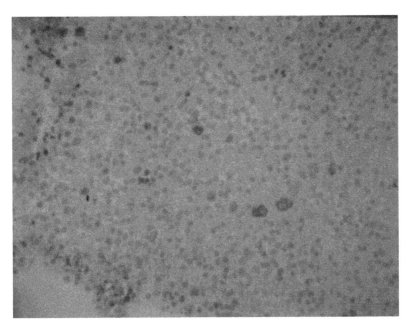

Figure 7 (*See color insert.*) Primary central nervous system lymphoma in an AIDS patient. Same patient as in Figure 6. Immunostained for the EBV-antigen LMP-1, which is a marker of latent infection. Note expression in the cytoplasm of the neoplastic cells. *Source*: Courtesy of Dr. William Kupsky, Division of Neuropathology, Harper University Hospital, Detroit, Michigan, U.S.A.

medical center, 289 (22%) had CNS involvement, but it is not known how many of these were EBV driven (88). In a series of 12 cases of primary CNS PTLD who developed the disease a mean of 31 months after solid organ transplantation, most showed multiple enhancing lesions within the CNS. The pathology of the disease was characterized by perivascular infiltration by large malignant lymphocytes that were positive for CD45 (leukocyte common antigen), CD20 (B-cell marker), and EBV, with light chain restriction or Ig gene rearrangement (89).

Any posttransplant patient with new clinical complaints involving the nervous system is at risk for CNS PTLD. The evaluation should include MRI of the brain, examination of the CSF for EBV by PCR, and probably also biopsy because the sensitivity and specificity of MRI and CSF alone are not known.

Other LPDs

A 14-year-old girl with a febrile illness and multifocal deficits, including ataxia and paraparesis was found to have diffuse areas of increased signal on T2-weighted images in the cerebral and cerebellar hemispheres and brainstem and initially improved with intravenous methylprednisolone (90). She had several relapses and remissions over the next few years. Four years later, a chest X-ray showed changes compatible with interstitial pneumonitis. Six years later, she had disseminated intravascular coagulation and hemophagocytic syndrome, which were treated with cyclophosphamide. A lung biopsy showed changes consistent with lymphomatoid granulomatosis. Her initial EBV titers were compatible with acute EBV infection, with positive EBV VCA IgG and VCA IgM, but negative EBNA antibodies. Later,

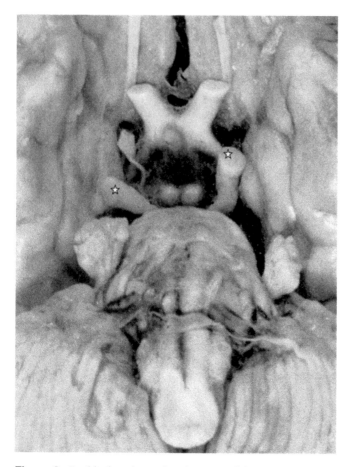

Figure 8 Burkitt lymphoma involvement of the oculomotor nerves (*star*). Note the enlargement of the nerve bilaterally. *Source*: From Ref. 84.

the EBV serology also became positive for EBNA antibodies, with no change in EBV VCA IgG and VCA IgM titers. In some proportion of cases of lymphomatoid granulomatosis in which there is a partly inflammatory and partly neoplastic pathogenetic involvement of multiple organ systems, particularly the lung and brain, atypical lymphocytes are found with staining for EBV antigens (91). Brain MRI in patients with lymphomatoid granulomatosis shows multiple diffusely scattered lesions in the white matter of the cerebral and cerebellar hemispheres with enhancement. These lesions can be distributed in the periventricular region and even be present in the corpus callosum (92). Some patients have appeared to respond to cyclophosphamide (90) and to rituximab (93). Other patients have apparently responded to full chemotherapy and radiation as in the case of lymphoma (90).

TREATMENT

There are no randomized, controlled trials of the use of any antiviral or immunosuppressive drugs for the treatment of neurological complications of EBV. Clearly, supportive care is important. Death due to neurological complications of EBV is uncommon, although residual deficits are not rare. The role of antiviral drugs in

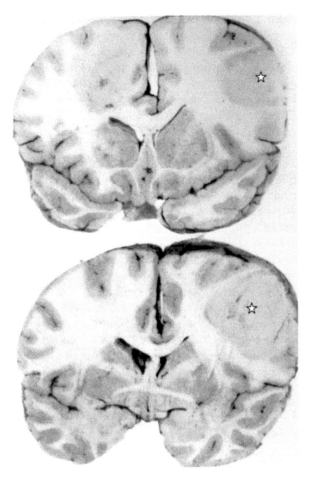

Figure 9 Burkitt lymphoma as a mass lesion (*star*) involving the left parietal lobe of the brain. *Source*: From Ref. 84.

the treatment of uncomplicated or complicated IM is unclear, because the pathogenesis of the disease and the neurological complications are not very clear. A brief discussion follows, with emphasis on neurological aspects of EBV disease; more details may be found in Chapters 6, 12, and 18.

Corticosteroids and acyclovir have been used to treat uncomplicated IM. Studies of the use of acyclovir alone in IM have shown little benefit apart from reduction of viral shedding in the treatment groups, although the studies tend to have small numbers of patients (94). Acyclovir inhibits EBV DNA polymerase in vitro, although viral production returns to control levels after discontinuing the drug, even after 11 months (95,96). Furthermore, while inhibiting viral (lytic) replication in productive infection, acyclovir did not affect latent viral burden, implying that latent virus replicates by host-dependent enzymes (95). The effects of latent virus are probably pathogenetically relevant, and therefore it is no surprise that acyclovir has little overall effect on acute EBV infection. Indeed, a meta-analysis of five randomized controlled clinical trials involving 339 patients found only a nonstatistically significant trend toward clinical improvement, and a significant reduction in viral shedding in the oropharynx (97). The role of ganciclovir, another nucleoside analog, is even less well established. Two cases of EBV encephalitis in transplant patients (one a renal transplant and another a bone marrow transplant), who were diagnosed by a positive EBV PCR in the CSF were treated with ganciclovir and had good clinical recoveries. One patient was given ganciclovir 100 mg intravenously twice a day for four weeks followed by four weeks of oral ganciclovir. The other patient was given ganciclovir 5 mg/kg intravenously for two weeks. Both patients had resolution of CSF and MRI abnormalities (98,99). While these reports are encouraging, the role of the drug in a disease the natural history of which is not completely known is unclear.

The combination of corticosteroids and acyclovir has been examined in one study in which 11 patients with fulminant IM requiring hospitalization were treated with a combination of acyclovir and prednisolone. There was a reduction in viral shedding and oropharyngeal symptoms compared to historical acyclovir and placebo-treated controls (100). In another study, it was demonstrated that acyclovir reduces oral viral shedding, but immortalized B-cells were still readily isolatable from the blood and there was little apparent effect on clinical symptoms (101). These results suggest that the pathogenesis of IM is due not simply to direct infection of B-cells, and that immunopathology plays a role in the pathogenesis of the disease. It is probably reasonable to treat significant EBV infections with acyclovir with the possible addition of prednisone, after a careful consideration of the risks and benefits of the use of these drugs. It must be emphasized, however, that there is no randomized controlled study that shows significant clinical benefit from the use of any drug or regimen in the neurological complications of EBV infection.

For the treatment of LPD which can rarely affect the nervous system, the optimal regimen is unknown. Reduction of immunosuppression can result in regression of disease (102). More recently, immune-based approaches have been explored in preliminary clinical trials (see Chapter 18), in particular the use of EBV-specific cytotoxic T-cells infused intravenously (103). In vitro proliferation of B-cells infected with EBV has been shown to be inhibited by mycophenolate, although there are no reports of its clinical use (104). Other modalities such as monoclonal antibodies, etoposide, and cyclosporine have been tried in individual cases of systemic LPD with apparent benefit (105). Rituximab is a promising therapeutic option for CNS LPD (see Chapters 12 and 18).

RELATION BETWEEN EBV AND MS

MS is an inflammatory demyelinating disease of the CNS. The etiology of MS is multifactorial, and may include infectious and genetic factors. The characteristic geographic distribution, nonfamilial clustering of cases, migration studies, and possible epidemics (e.g., the appearance of MS in the Faroe Islands after British troops were stationed there in World War II) suggest an infectious etiology (106,107). Studies of identical twins show concordance of 30%, which indicates more than simply genetic susceptibility. Finally, infectious demyelination is not unprecedented: progressive multifocal encephalopathy is a viral infection of oligodendrocytes. Recent studies have focused on infectious agents such as measles, herpes simplex virus, varicella-zoster virus, human herpesvirus 6, human T-cell lymphotropic virus (HTLV)-1, and EBV, each of which is recognized to interact strongly with the immune system. A role for EBV in MS was first suggested by Warner and Carp, based on these considerations (108).

Interestingly, several cases of postinfectious demyelinating disease, which would satisfy the criteria for MS following neurologically complicated primary EBV infection, have been described. Bray et al. (16) reported five patients with acute neurological syndromes over a six-year period presenting with laboratory evidence of primary EBV infection. Four of these patients went on to develop relapsing neurological deficits over the next 4 to 12 years and were ultimately diagnosed with MS. The fifth patient had a neurological syndrome akin to acute disseminated encephalomyelitis.

We give here a brief personal survey of the evidence linking EBV to MS. This is intended to convey the flavor of the arguments given, but the whole notion of the etiologic relation between the virus and disease is subtle and nuanced (see Chapter 17). This is well illustrated by a study of pediatric MS patients, in which children with MS were more likely to show evidence of remote EBV infection than controls, suggesting a link, but in which five MS patients had no antibodies to any of EBV VCA, EBNA, or EA (109).

Epidemiologic Evidence for the Role of EBV in MS

MS patients are more likely to have had symptomatic IM than non-MS controls, even if years before the onset of MS. In a case–control study, Marrie et al. (110) found that MS patients had a prior history of symptomatic IM more commonly than controls (odds ratio 5). Operskalski et al. (111) found a higher proportion of prior IM in MS patients (13%) compared to controls (2%). Haahr et al. (112) compared a list of all Danish patients with sera positive for heterophile antibody and matched them with the Danish MS registry. Subjects who were positive for heterophile antibody, which indicates acute IM, were about three times more likely to eventually be listed in the MS registry than those who were negative for heterophile antibody. Lindberg et al. (113) reported similar findings in Swedish patients. The odds ratio for subsequent development of MS in IM cases was 3.7, which was statistically significant when compared to those who did not have IM. Thus, symptomatic IM frequently precedes the onset of MS.

EBV-seropositive status is more common among MS patients than among controls. Several studies show that the frequency and titers of antibodies to EBV are higher among MS patients than among controls (114–117). In an interesting study that compared antibody prevalence and titers in the serum and CSF of MS patients and controls, Sumaya et al. (118) found that these were higher in MS patients than in controls, both in the serum and (in a limited number of subjects) in the CSF. Ascherio and Munch (119), in a meta-analysis, identified 1005 MS cases and 1060 controls who were studied for EBV seropositivity. Less than 1% (8 out of 1005) of the cases were seronegative compared to 10% (103 out of 1060) of controls, with an odds ratio of more than 13. This relationship between EBV seropositivity and MS was affirmed in a study of pediatric MS patients, in which 83% of 30 patients and only 42% of 90 matched controls (all 4–18 years of age), while positivity to control viruses were the same (120).

Higher titers of EBV antibodies in healthy persons appear to be a risk factor for the development of MS in the future. Ascherio et al. (17) found that increased baseline titers of EBNA-2 were significantly predictive of the development of MS among participants in a Nurses' Health Study. High titers of EBNA-1 and EA were found among those who subsequently developed MS, but these trends were not statistically significant. Levin et al. (121) reported a case–control study of U.S. military personnel whose blood samples had been collected every two years between 1988 and

2000. Serum antibody titers to EBV VCA and EBNA were significantly and consistently higher among individuals who later developed MS, when compared to matched controls, and with the risk increasing as the titers increased. Some errors were later noted in this paper, but a reanalysis confirmed the results (122).

Several studies suggest that reactivation of EBV occurs during a relapse of MS. Wandinger et al. (123) followed 19 MS patients serially over a year. Eleven of these patients had active MS disease with relapses or progression, while eight were clinically stable. All the patients with active MS had "EBV reactivation," as defined by either positive EA IgM or EA IgA, positive serum EBV PCR, or either threefold increase in EA IgG or threefold decrease in EBNA IgG, while only half of the stable patients did so.

Biological Evidence

The biological evidence for the involvement of EBV in MS is indirect and conflicting, and often involves some speculation. There are some interesting and suggestive observations regarding the involvement of EBV in MS pathogenesis.

In many MS patients, there is a humoral immune reaction against EBV antigens in the CNS. OCBs develop in the CSF of over 95% of clinically definite MS patients. Such bands are usually seen in viral infections of the brain, such as subacute sclerosing panencephalitis, HIV disease, HTLV-associated myelopathy or tropical spastic paraparesis, and HSV encephalitis, as well as bacterial infections such as neurosyphilis, Lyme neuroborreliosis, and neurotuberculosis. The OCBs are intrathecally synthesized antibodies directed against the offending infective agent. The target of the OCBs associated with MS is not well characterized; however, OCBs in MS have usually been considered as "nonsense antibodies," which are not specifically directed to any particular agent but may be found acting against several agents simultaneously (124,125). Some of these antibodies are directed against EBV antigens. Rand et al. (126,127) showed that the OCBs found in 5 of the 15 MS patients were targeted toward a specific RRPFF sequence found on the EBNA-1 molecule. Because EBNA-1 and myelin basic protein (MBP), a major component of myelin, have sequence homologies in at least two pentapeptide sequences (128), a role for the EBV in the pathogenesis of MS suggests itself. CSF antibodies to EBV EBNA-1 are not the whole story because they are seen only in 30% of MS patients. Because the antibody indices in these patients were extremely high, reminiscent of other viral CNS infections, this suggests an etiologic role of EBV in at least some MS patients (127).

Cell-mediated immunity against myelin antigens is also seen in MS patients. T-cell–mediated immune reactivity is an important aspect of MS pathogenesis (129). T-cell clones specific for myelin antigens are obtained more easily from MS patients than controls (130). There are several lines of evidence suggesting involvement of EBV in this process. The proposed mechanisms are not mutually exclusive, of course.

First, there may be cross-reactivity between EBV and myelin antigens. Epitopes obtained from EBV DNA polymerase expressed during the lytic phase of the virus life cycle can effectively activate MBP-specific T-cell clones, allowing them to cross the blood–brain barrier (131). Sequence homology between several regions of MBP and epitopes on EBV, as well as measles and influenza A and B viruses have also been demonstrated (132). Lang et al. (133) have shown significant structural similarity between a major histocompatibility complex (MHC) class 2 molecule EBV-peptide fragment and another MHC class 2 molecule MBP-peptide fragment. T-cells obtained from an MS patient were highly cross-reactive with the structurally similar areas on the MBP class 2 and the EBV DNA polymerase class 2 complexes, thereby providing evidence of functional as well as structural cross-reactivity. EBV-specific CD4 T-cells may be concentrated in the CSF. In one patient, T-cells cross-recognizing an MBP epitope and an EBV polymerase-peptide epitope were present in the CSF (1:10,000) at a 10-fold higher concentration than in the blood (1:100,000) (134).

Second, EBV may induce synthesis of a myelin antigen in such a manner as to stimulate a cell-mediated response. After infection with EBV, human B-cells express a group of small stress proteins called αB-crystallin, which is normally absent from lymphoid tissue in humans but present in many other species (135). αB-crystallin has previously been shown to be a dominant CNS myelin antigen for T-cells in MS patients (136). This is a potential mechanism whereby a viral infection such as EBV could trigger myelin-directed autoimmunity and may explain why humans, but not other species, develop MS.

It is not likely that EBV directly invades the CNS in patients with MS. Martin et al. (137) from Sweden report on the CSF and serum studies on patients with MS and optic neuritis using nested PCR for detection of viral DNA. They found no evidence of EBV or any other herpesvirus. Morre et al. (138) reported similar negative findings not only in the CSF, but also in active demyelinating lesions obtained from autopsied brain specimens of clinically definite MS patients. They found no evidence of EBV DNA in any of the specimens.

Thus, there is considerable evidence to suggest that MS is an autoimmune disease that may be triggered or accentuated by viruses such as EBV. The epidemiological evidence linking MS to EBV includes the high seropositivity, which is virtually 100% in MS patients. However, EBV probably does not directly infect brain cells to cause MS. It is more likely that any role that EBV plays is a more indirect role in the pathogenesis of MS by way of triggering an aberrant immune response, possibly due to molecular mimicry.

CONCLUSION

EBV plays a role in a spectrum of neurological illnesses, spanning all of the components of the central and peripheral nervous systems. Although uncommon, involvement of EBV in acute and subacute neurological illnesses of unknown nature must always be considered. For acute infectious and parainfectious illnesses, the outlook is generally favorable, but EBV-associated LPDs (e.g., XLPD, PCNSL) present a greater challenge. This is especially true in the era of iatrogenic immunosuppression for cancer chemotherapy and transplantation. The full spectrum of neurological illnesses associated with EBV and their pathogenee still awaits elucidation of their mechanisms.

REFERENCES

1. Epstein S, Dameshek W. Involvement of the central nervous system in a case of glandular fever. N Engl J Med 1931; 205(26):1238–1241.
2. Johansen A. Serous meningitis and infectious mononucleosis. Acta Med Scand 1931; 76:269.
3. Gautier-Smith P. Neurological complications of glandular fever (infectious mononucleosis). Brain 1965; 88:323–334.

4. Silverstein A, Steinberg G, Nathanson M. Nervous system involvement in infectious mononucleosis. The heralding and/or major manifestation. Arch Neurol 1972; 26:353–358.

5. Schnell R, Dyck P, Walter Bowie E, Klass D, Taswell H. Infectious mononucleosis: neurologic and EEG findings. Medicine 1966; 45(1):51–63.

6. Hausler M, Ramaekers V, Doenges M, et al. Neurological complications due to acute and persistent Epstein–Barr virus infection in pediatric patients. J Med Virol 2002; 68:253–263.

7. Bernstein T, Wolfe H. Involvement of the nervous system in infectious mononucleosis. Ann Intern Med 1950; 33:1120–1138.

8. Walsh F, Poser C, Carter S. Infectious mononucleosis encephalitis. Pediatrics 1954; 13:536–543.

9. Tselis A, Duman R, Storch G, Lisak R. Epstein–Barr virus encephalomyelitis diagnosed by polymerase chain reaction: detection of the genome in the CSF. Neurology 1997; 48:1351–1355.

10. Schellinger P, Sommer C, Leithauser F, et al. Epstein–Barr virus meningoencephalitis with a lymphoma-like response in an immunocompetent host. Ann Neurol 1999; 45(5):659–662.

11. Thomson D. Focal encephalitis in infectious mononucleosis simulating herpes simplex encephalitis: case report. Mil Med 1975; 140:188–189.

12. Shian W, Chi C. Fatal brainstem encephalitis caused by Epstein–Barr virus. Pediatr Radiol 1994; 24:596–597.

13. North K, de Silva L, Procopis P. Brain-stem encephalitis caused by Epstein–Barr virus. J Child Neurol 1993; 8:40–42.

14. Angelini L, Bugiani M, Zibordi F, Cinque P, Bizzi A. Brainstem encephalitis resulting from Epstein–Barr virus mimicking an infiltrating tumor in a child. Pediatr Neurol 2000; 22(2):130–132.

15. Caruso J, Tung G, Gascon G, Rogg J, Davis L, Brown W. Persistent preceding focal neurologic deficits in children with Epstein–Barr encephalitis. J Child Neurol 2000; 15:791–796.

16. Bray P, Culp K, McFarlin D, Panitch H, Torkelson R, Schlight J. Demyelinating disease after neurologically complicated primary Epstein–Barr virus infection. Neurology 1992; 42:278–282.

17. Ascherio A, Munger K, Lennette E, et al. Epstein–Barr virus antibodies and risk of multiple sclerosis. A prospective study. JAMA 2001; 286:3083–3088.

18. Verma A, Brozman B. Opsoclonus-myoclonus syndrome following Epstein–Barr virus infection. Neurology 2002; 58:1131–1132.

19. Sworn M, Urich H. Acute encephalitis in infectious mononucleosis. J Pathol 1970; 100:201–205.

20. Ambler M, Stoll J, Tzamaloukas A, Albala M. Focal encephalomyelitis in infectious mononucleosis. A report with pathological description. Ann Intern Med 1971; 75(4):579–583.

21. Paskavitz J, Anderson C, Filley C, Kleinschmidt-DeMasters B, Tyler K. Acute arcuate fiber demyelinating encephalopathy following Epstein–Barr virus infection. Ann Neurol 1995; 38(1):127–131.

22. Lehrnbecker T, Chittka B, Nanan R, et al. Activated T lymphocytes in the cerebrospinal fluid of a patient with Epstein–Barr virus associated meningoencephalitis. Pediatr Infect Dis J 1996; 15:631–633.

23. Bergin J. Fatal encephalopathy in glandular fever. J Neurol Neurosurg Psychiatr 1960; 23:69–73.

24. Tselis A, Lisak R. Acute disseminated encephalomyelitis. In: Antel J, Birnbaum G, Hartung H-P, eds. Clinical Neuroimmunology. London: Blackwell, 1997.

25. Greenberg D, Weinkle D, Aminoff M. Periodic EEG complexes in infectious mononucleosis encephalitis. J Neurol Neurosurg Psychiatr 1982; 45:648–651.

26. Russell J, Fisher M, Zivin J, Sullivan J, Drachman D. Status epilepticus and Epstein–Barr virus encephalopathy. Diagnosis by modern serologic techniques. Arch Neurol 1985; 42:789–792.

27. Hollister L, Houck G, Dunlap W. Infectious mononucleosis of the central nervous system. Demonstration of atypical lymphocytes in the cerebrospinal fluid. Am J Med 1956; 20:643–646.

28. Joncas J, Chicoine L, Thiverge R, Bertrand M. Epstein–Barr virus antibodies in the cerebrospinal fluid. Am J Dis Child 1974; 127:282–285.

29. Halsted C, Chang R. Infectious mononucleosis and encephalitis: recovery of EB virus from spinal fluid. Pediatrics 1979; 64(2):257–258.

30. Schiff J, Schaefer J, Robinson J. Epstein–Barr virus in cerebrospinal fluid during infectious mononucleosis encephalitis. Yale J Bio Med 1982; 55:59–63.

31. Landgren M, Kyllerman M, Bergstrom T, Dotevall L, Ljungstrom L, Ricksten A. Diagnosis of Epstein–Barr virus-induced central nervous system infections by DNA amplification from cerebrospinal fluid. Ann Neurol 1994; 35(5):631–635.

32. Weinberg A, Li S, Palmer M, Tyler K. Quantitative CSF PCR in Epstein–Barr virus infections of the central nervous system. Ann Neurol 2002; 52:543–548.

33. Grose C, Feorino P, Dye L, Rand J. Bell's palsy and infectious mononucleosis. Lancet 1973; 2:231–232.

34. Snyder R. Bell's palsy and infectious mononucleosis. Lancet 1973; 2:917–918.

35. Egan R. Facial diplegia in infectious mononucleosis in the absence of Landry–Guillain–Barre syndrome. N Engl J Med 1960; 262(23):1178–1179.

36. Taylor L, Parsons-Smith G. Infectious mononucleosis, deafness and facial paralysis. J Laryngol Otol 1969; 83:613–616.

37. DeSimone P, Snyder D. Hypoglossal nerve paralysis in infectious mononucleosis. Neurology 1978; 28:844–847.

38. Ashworth J, Motto S. Infectious mononucleosis complicated by papilloretinal edema. N Engl J Med 1947; 237:544–545.

39. Blaustein A, Caccavo A. Infectious mononucleosis complicated by bilateral papilloretinal edema. Arch Ophthalmol 1950; 43:853–856.

40. Bonynge T, Van Hagen K. Severe optic neuritis in infectious mononucleosis. J Am Med Assoc 1952; 145:933–934.

41. Cotton P, Webb-Peploe M. Acute transverse myelitis as a complication of glandular fever. Br Med J 1966; 1:654–655.

42. Grose C, Feorino p. Epstein–Barr virus and transverse myelitis. Lancet 1973; 1:892.

43. Clevenbergh R, Brohee P, Velu T, et al. Infectious mononucleosis complicated by transverse myelitis: detection of the viral genome by polymerase chain reaction in the cerebrospinal fluid. J Neurol 1997; 244:592–594.

44. Bergen D, Grossman H. Acute cerebellar ataxia of childhood associated with infectious mononucleosis. J Pediatr 1975; 87:832–833.

45. Cleary T, Henle W, Pickering L. Acute cerebellar ataxia associated with Epstein–Barr virus infection. J Am Med Assoc 1980; 243:148–149.

46. Bennett D, Peters H. Acute cerebellar syndrome secondary to infectious mononucleosis in a fifty-two year old man. Ann Intern Med 1961; 55(1):147–149.

47. Gilbert J, Culebras A. Cerebellitis in infectious mononucleosis. J Am Med Assoc 1972; 220(5):727.

48. Lascelles R, Johnson P, Longson M, Chiang A. Infectious mononucleosis presenting as acute cerebellar syndrome. Lancet 1973:707–709.

49. Shoji H, Goto Y, Yanase Y, et al. Recurrent cerebellitis. A case report of a possible relationship with Epstein–Barr virus infection. Kurume Med J 1983; 30:23–26.

50. Schmahmann J. Plasmapheresis improves outcome in postinfectious cerebellitis induced by Epstein–Barr virus. Neurology 2004; 62:1443.

51. Raymond R, Williams R. Infectious mononucleosis with psychosis. Report of a case. N Engl J Med 1948; 239(15):542–544.

52. Hendler N, Leahy W. Psychiatric and neurologic sequelae of infectious mononucleosis. Am J Psychiat 1978; 135(7):842–844.
53. White P, Lewis S. Delusional depression after infectious mononucleosis. Br Med J 1987; 295:97–98.
54. Copperman S. "Alice in Wonderland" syndrome as a presenting symptom of infectious mononucleosis in children. Clin Pediatr 1977; 16:143–146.
55. Eshel G, Eyov A, Lahat E, Brauman A. Alice-in-Wonderland syndrome, a manifestation of acute Epstein–Barr virus infection. Pediatr Infect Dis J 1987; 6:68.
56. Lahat E, Berkovitch M, Barr J, Peret G, Barzilai A. Abnormal visual evoked potentials in children in "Alice-in-Wonderland" syndrome due to infectious mononucleosis. J Child Neurol 1999; 14:732–735.
57. Kuo Y, Chiu N, Shen C, et al. Cerebral perfusion in children with Alice-in-Wonderland syndrome. J Child Neurol 1998; 19:105–108.
58. Leavell R, Ray CG, Ferry P, Minnich LL. Unusual acute neurological presentations with Epstein–Barr virus infection. Arch Neurol 1986; 43:186–188.
59. Baker F, Kotchmar G, Foshee W, Sumaya C. Acute hemiplegia of childhood associated with Epstein–Barr virus infection. Pediatr Infect Dis J 1983; 2:136–138.
60. Adamson D, Gordon P. Hemiplegia – a rare complication of acute Epstein–Barr virus (EBV) infection. Scand J Infect Dis 1992; 24:379–380.
61. Zohman B, Silverman E. Infectious mononucleosis and encephalomyelitis. Ann Intern Med 1942; 16:1233–1239.
62. Grose C, Feorino P. Epstein–Barr virus and Guillain–Barre syndrome. Lancet 1972; 2:1285–1287.
63. Davie J, Ceballos R, Little S. Infectious mononucleosis with fatal neuronitis. Arch Neurol 1963; 9:265–272.
64. Sharma K, Sriram S, Fries T, Bevan H, Bradley W. Lumbosacral radiculoplexopathy as a manifestation of Epstein–Barr virus infection. Neurology 1993; 43:2550–2554.
65. Watson P, Ashby P. Brachial plexus neuropathy associated with infectious mononucleosis. Can Med Assoc J 1976; 114:758–759.
66. Mohanaruban K, Fisher D. A combination of cranial and peripheral nerve palsies in infectious mononucleosis. Postgrad Med J 1986; 62:1129–1130.
67. Tsao B, Avery R, Shields R. Neuralgic amyotrophy precipitated by Epstein–Barr virus. Neurology 2004; 62:1234–1235.
68. Majid A, Galetta S, Sweeney C, et al. Epstein–Barr virus with myeloradiculitis and encephalomyeloradiculitis. Brain 2002; 125:159–165.
69. Bennett J, Mahalingam R, Wellish M, Gilden D. Epstein–Barr virus-associated acute autonomic neuropathy. Ann Neurol 1996; 40(3):453–455.
70. Besnard M, Faure C, Fromont-Hankard G, et al. Intestinal pseudoobstruction and acute pandysautonomia associated with Epstein–Barr virus infection. Am J Gastroenterol 2000; 95:280–284.
71. Hauptmann S, Meru N, Schewe C, et al. Fatal T-cell proliferation associated with Epstein–Barr virus infection. Br J Haematol 2001; 112:377–380.
72. Calnek B. Pathogenesis of Marek's disease virus infection. In: Hirai K, ed. Marek's disease. Berlin: Springer Verlag, 2001:25–55.
73. So Y, Beckstead J, Davis R. Primary central nervous system lymphoma in acquired immune deficiency syndrome: a clinical and pathological study. Ann Neurol 1986; 20:566–572.
74. MacMahon E, Glass J, Hayward S, et al. Epstein–Barr virus in AIDS-related primary CNS lymphoma. Lancet 1991; 338:969–973.
75. Larocca L, Capello D, Rinelli A, et al. The molecular and phenotypic profile of primary central nervous system lymphoma identifies distinct categories of the disease and is consistent with histogenetic derivation from germinal center-related B-cells. Blood 1998; 92:1011–1019.

76. Hochberg F, Miller G, Schooley R, Hirsch M, Feorino P, Henle G. Central nervous system lymphoma related to Epstein–Barr virus. N Engl J Med 1983; 309:745–748.

77. Ruiz A, Post M, Bundschu C, Ganz W, Georgiou M. Primary central nervous system lymphoma in patients with AIDS. In: Post M, ed. Neuroimaging of AIDS 1. Philadelphia: WB Saunders, 1997:281–296.

78. Cinque P, Brytting M, Vago L, et al. Epstein–Barr virus DNA in cerebrospinal fluid from patients with AIDS-related primary lymphoma of the central nervous system. Lancet 1993; 342:398–401.

79. Formenti S, Gill P, Lean E, et al. Primary central nervous system lymphoma in AIDS. Results of radiation therapy. Cancer 1989; 63:1101–1107.

80. Slobod K, Taylor G, Sandlund J, Furth P, Helton K, Sixbey J. Epstein–Barr virus targeted therapy for AIDS-related primary lymphoma of the central nervous system. Lancet 2000; 356:1493–1494.

81. McGowan J, Shah S. Long-term remission of AIDS-related primary central nervous system lymphoma associated with highly active antiretroviral therapy. AIDS 1998; 12:952–954.

82. Antinori A, Cingolani A, DeLuca A, et al. Epstein–Barr virus in monitoring the response to therapy of acquired immunodeficiency syndrome-related primary central nervous system lymphoma. Ann Neurol 1999; 5:259–261.

83. Burkitt D. Lesions outside the jaws. In: Burkitt D, Wright D, eds. Burkitt's lymphoma. Edinburgh: E. and S Livingstone, 1970:16–22.

84. Mwanda O. Clinical characteristics of Burkitt's lymphoma seen in Kenyan patients. East Afr Med J 2004; 8(suppl):S78–S89.

85. Bar R, DeLor C, Clausen K, et al. Fatal infectious mononucleosis in a family. N Engl J Med 1974; 290:363–367.

86. Purtilo D, Yang J, Cassel C, et al. X-linked recessive progressive combined variable immunodeficiency (Duncan's disease). Lancet 1975; 1:935–940.

87. Swinnen L. Posttransplant lymphoproliferative disorder. In: Goedert J, ed. Infectious Causes of Cancer. Targets for Intervention. Totowa: Humana Press, 2000.

88. Penn I, Porat G. Central nervous system lymphomas in organ allograft recipients. Transplantation 1995; 59:240–244.

89. Castellano-Sanchez A, Li S, Qian J, Lagoo A, Weir E, Brat D. Primary central nervous system post-transplant lymphoproliferative disorders. Am J Clin Pathol 2004; 121:246–253.

90. Mizuno T, Takanashi Y, Onodera H, et al. A case of lymphomatoid granulomatosis/angiocentric immunoproliferative lesion with long clinical course and diffuse brain involvement. J Neurol Sci 2003; 213:67–76.

91. Taniere P, Thivolet-Bejui F, Vitrey D, et al. Lymphomatoid granulomatosis-a report on four cases: evidence for B phenotype of tumoral cells. Eur Resp J 1998; 12:102–106.

92. Tateishi U, Terai S, Ogata A, et al. MR imaging of the brain in lymphomatoid granulomatosis. Am J Neuroradiol 2001; 22:1283–1290.

93. Zaidi A, Kampalath B, Peltier W, Viesole D. Successful treatment of systemic and central nervous system lymphomatoid granulomatosis with rituximab. Leuk Lymphoma 2004; 45:777–780.

94. Straus S, Cohen J, Tosato G, Meier J. Epstein–Barr virus infection: biology, pathogenesis and management. Ann Intern Med 1993; 18:45–58.

95. Colby B, Shaw J, Elion G, Pagano J. Effect of acyclovir on Epstein–Barr virus DNA replication. J Virol 1980; 34:560–568.

96. Colby B, Shaw J, Datta A, Pagano J. Replication of Epstein–Barr virus DNA in lymphblastoid cells treated for extended periods with acyclovir. Am J Med 1982; 73(1A):77–81.

97. Torre D, Tambini R. Acyclovir for treatment of infectious mononucleosis: a meta-analysis. Scand J Infect Dis 1999; 31:543–547.

98. Dellemijn P, Brandenburg A, Niesters H, van den Bent M, Rothbarth P, Vlasveld L. Successful treatment with ganciclovir of presumed Epstein–Barr meningo-encephalitis following bone marrow transplant. Bone Marrow Transplant 1995; 16:311–312.

99. Garamendi I, Montejo M, Cancelo L, et al. Encephalitis caused by Epstein–Barr virus in a renal transplant recipient. Clin Infect Dis 2002; 34:287–288.
100. Andersson J, Emberg I. Management of Epstein–Barr virus infections. Am J Med 1988; 85(suppl 2A):107–115.
101. Pagano J, Sixbey J, Lin JC. Acyclovir and Epstein–Barr virus infection. J Antimicrob Chemother 1983; 12(suppl B):113–121.
102. Nalesnik M, Makowka L, Starzl T. The diagnosis and treatment of posttransplant lymphoproliferative disorders. Curr Probl Surg 1988; 25:367–472.
103. Papadopoulos E, Ladanyi M, Emanuel D, et al. Infusions of donor leukocytes to treat Epstein–Barr virus-associated lymphoproliferative disorders after allogeneic bone marrow transplantation. N Engl J Med 1994; 330(17):1185–1191.
104. Alfieri C, Allison A, Kieff E. Effect of mycophenolic acid on Epstein–Barr virus infection of human B lymphocytes. Antimicrob Agents Chemother 1994; 38:126–129.
105. Okano M. Epstein–Barr virus in patients with immunodeficiency disorders. Biomed Pharmacother 2001; 55:353–361.
106. Kurtzke J. Epidemiologic evidence for multiple sclerosis as an infection. Clin Microbiol Rev 1993; 6:382–427.
107. Kurtzke J, Hyllested K. Multiple sclerosis in the Faroe Islands: I. Clinical and epidemiological features. Ann Neurol 1979; 5:6–21.
108. Warner H, Carp R. Multiple sclerosis and Epstein–Barr virus. Lancet 1981; 2:1290.
109. Alotaibi S, Kennedy J, Tellier R, Stephens D, Banwell B. Epstein–Barr virus in pediatric multiple sclerosis. JAMA 2004; 291:1875–1879.
110. Marrie R, Wolfson C, Sturkenboom M, et al. Multiple sclerosis and antecedent infections: a case control study. Neurology 2000; 27:2307–2310.
111. Operskalski E, Visscher B, Malmgren R, Detels R. A case-control study of MS. Neurology 1989; 39:825–829.
112. Haahr S, Koch-Henriksen N, Moller-Larsen A, Eriksen L, Andersen H. Increased risk of multiple sclerosis after late Epstein–Barr virus infection. A historical prospective study. Mult Scler 1995; 1(2):73–77.
113. Lindberg C, Andersen O, Vahlne A, Dalton M, Runmarker B. Epidemiological investigation of the association between infectious mononucleosis and multiple sclerosis. Neuroepidemiology 1991; 10:62–65.
114. Sumaya C, Myers L, Ellison G. Epstein–Barr virus antibodies in multiple sclerosis. Arch Neurol 1980; 37:94–96.
115. Bray P, Bloomer L, Salmon V, Bagley M, Larsen P. Epstein–Barr virus infection and antibody synthesis in patients with multiple sclerosis. Arch Neurol 1983; 40:406–408.
116. Larsen P, Bloomer L, Bray P. Epstein–Barr nuclear antigen and viral capsid antigen antibody titers in multiple sclerosis. Neurology 1985; 35:435–438.
117. Myhr K, Riise T, Barrett-Connor E, et al. Altered antibody pattern to Epstein–Barr virus but not to other herpesviruses in multiple sclerosis: a population based case-control study from western Norway. J Neurol Neurosurg Psychiatry 1998; 64:539–542.
118. Sumaya C, Myers L, Ellison G, Ench Y. Increased prevalence and titer of Epstein–Barr virus antibodies in patients with multiple sclerosis. Ann Neurol 1985; 17:371–377.
119. Ascherio A, Munch M. Epstein–Barr virus and multiple sclerosis. Epidemiology 2000; 11:220–224.
120. Banwell B, Al-Otaibi S, Heurter H, Tellier R. Viral studies in pediatric multiple sclerosis. Neurology 2003; 60(suppl 1):A334–A335.
121. Levin L, Munger K, Rubertone M, et al. Multiple sclerosis and Epstein–Barr virus. JAMA 2003; 289:1533–1536.
122. Levin L, Munger K, Rubertone M, et al. Temporal relationship between elevation of Epstein–Barr virus antibody titers and initial onset of neurological symptoms in multiple sclerosis. JAMA 2005; 293:2496–2500.
123. Wandinger K, Jabs W, Siekhaus A, et al. Association between clinical disease activity and Epstein–Barr virus reactivation in MS. Neurology 2000; 55:178–184.

124. Vartdal F, Norrby E. Viral and bacterial antibody responses in multiple sclerosis. Ann Neurol 1980; 8:248–255.

125. Rostrom B, Link H, Laurenzi MA, Kam-Hansen S, Norrby E, Wahren B. Viral antibody activity of oligoclonal and polyclonal immunoglobulins synthesized within the central nervous system in multiple sclerosis. Ann Neurol 1981; 9:569–574.

126. Rand K, Houck H, Denslow N, Heilman K. Molecular approach to find targets for oligoclonal bands in multiple sclerosis. J Neurol Neurosurg Psychiat 1998; 65:48–55.

127. Rand K, Houck H, Denslow N, Heilman K. Epstein–Barr virus nuclear antigen-1 (EBNA-1) associated oligoclonal bands in patients with multiple sclerosis. J Neurol Sci 2000; 173:32–39.

128. Bray P, Luka J, Culp K, Sehlight J. Antibodies against Epstein–Barr nuclear antigen in multiple sclerosis CSF and two pentapeptide sequence between EBNA and myelin basic protein. Neurology 1992; 42:1798–1804.

129. Raine C. Multiple sclerosis: a pivotal role for the T-cell in lesion development. Neuropathol Appl Neurobiol 1991; 17:265–274.

130. Zhang J, Markovic-Plese S, Lacet B, et al. Increased frequency of interleukin 2-responsive T-cells specific for myelin basic protein and proteolipid protein in peripheral blood and cerebrospinal fluid of patients with multiple sclerosis. J Exp Med 1994; 179:973–984.

131. Wucherpfennig K, Strominger J. Molecular mimicry in cell-mediated autoimmunity: viral peptides activate human cell clones specific for myelin basic protein. Cell 1995; 80:695–705.

132. Jahnke U, Fischer EH, Alvord EC Jr. Sequence homology between certain viral proteins and proteins related to encephalomyelitis and neuritis. Science 1985; 229:282–284.

133. Lang H, Jacobsen H, Ikemizu S, et al. A functional and structural basis for TCR cross-reactivity in multiple sclerosis. Nat Immunol 2002; 3:940–943.

134. Holmoy T, Vartdal F. Cerebrospinal fluid T-cells from multiple sclerosis patients recognize autologous Epstein–Barr virus-transformed cells. J Neurovirol 2004; 10:52–56.

135. van Sechel A, Bajramovic J, van Stipdonk M, Persoon-Deen C, Geutskens SB, van Noort JM. EBV-induced expression and HLA-DR restricted presentation by human B-cells of aB-crystallin, a candidate autoantigen in multiple sclerosis. J Immunol 1999; 162:129–135.

136. van Noort J, van Sechel A, Bajramovic J, et al. The small heat-shock protein alpha B-crystallin as candidate autoantigen in multiple sclerosis. Nature 1995; 375:798–801.

137. Martin C, Enbom M, Soderstrom M, et al. Absence of seven human herpesviruses including HHV-6 by polymerase chain reaction in CSF and blood from patients with multiple sclerosis and optic neuritis. Acta Neurol Scand 1997; 95:280–283.

138. Morre S, Van Beck J, De Groot C, et al. Is Epstein–Barr virus present in the CNS of patients with MS? Neurology 2001; 56:692.

9

Epstein–Barr Virus and HIV

Richard F. Ambinder

Department of Oncology, Johns Hopkins School of Medicine, Baltimore, Maryland, U.S.A.

INTRODUCTION

The gammaherpesviruses play a key role in the malignancies that led to the recognition of HIV infection. The occurrence of rare cancers—Kaposi's sarcoma and aggressive B-cell lymphoma—in men who have sex with men and who also developed opportunistic infections attracted attention to the acquired immunodeficiency syndrome (AIDS) and ultimately gave it a definition (1–6). Among the aggressive B-cell lymphomas that were recognized early on as AIDS defining, primary central nervous lymphoma was ultimately recognized to be nearly uniformly associated with Epstein–Barr virus (EBV). Since that time, much has been learned about EBV in HIV-infected patients. EBV is linked with benign and malignant diseases. The associations are often not what might be predicted. This chapter summarizes what is known about EBV and EBV-associated disease in HIV-infected patients (Table 1).

HIV INFECTION, EBV ANTIBODY RESPONSES, AND EBV COPY NUMBER

HIV infection leads to an increase in EBV antibody titers even before HIV seroconversion (7). This increase in titers is distinct from, and does not correlate with, the generalized hypergammaglobulinemia and polyclonal B-cell activation associated with HIV infection. EBV titers also vary independently of titers to cytomegalovirus antigens. With HIV disease progression, titers to viral capsid antigen (VCA) rise and titers to EBV nuclear antigen (EBNA) fall (8). In infants congenitally infected with HIV, antibodies to EBNA2 arise after antibodies to EBNA1 appear and tend to persist; whereas in HIV-uninfected infants, antibodies to EBNA2 often appear before antibodies to EBNA1 (9). In adults, with the initiation of highly active antiretroviral therapy (HAART), antibody levels against EBV antigens rise further, often accompanied by a rise in EBV copy number as measured in peripheral blood mononuclear cells, while antibodies directed against HIV antigens fall (10).

EBV copy number, as measured by limiting dilution spontaneous outgrowth studies or by quantitative polymerase chain reaction, is increased in HIV-infected

Table 1 Epstein–Barr Virus–Associated Diseases in the Setting of HIV Infection

Disease or tumor	AIDS defining condition	% Associated (approx.)	Cells affected	Comparable disease in non-AIDS setting
Oral hairy leukoplakia	No	100	Lingual epithelium	Organ transplant recipients (also EBV associated)
Primary central nervous system lymphoma	Yes	>95	B-cells	Organ transplant recipients (also EBV associated) Nonimmunocompromised (not EBV associated)
Diffuse large B-cell lymphoma	Yes	40–75	B-cells	Organ transplant recipients (also EBV associated) Nonimmunocompromised individuals (not EBV associated)
Immunoblastic B-cell lymphoma	Yes	>75	B-cells	Mainly in immunocompromised populations (also EBV associated)
Hodgkin's lymphoma	No	>90	B lineage	Occurs worldwide but is less commonly associated with EBV in Caucasian nonimmunocompromised populations
Leiomyosarcoma	No	>90	Smooth muscle	Leiomyosarcomas in organ transplant recipients are also associated with EBV Smooth muscle tumors in other populations are not EBV associated

Abbreviation: EBV, Epstein–Barr virus.

patients (11,12). Viral load in whole blood is highest in patients with high immuno-globulin G (IgG) anti-VCA and low IgG anti-EBNA1 titers, perhaps owing to poor control of lytic infection (13). In contrast to the situation with solid organ and bone marrow or hematopoietic stem cell transplant recipients, EBV copy number in per-ipheral blood mononuclear cells does not predict the development of non-Hodgkin's lymphoma in AIDS patients (12). In patients with other cancers such as nasophar-yngeal cancer and EBV-associated nasal lymphoma, viral copy number in serum or plasma has been useful as a marker of clinical disease and prognosis (14,15). In nasopharyngeal carcinoma, evidence has been presented that the viral DNA detected is free DNA that is released from apoptotic tumor cells rather than being packaged in virions (16). The character of DNA detected in HIV patients has not yet been reported, but detection of a combination of circulating virions and viral DNA released from cells undergoing apoptosis would not be surprising.

VIRAL STRAINS IN HIV-INFECTED PATIENTS

Type 1 (or A) EBV infection predominates in most EBV-associated malignancies including nasopharyngeal carcinoma, Hodgkin's lymphoma, and posttransplant lymphoma (17). However, type 2 (or B) infection is detected in tumors, particularly those arising in men who have sex with men and are HIV infected (18). Although initially the increased relative frequency of type 2 virus in AIDS lymphomas was pre-sumed to reflect HIV immunocompromise, study of HIV-infected patients with hemophilia showed that type 2 virus is less common in this population than in men who have sex with HIV positive men (19). Furthermore, the risk of type 2 virus infection in men who have sex with men can be expressed as a function of the num-ber of sexual partners (20). Men with more than 500 partners have greater risk of infection with type 2 virus than men with fewer partners. In this context, it is perhaps worth noting that EBV has been detected in anal swabs, and transmission by anal penetration or oral–anal sexual activities has been suggested (21).

The seroprevalence of Kaposi's sarcoma–associated herpesvirus (KSHV) is much higher among men who have sex with men than in the general population. The incidence of Kaposi's sarcoma is also much higher among men who have sex with men than in other risk groups in North America and Europe (22).

NON-NEOPLASTIC MANIFESTATIONS OF EBV INFECTION IN HIV-INFECTED PATIENTS

Several non-neoplastic manifestations of EBV infection in HIV patients are well recognized (Table 1). Oral hairy leukoplakia affects the lingual epithelium and is characterized by white patches typically occurring along the lateral margins of the tongue and is associated with intense replication of EBV (23). The absence of EBV encoded RNA expression, the frequent presence of intertypic recombinants, and the coexpression of lytic and latent genes in the lesion have attracted particular attention (24–26). Nonetheless, the pathogenesis of oral hairy leukoplakia remains poorly understood. In particular, the possible contributions of immunodeficiency per se versus specific interactions with HIV are essentially unknown. The condition is not often symptomatic, but usually responds to acyclovir or valacyclovir therapy (Table 2) (23). Therapy is suppressive rather than curative and recurrence following discontinuation of therapy is common. Lymphoid interstitial pneumonia is another process that is more common in HIV-infected patients, particularly children, that has also been linked with EBV although the relationship remains ill defined (27).

HIV AND LYMPHOMA

Aggressive B-cell lymphomas occur in all populations of HIV-infected people worldwide (28,29). The HIV-associated lymphomas include Burkitt lymphoma, diffuse large B-cell lymphoma, immunoblastic B-cell lymphoma, primary central nervous system lymphoma, primary effusion lymphoma, plasmablastic lymphoma, and Hodgkin's lymphoma. Primary central nervous system lymphoma occurred with a 3600-fold greater incidence among people with a diagnosis of AIDS than in the general population in the era before effective antiretroviral therapy (30). With the advent of effective antiretroviral therapy, the incidence of many HIV-associated lymphomas and Kaposi's sarcoma has declined (31–35).

Roughly 50% of lymphomas arising in HIV patients are EBV associated (36–39). EBV is present in the tumor cells of virtually all primary central nervous system lymphomas in HIV patients, most immunoblastic lymphomas, some diffuse large B-cell lymphomas, most primary effusion lymphomas, and most Hodgkin's lymphomas. The primary effusion lymphomas also harbor KSHV (40). Curiously, Burkitt lymphomas arising in AIDS patients are less likely to be EBV associated than other B-cell lymphomas (41,42).

Immunocompromise must be an important contributing factor to EBV-driven lymphomagenesis in HIV-infected patients. Primary central nervous system lymphomas typically present in the end stages of AIDS in patients with CD4+ T-cell counts less than $20/\mu L$ (43). In AIDS patients with marked CD4+ T-cell lymphopenia, the EBV-associated lymphoma cells tend to express the full spectrum of EBV latency genes (39,44–46). However, progressive immunocompromise may not be the sole contribution of HIV to lymphomagenesis in EBV-associated tumors. Some EBV-associated lymphomas in HIV patients such as Hodgkin's lymphoma are not associated with marked CD4+ T-cell lymphopenia (38).

Table 2 Epstein–Barr Virus–Targeted Therapies Suggested in HIV Patients

Intervention	Suggested mechanism	Status
Acyclovir, valacyclovir for oral hairy leukoplakia	Effective	Accepted
Acyclovir, ganciclovir for lymphoma prevention	Inhibition of EBV DNA polymerase	Conflicting data
Azidothymidine, interferon, and ganciclovir	Activation of cellular apoptotic pathways in lymphoma	Limited anecdotal data
Hydroxyurea	Disruption of episomal maintenance in lymphoma	Limited anecdotal data
Allo or auto EBV-specific T-cell infusion	Immune-mediated killing	Not yet tested
Azacytidine for EBV lymphoma	Reactivation of lytic or latency genes to increase susceptibility to immune surveillance	Failed in anecdotal report

Those lymphomas that are associated with profound CD4+ T-cell lymphopenia such as primary central nervous system lymphomas are those that have declined most with HAART. Among patients receiving antiretroviral therapy, the highest incidence of lymphoma was reported in those with a poor "immunologic response" to antiviral therapy as measured by CD4+ T-cell count and a poor "viral response" as measured by HIV load (31).

Despite the evidence that immunocompromise contributes to the pathogenesis of AIDS lymphoma, these lymphomas only very rarely regress in response to restoration of immune function and in this regard must be regarded as quite distinct from lymphomas that develop in organ transplant recipients. In patients with AIDS and Kaposi's sarcoma, the paradigm of using organ transplant for restoration of immunity as the first therapeutic intervention (rather than cytotoxic chemotherapy) is appropriate, although it is not appropriate in AIDS lymphoma.

HIV AND OTHER MALIGNANCIES

Leiomyosarcomas have been reported in HIV-infected patients and in organ transplant recipients, mostly but not exclusively in children (see Chapter 15) (47). Plasma cell and related B-cell malignancies may also occur with increased frequency in HIV patients (48). U.S. and Australian registry linkage studies suggest that multiple myeloma is increased in HIV patients (49,50). The U.S. linkage study found an odds ratio in AIDS patients of 2.6-fold, whereas Italian and South African studies involving an AIDS and cancer registry linkage did not find an increased risk of myeloma. Although these malignancies are often EBV associated in immunocompromised populations, they are not so in nonimmunocompromised populations.

Although several very different malignancies are associated with EBV in HIV-infected patients, other EBV malignancies do not seem to occur with increased frequency. Thus nasopharyngeal carcinoma, gastric carcinoma, EBV-associated peripheral T-cell lymphoma, and nasal type natural killer cell lymphomas have not been reported to occur with increased incidence.

EBV DETECTION AND CLINICAL DECISION MAKING

In two instances, EBV detection in HIV patients has specific clinical significance. The first and best studied is the detection of viral DNA in the cerebrospinal fluid of HIV-infected patients with intracranial masses (43,51–53). Many etiologies of such masses have been recognized but the majority are associated with toxoplasmosis—a disease treated with antibacterial antibiotics. A large fraction of the masses that are not caused by toxoplasmosis are primary central nervous system lymphomas, which are treated with radiation therapy or possibly chemotherapy or combined modality therapy. The most widely available imaging techniques, magnetic resonance imaging or computed tomography, do not reliably distinguish among these processes although thallium-201 scanning of the brain may help (see Chapter 8). Thus brain biopsy, typically stereotactic, is often required (43). This is a procedure associated with some morbidity and occasional mortality in AIDS patients, particularly those with primary central nervous system lymphoma. Detection of EBV DNA in the cerebrospinal fluid provides an alternative diagnostic modality. In AIDS patients with primary central nervous system lymphomas, more than 80% will have EBV DNA detectable in the cerebrospinal fluid. In contrast, EBV DNA is almost never found in the cerebrospinal fluid of patients with toxoplasmosis. When viral DNA is detected, its precise origin is not yet entirely clear (Fig. 1). Primary central nervous system lymphomas are typically located deep in brain parenchyma often in close proximity to the ventricles. How often viral DNA detected in cerebrospinal fluid reflects the presence of intact tumor cells (which are rarely detected by cytologic techniques), DNA shed by apoptotic tumor cells or free virions has not been characterized. However, it is clear that with tumor response, viral DNA generally clears from the cerebrospinal fluid.

EBV is usually associated with other lymphomas that spread to the central nervous system in AIDS patients (54). Detection of EBV in the systemic tumor or viral DNA in the cerebrospinal fluid appear to identify patients at high risk for central nervous system involvement and suggest the need for intrathecal prophylaxis with methotrexate or cytosine arabinoside.

PREVENTION OF EBV-ASSOCIATED LYMPHOMA

Several investigators have considered the possibility that antiherpesviral agents might prevent non-Hodgkin's lymphoma. In a retrospective study, HIV patients with lymphoma were matched with control subjects with HIV but without lymphoma (55). Cases were much less likely to have used high-dose acyclovir than the controls did. However, attempts to replicate the findings in a larger and different cohort were unsuccessful (56). Meta-analysis of studies also failed to suggest a protective effect of antiviral therapy (57). Thus, the case for the use of acyclovir or ganciclovir to prevent EBV-associated malignancies remains weak at best.

TREATMENT OF EBV-ASSOCIATED LYMPHOMA

In contrast to the uncertainty with regard to prevention, there is no uncertainty with regard to established malignancy. EBV-associated tumor cell lines and tumors will

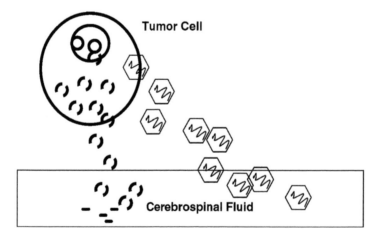

Figure 1 Sources of Epstein–Barr virus DNA detected in cerebrospinal fluid. At least two sources must be considered: virions produced by infected cells and free DNA released from cells. In addition tumor cells may also be present in cerebrospinal fluid in some instances. Free DNA is indicated as fragmented consistent with an origin in apoptotic cells.

proliferate in the presence of acyclovir, ganciclovir, and their congeners. None of these agents is appropriate as an alternative to aggressive cytotoxic chemotherapy.

Therapies that target EBV, such as adoptive cellular immunotherapy, have been extensively studied in the bone marrow transplant setting and studied to a lesser extent in organ transplant recipients (58,59). There has been considerably less work in HIV-infected patients with lymphoma. This in part reflects the difficulties in identifying an appropriate source for EBV-specific T-cell expansion and difficulties in achieving long-term survival of infused cells. Expansion of patient cells is sometimes problematic, perhaps reflecting the ravages of HIV on immune function. Adoptive cellular transfer in the absence of myeloablative chemotherapy to make "space" for the infused cells has also been disappointing.

There have been anecdotal reports of successful therapy with combinations of zidovudine, ganciclovir, and interferon, which may activate cellular apoptotic pathways, as well as with hydroxyurea, which may interfere with episomal maintenance (60–64). A demethylating agent, 5-azacytidine, has also been used in an attempt to reactivate EBV genes silenced by CpG methylation (65). Although target viral genes were demethylated, no clinical response was observed. Reactivation of the repressed thymidine kinase gene by treatment with butyrate followed by ganciclovir therapy has also been proposed (66). Finally, several gene therapy approaches relying on selective expression in EBV-infected cells have been proposed, but have not yet been assessed clinically (67–69).

Monoclonal antibodies now have a well-established role in the management of lymphomas in the general population (70). Studies on rituximab, an antibody directed against the CD20 B-cell antigen, suggest a role for it in the management of a broad spectrum of B-cell lymphomas including EBV-associated lymphomas arising in organ transplant patients (see Chapter 12) (71,72). Rituximab is being actively studied in combination with conventional cytotoxic chemotherapy in AIDS lymphomas. This antibody leads to a depletion of circulating B-cells for approximately six months. There is little or no impact on immunoglobulin levels because long-lived plasma cells that secrete most of the immunoglobulins do not express CD20. Given the evidence that EBV requires a B-cell latency compartment for persistence, there is the possibility that patients at high risk for developing EBV-associated B-cell malignancies might be treated with rituximab as prophylaxis similar to that done in organ transplant recipients (73).

CONCLUSION

EBV-associated problems remain an important issue for HIV-infected patients, particularly EBV-associated malignancies. Most are B lineage malignancies including non-Hodgkin's lymphomas, Hodgkin's lymphoma, and plasma cell–related neoplasms. Their annual incidence has declined in the wake of antiretroviral therapy, particularly those lymphomas associated with profound lymphopenia such as primary central nervous system lymphoma. The impact of HAART on lifetime incidence of EBV-associated malignancies remains uncertain. At present, measurements of EBV antibody titer and EBV copy number in peripheral blood mononuclear cells have not been shown to identify HIV patients at risk for EBV-associated malignancies. However, the possibility remains that monitoring viral copy number in plasma or serum may be useful. Several strategies for specifically targeting EBV-associated tumors in HIV patients have been suggested but none has yet become a standard therapy, nor is there general agreement as to their efficacy in the HIV setting.

ACKNOWLEDGMENTS

Supported by the Johns Hopkins Lymphoma Special Programs of Research Excellence (SPORE) (P50 CA96888) and the AIDS Malignancy Consortium (UO1 CA70062).

REFERENCES

1. Hymes KB, Cheung T, Greene JB, et al. Kaposi's sarcoma in homosexual men—a report of eight cases. Lancet 1981; 2:598–600.
2. Kaposi's sarcoma and pneumocystis pneumonia among homosexual men—New York City and California. Morb Mortal Wkly Rep 1981; 30:305–308.
3. Ziegler JL, Drew WL, Miner RC, et al. Outbreak of Burkitt's-like lymphoma in homosexual men. Lancet 1982; 2:631–633.
4. Diffuse, undifferentiated non-Hodgkin's lymphoma among homosexual males—United States. Morb Mortal Wkly Rep 1982; 31:277–279.
5. Doll DC, List AF. Burkitt's lymphoma in a homosexual. Lancet 1982; 1:1026–1027.
6. Ziegler JL, Beckstead JA, Volberding PA, et al. Non-Hodgkin's lymphoma in 90 homosexual men. Relation to generalized lymphadenopathy and the acquired immunodeficiency syndrome. N Engl J Med 1984; 311:565–570.
7. Rahman MA, Kingsley LA, Breinig MK, et al. Enhanced antibody responses to Epstein–Barr virus in HIV-infected homosexual men. J Infect Dis 1989; 159:472–479.
8. Quesnel A, Pozzetto B, Touraine F, et al. Antibodies to Epstein–Barr virus and cytomegalovirus in relation to CD4 cell number in human immunodeficiency virus 1 infection. J Med Virol 1992; 36:60–64.
9. Pedneault L, Lapointe N, Alfieri C, et al. Antibody responses to two Epstein–Barr virus (EBV) nuclear antigens (EBNA-1 and EBNA-2) during EBV primary infection in children born to mothers infected with human immunodeficiency virus. Clin Infect Dis 1996; 23:806–808.
10. O'Sullivan CE, Peng R, Cole KS, et al. Epstein–Barr virus and human immunodeficiency virus serological responses and viral burdens in HIV-infected patients treated with HAART. J Med Virol 2002; 67:320–326.
11. Birx DL, Redfield RR, Tosato G. Defective regulation of Epstein–Barr virus infection in patients with acquired immunodeficiency syndrome (AIDS) or AIDS-related disorders. N Engl J Med 1986; 314:874–879.
12. Van Baarle D, Wolthers KC, Hovenkamp E, et al. Absolute level of Epstein–Barr virus DNA in human immunodeficiency virus type 1 infection is not predictive of AIDS-related non-Hodgkin lymphoma. J Infect Dis 2002; 186:405–409.
13. Stevens SJ, Blank BS, Smits PH, Meenhorst PL, Middeldorp JM. High Epstein–Barr virus (EBV) DNA loads in HIV-infected patients: correlation with antiretroviral therapy and quantitative EBV serology. AIDS 2002; 16:993–1001.
14. Lo YM, Chan WY, Ng EK, et al. Circulating Epstein–Barr virus DNA in the serum of patients with gastric carcinoma. Clin Cancer Res 2001; 7:1856–1859.
15. Lo YM. Quantitative analysis of Epstein–Barr virus DNA in plasma and serum: applications to tumor detection and monitoring. Ann NY Acad Sci 2001; 945:68–72.
16. Chan KC, Zhang J, Chan AT, et al. Molecular characterization of circulating EBV DNA in the plasma of nasopharyngeal carcinoma and lymphoma patients. Cancer Res 2003; 63:2028–2032.
17. Tao Q, Yang J, Huang H, Swinnen LJ, Ambinder RF. Conservation of Epstein–Barr virus cytotoxic T-cell epitopes in posttransplant lymphomas: implications for immune therapy. Am J Pathol 2002; 160:1839–1845.

18. Sculley TB, Apolloni A, Hurren L, Moss DJ, Cooper DA. Coinfection with A- and B-type Epstein–Barr virus in human immunodeficiency virus-positive subjects. J Infect Dis 1990; 162:643–648.
19. Yao QY, Croom-Carter DS, Tierney RJ, et al. Epidemiology of infection with Epstein–Barr virus types 1 and 2: lessons from the study of a T-cell-immunocompromised hemophilic cohort. J Virol 1998; 72:4352–4363.
20. van Baarle D, Hovenkamp E, Dukers NH, et al. High prevalence of Epstein–Barr virus type 2 among homosexual men is caused by sexual transmission. J Infect Dis 2000; 181:2045–2049.
21. Naher H, Lenhard B, Wilms J, Nickel P. Detection of Epstein–Barr virus DNA in anal scrapings from HIV-positive homosexual men. Arch Dermatol Res 1995; 287:608–611.
22. Moore PS. The emergence of Kaposi's sarcoma-associated herpesvirus (human herpesvirus 8). N Engl J Med 2000; 343:1411–1413.
23. Walling DM, Flaitz CM, Nichols CM. Epstein–Barr virus replication in oral hairy leukoplakia: response, persistence, and resistance to treatment with valacyclovir. J Infect Dis 2003; 188:883–890.
24. Gilligan K, Rajadurai P, Resnick L, Raab-Traub N. Epstein–Barr virus small nuclear RNAs are not expressed in permissively infected cells in AIDS-associated leukoplakia. Proc Natl Acad Sci USA 1990; 87:8790–8794.
25. Cruchley AT, Murray PG, Niedobitek G, Reynolds GM, Williams DM, Young LS. The expression of the Epstein–Barr virus nuclear antigen (EBNA-I) in oral hairy leukoplakia. Oral Dis 1997; 3(suppl 1):S177–S179.
26. Webster-Cyriaque J, Middeldorp J, Raab-Traub N. Hairy leukoplakia: an unusual combination of transforming and permissive Epstein–Barr virus infections. J Virol 2000; 74:7610–7618.
27. Swigris JJ, Berry GJ, Raffin TA, Kuschner WG. Lymphoid interstitial pneumonia: a narrative review. Chest 2002; 122:2150–2164.
28. Goedert JJ, Cote TR, Virgo P, et al. Spectrum of AIDS-associated malignant disorders. Lancet 1998; 351:1833–1839.
29. Franceschi S, Dal Maso L, La Vecchia C. Advances in the epidemiology of HIV-associated non-Hodgkin's lymphoma and other lymphoid neoplasms. Int J Cancer 1999; 83:481–485.
30. Cote TR, Biggar RJ, Rosenberg PS, et al. Non-Hodgkin's lymphoma among people with AIDS: incidence, presentation and public health burden. AIDS/Cancer Study Group. Int J Cancer 1997; 73:645–650.
31. Kirk O, Pedersen C, Cozzi-Lepri A, et al. Non-Hodgkin lymphoma in HIV-infected patients in the era of highly active antiretroviral therapy. Blood 2001; 98:3406–3412.
32. Jones JL, Hanson DL, Dworkin MS, Ward JW, Jaffe HW. Effect of antiretroviral therapy on recent trends in selected cancers among HIV-infected persons Adult/Adolescent Spectrum of HIV Disease Project Group. J AIDS 1999; 21(suppl 1):S11–S17.
33. Jacobson LP, Yamashita TE, Detels R, et al. Impact of potent antiretroviral therapy on the incidence of Kaposi's sarcoma and non-Hodgkin's lymphomas among HIV-1-infected individuals. Multicenter AIDS Cohort Study. J AIDS 1999; 21(suppl 1):S34–S41.
34. Rabkin CS. AIDS and cancer in the era of highly active antiretroviral therapy (HAART). Eur J Cancer 2001; 37:1316–1319.
35. Grulich AE, Li Y, McDonald AM, Correll PK, Law MG, Kaldor JM. Decreasing rates of Kaposi's sarcoma and non-Hodgkin's lymphoma in the era of potent combination anti-retroviral therapy. AIDS 2001; 15:629–633.
36. Knowles DM. Immunodeficiency-associated lymphoproliferative disorders. Mod Pathol 1999; 12:200–217.
37. MacMahon EM, Glass JD, Hayward SD, et al. Epstein–Barr virus in AIDS-related primary central nervous system lymphoma. Lancet 1991; 338:969–973.

38. Glaser SL, Clarke CA, Gulley ML, et al. Population-based patterns of human immuno-deficiency virus-related Hodgkin lymphoma in the Greater San Francisco Bay Area, 1988–1998. Cancer 2003; 98:300–309.
39. Gabarre J, Raphael M, Lepage E, et al. Human immunodeficiency virus-related lymphoma: relation between clinical features and histologic subtypes. Am J Med 2001; 111:704–711.
40. Horenstein MG, Nador RG, Chadburn A, et al. Epstein–Barr virus latent gene expression in primary effusion lymphomas containing Kaposi's sarcoma-associated herpes-virus/human herpesvirus-8. Blood 1997; 90:1186–1191.
41. Knowles DM, Chamulak GA, Subar M, et al. Lymphoid neoplasia associated with the acquired immunodeficiency syndrome (AIDS). The New York University Medical Center experience with 105 patients (1981–1986). Ann Intern Med 1988; 108:744–753.
42. Subar M, Neri A, Inghirami G, Knowles DM, Dalla-Favera R. Frequent c-myc onco-gene activation and infrequent presence of Epstein–Barr virus genome in AIDS-associated lymphoma. Blood 1988; 72:667–671.
43. Ambinder RF, Lee S, Curran WJ, et al. Phase II intergroup trial of sequential chemo-therapy and radiotherapy for AIDS-related primary central nervous system lymphoma. Cancer Ther 2003; 1:215–221.
44. Pedersen C, Gerstoft J, Lundgren JD, et al. HIV-associated lymphoma: histopathology and association with Epstein–Barr virus genome related to clinical, immunological and prognostic features. Eur J Cancer 1991; 27:1416–1423.
45. Kersten MJ, Van Gorp J, Pals ST, Boon F, Van Oers MH. Expression of Epstein–Barr virus latent genes and adhesion molecules in AIDS-related non-Hodgkin's lymphomas: correlation with histology and CD4-cell number. Leuk Lymphoma 1998; 30:515–524.
46. Davi F, Delecluse HJ, Guiet P, et al. Burkitt-like lymphomas in AIDS patients: character-ization within a series of 103 human immunodeficiency virus-associated non-Hodgkin's lymphomas. Burkitt's Lymphoma Study Group. J Clin Oncol 1998; 16:3788–3795.
47. McClain KL, Leach CT, Jenson HB, et al. Association of Epstein–Barr virus with leio-myosarcomas in children with AIDS. N Engl J Med 1995; 332:12–18.
48. Carraway H, Ambinder RF. Plasma cell dyscrasia, Hodgkin lymphoma, HIV, and Kaposi sarcoma-associated herpesvirus. Curr Opin Oncol 2002; 14:543–545.
49. Grulich AE, Li Y, McDonald A, Correll PK, Law MG, Kaldor JM. Rates of non-AIDS-defining cancers in people with HIV infection before and after AIDS diagnosis. 2002; 16:1155–1161.
50. Frisch M, Smith E, Grulich A, Johansen C. Cancer in a population-based cohort of men and women in registered homosexual partnerships. Am J Epidemiol 2003; 157:966–972.
51. Lechowicz MJ, Lin L, Ambinder RF. Epstein–Barr virus DNA in body fluids. Curr Opin Oncol 2002; 14:533–537.
52. De Luca A, Antinori A, Cingolani A, et al. Evaluation of cerebrospinal fluid EBV-DNA and IL-10 as markers for in vivo diagnosis of AIDS-related primary central nervous system lymphoma. Br J Haematol 1995; 90:844–849.
53. Roberts TC, Storch GA. Multiplex PCR for diagnosis of AIDS-related central nervous system lymphoma and toxoplasmosis. J Clin Microbiol 1997; 35:268–269.
54. Cingolani A, Gastaldi R, Fassone L, et al. Epstein–Barr virus infection is predictive of CNS involvement in systemic AIDS-related non-Hodgkin's lymphomas. J Clin Oncol 2000; 18:3325–3330.
55. Fong IW, Ho J, Toy C, Lo B, Fong MW. Value of long-term administration of acyclovir and similar agents for protecting against AIDS-related lymphoma: case-control and historical cohort studies. Clin Infect Dis 2000; 30:757–761.
56. Grulich AE, Law MG. Long-term high-dose acyclovir and AIDS-related non-Hodgkin's lymphoma. Clin Infect Dis 2001; 32:989–990.
57. Ioannidis JP, Collier AC, Cooper DA, et al. Clinical efficacy of high-dose acyclovir in patients with human immunodeficiency virus infection: a meta-analysis of randomized individual patient data. J Infect Dis 1998; 178:349–359.

58. Wagner HJ, Rooney CM, Heslop HE. Diagnosis and treatment of posttransplantation lymphoproliferative disease after hematopoietic stem cell transplantation. Biol Blood Marrow Transplant 2002; 8:1–8.

59. Moss DJ, Khanna R, Sherritt M, Elliott SL, Burrows SR. Developing immunotherapeutic strategies for the control of Epstein–Barr virus-associated malignancies. J AIDS 1999; 21(suppl 1):S80–S83.

60. Chodosh J, Holder VP, Gan YJ, Belgaumi A, Sample J, Sixbey JW. Eradication of latent Epstein–Barr virus by hydroxyurea alters the growth-transformed cell phenotype. J Infect Dis 1998; 177:1194–1201.

61. Slobod KS, Taylor GH, Sandlund JT, Furth P, Helton KJ, Sixbey JW. Epstein–Barr virus-targeted therapy for AIDS-related primary lymphoma of the central nervous system. Lancet 2000; 356:1493–1494.

62. Lee RK, Cai JP, Deyev V, et al. Azidothymidine and interferon-alpha induce apoptosis in herpesvirus-associated lymphomas. Cancer Res 1999; 59:5514–5520.

63. Toomey NL, Deyev VV, Wood C, et al. Induction of a TRAIL-mediated suicide program by interferon alpha in primary effusion lymphoma. Oncogene 2001; 20:7029–7040.

64. Ghosh SK, Wood C, Boise LH, et al. Potentiation of TRAIL-induced apoptosis in primary effusion lymphoma through azidothymidine-mediated inhibition of NF-kappa B. Blood 2003; 101:2321–2327.

65. Chan AT, Tao Q, Robertson KD, et al. Azacitidine induces demethylation of the Epstein–Barr virus genome in tumors in patients. J Clin Oncol 2004.

66. Faller DV, Mentzer SJ, Perrine SP. Induction of the Epstein–Barr virus thymidine kinase gene with concomitant nucleoside antivirals as a therapeutic strategy for Epstein–Barr virus-associated malignancies. Curr Opin Oncol 2001; 13:360–367.

67. Franken M, Estabrooks A, Cavacini L, Sherburne B, Wang F, Scadden DT. Epstein–Barr virus-driven gene therapy for EBV-related lymphomas. Nat Med 1996; 2:1379–1382.

68. Rogers RP, Ge JQ, Holley-Guthrie E, et al. Killing Epstein–Barr virus-positive B-lymphocytes by gene therapy: comparing the efficacy of cytosine deaminase and herpes simplex virus thymidine kinase. Hum Gene Ther 1996; 7:2235–2245.

69. Gutierrez MI, Judde JG, Magrath IT, Bhatia KG. Switching viral latency to viral lysis: a novel therapeutic approach for Epstein–Barr virus-associated neoplasia. Cancer Res 1996; 56:969–972.

70. Maloney DG, Grillo-Lopez AJ, White CA, et al. IDEC-C2B8 (Rituximab) anti-CD20 monoclonal antibody therapy in patients with relapsed low-grade non-Hodgkin's lymphoma. Blood 1997; 90:2188–2195.

71. Yang J, Tao Q, Flinn IW, et al. Characterization of Epstein–Barr virus-infected B-cells in patients with posttransplantation lymphoproliferative disease: disappearance after rituximab therapy does not predict clinical response. Blood 2000; 96:4055–4063.

72. Verschuuren EA, Stevens SJ, van Imhoff GW, et al. Treatment of posttransplant lymphoproliferative disease with rituximab: the remission, the relapse, and the complication. Transplantation 2002; 73:100–104.

73. Gruhn B, Meerbach A, Hafer R, Zell R, Wutzler P, Zintl F. Pre-emptive therapy with rituximab for prevention of Epstein–Barr virus-associated lymphoproliferative disease after hematopoietic stem cell transplantation. Bone Marrow Transplant 2003; 31:1023–1025.

10

Burkitt Lymphoma

Jeffery T. Sample
Department of Biochemistry, St. Jude Children's Research Hospital,
Memphis, Tennessee, U.S.A.

Ingrid K. Ruf
Department of Molecular Biology and Biochemistry, University of California,
Irvine, California, U.S.A.

INTRODUCTION

Burkitt lymphoma (BL) is a tumor of B-lymphocytes that, by definition, carries one of three reciprocal chromosomal translocations that juxtapose the coding region of the *MYC* proto-oncogene located on chromosome 8 to an immunoglobulin (Ig) gene locus from either chromosome 2, 14, or 22 (1). The consequence of these translocations is constitutive transcription of the affected *MYC* allele, ultimately resulting in malignant transformation of the B-cell. In addition to the classic endemic, or African, form of BL (eBL) initially described by Dr. Dennis Burkitt in 1958 (2), which is virtually always associated with latent (nonproductive) Epstein–Barr virus (EBV) infection, at least two additional forms of BL, sporadic (sBL) and HIV or AIDS associated, are formally recognized by the World Health Organization (1,3). Unlike eBL, nonendemic forms are less frequently associated with EBV. Because the distribution of eBL coincides with the malarial belt of Central Africa, infection with malarial parasites has long been believed to be an important cofactor for the development of EBV-positive BL in this region.

Although it has been four decades since the discovery by Epstein and colleagues of EBV particles within cultured BL cells (4), the etiologic role of EBV in BL is far from being fully understood. On the one hand, the high association of clonal EBV infection with EBV-positive cases of BL (5), in conjunction with the potent B-cell immortalizing capability of the virus, provides a strong argument for a causal role. Yet, the absence of EBV infection in a majority of the cases of nonendemic forms of the disease and the general lack of expression of the so-called "transforming" genes of the virus in EBV-positive cases of BL have raised the possibility that while EBV may be an important factor in the development of BL, particularly eBL, it is not necessarily an essential one. Ongoing analyses employing transgenic mouse models of c-*myc*–induced lymphomagenesis, which obviously lack an EBV component, have revealed some striking similarities between human BL and the

B-cell tumors that arise in mice as a consequence of deregulated c-*myc* expression. However, at least one specific difference has been noted. Moreover, recent studies have indicated that EBV genes expressed in BL, but which are not essential for B-cell immortalization by the virus in vitro, can contribute significantly to the tumorigenic potential of BL cells. It is evident, therefore, that BL should not be considered a single entity, but a family of similar but distinct tumors for which the role of EBV varies and is linked to other cofactors of infectious, genetic, or environmental nature.

CLASSIFICATION AND CHARACTERISTICS OF BL

BL is defined as a small noncleaved cell lymphoma of B-cell origin that contains a reciprocal chromosomal translocation that joins an *MYC* allele located on the long arm of chromosome 8 (q24) with either an Ig heavy chain (IgH) locus (chromosome 14), or a κ or λ light chain locus (chromosomes 2 and 22, respectively) [Fig. 1; reviewed in Ref. (1)]. The t(8;14) is the most frequently occurring translocation (80%), and results in transfer of at least the protein-coding portion of the *MYC* gene (exons 2 and 3) to the IgH locus on chromosome 14. By contrast, the variant translocations t(2;8) and t(8;22) occur at frequencies of approximately 15% and 5%, respectively, and result in placement of an Ig light chain (IgL) locus onto chromosome 8,

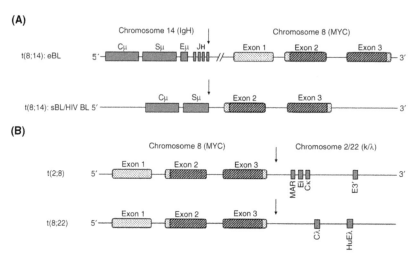

Figure 1 Chromosomal translocations that target the *MYC* gene in BL. (**A**) Positions of typical breakpoints (*vertical arrows*) that involve the IgH locus in t(8;14) translocations within eBL (J_H) and in sBL and HIV-associated BLs ($S\mu$). Transcriptional orientation is shown relative to the *MYC* gene on chromosome 8; note that within t(8;14), the transcriptional orientation of the IgH locus is opposite to that of *MYC*. Breakpoints within chromosome 8 in eBL commonly occur 100 kbp or more upstream of the *MYC* gene, which consists of three exons, of which only exons 2 and 3 encode for MYC as indicated by the dark fill. The Eμ heavy chain enhancer is believed to promote *MYC* transcription in such translocations, whereas translocations that involve the Sμ locus result in loss of Eμ, and presumably transcriptional regulation of *MYC* through a 3' Ig enhancer (e.g., Eα). (**B**) Variant translocations involving either the κ or λ IgL loci on chromosomes 2 and 22, respectively, that can occur in any of the BL classifications. These translocations place IgL enhancers, such as Ei, E3', or HuEλ, downstream of the *MYC* gene. Figure is not to scale. *Abbreviations*: BL, Burkitt lymphoma; eBL, endemic Burkitt lymphoma; Ig, immunoglobulin; sBL, sporadic Burkitt lymphoma. *Source*: From Ref. 6.

downstream of the MYC gene (6). Regardless of the translocation involved, the outcome is a deregulated expression of MYC, which is now under the influence of an Ig gene transcriptional enhancer. The disruption of the normally tightly regulated transcription of this proto-oncogene is without doubt the critical founding event in the development of BL, though as discussed below, it alone is not sufficient to cause BL.

BL Subgroups, Clinical Presentation, and Geographical Distribution

As indicated above, there are three formally recognized classifications of BL: endemic, sporadic, and HIV or AIDS associated. These subgroup classifications primarily take into consideration the presence of EBV within tumor cells, clinical presentation, geographic location, and the HIV status of the patient. However, there is certainly some overlap among the BL subgroups with respect to these criteria. For instance, while the majority of sBL and HIV-associated BL are EBV-negative, approximately 10% to 30% of sBL and a slightly higher percentage of HIV/AIDS-associated BL are in fact EBV-positive (6,7). Additionally, the clinical presentation of BL most commonly seen in Northeastern Brazil (abdominal tumors) is similar to sBL; yet these tumors have a much higher association with EBV infection (70–90%) than typical sBL in the United States and Western Europe (8–10). There are also nonclinical characteristics that tend to be characteristic of one form of BL over another, e.g., a general difference between eBL and sBL in the breakpoint position within the MYC gene in t(8;14) (Fig. 1) (1,11,12).

The most common clinical descriptors of BL are the anatomical site of the primary tumor mass (e.g., jaw-associated or abdominal), and the involvement of bone marrow and the central nervous system (CNS). While abdominal tumors are not infrequently associated with eBL, jaw-associated tumors are the most common (1,2,13). This is in stark contrast to sBL and HIV-associated BL, which rarely present as a jaw tumor (13–16). Furthermore, even between sBL and eBL tumors occurring within the abdomen, differences have been noted in the organ sites at which the tumors predominately occur (1). Involvement of bone marrow, as opposed to the CNS, is less frequent in eBL (though not uncommon), whereas among sBL patients a higher frequency (perhaps as many as two-thirds) present with marrow involvement, and bone marrow and CNS involvement is common in HIV-associated BL (1,6,17).

The study of BL has historically focused on eBL, perhaps in large part due to its long-known association with a transforming virus. Additionally, there has been increasing attention on sBL as a subset of non-Hodgkin's lymphoma in patients within the United States and Western Europe, as well as immunodeficiency-associated BL in response to the worldwide rise in AIDS. Our knowledge of other potential forms of BL, particularly in developing countries outside of Africa, is relatively limited. The most detailed information for such cases comes from analyses of BL from Northeastern Brazil, a region with socioeconomic and climatic conditions similar to Central Africa. Of 54 cases of BL from Bahia studied by Stein and colleagues (8), 87% were found to be positive for EBV, slightly lower than the frequency of EBV association with classic eBL. Unlike eBL, however, the predominant anatomical site of these tumors was abdominal (90%), and therefore similar to sBL. A similar frequency of EBV association (i.e., intermediate between sBL and eBL) and a prevalence of abdominal tumors have also been observed for BL in Northern Africa (i.e., outside of the malaria belt) (18), perhaps suggesting a common biology that is distinct from currently recognized BL classifications. Among the Bahia cases, EBV gene expression was found to be identical to that seen in other cases of EBV-positive BL. Unlike classic eBL, the high association with EBV infection among the Brazilian cases could not be linked to a regional prevalence of malaria (8). However, all of the cases evaluated were from areas in which *Schistosoma mansoni* infection is endemic, raising the possibility that, as for eBL, chronic parasitic infection may be a predisposing factor. It will be interesting to learn if a similar trend of increased EBV association is observed for BL within other developing countries with comparable socioeconomic and climatic conditions, e.g., India (19), that favor infection with EBV early in life [a factor long known to correlate with EBV involvement in BL (1)] and exposure to chronic parasitic infections.

INFECTIOUS COFACTORS

Even before the association between eBL and EBV was identified, it was clear that the distribution of BL in Africa corresponded to climatic conditions favorable to arthropod vectors of malaria parasites, primarily *Plasmodium falciparum*, suggesting that malaria is a predisposing factor in the development of BL (20–22). A causative connection between malaria and EBV in the development of eBL is strongly favored to this day, and though it is well supported by epidemiological studies (1,23), there is yet no direct evidence that malaria predisposes one to BL as a consequence of EBV infection. The absence of scientific evidence to either support or dispel cooperation between malaria and EBV infection, however, can be attributed to the unavailability of an appropriate animal model to test the validity of this proposal. This is also true for BL in other geographic regions in which EBV positivity may be linked to non-malarial parasitic infections endemic to these locales, e.g., *S. mansoni* infection in Northeastern Brazil (8). The relatively recent development of nonhuman primate models representative of human malaria and EBV infection could be used to address this question.

Immune Suppression as a Predisposing Factor for EBV Involvement

Given the strong epidemiological link between malaria and the presence of EBV in eBL, how might malaria and potentially other parasitic infections promote an etiologic role for EBV in BL? The most attractive theory is that as a consequence of the immunosuppressive effects of these parasitic infections, there is a breakdown in the maintenance of an effective anti-EBV immunosurveillance (24–26). Therefore, if one assumes that the BL progenitor is a cell that is at increased risk for chromosomal translocation or subsequent outgrowth as a consequence of EBV infection, a breakdown in immunosurveillance would, logically speaking, result in an increase in the pool of potential BL precursors—namely EBV-infected B-cells. Consistent with this prediction, a study on children with acute malaria in Gambia found that the levels of EBV-positive cells in peripheral blood was five times higher than in convalescent malaria patients and normal healthy adult controls from the United Kingdom (27). The potential for an increase in EBV load associated with immunodeficiency is of course well established in AIDS and in patients undergoing immunosuppressive therapy related to solid organ or hematopoietic cell transplantation (28), and almost certainly accounts for HIV infection as a predisposing factor for development of AIDS-associated BL, a variable but significant percentage (30–80%) being EBV-positive. Additionally, a general B-cell expansion in acute malaria (29) could randomly add to the expanding pool of EBV-positive B-cells to further increase the risk for a critical lymphomagenic event, presumably the translocation of *MYC*.

MOLECULAR PATHOGENESIS OF BL

Historically, elucidation of the molecular pathogenesis of BL, i.e., the sum of events both genetic and biochemical that give rise to BL, has been approached from two basic directions. First are studies that have primarily focused on delineating functions of the *MYC* proto-oncogene (or its mouse equivalent, c-*myc*) and its contributions to cell transformation and lymphoma development. The second approach comprises complementing studies seeking to define the natural biology of persistent (latent) EBV infection and the specific contributions of EBV latency to BL. To better understand known and potential roles of EBV in BL, it is important to have an appreciation for the specific cellular environment of BL. It is in this context that the virus presumably makes its contributions, and it may also be true that the specific genetic and biochemical milieu of the BL cell, or its progenitor, dictates whether EBV will be required to progress to an actual tumor. Therefore, in this section we will review the current status of our collective understanding of the role of *MYC* in BL, as well as the contribution of a number of other cellular genes, i.e., components of the p53 and retinoblastoma protein (pRb) tumor suppressor pathways, following their altered expression, deletion, or mutation. The involvement of these "accessory" genes to *MYC*, particularly those within the p53 pathway, has been realized primarily from studies of a mouse model of c-*myc*–induced lymphomagenesis— the Eμ-*myc* transgenic mouse—which has provided enormous insight in recent years that is directly relevant to BL in man.

The MYC Oncoprotein

MYC is one of three members of the MYC family of oncoproteins (the others being MYCN and MYCL), and is the cellular homolog of the viral Myc oncoprotein (v-Myc) encoded by the avian MC29 myelocytomatosis transforming virus (30,31). It is one of the most intensely studied transforming proteins, and at current count activation of *MYC* family members (through translocation, amplification, enhanced translation, or protein stability) occurs in nearly 70% of human cancers (32). MYC (c-Myc in the mouse) belongs to the basic helix-loop-helix leucine zipper (bHLH-Zip) family of transcription factors and binds to the DNA element CAYGTG (the so-called E-box) as a heterodimer with MAX, another member of the bHLH-Zip family (33–37). MYC:MAX heterodimers activate gene expression by targeting transcriptional coactivators and their associated histone acetyltransferases and/or ATPase/helicases to MYC-responsive genes containing an E-box within their promoter (38–42). However, as is true for a growing number of transcriptional activators, MYC can also contribute to repression of transcription [for a discussion of the transcriptional properties of MYC, see Ref. (32)]. The number of genes whose expression is affected by MYC continues to grow and is substantial [currently approximately 1400, though most of these are indirect targets (43)]. Thus, it is highly unlikely that the list of MYC-responsive genes can be reduced to a limited number of candidate genes that are most important for MYC's role in transformation, because these genes contribute to a vast array of cellular processes important for tumorigenesis, not the least of which are those that directly promote cell proliferation (6).

Activation of MYC in BL

Cell proliferation and the transformed state in BL are, without doubt, the direct result of activated *MYC* expression, initiated by chromosomal translocations that place *MYC* under the control of B-cell specific transcriptional regulatory elements, namely Ig gene enhancers. Although mutations within *MYC* and increased protein half-life (the latter a consequence of a subset of these mutations) in some BL tumors may contribute additionally to the oncogenic potential of MYC (44–47), it is the deregulated expression of *MYC* that is central to the pathogenesis of all forms of BL. Identification of the factors that predispose a *MYC* allele to translocation and the mechanism through which this occurs is, therefore, of great interest.

Within BLs containing t(8;14), the breakpoint positions within both chromosomes involved tend to correlate with clinical classification (1,11,48–52). Specifically, in eBL the breakpoint on chromosome 8 most often occurs at a considerable distance (as much as 100 kb or more) upstream of the *MYC* exons, and commonly within the IgH joining (J$_H$) regions on chromosome 14 (Fig. 1). Within sBL and HIV-associated BL, breakpoints generally fall between the first and second exons of *MYC* (only exons 2 and 3 encode protein), and the IgH Sμ region. In the variant translocations, breakpoints within chromosome 8 occur downstream of the *MYC* gene, and upstream of the κ and λ gene constant region segments on chromosomes 2 and 22, respectively (Fig. 1) (1,6,12,53).

Breakpoints within the IgH switch locus in sBL and HIV-associated tumors suggest that these translocations are a consequence of attempted Ig class switching. Because Ig class switching is a normal occurrence only within germinal centers (GCs), this is viewed as further evidence of a GC-cell origin for BL. Another form of Ig remodeling that occurs specifically in GC B-cells is somatic hypermutation of Ig variable (V) regions during affinity maturation of the B-cell antigen receptor. A consequence of hypermutation is the generation of deletions/duplications that appear to be associated with double-strand breaks in DNA that are potentially recombinogenic (54,55). Within BL, IgH and IgL breakpoints often occur throughout the regions targeted by hypermutation (56), suggesting that somatic hypermutation may also contribute to the generation of *MYC*/Ig translocations, particularly those involving the IgL loci (class switching only occurs within the IgH locus).

The mechanism by which the IgH breakpoints involved in eBL are targeted is less clear. While it has been noted that these sometimes have characteristics of Ig V(D)J recombination (57,58), GC B-cells as a rule do not express the recombination activating genes (RAG) 1 and 2 that mediate V(D)J recombination (an event normally confined to immature B-cells), and breakpoints are rarely flanked by the canonical recombination signal sequences recognized by RAG proteins (56). However, there have been reports of "reactivated" RAG expression in GC cells (59–61), which could conceivably promote inappropriate V(D)J recombination, leading to breakpoints seen in eBL containing the t(8;14) translocation. Alternatively, it has been proposed that these translocations could occur in immature B-cells, i.e., RAG-positive cells, prior to their arrival within GCs (6). Of particular interest with respect to a reactivation of RAG expression and potentially variant V(D)J recombination leading to t(8;14) in eBL are earlier reports that EBV and, specifically, the viral protein EBV nuclear antigen (EBNA)-1 can induce *RAG* gene expression in B-cells (62,63). Although one group found no detectable *RAG* gene expression in eBL (64), increased *RAG* expression has been observed in preneoplastic lymphoid samples but not tumors in EBNA-1 transgenic mice (see below) that develop B-cell lymphoma (65). Induction of *RAG* gene expression by EBNA-1, therefore, may be restricted to the early stages of lymphomagenesis.

Unlike for the Ig breakpoints, the mechanisms that result in the chromosomal breaks on chromosome 8 are less clear because they do not exhibit hallmarks of V(D)J recombination, class switching, or somatic hypermutation. In addition to the question of what events predispose *MYC* for translocation, the equally perplexing question is "What determines the selection and frequency of translocation to the three different Ig loci?" A provocative answer to the latter question may have been provided by a recent report from Misteli and coworkers (66), who contest that gene loci frequently have nonrandom and gene-specific distribution patterns within the nucleus, and that proximity of translocation-prone genes may influence the frequency at which certain alleles are involved in translocation—basically, the closer the two alleles, the greater the possibility that they will be recurrently translocated. With respect to *MYC*/Ig translocations in BL, the mean separation values determined in B-cells (this apparently does not hold true for all cell types) for *MYC* alleles and the three Ig loci reflected the frequency of the *MYC*/Ig translocations for the population of BL tumors cited in this report: IgH > Igλ > Igκ. One caveat is that the relative frequencies of the two variant translocations as reported (8% Igλ, 3% Igκ) differ from commonly reported values of either equivalent frequencies (10%) or a preference for Igκ (15%) over Igλ (5%). However, this discrepancy could be due to the relatively low number of BLs containing either variant translocation in a single sample population. If the conclusions of this study are correct, then one could predict that the combination of increased recombinogenic potential associated with Ig gene remodeling and active *MYC* gene transcription (and thus an open chromatin configuration) occurring in close proximity within vigorously proliferating GC B-cells underlies the propensity for the characteristic *MYC*/Ig translocations in BL.

MYC—Purveyor of Cell Proliferation, Immortality, and Death

As would be expected of an oncoprotein, MYC has a dominant influence on cell-cycle progression and is required for sustained cell proliferation in tumors in which it is activated (67,68). Often referred to as the "master regulator" of the cell cycle, MYC drives cell proliferation through its effects on genes that directly regulate the cell cycle. This includes, for example, upregulation of D cyclins, their associated cyclin-dependent kinases (CDKs) 4 and 6, and cdc25A (a protein phosphatase that activates CDK2 and CDK4), and downregulation of the CDK inhibitors p21^{Cip1} and p27^{Kip1} (6,43,69–72). MYC also influences a number of ancillary processes central to tumorigenesis, e.g., inhibition of terminal differentiation and the induction of telomerase activity and angiogenesis (68,73–75). Additionally, overexpression of MYC in B-cells can impose a nonimmunogenic phenotype as a result of reduced expression of human leukocyte antigen (HLA) class I and II molecules and several components of the class I antigen processing and presentation pathway (76). This has obvious implications for the evasion of anti-tumor and -EBV immunity by preneoplastic and neoplastic B-cells that overexpress MYC.

Despite the many positive influences of MYC on processes that directly and indirectly promote cell proliferation and tumorigenesis, MYC is also a potent inducer of programmed cell death (apoptosis) (77,78). This apparent paradox to MYC's role in cell transformation actually represents a safeguard mechanism in the host to eliminate those cells that support inappropriate expression of potentially oncogenic proteins, of which MYC is a prototypical example. Not surprisingly, disablement of

MYC-activated apoptotic pathways has proven to be critical for the progression to malignancy. This now common theme in tumorigenesis has been most effectively demonstrated in mouse models of c-Myc–induced cancer.

Mouse Models of c-Myc–Induced Lymphomagenesis

Given the timing of the identification of MYC as a likely transforming protein in human tumors, it was one of the first proteins evaluated for its oncogenic potential in transgenic mouse models of cancer (79–81). Of these, the Eµ-*myc* mouse in which a mouse c-*myc* transgene is under transcriptional control of the Eµ IgH enhancer (79) has been a particularly insightful model of MYC-induced lymphomagenesis. More recently, an alternative mouse model of BL has been described (λ-*MYC*) in which a *MYC* transgene is under the control of an Igλ transcriptional regulatory domain [mimicking t(8;22)] (82). This model appears to accurately recapitulate features of BL-specific *MYC* activation, perhaps more so than the Eµ-*myc* mouse, though it is yet to be as thoroughly studied.

At approximately four to six months of age, Eµ-*myc* mice develop clonal pre-B and B-cell lymphoma (tumor latency varies among mouse litters, but within a litter spans approximately two weeks), similar to BLs bearing the t(8;14) translocation (79). Crosses of Eµ-*myc* with either Eµ-*bcl-2* transgenic (83) or *p53*$^{-/+}$ mice significantly accelerates lymphoma development, suggesting that inactivation of proapoptotic mechanisms is critical for MYC-induced lymphomagenesis (84,85). Concordantly, within tumors that arise in Eµ-*myc* mice, there is a selection for disruption of the p53-mediated pathway of apoptosis (see below) in a majority of tumors. This occurs by loss of either p53 function through mutation or (rarely) deletion (28%), bi-allelic deletion of the *p19*^{ARF} locus (24%) (ARF is an antagonist of murine double minute 2 (Mdm2), a negative regulator of p53), and frequent overexpression of Mdm2, notably in tumors that retain a wild-type (wt) *p53* gene (86). The importance of inactivation of the ARF-Mdm2-p53 tumor suppressor pathway to c-Myc–induced lymphomagenesis is further highlighted by Eµ-*myc* crosses with mice deficient in ARF or Mdm2—on an *ARF*$^{-/-}$ background lymphomagenesis is rapidly accelerated (86), whereas it is profoundly inhibited by Mdm2 haplo-insufficiency (87). Moreover, loss of the proapoptotic protein Bax, which is important for p53-dependent and c-Myc–induced apoptosis, circumvents the selection of p53 mutations during lymphomagenesis in Eµ-*myc* mice (88).

Undoubtedly, significant insight into c-Myc–induced lymphomagenesis has been obtained from studies of the Eµ-*myc* mouse, but with a question of "how much of this information is relevant to human BL?" The Eµ-*myc* mouse model has proven to be remarkably representative of BL in general, particularly with respect to the status of the ARF-HDM2-p53 pathway (HDM2 is the human equivalent of the mouse Mdm2 protein). However, whereas the frequencies of p53 loss-of-function and overexpression of HDM2 in BL tumors are very similar to those observed in Eµ-*myc* lymphomas, *ARF* is targeted to a much lesser degree (see below). The frequent deletion of the *ARF* locus in the Eµ-*myc* system may reflect the absence of EBV, which has been demonstrated to provide a survival function in maintenance of the BL tumor phenotype (89,90). Thus, this function of the virus may potentially supplant a need to target *ARF*, though it is unclear how this may be accomplished. Unfortunately, insufficient numbers of BL tumors (adequately classified according to subtype and EBV status) have been assessed to date to permit definitive identification (by comparative analyses) of features common among or unique to the three subgroups of BL and Eμ-*myc* tumors and to find if there are properties that are more likely to occur in EBV-positive versus EBV-negative cases of BL. Nonetheless, the Eμ-*myc* mouse model has proven immensely valuable in demonstrating the need for inactivation of apoptotic pathways to promote the tumorigenic properties of c-Myc, which is certainly applicable to BL.

Alterations in the p53 Tumor Suppressor Pathway and Its Modifiers in BL

The p53 protein is a transcription factor that is active in response to numerous pro-apoptotic stimuli, notably DNA damage (and thus potential genome instability) and inappropriate expression of proto-oncogenes such as *MYC*, which can contribute to tumorigenesis. Depending on the nature and severity of the insult to the cell, p53 either enforces a cell-cycle arrest until the damage to the cell can be repaired (i.e., in the case of DNA damage) or initiates apoptosis. At least 50% of all human tumors have acquired mutations in p53. Most commonly, these mutations cluster in the so-called core domain, resulting in loss of DNA binding capability and thus inhibition of p53 target gene transactivation. Mutations in p53 have been reported to occur in approximately 30% of BL tumors (28% in the Eμ-*myc* mouse) (91–93), and these mutations cluster at a number of "hot spot" residues and result in functional inactivation of p53 (94). In addition to eBL, mutations in p53 were found in 50% to 60% of HIV-associated cases of BL (95). The mutation rate of p53 among BL-derived cell lines, regardless of EBV status, is even higher–70% to 80% of lines analyzed (92,96–99)–suggesting that there is continual selection for disruption of p53 function, even when other components of this tumor suppressor pathway are inactivated (see below). However, this may be viewed as a consequence of long-term growth in culture, and not necessarily critical to lymphomagenesis.

In addition to mutation of p53 itself, other components of the p53 tumor suppressor pathway are commonly altered in BL (Fig. 2). Specifically, the ARF protein, which binds to and inhibits the p53 antagonist HDM2 (an E3 ubiquitin ligase that targets p53 for degradation via the 26S proteosome) (100), is lost as a consequence of homozygous deletion of the genetic locus encoding ARF in 12.5% of BL tumors and 6% to 7% of BL cell lines analyzed (98,101,102). In Germany, a recent analysis of sBL tumors, however, found no loss of ARF expression (103). Interestingly, in cases in which *ARF* is deleted, p53 is wt, a situation also found in tumors within Eμ-*myc* mice, though the frequency of *ARF* deletion in the mouse tumors is notably higher (24%) (86). Likewise, BL lines that are found to harbor wt p53 and to retain the *ARF* locus are prone to overexpression of HDM2 (16–20%) (96,98), similar to Mdm2 in tumors from Eμ-*myc* mice. HDM2 overexpression in these cell lines is apparently due to enhanced translation. Thus, while alterations in either ARF or HDM2 expression in BL are less frequent than mutations in p53, together they may account for an equivalent number of known hits within this tumor suppressor pathway in BLs in which p53 is wt. In summary, therefore, the ARF-HDM2-p53 tumor suppressor pathway is inactivated in approximately 55% to 65% of BLs (approximately 90% in BL cell lines), and is impacted by p53 mutation, homozygous deletion of *ARF*, or overexpression of HDM2, which appear to be mutually exclusive events within the primary tumor. Inactivation of this pathway leads to inhibition of p53-dependent apoptosis in response to MYC overexpression and, as demonstrated in the Eμ-*myc* mouse model, undoubtedly provides a strong selective advantage during development of BL.

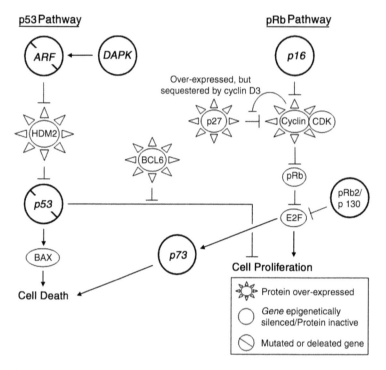

Figure 2 Disruption of proapoptotic and cell-cycle–regulatory networks in Burkitt lymphoma. Shown are common events resulting in inactivation of the p53 and pRb tumor suppressor pathways in BL. See text for discussion. *Abbreviations*: ARF, p14^{ARF} (human homolog of murine p19^{ARF}); BCL6, B-cell lymphoma gene 6; CDK, cyclin-dependent kinase; DAPK, death-associated protein kinase; E2F, adenovirus E2 gene regulatory factor; HDM2, human homolog of murine double minute 2 protein (Mdm2); pRb, retinoblastoma protein.

In addition to events that directly target components of the p53 pathway, mutations also occur within BL in genes that modulate the activity of this pathway (Fig. 2). These include deregulation of B-cell lymphoma gene 6 (BCL-6), a transcriptional repressor and multifunctional regulator of cell-cycle control, B-cell activation and differentiation, apoptosis, and inflammation (104). In 29% of sBL and 50% of eBL, BCL-6 expression is reported to be upregulated as a consequence of point mutations within the first intron that are believed to arise during B-cell transit through the GC (105,106). This may lead to inhibition of p53-induced senescence, in addition to influencing other aspects of BCL-6 function. However, others have reported that although mutations do occur within the *BCL-6* gene in BL cells (71.4%), there is no obvious correlation between the presence of mutations and protein levels or clinical outcome (107). Death-associated protein kinase (DAP-kinase) and p73 (see below) have been shown to be targets of epigenetic silencing in BL. DAP-kinase is a novel proapoptotic serine/threonine kinase whose expression is necessary for interferon-γ–induced apoptosis (108). The tumor suppressive properties of DAP-kinase appear to act at two apoptotic checkpoints: an early oncogene-activated apoptotic checkpoint mediated by the ARF-p53 pathway, as well as a p53-independent checkpoint (109,110). The DAP-kinase gene has been found to have hypermethylated CpG islands in 100% of BL tumors examined (111,112). This is in contrast to normal B-cells and those immortalized in vitro that show no evidence of DNA hypermethylation. p73 encodes a protein with structural homology to p53 and similar functional characteristics, including the ability to promote apoptosis upon its overexpression and to transactivate p53-responsive genes (113). Epigenetic silencing of p73 via DNA methylation of a 5′ CpG island has been demonstrated in 30% of BL tumors (114). As mutation of p53 has a lower than average incidence in BL as compared to other tumors, silencing of p73 may serve as an alternative event that contributes to abnormal cell cycle and apoptotic regulation in BL.

Mutation of the pRb Pathway

The retinoblastoma tumor suppressor protein pRb and the related p107 and p130 (also referred to as pRb2) interact with specific members of the E2F family of proteins to negatively regulate E2F-mediated transcription of genes important for entry into and progression through the cell cycle (115,116). Direct regulation of E2F members by these proteins is coordinated primarily through their phosphorylation by CDKs—hypophosphorylated forms of pRb inhibit E2F function, whereas hyperphosphorylation of pRb releases E2F factors from this negative regulation. Given the integral role played by pRb proteins in regulating cell-cycle progression, it is not surprising that components within the pRb regulatory pathway (p16^{INK4a}-CDK4,6/cyclin D-pRb-E2F) are frequently compromised in human cancers, including BL (Fig. 2). One target of alterations is the cyclin-dependent kinase inhibitor 2A (CDKN2A) locus that encodes the tumor suppressors ARF (see above) and p16^{INK4a} (p16). p16 inhibits the phosphorylation of pRb by the cyclin D/CDK4 complex. Homozygous deletion of this locus has been reported in a wide variety of human primary tumors (117), and deletion of this locus dually impacts both the p53 and pRb pathways (118). Though deletion and mutation of the *p16* locus is a relatively rare event in BL (101,102,119), silencing of the *p16* gene by DNA methylation of exon 1 occurs in 42% of primary BL tumors and in the majority of BL cell lines (101,119).

Alterations in this pathway leading to dysregulation of cell-cycle control also occur downstream of p16. Downregulation of the CDK inhibitor p27^{Kip1} is an essential step in the transition of cycling cells into S phase. Consequently, proliferating lymphoid cells typically exhibit undetectable levels of p27. Additionally, the degree of malignancy of a variety of tumors, including numerous B-cell lymphomas, has been shown to be in inverse correlation with the level of p27 expression, such that low p27 levels correlate with a high degree of malignancy (120). BL represents an exception to this in that anomalously high levels of p27 are present in cells despite their high proliferative index. In BL, it appears that elevated p27 levels are accompanied by overexpression of cyclin D3. Further work has demonstrated that p27 is sequestered within an inactive complex, likely in part by cyclin D3, resulting in the ability of these tumor cells to overcome a potential p27-mediated growth arrest (121,122).

Frequent mutations in the pRb-related tumor suppressor *pRb2/p130* gene have also been reported in both BL tumors and cell lines (Fig. 2) (123). Under normal conditions, quiescent cells in G$_0$ contain an E2F-pRb2/p130 complex in the nucleus that is responsible for active repression of a number of cellular gene promoters. Upon entry into the cell cycle, pRb2 is phosphorylated by the G$_1$ CDKs, resulting in degradation of pRb2 through the proteosomal pathway and derepression of E2F-responsive promoters. Often in BL, the nuclear localization signal (NLS) in pRb2 is mutated, resulting in a cytoplasmic localization of pRb2 and thus functional inactivation of the protein (124). Mutations in the NLS are most common in eBL, occurring in 84% of studied cases. Mutation of pRb2 in sBL is also fairly common, but appears to occur at a lower frequency (46%). Interestingly, mutations in pRb2 have not been found in HIV-associated BL (3). It has been postulated that in these cases, functional inactivation of pRb2 occurs as a result of the physical interaction of the HIV-1 transactivating (Tat) protein with the pocket domain of pRb2/p130 (125). Despite the finding that HIV-1 is not commonly found in B-cells in AIDS-associated lymphoma, a diffuse nuclear stain has been observed in tissue sections probed with an anti-Tat monoclonal antibody. This is likely the result of soluble Tat, which can be released from infected cells and subsequently taken up by uninfected cells (125,126).

EBV IN BL—CAUSAL ROLE OR B-CELL COHABITATION?

Two theories, not mutually exclusive, are currently favored to explain the contributions of EBV to BL. One provides for a direct role of the virus in maintenance of the tumor phenotype and is supported by observations that in at least one commonly studied BL cell line (Akata, see below), tumorigenic potential is dependent on EBV infection despite absence of the expression of viral genes critical to the growth-transforming properties of EBV. The second theory invokes the active establishment of a persistent latent infection as a process that, though not tumorigenic by itself, predisposes the infected B-cell to a lymphomagenic event, notably the chromosomal translocations that juxtapose *MYC* and an *Ig* locus. This is predicated on the belief (for which there is ample scientific evidence) that EBV, to sustain a lifelong infection of its host, must gain entry into a pool of memory B-cells that serve as the primary reservoir of latent EBV within healthy virus carriers (127,128). To effectively establish a critical mass of this long-lived population of latently infected B-cells, it has been proposed that the virus is able to drive, through the actions of its latency-associated genes, a GC reaction that functionally mimics this normally antigen-driven process leading to establishment of long-lived B-cell memory (129). The critical connection to BL here is the observation that BL cells have characteristics of a GC cell, namely, they express GC-specific cell-surface markers and have either undergone or continue to undergo somatic hypermutation of their *Ig* variable–region loci (130,131). An illustration linking the establishment of EBV latency to development of BL is shown in Figure 3.

Is Viral Latency a Prerequisite for EBV-Induced Lymphomagenesis?

EBV-associated tumors characteristically maintain a latent EBV infection that is associated with the expression of a distinct set of viral genes, and effectively repress virus replication, which is cytolytic and thus incompatible with long-term cell growth and survival. Further, within BL and other tumor cells, the episomal or latency-associated configuration of the EBV genome is present in clonal form (5). This suggests that latency is established prior to the outgrowth of the BL progenitor cell, and thus any direct contribution of EBV to BL would appear to require the establishment of a latent infection. Although the establishment and maintenance of latency within B-lymphocytes was once believed to closely mimic that which occurs in in vitro infections, it is now evident that this is a more complex and multistep process that is influenced as much by the B-cell as it is by the virus.

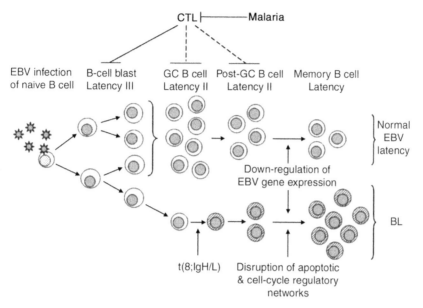

Figure 3 Model for establishment of long-term EBV latency in B lymphocytes and consequential initiation of lymphomagenesis leading to BL. Dashed lines depict limited ability of
CTLs to kill B-cells maintaining the EBV latency II program relative to those maintaining
the latency III or growth program. *Abbreviations*: CTLs, cytotoxic T-lymphocytes; BL, Burkitt
lymphoma; EBV, Epstein–Barr virus. *Source*: From Refs. 158, 159.

In vitro, EBV infection of B-lymphocytes (predominantly resting cells, commonly isolated from umbilical cord or peripheral blood) induces cell proliferation
and immortalization through the concerted actions of several of the 12 known viral
latency genes (28). The resulting B lymphoblastoid cell lines (LCLs) sustain expression
of the full complement of EBV latency–associated genes (Table 1). However, this
pattern of EBV gene expression, referred to as either the growth or type III program
of latency, cannot normally be sustained in vivo as it predisposes the infected B-cell to
elimination by the host cellular immune response, primarily through the actions of
$CD8^+$ T-cells directed toward peptide epitopes within several of the latency proteins
(see Chapter 5). Not surprisingly, then, B-cells that serve as the long-term reservoir of
EBV within the persistently infected host express a very limited repertoire of EBV
proteins (129,132,133).

EBV Latency in BL

The first indication that EBV-infected B-cells might actually restrict viral latency-gene
expression in vivo came from analyses by Rickinson and coworkers of the cytotoxic
T-lymphocyte (CTL) response to BL cells (134). Specifically, in ^{51}Cr-release assays,
some BL lines, often derived from the same tumor, demonstrated intermediate (group
II) or complete resistance to CTL killing (group I), whereas other early-passage BL
cell lines (group III) were comparable to HLA-matched LCLs in their sensitivity to
CTL lysis. The group III BL lines, furthermore, displayed the same propensity as
LCLs to form large multicellular aggregates in culture, with group II lines being
intermediate in this regard [a phenotype subsequently attributed to EBV-induced
expression of cellular adhesion molecules (135)]. A comparative analysis of the

Table 1 Epstein–Barr Virus Latency–Gene Expression Within B Lymphocytes and B Cell–Derived Tumors

Latency program[a]	EBNAs	LMPs	BARTs[b]	EBERs	B-cell type/tumor
Latency	±1[c]	2A	+	+	Memory B-cells in peripheral blood
Latency I	1	–	+	+	BL
Latency II/ default	1	1/2A/2B	+	+	Tonsillar GC and memory B-cells; HL
Latency III/ growth	1/2/3A/3B/ 3C/LP	1/2A/2B	+	+	Naive B-cells; immunoblastic lymphoma; LCL

[a]Latency I, II, and III are alternative designations for type I, II, and III latency programs, respectively.
[b]BART expression has been confirmed in peripheral blood B-cells (CD19$^+$ CD23$^-$; 211) and EBV-associated tumors, but has not been specifically determined for specific B-cell populations.
[c]EBNA-1 expression is activated upon division of infected memory B-cells within the peripheral blood (132).
Abbreviations: BL, Burkitt lymphoma; HL, Hodgkin's lymphoma; LCL, lymphoblastoid cell line; EBNAs, EBV nuclear antigens; LMPs, latent membrane proteins; BARTs, *Bam*HI-A rightwards transcripts; EBER, EBV encoded RNA; GC, germinal centers.

expression of known latency proteins (for which antibody reagents were available) revealed that little or no EBNA-2 and latent membrane protein (LMP)-1 could be detected in the BL lines resistant to CTL killing, whereas EBNA-1 expression was evident in all BL groups (136,137). Subsequent analyses indicated that the other members of the EBNA (EBNA-LP, EBNA-3A, EBNA-3B, and EBNA-3C) and LMP (LMP-2A and LMP-2B) latency-gene families were likewise downregulated in the group I BL cells (138,139). Thus, the only latency-associated genes of EBV consistently expressed in BL tumors and group I BL cell lines, commonly referred to as the type I latency program, are the genome-maintenance protein EBNA-1, the small noncoding RNAs [EBV encoded RNA (EBER)-1 and EBER-2] and the *Bam*HI-A rightwards transcripts (BARTs) (Table 1). Other EBV-associated tumors, most notably nasopharyngeal carcinoma and Hodgkin's lymphoma, display a similar but less restricted program of latency-gene expression that includes the LMP genes and is often referred to as the type II latency program (not to be confused with the group II classification described above) (140–146). Although these tumors at least express the oncogenic LMP-1, none of the viral genes expressed within the type I latency program in BL had been shown to possess either overt transforming activity or be essential for B-cell immortalization by EBV—the exception being EBNA-1, required for replication and maintenance of the EBV episome in dividing cells (147–150).

Is Establishment of Latency a Potentially Lymphomagenic Event?

B-lymphocytes that serve as the long-term reservoir of EBV in the periphery are predominantly resting memory B-cells (IgD$^-$/CD20$^+$) (127,128,132). These B-cells, similar to their BL-cell counterparts, express a very limited repertoire of the latency-associated genes (Table 1), which undoubtedly contributes to immune evasion (132). The elucidation of how EBV gains entry into this long-lived population of B-cells promises to provide substantial insight into EBV biology, and may also provide significant clues to the role of EBV in BL (151). As stated above, a currently favored hypothesis is that EBV gains entry into the memory B-cell pool by directly promoting a GC reaction. Given that BL cells have features common to a GC cell, it is presumed that the founding event in BL—the translocation and consequential deregulated expression of a *MYC* allele—most likely occurs within a GC B-cell (130,151). Therefore, EBV in its quest to establish a long-lived persistent infection within the memory B-cell population may simply promote BL by increasing the pool of BL progenitor cells. Additionally, as discussed earlier, this target pool of EBV-infected B-cells may be further expanded as a consequence of immunosuppressive parasitic infections, e.g., malaria, possibly explaining the much higher incidence of EBV involvement in BL in geographical locations where such infections are prevalent.

An alternative (or complementary) role to the indirect one in which EBV simply expands the pool of BL progenitors would be the direct influence of a viral gene product(s) on a potentially lymphomagenic event or process. The reported induction of RAG 1 and 2 expression by the EBV EBNA-1 protein suggested a scenario in which EBV may contribute to BL by directly promoting translocation and, thus, activation of the *MYC* gene (62,65). However, this currently seems unlikely given that translocations in BL involving *MYC* and *Ig* loci typically do not bear the hallmarks of classic RAG-mediated V(D)J recombination, but that of Ig class switching and recombinogenic events associated with somatic hypermutation of *Ig* V regions (56). Alternatively, survival functions provided by EBV during primary infection may indirectly increase the chance for a *MYC*/Ig translocation by merely expanding the window of opportunity for this event in a GC cell that is programmed for recombination and is prone to mistakes. In this respect it is interesting to note that *MYC*/ *Ig* translocations have been detected within the blood of mice and 2% of healthy humans, suggesting that mistakes normally occur during Ig remodeling, and that cells carrying these inappropriate translocations can survive (152,153). This raises the possibility that EBV infection of a B-cell that already carries a translocated *MYC* allele may provide a critical step needed to advance the targeted cell along the lymphomagenesis pathway. However, given the extremely low frequency of these *MYC*/Ig-bearing cells, this particular mechanism would seem unlikely to be a viable means for EBV to contribute to BL.

The current "working" model for the establishment of a normal persistent infection is that upon infection of a naive B-cell, the growth or type III program of EBV latency (Table 1) drives an expansion of infected B-cells, which subsequently are able to enter a GC reaction (Fig. 3). This would enable further expansion of the infected-cell pool, perhaps upon downregulation of growth-promoting EBV genes, as expression of the LMP-1 protein appears to be incompatible with GC formation (154). Ultimately, establishment of latency within a long-lived B-cell population would occur upon differentiation of infected GC B-cells into memory B-cells, which limit EBV gene expression to LMP-2A and the EBER RNAs, though upon periodic division, activation of EBNA-1 expression ensures against loss of the EBV genome (Table 1) (127,132,133).

Conclusive evidence that EBV primarily enters the memory cell pool by promoting a GC reaction, however, has been elusive, and is confounded by several observations that are inconsistent with such a function mediated by EBV. This problem has been addressed primarily by assessment of EBV gene expression and the B-cell type infected within tonsils obtained from acute infectious mononucleosis (IM) and non-IM patients (129,155–157). First, it is clear that naive cells are not the only B-cells infected by EBV during primary infection, and that the resulting pattern of EBV latency–gene expression is complex and depends on the differentiation state of the infected cell, with the growth program of latency probably occurring only upon infection of a resting naïve (IgD$^+$) B-cell (158,159). Further, two observations argue against direct involvement of EBV in a GC reaction: (i) EBV-positive B-cells infrequently appear within the GCs themselves, but instead predominate within the interfollicular region and (ii) those that are present and expanding within GCs are not undergoing somatic hypermutation of Ig V genes (156), and thus are not participating in a classic GC reaction (151). Despite the observation that EBV-positive B-cells within the GC do not support ongoing hypermutation, they do harbor somatically mutated V gene rearrangements, suggesting at least that EBV may gain entry into GC (or memory) B-cells by direct infection, and that this pool of infected cells expands without further hypermutation (156). The latter observation also suggests that EBV may actually interfere with the GC reaction by suppressing somatic hypermutation, though one study employing BL cell lines that constitutively hypermutate their Ig gene V regions has demonstrated that EBV is unable to inhibit this process (131). An obvious caveat to these interpretations is that EBV infection of such tonsillar B-cells during either acute IM or the tonsillitis that prompted their resection may not be representative of the normal pathway through which EBV gains entry into the memory B-cell pool, if that is indeed through direct participation in a GC reaction.

Evidence for Direct Contribution to the Tumorigenic Phenotype

Active participation of EBV in lymphomagenesis leading to BL would, by definition, require the action of at least one EBV gene product, presumably one that is expressed during latent infection. Although BL cells themselves express a limited repertoire of EBV genes, this does not necessarily exclude important contributions from other viral genes that may have contributed to the founding events of lymphomagenesis, e.g., inhibition of MYC-induced apoptosis prior to inactivation of the p53 tumor suppressor pathway, but whose expression is ultimately silenced. Because the identity of the true BL progenitor cell and the EBV genes that are expressed within it are currently unclear, evaluation of the direct contribution of EBV to BL has focused on those genes expressed in group I BL cell lines, namely, EBNA-1, the EBERs, and the BARTs.

The Akata BL Cell System

Some of the most informative studies of late to address the role of EBV and individual EBV genes in BL have come from analyses of the Akata BL cell line. For reasons unknown, Akata cells spontaneously lose the EBV genome and their tumorigenic potential (160). Importantly, upon reinfection and establishment of a type I latency program in EBV-negative Akata cells, tumorigenicity is restored, providing definitive evidence that this subgroup of EBV genes thought not to directly contribute to growth transformation of B-cells in vitro can contribute to oncogenic potential, at least in the setting of BL (89,90). The Akata cell system, therefore, offers a unique cell model to directly address contributions of the EBV genes expressed during type I latency to the malignant phenotype of BL.

Two events, both with antiapoptotic consequences, have been identified in analyses of Akata BL cells that could contribute to their EBV-dependent tumorigenic potential. These are an apparent virus-mediated upregulation of Bcl-2 expression, and a downregulation of MYC levels under growth-restrictive conditions (89,90). Stable expression of higher levels of Bcl-2 in EBV-negative Akata cells at levels comparable to that seen in their EBV-positive counterparts increases tumorigenic potential (161) (Ruf IK, Sample JT, unpublished observation). However, the tumorigenic potential of these cells does not rise to the level maintained by their EBV-positive counterparts, suggesting that an additional event(s) (perhaps the downregulation of MYC expression under proapoptotic conditions) is required to obtain their full tumorigenic potential associated with EBV infection. Increased tumorigenic potential of BL cells as a result of Bcl-2 overexpression is consistent with the early observations of Strasser et al. (83) that the antiapoptotic Bcl-2 protein can complement c-Myc in B-cell tumorigenesis in vivo. Whereas one group has reported that reinfection of EBV-negative Akata cells promotes higher Bcl-2 expression (90), we have found that reinfection does not consistently result in higher Bcl-2 levels, though it does regularly increase their resistance to apoptosis induced by serum withdrawal, even in the absence of an apparent Bcl-2 induction (89). Further, Akata cells are somewhat unique in this respect as Bcl-2 levels within group I BL lines are typically very low or undetectable. Thus, it would seem unlikely that induction of Bcl-2 expression is a mechanism through which EBV consistently contributes to maintenance of the tumorigenic phenotype of BL.

The EBV-dependent downregulation of MYC levels in Akata and other group I BL cell lines under growth-restrictive culture conditions (88) could contribute to tumorigenic potential by limiting the proapoptotic tendencies of MYC under conditions, such as those in a growing tumor, that would otherwise favor apoptosis. Although the mechanism through which the virus accomplishes this has yet to be defined, it does appear to be mediated post-transcriptionally and is not the result of a decrease in the $t_{1/2}$ of MYC (89). Directly targeting MYC expression to reduce its apoptotic potential, as opposed to upregulating antiapoptotic proteins, e.g., Bcl-2 family members, would clearly be a novel mechanism to promote the tumorigenic phenotype, though the finding that the ARF-HDM2-p53 pathway is frequently disrupted in BL indicates that this may be more of a fine-tuning mechanism than a pivotal event in BL lymphomagenesis. Nonetheless, due to a missense mutation, Akata cells are null for p53 (97), and, thus, inhibition of p53-independent mechanisms of apoptosis would also appear to be critical to development of BL.

EBNA-1

Of the six-member family of EBNAs, EBNA-1 is the only one that is routinely expressed in BL. Furthermore, it is the only known EBV protein expressed in all EBV-associated tumors, potentially implicating a role for EBNA-1 in tumorigenesis. While the genome-maintenance functions of EBNA-1 are unquestionably essential for sustaining latent infection in BL cells, whether EBNA-1 contributes directly to the oncogenic potential of EBV has been a longstanding question within the field, and one with often-conflicting answers. Through its ability in part to bind to DNA in a sequence-specific manner within the EBV origin of episomal DNA replication (*oriP*) (162), EBNA-1 is also able to activate transcription of latency-gene promoters, including the promoter Cp that regulates transcription of the multicistronic EBNA gene (163–165). EBNA-1 is also able to negatively regulate its own expression through two EBNA-1 binding sites within the EBNA-1–specific promoter Qp that is silent during the type III or growth program of EBV latency (Cp active), but responsible for driving EBNA-1 expression in all EBV-associated tumors and proliferating normal B-cells in which Cp has been silenced (166–168). Theoretically, as a transcription factor, EBNA-1 could contribute to tumorigenesis by either positively or negatively regulating cellular gene expression. There are conflicting reports, however, of whether EBNA-1 is able to directly activate transcription of nonepisomal templates (i.e., cellular genes) (169,170), and recent mRNA profiling experiments have failed to identify significant effects of EBNA-1 on cellular gene expression (170), though EBNA-1 has been demonstrated to increase expression of RAG, Bcl-X_L, and CD25 (note that RAG and CD25 genes were not represented on the arrays used in the profiling study quoted) (62,65,170).

In EBV-negative Akata BL cells, stable expression of EBNA-1 fails to confer the survival functions associated with EBV infection of these cells and, perhaps consequently, does not enhance their tumorigenic potential (89,90). Thus, it would seem that EBNA-1 alone does not contribute significantly to the EBV-dependent tumorigenic potential of Akata BL cells through antiapoptotic or other means. A recent report from Sugden and coworkers, however, suggests that EBNA-1 can provide a survival (antiapoptotic) signal to Akata and other BL cell lines (172). These effects of EBNA-1 were observed following ectopic expression of a dominant negative form of the protein that interferes with EBNA-1 activation of transcription. Although it seems unlikely that this survival function contributes significantly to the tumorigenicity of BL cells given previous demonstrations that EBNA-1 does not increase the tumorigenic potential of EBV-negative Akata cells, it could conceivably play an important role earlier in lymphomagenesis.

The strongest evidence to date to support a direct role of EBNA-1 in tumorigenesis would appear to come from the analyses of EBNA-1 transgenic mice by Wilson and coworkers (173,174). In 10 lines of mice generated on the C57BL/6 background in which B-cell–specific expression of EBNA-1 is under control of the Eμ heavy chain enhancer, two lines developed B-cell lymphomas at 4 to 24 months of age (the remaining eight lines did not detectably express the transgene, and exhibited no pathology) (174). The two transgenic lines that did develop tumors (designated 26 and 59) were considerably different in terms of penetrance and latency period prior to onset of disease: line 26 was fully penetrant with mice succumbing to lymphoma within 4 to 12 months (mean: 200 days, median: 235 days), whereas within line 59, 43% of all mice developed lymphoma by 24 months (6% of control mice also developed lymphoma during this time interval). Notably, while levels of steady-state transgene RNA correlated with the degree of the neoplastic phenotype, an inverse relationship between the levels of EBNA-1 protein and the penetrance of the disease was found to exist, raising the possibility that lymphomas were not a direct consequence of EBNA-1 function but of transgene insertion. Subsequent studies performed to investigate potential oncogenic mechanisms in these EBNA-1 transgenic mice found that while EBNA-1 and Bcl-2 are redundant in lymphomagenesis, EBNA-1 and c-Myc appear to cooperate, implying a survival role for EBNA-1 that is consistent with the apparent upregulation of Bcl-X_L in these studies (65,173). Evidence of an oncogenic role for EBNA-1, however, has not been observed in three independently derived transgenic lines (on the FVB genetic background) that express EBNA-1 in mature B-cells near levels seen in latently infected B-cell lines (Kieff E, personal communication, 2003). Thus, whether EBNA-1 plays any role in BL other than through its requirement for maintaining the EBV genome within tumor cells is an unresolved question.

EBER-1 and EBER-2

EBER-1 and EBER-2 are small noncoding RNAs of 167 and 172 nucleotides, respectively, whose tandemly arranged genes are transcribed by cellular RNA polymerase III (Pol III) (175–177). They are expressed within latently infected cells at approximately 10^7 copies per cell (EBER-1 levels are roughly 10-fold EBER-2 levels) and are present predominantly within the cell nucleus in complexes with the cellular protein La/SS-B (175,178). The EBERs are expressed in all latently infected cell lines and tumors, and are detectable as well within the memory B-cell pool that normally serves as the long-term reservoir of EBV in healthy individuals (132,179). Most importantly, the EBERs are able to significantly enhance the tumorigenic potential of EBV-negative Akata BL cells (180,181), as well as the EBV-negative B-lymphoma cell line BJAB (182). Whether one or both EBER species are required to achieve this effect has not been determined, and the mechanism(s) through which these small RNAs contribute to tumorigenic potential is currently unclear.

There are conflicting reports as to whether the EBERs enhance tumorigenic potential by promoting cell survival. One group has attributed the higher levels of Bcl-2 expression and enhanced cell survival demonstrated by EBV-positive relative to EBV-negative Akata cells to expression of the EBERs (180). These conclusions are based on the observation of these apparent EBV-dependent effects in two EBV-negative Akata cell lines that stably express both EBERs. In contrast, after examining approximately one dozen independently derived EBV–/EBER+ Akata cell lines, we found no consistent upregulation of Bcl-2 that could be attributed to the EBERs, because vector-control lines were as likely as the EBER-expressing lines to have elevated levels of Bcl-2 (181). Although modest upregulation of Bcl-2 as observed in EBV-positive versus EBV-negative Akata cells can promote cell survival and tumorigenic potential (see above), whether this is an EBER-dependent mechanism seems doubtful. Perhaps consistent with this conclusion is the finding that the EBERs, when expressed in EBV-negative Akata cells, do not affect MYC levels or enhance cell survival under growth-restrictive conditions as demonstrated for EBV infection (181). Moreover, the effect of EBER expression on the tumorigenic potential of EBV-negative Akata cells, like that of elevated Bcl-2 levels, is partial relative to EBV infection (181). Thus, multiple EBV gene products likely contribute to maintenance of the tumorigenic phenotype of Akata and presumably other EBV-positive BLs.

If the EBERs do not contribute to tumorigenic potential by promoting cell survival, upregulation of Bcl-2, modulation of MYC expression, or through other means, then what might their contribution be? Three EBER–protein interactions have been described that may shed light on this question. The cellular proteins targeted are the nuclear protein La/SS-B (178), the ribosomal protein L22, also known as EBER-associated protein (183–185), and the double-stranded RNA (dsRNA)-dependent/activated protein kinase, PKR (186,187). La is critical for the nuclear processing of small cellular transcripts generated by Pol III, e.g., transfer RNAs (tRNAs) (188–190). By binding to the UUU-OH component at the $3'$ termini of these RNAs, the transcripts are protected from exonucleolytic digestion and retained within the nucleus until processing is complete. Unlike some cellular Pol III transcripts bound by La (e.g., tRNAs), the EBER transcripts stably associate with La, which presumably serves to retain the EBERs within the nucleus (175,191). La, a fraction of which is believed to shuttle to the cell cytoplasm, has also been implicated in translation of several cellular and viral messenger RNAs (mRNAs) (188), e.g., cellular Mdm2 and X-linked inhibitor of apoptosis (XIAP) synthesis is enhanced through the interaction of La with the 5′ untranslated region (UTR) of the *mdm2* mRNA and promotion of internal ribosome entry–mediated translation of XIAP, respectively (192,193). It has also been proposed that La enhances the synthesis of ribosomal and other proteins involved in protein synthesis through an interaction with the 5′-terminal oligopyrimidine motif in their mRNAs (194). Whether EBER interaction with La significantly affects La-mediated cellular processes is unknown, though we have observed no effect on XIAP expression in the presence of the EBERs under conditions reported to influence XIAP regulation by La (Ruf IK, Sample JT, unpublished observations).

The ability of the EBERs, which have extensive secondary structure (175), to interact with PKR and inhibit its activation in vitro is well documented (186,187,195,196). However, it is unclear whether EBERs significantly influence PKR activity in vivo. Specifically, the predominantly nuclear localization of the EBERs during latent infection (191) would argue against significant inhibition of the activation and thus function of PKR, which is primarily cytoplasmic and requires a relatively high concentration of dsRNA to saturate its dsRNA-binding sites to prevent dsRNA-mediated autoactivation. Recent experiments have demonstrated that within cell lysates or in cells transiently overexpressing PKR following transfection by electroporation, EBERs are able to inhibit PKR activation and phosphorylation of its primary known target, the translation initiation factor eukaryotic initiation factor 2α (eIF-2α) (182,197). Unfortunately, interpretation of these results is confounded by either an obvious (in cell lysates) or likely (following electroporation) corruption within these assays of the nuclear localization of the EBERs.

As dominant negative forms of PKR are tumorigenic (198,199), the promotion of tumorigenic potential by the EBERs could occur through their inhibition of PKR function. PKR is best known for its antiviral role, mediated through inhibition of cap-dependent initiation of mRNA translation as a consequence of eIF-2α phosphorylation (200). PKR expression and activation are also inducible with interferon (201). EBER inhibition of PKR activation during an antiviral interferon response to latent EBV infection, therefore, could have important implications for EBV persistence, in addition to maintenance of a tumor phenotype. However, replication of vesicular stomatitis virus, which is sensitive to the actions of PKR and interferon-alpha, is equivalent within LCLs that carry either a latent infection with wt EBV or a recombinant EBV that lacks the EBER genes, in either the absence or presence of interferon-alpha (202). Thus, whether the EBERs truly inhibit PKR function in vivo, either in response to interferon or during normal latency within BL cells, awaits definitive demonstration.

Within latently infected B-cell lines, interaction of the L22 ribosomal protein with the EBER-1 RNA results in redistribution of approximately 50% of the cellular pool of L22 from the cytoplasm and nucleolus (the site of ribosome biogenesis) to the nucleoplasm (185). Because this is a selective interaction of L22 with the third and possibly fourth stem-loop of the EBER-1 molecule, i.e., it is sequence and/or secondary-structure specific (184,203), it would appear that this EBV RNA has evolved to specifically target L22. Presumably, this would affect the ability of L22 to perform its normal function in protein synthesis, though attempts thus far to consistently demonstrate a significant decrease in polysome-associated L22 within latently infected B-cells have been inconclusive (185). L22 lies within the exit tunnel of mature ribosomes, and within the *Escherichia coli* ribosome, acts as a discriminating gate to regulate the passage of nascent polypeptides containing the amino acid sequence FXXXXWIXXXXGIRAGP (X is any amino acid) in the secretion monitor protein, secM (204,205). An attractive hypothesis, therefore, is that redistribution of L22 (from the ribosome fraction) by EBER-1 results in altered synthesis of a subgroup of cellular proteins, the collective consequence of which is an enhanced tumorigenic potential in the setting of BL and perhaps other EBV-associated tumors. Although searches of the protein database have failed to identify mammalian polypeptides containing the motif present in the *E. coli* secM protein targeted by L22, this is not entirely unexpected given the evolutionary divergence between mammalian and prokaryotic L22 proteins, and predictably their respective target polypeptides.

Alternatively, interaction of EBER-1 with a subfraction of the cellular L22 pool may serve to influence a nonribosomal function of L22. In this respect, it is interesting to note that L22 also interacts with the immediate-early proteins ICP4 and ICP22 of the alphaherpesvirus herpes simplex virus-1 (HSV-1) and the ICP4 homolog encoded by the equine herpesvirus 1 (206–208). Because of the transcriptional regulatory nature of these viral proteins, these interactions may imply that L22 has functions distinct from its role in protein synthesis. It is also conceivable that an interaction of a viral gene product with L22 could impart a gain-of-function upon L22. Regardless, the fact that L22 is specifically targeted by at least four herpesvirus gene products—three of which are proteins and one an RNA—suggests that modulation of L22 function(s) plays biologically relevant, though likely distinct, roles in herpesvirus lifecycles. For EBV, this role may influence the tumorigenic potential of BL and other EBV-associated tumors.

BARTs

The BARTs are a family of alternatively spliced, polyadenylated RNAs, whose protein-coding potential is currently a matter of some debate. Although they appear to be most highly expressed within nasopharyngeal carcinoma cells, in which they were first identified (209,210), they are detectable in all latently infected cell lines, EBV-positive tumors, and normal peripheral-blood B-cells that harbor EBV (139,211–213). Like the EBERs, they are nonessential for EBV immortalization of B-cells in vitro (214) and thus a contribution of the BARTs to tumorigenesis is not necessarily intuitive. The finding that the EBERs and EBNA-1 together do not confer the same degree of tumorigenic potential as EBV infection on Akata BL cells (181) suggests the contribution of an additional EBV gene product. Because the BARTs are the only other EBV gene products known to be consistently expressed in BL, they are obvious candidates.

The fact that these transcripts encode protein is supported indirectly by two forms of experimental data. First, antibodies have been detected in the serum of nasopharyngeal carcinoma (NPC) patients to a polypeptide encoded by the BARF0 open reading frame (ORF) within the common 3′ termini of the BARTs (215). Unfortunately, it has not been possible to definitively identify this or other endogenous BART-encoded proteins within infected cells, and attempts thus far to stably express these proteins in EBV-negative Akata cells have not been successful, as they appear to not be tolerated at levels readily detected by standard immunodetection techniques. Second, studies employing two-hybrid screens to identify cellular proteins that interact with the putative protein products of three BART ORFs have demonstrated that two, RPMS1 and RK-BARF0, interact with components of the Notch signaling pathway: RBP-Jκ and its associated corepressor CIR, and Notch4, respectively (216–218). The third BART protein, encoded by the A73 ORF, interacts with the cellular protein receptor for activated protein kinase C (RACK1), a scaffolding protein that serves as the cytoplasmic receptor for protein kinase C (216).

While demonstration of a protein–protein interaction itself does not confirm that any of these proteins are actually expressed during EBV infection, the interaction of BART-encoded proteins with components of the Notch pathway may be particularly relevant given that it is targeted by four known EBV latency–associated proteins. The EBNA-2, EBNA-3A, EBNA-3B, and EBNA-3C proteins all interact with the DNA-binding protein RBP-Jκ (alternatively known as CBF1 (219–222), which targets transcriptional coactivators and corepressors to the promoters of Notch-regulated genes. Analogously, interaction of these EBNA proteins with RBP-Jκ permits positive and negative regulation of transcription of the EBNA and LMP genes (the promoters for which have RBP-Jκ binding sites) by EBNA-2 and the EBNA-3 proteins, respectively, during the growth or type III program of EBV latency (220,221,223–227). Based on promoter studies in transient transfection assays (228), EBNA–RBP-Jκ interactions are also likely to regulate cellular target genes of the Notch pathway, though this largely awaits the identification of Notch-regulated genes.

First described as a developmental network in *Drosophila*, the Notch pathway is now known to control diverse aspects of mammalian cell development and tissue homeostasis, including a role in antiapoptosis, and is often subverted in cancer (229,230). Various signaling components within this pathway are targeted by no less than four EBV latency proteins, strongly suggesting that regulation by EBV is critical to latency. This lends credence to the likelihood that the RPMS1 and RK-BARF0 ORFs do indeed encode proteins and that they may be critical for regulation of events within the Notch pathway. The interaction of the RPMS1 protein with RBP-Jκ and CIR has been proposed to repress promoters containing RBP-Jκ binding sites by stabilizing this repressor complex on the DNA (217). By contrast, EBNA-3 proteins are believed to repress transcription by interfering with RBP-Jκ binding to the promoter (220,221), thus preventing recruitment of activators, e.g., EBNA-2 and its associated coactivators, to the promoter. The interaction between RK-BARF0 and Notch4 results in translocation of the unprocessed form of Notch4 directly into the nucleus (218). This complex is believed to bind to and activate the LMP-1 promoter in the absence of EBNA-2, e.g., in tumors such as Hodgkin's lymphoma and nasopharyngeal carcinoma, which must express LMP-1 independently of EBNA-2 during type II latency. Although the capacity of the BARTs to encode proteins that interact with and usurp or redirect the function of cellular proteins in the Notch pathway may underlie their potential contribution to tumorigenesis, this awaits formal confirmation. Finally, the normal cellular pathways mediated through RACK1, a scaffold protein that links protein kinase C to many of its substrates, may be disrupted as a result of the demonstrated interaction between the BART-encoded A73 protein and RACK1 (216). Furthermore, RACK1 has been shown to interact with the tyrosine kinases Lck and Src and to inhibit their activities (231), suggesting a possible mechanism for A73 promotion of BL tumorigenic potential.

Alternatively, it has been proposed that the BARTs may negatively regulate, through transcriptional interference or an antisense mechanism, the expression of EBV transcripts that originate from the DNA strand complementary to that which encodes the BARTs—hence their alternative designation of complementary-strand transcripts (232). These potential gene targets of the BARTs are characteristically expressed during the EBV lytic cycle, implying that any negative effect on their expression by the BARTs is for the purpose of interfering with reactivation of the virus in latently infected cells that would be counterproductive to tumorigenesis. However, currently there are no published studies to support such a mechanism of BART function.

PROSPECTS FOR FUTURE DISCOVERY

Clearly there is still much to learn about the biology of BL—from the role of EBV and other infectious agents that most certainly play a part in pathogenesis, to the factors that underlie the differences among the various BL subtypes. From the perspective of EBV infection, the elucidation of EBER functions promises to provide significant insight into EBV's unexpected role in maintenance of the tumorigenic phenotype and whether this role will be important in EBV-positive BLs as a rule, or only in a subset of these tumors. Furthermore, there is good reason to believe that additional EBV genes play significant roles. Will these prove to be the BARTs—long studied but poorly understood—or a latency gene, possibly a novel one, whose expression in BL has thus far gone unrecognized? Moreover, this need not be a strictly latency-associated gene, but perhaps an aberrantly expressed gene of the EBV lytic cycle. Through the use of viral DNA microarrays, it should be a relatively straightforward endeavor to address these possibilities by screening the entire EBV genome for expression within group I BL lines and tumor biopsies.

Another area of research that could potentially yield significant insight into the role of EBV involves an innovative use of two available animal models that have not been previously exploited for this purpose. Firstly, the Eμ-*myc* transgenic mouse has provided a wealth of information on the genetic and biochemical pathways critical for c-Myc–induced B-cell lymphomagenesis. Importantly, much of this information acquired thus far is consistent with human BL given the striking parallels, for example, in the frequency and manner in which the ARF-HDM2/Mdm2-p53 tumor suppressor pathway is targeted. However, as we have discussed, there are differences that, potentially, could reflect the absence of the EBV component of BL in mouse tumors. It is technically feasible to test this by introducing the candidate EBV genes into the B-cells of this mouse model or into the more recently described Igλ-*MYC* transgenic mouse model of BL (82). Although there is the possibility that EBV genes will not function appropriately in the context of a mouse B-cell, the opportunity for a significant payoff is inviting. Secondly, a combination of the rhesus macaque models of malaria and EBV infection could test the long-standing hypothesis that malaria and EBV infection are important cofactors in the development of eBL. This model of EBV infection employs the endogenous *Lymphocryptovirus* of macaques (Cercopithecine herpesvirus 15), which is the biological equivalent to EBV in this primate model (233). Although macaque models of malaria that employ various simian *Plasmodium* species may not display clinical courses completely identical to *P. falciparum* malaria in man (234), and the cost of such studies could be substantial given the number of animals that may have to be coinfected to establish whether there is a significant correlation, a successful test of this hypothesis would be particularly satisfying given the 40 or so years that have passed since the link between malaria and EBV infection in eBL was first conceived.

Finally, what is the basis for the different subtypes of BL? The collective answer to this question will likely provide the "big picture" of BL pathogenesis, and will only come from a much better understanding of the contributions of

EBV and other environmental cofactors, and a thorough knowledge of the genetic and biochemical differences exhibited by the different tumor subtypes. As has now been demonstrated for a number of human cancers, much of the latter information could be extracted through the use of mRNA (and also protein) profiling of actual tumor material. A thorough evaluation of all BL subtypes for the alterations in tumor suppressor pathways previously noted in BL is also warranted, because this information is currently incomplete, particularly for the nonendemic BLs. Moreover, many of these analyses have been primarily restricted to cell lines that are not necessarily representative of the tumors from which they had been derived. We expect, furthermore, that the mouse models of c-Myc–induced B lymphomagenesis will continue to play an important role here, particularly in defining the contributions of newly implicated disease mechanisms and molecular networks in BL.

FURTHER READING

This chapter represents our attempt to cover what we believe are currently the most salient aspects of BL, with an emphasis on the role of EBV. We suggest the following works for additional reading, as they cover in considerable detail a number of points of interest and importance to BL that could only be touched upon here.

Hecht JL, Aster JC. Molecular biology of Burkitt's lymphoma. J Clin Oncol 2000; 18:3707–3721.
Küppers R, Dalla-Favera R. Mechanisms of chromosomal translocations in B-cell lymphomas. Oncogene 2001; 20:5580–5594.
Magrath I. The pathogenesis of Burkitt lymphoma. Adv Cancer Res 1990; 55:133–270.
Nilsson JA, Cleveland JL. Myc pathways provoking cell suicide and cancer. Oncogene 2003; 22:9007–9021.

REFERENCES

1. Magrath I. The pathogenesis of Burkitt's lymphoma. Adv Cancer Res 1990; 55:133–270.
2. Burkitt DP. A sarcoma involving the jaws in African children. Br J Surg 1958; 45: 218–223.
3. Bellan C, Lazzi S, De Falco G, Nyongo A, Giordano A, Leoncini L. Burkitt's lymphoma: new insights into molecular pathogenesis. J Clin Pathol 2003; 56(3):188–192.
4. Epstein MA, Achong BG, Barr YM. Virus particles in cultured lymphoblasts from Burkitt's lymphoma. Lancet 1964; 1:702–703.
5. Neri A, Barriga F, Inghirami G, et al. Epstein–Barr virus infection precedes clonal expansion in Burkitt's and acquired immunodeficiency syndrome-associated lymphoma [see comments]. Blood 1991; 77(5):1092–1095.
6. Hecht JL, Aster JC. Molecular biology of Burkitt's lymphoma. J Clin Oncol 2000; 18(21):3707–3721.
7. Karajannis MA, Hummel M, Oschlies I, et al. Epstein–Barr virus infection in Western European pediatric non-Hodgkin lymphomas. Blood 2003; 102(12):4244.
8. Araujo I, Foss HD, Bittencourt A, et al. Expression of Epstein–Barr virus-gene products in Burkitt's lymphoma in Northeast Brazil. Blood 1996; 87(12):5279–5286.
9. Sandlund JT, Fonseca T, Leimig T, et al. Predominance and characteristics of Burkitt lymphoma among children with non-Hodgkin lymphoma in northeastern Brazil. Leukemia 1997; 11:743–746.

10. Bacchi MM, Bacchi CE, Alvarenga M, Miranda R, Chen YY, Weiss LM. Burkitt's lymphoma in Brazil: strong association with Epstein–Barr virus. Mod Pathol 1996; 9:63–67.
11. Gutierrez MI, Bhatia K, Barriga F, et al. Molecular epidemiology of Burkitt's lymphoma from South America: differences in breakpoint location and Epstein–Barr virus association from tumors in other world regions. Blood 1992; 79:3261–3266.
12. Blum KA, Lozanski G, Byrd JC. Adult Burkitt leukemia and lymphoma. Blood 2004; 104(10):3009–3020.
13. Magrath IT, Sariban E. Clinical features of Burkitt's lymphoma in the U.S.A. IARC Sci Publ 1985:119–127.
14. Davi F, Delecluse HJ, Guiet P, et al. Burkitt-like lymphomas in AIDS patients: characterization within a series of 103 human immunodeficiency virus-associated non-Hodgkin's lymphomas. Burkitt's Lymphoma Study Group. J Clin Oncol 1998; 16(12):3788–3795.
15. Diebold J, Raphael M, Prevot S, Audouin J. Lymphomas associated with HIV infection. Cancer Surv 1997; 30:263–293.
16. Spina M, Tirelli U, Zagonel V, et al. Burkitt's lymphoma in adults with and without human immunodeficiency virus infection: a single-institution clinicopathologic study of 75 patients. Cancer 1998; 82:766–774.
17. Sariban E, Edwards B, Janus C, Magrath I. Central nervous system involvement in American Burkitt's lymphoma. J Clin Oncol 1983; 1:677–681.
18. Ladjadj Y, Philip T, Lenoir GM, et al. Abdominal Burkitt-type lymphomas in Algeria. Br J Cancer 1984; 49:503–512.
19. Rao CR, Gutierrez MI, Bhatia K, et al. Association of Burkitt's lymphoma with the Epstein–Barr virus in two developing countries. Leuk Lymphoma 2000; 39(3–4): 329–337; 2000; 39:329–337.
20. Burkitt DP. A children's cancer dependent upon climatic factors. Nature 1962; 194: 232–234.
21. Burkitt DP. Epidemiology of Burkitt's lymphoma. Proc R Soc Med JID-7505890 1971; 64(9):909–910.
22. Burkitt DP. Etiology of Burkitt's lymphoma—an alternative hypothesis to a vectored virus. J Natl Cancer Inst 1969; 42:19–28.
23. Facer CA, Playfair JH. Malaria, Epstein–Barr virus, and the genesis of lymphomas. Adv Cancer Res 1989; 53:33–72.
24. Whittle HC, Brown J, Marsh K, et al. T cell control of Epstein–Barr virus-infected B cells is lost during *P. falciparum* malaria. Nature 1984; 312:449–450.
25. Urban BC, Roberts DJ. Inhibition of T cell function during malaria: implications for immunology and vaccinology. J Exp Med 2003; 197(2):137–141.
26. Hisaeda H, Maekawa Y, Iwakawa D, et al. Escape of malaria parasites from host immunity requires CD4(+)CD25(+) regulatory T cells. Nat Med 2004; 10(1):29–30; Epub 2003 Dec 21, 2004; 10:29–30.
27. Lam KM, Syed N, Whittle H, Crawford DH. Circulating Epstein–Barr virus-carrying B-cells in acute malaria. Lancet 1991; 337(8746):876–878.
28. Rickinson A, Kieff E. Epstein–Barr virus. In: Knipe DM, et al. eds. Fields Virology. 4th[2] ed. Philadelphia, PA: Lippincott Williams & Wilkins, 2001:2575–2628.
29. Greenwood BM, Vick RM. Evidence for a malaria mitogen in human malaria. Nature 1975; 257:592–594.
30. Alitalo K, Bishop JM, Smith DH, Chen EY, Colby WW, Levinson AD. Nucleotide sequence to the v-myc oncogene of avian retrovirus MC29. Proc Natl Acad Sci USA 1983; 80:100–104.
31. Sheiness D, Bishop JM. DNA and RNA from uninfected vertebrate cells contain nucleotide sequences related to the putative transforming gene of avian myelocytomatosis virus. J Virol 1979; 31:514–521.
32. Nilsson JA, Cleveland JL. Myc pathways provoking cell suicide and cancer. Oncogene 2003; 22(56):9007–9021.

33. Blackwell TK, Huang J, Ma A, et al. Binding of myc proteins to canonical and noncanonical DNA sequences. Mol Cell Biol 1993; 13:5216–5224.
34. Blackwell TK, Kretzner L, Blackwood EM, Eisenman RN, Weintraub H. Sequence-specific DNA binding by the c-Myc protein. Science 1990; 250:1149–1151.
35. Prendergast GC, Ziff EB. Methylation-sensitive sequence-specific DNA binding by the c-Myc basic region. Science 1991; 251:186–189.
36. Blackwood EM, Luscher B, Eisenman RN. Myc and Max associate in vivo. Genes Dev 1992; 6:71–80.
37. Blackwood EM, Eisenman RN. Max: a helix-loop-helix zipper protein that forms a sequence-specific DNA-binding complex with Myc. Science 1991; 251:1211–1217.
38. Dugan KA, Wood MA, Cole MD. TIP49, but not TRRAP, modulates c-Myc and E2F1 dependent apoptosis. Oncogene 2002; 21(38):5835–5843.
39. Park J, Wood MA, Cole MD. BAF53 forms distinct nuclear complexes and functions as a critical c-Myc-interacting nuclear cofactor for oncogenic transformation. Mol Cell Biol 2002; 22:1307–1316.
40. Park J, Kunjibettu S, McMahon SB, Cole MD. The ATM-related domain of TRRAP is required for histone acetyltransferase recruitment and Myc-dependent oncogenesis. Genes Dev 2001; 15:1619–1624.
41. McMahon SB, Wood MA, Cole MD. The essential cofactor TRRAP recruits the histone acetyltransferase hGCN5 to c-Myc. Mol Cell Biol 2000; 20:556–562.
42. McMahon SB, Van Buskirk HA, Dugan KA, Copeland TD, Cole MD. The novel ATM-related protein TRRAP is an essential cofactor for the c-Myc and E2F oncoproteins. Cell 1998; 94:363–374.
43. http://www.myc-cancer-gene.org.
44. Bhatia K, Spangler G, Gaidano G, Hamdy N, Dalla-Favera R, Magrath I. Mutations in the coding region of c-myc occur frequently in acquired immunodeficiency syndrome-associated lymphomas. Blood 1994; 84:883–888.
45. Bhatia K, Huppi K, Spangler G, Siwarski D, Iyer R, Magrath I. Point mutations in the c-Myc transactivation domain are common in Burkitt's lymphoma and mouse plasmacytomas. Nat Genet 1993; 5:56–61.
46. Gregory MA, Hann SR. c-Myc proteolysis by the ubiquitin-proteasome pathway: stabilization of c-Myc in Burkitt's lymphoma cells [In Process Citation]. Mol Cell Biol 2000; 20(7):2423–2435.
47. Bahram F, von der LN, Cetinkaya C, Larsson LG. c-Myc hot spot mutations in lymphomas result in inefficient ubiquitination and decreased proteasome-mediated turnover. Blood 2000; 95(6):2104–2110.
48. Pelicci PG, Knowles DM, Magrath I, Dalla-Favera R. Chromosomal breakpoints and structural alterations of the c-myc locus differ in endemic and sporadic forms of Burkitt lymphoma. Proc Natl Acad Sci USA 1986; 83:2984–2988.
49. Neri A, Barriga F, Knowles DM, Magrath IT, Dalla-Favera R. Different regions of the immunoglobulin heavy-chain locus are involved in chromosomal translocations in distinct pathogenetic forms of Burkitt lymphoma. Proc Natl Acad Sci USA 1988; 85:2748–2752.
50. Shiramizu B, Barriga F, Neequaye J, et al. Patterns of chromosomal breakpoint locations in Burkitt's lymphoma: relevance to geography and Epstein–Barr virus association. Blood 1991; 77:1516–1526.
51. Joos S, Haluska FG, Falk MH, et al. Mapping chromosomal breakpoints of Burkitt's t(8;14) translocations far upstream of c-myc. Cancer Res 1992; 52:6547–6552.
52. Joos S, Falk MH, Lichter P, et al. Variable breakpoints in Burkitt lymphoma cells with chromosomal t(8;14). translocations for upstream of c-myc. Cancer Res 1992; 1:625–632.
53. Gerbitz A, Mautner J, Geltinger C, et al. Deregulation of the proto-oncogene c-myc through t(8;22) translocation in Burkitt's lymphoma. Oncogene 1999; 18:1745–1753.

54. Bross L, Fukita Y, McBlane F, Demolliere C, Rajewsky K, Jacobs H. DNA double-strand breaks in immunoglobulin genes undergoing somatic hypermutation. Immunity 2000; 13(5):589–597.

55. Papavasiliou FN, Schatz DG. Cell-cycle-regulated DNA double-stranded breaks in somatic hypermutation of immunoglobulin genes. Nature 2000; 408(6809):216–221.

56. Kuppers R, Dalla-Favera R. Mechanisms of chromosomal translocations in B cell lymphomas. Oncogene 2001; 20(40):5580–5594.

57. Haluska FG, Tsujimoto Y, Croce CM. The t(8;14) chromosome translocation of the Burkitt lymphoma cell line Daudi occurred during immunoglobulin gene rearrangement and involved the heavy chain diversity region. Proc Natl Acad Sci USA 1987; 84:6835–6839.

58. Haluska FG, Finver S, Tsujimoto Y, Croce CM. The t(8; 14) chromosomal translocation occurring in B-cell malignancies results from mistakes in V-D-J joining. Nature 1986; 324:158–161.

59. Hikida M, Mori M, Takai T, Tomochika K, Hamatani K, Ohmori H. Reexpression of RAG-1 and RAG-2 genes in activated mature mouse B cells. Science 1996; 274:2092–2094.

60. Han S, Dillon SR, Zheng B, Shimoda M, Schlissel MS, Kelsoe G. V(D)J recombinase activity in a subset of germinal center B lymphocytes. Science 1997; 278(5336):301–305.

61. Ohmori H, Hikida M. Expression and function of recombination activating genes in mature B cells. Crit Rev Immunol 1998; 18:221–235.

62. Srinivas SK, Sixbey JW. Epstein–Barr virus induction of recombinase-activating genes RAG1 and RAG2. J Virol 1995; 69(12):8155–8158.

63. Kuhn-Hallek I, Sage DR, Stein L, Groelle H, Fingeroth JD. Expression of recombination activating genes (RAG-1 and RAG-2) in Epstein–Barr virus-bearing B cells. Blood 1995; 85:1289–1299.

64. Meru N, Jung A, Lisner R, Niedobitek G. Expression of the recombination activating genes (RAG1 and RAG2) is not detectable in Epstein–Barr virus-associated human lymphomas. Int J Cancer 2001; 92(1):75–78.

65. Tsimbouri P, Drotar ME, Coy JL, Wilson JB. bcl-xL and RAG genes are induced and the response to IL-2 enhanced in EmuEBNA-1 transgenic mouse lymphocytes. Oncogene 2002; 21(33):5182–5187.

66. Roix JJ, McQueen PG, Munson PJ, Parada LA, Misteli T. Spatial proximity of translocation-prone gene loci in human lymphomas. Nat Genet 2003; 34(3):287–291.

67. Jain M, Arvanitis C, Chu K, et al. Sustained loss of a neoplastic phenotype by brief inactivation of MYC. Science 2002; 297(5578):102–104.

68. Felsher DW, Bishop JM. Reversible tumorigenesis by MYC in hematopoietic lineages. Mol Cell 1999; 4:199–207.

69. Hermeking H, Rago C, Schuhmacher M, et al. Identification of CDK4 as a target of c-MYC. Proc Natl Acad Sci USA 2000; 97(5):2229–2234.

70. Mateyak MK, Obaya AJ, Sedivy JM. c-Myc regulates cyclin D-Cdk4 and -Cdk6 activity but affects cell cycle progression at multiple independent points. Mol Cell Biol 1999; 19:4672–4683.

71. Muller D, Bouchard C, Rudolph B, et al. Cdk2-dependent phosphorylation of p27 facilitates its Myc-induced release from cyclin E/cdk2 complexes. Oncogene 1997; 15: 2561–2576.

72. Galaktionov K, Chen X, Beach D. Cdc25 cell-cycle phosphatase as a target of c-myc. Nature 1996; 382:511–517.

73. Baudino TA, McKay C, Pendeville-Samain H, et al. c-Myc is essential for vasculogenesis and angiogenesis during development and tumor progression. Genes Dev 2002; 16(19):2530–2543.

74. Wang J, Xie LY, Allan S, Beach D, Hannon GJ. Myc activates telomerase. Genes Dev 1998; 12(12):1769–1774.

75. Wu KJ, Grandori C, Amacker M, et al. Direct activation of TERT transcription by c-MYC. Nat Genet 1999; 21:220–224.

76. Staege MS, Lee SP, Frisan T, et al. MYC overexpression imposes a nonimmunogenic phenotype on Epstein–Barr virus-infected B cells. PNAS 2002;072495599.

77. Askew DS, Ashmun RA, Simmons BC, Cleveland JL. Constitutive c-myc expression in an IL-3-dependent myeloid cell line suppresses cell cycle arrest and accelerates apoptosis. Oncogene 1991; 6(10):1915–1922.

78. Evan GI, Wyllie AH, Gilbert CS, et al. Induction of apoptosis in fibroblasts by c-myc protein. Cell 1992; 69(1):119–128.

79. Adams JM, Harris AW, Pinkert CA, et al. The c-myc oncogene driven by immunoglobulin enhancers induces lymphoid malignancy in transgenic mice. Nature 1985; 318(6046):533–538.

80. Leder A, Pattengale PK, Kuo A, Stewart TA, Leder P. Consequences of widespread deregulation of the c-myc gene in transgenic mice: multiple neoplasms and normal development. Cell 1986; 45:485–495.

81. Schmidt EV, Pattengale PK, Weir L, Leder P. Transgenic mice bearing the human c-myc gene activated by an immunoglobulin enhancer: a pre-B-cell lymphoma model. Proc Natl Acad Sci USA 1988; 85:6047–6051.

82. Kovalchuk AL, Qi CF, Torrey TA, et al. Burkitt lymphoma in the mouse. J Exp Med 2000; 192(8):1183–1190.

83. Strasser A, Harris AW, Bath ML, Cory S. Novel primitive lymphoid tumours induced in transgenic mice by cooperation between myc and bcl-2. Nature 1990; 348(6299): 331–333.

84. Hsu B, Marin MC, el Naggar AK, Stephens LC, Brisbay S, McDonnell TJ. Evidence that c-myc mediated apoptosis does not require wild-type p53 during lymphomagenesis. Oncogene 1995; 11:175–179.

85. Schmitt CA, McCurrach ME, de Stanchina E, Wallace-Brodeur RR, Lowe SW. INK4a/ARF mutations accelerate lymphomagenesis and promote chemoresistance by disabling p53. Genes Dev 1999; 13(20):2670–2677.

86. Eischen CM, Weber JD, Roussel MF, Sherr CJ, Cleveland JL. Disruption of the ARF-Mdm2-p53 tumor suppressor pathway in Myc-induced lymphomagenesis. Genes Dev 1999; 13(20):2658–2669.

87. Alt JR, Greiner TC, Cleveland JL, Eischen CM. Mdm2 haplo-insufficiency profoundly inhibits Myc-induced lymphomagenesis. EMBO J 2003; 22(6):1442–1450.

88. Eischen CM, Roussel MF, Korsmeyer SJ, Cleveland JL. Bax loss impairs Myc-induced apoptosis and circumvents the selection of p53 mutations during Myc-mediated lymphomagenesis. Mol Cell Biol 2001; 21(22):7653–7662.

89. Ruf IK, Rhyne PW, Yang H, et al. Epstein–Barr virus regulates c-MYC, apoptosis, and tumorigenicity in Burkitt lymphoma. Mol Cell Biol 1999; 19(3):1651–1660.

90. Komano J, Sugiura M, Takada K. Epstein–Barr virus contributes to the malignant phenotype and to apoptosis resistance in Burkitt's lymphoma cell line Akata. J Virol 1998; 72(11):9150–9156.

91. Bhatia KG, Gutierrez MI, Huppi K, Siwarski D, Magrath IT. The pattern of p53 mutations in Burkitt's lymphoma differs from that of solid tumors. Cancer Res 1992; 52:4273–4276.

92. Gaidano G, Ballerini P, Gong JZ, et al. p53 mutations in human lymphoid malignancies: association with Burkitt lymphoma and chronic lymphocytic leukemia. Proc Natl Acad Sci USA 1991; 88(12):5413–5417.

93. Preudhomme C, Dervite I, Wattel E, et al. Clinical significance of p53 mutations in newly diagnosed Burkitt's lymphoma and acute lymphoblastic leukemia: a report of 48 cases. J Clin Oncol 1995; 13:812–820.

94. Vousden KH, Crook T, Farrell PJ. Biological activities of p53 mutants in Burkitt's lymphoma cells. J Gen Virol 1993; 74(Pt 5):803–810.

95. Carbone A. Emerging pathways in the development of AIDS-related lymphomas. Lancet Oncol 2003; 4(1):22–29.

96. Capoulade C, Bressac-de PB, Lefrere I, et al. Overexpression of MDM2, due to enhanced translation, results in inactivation of wild-type p53 in Burkitt's lymphoma cells. Oncogene 1998; 16(12):1603–1610.

97. Farrell PJ, Allan GJ, Shanahan F, Vousden KH, Crook T. p53 is frequently mutated in Burkitt's lymphoma cell lines. EMBO J 1991; 10(10):2879–2887.

98. Lindstrom MS, Klangby U, Wiman KG. p14ARF homozygous deletion or MDM2 overexpression in Burkitt lymphoma lines carrying wild type p53. Oncogene 2001; 20(17):2171–2177.

99. Wiman KG, Magnusson KP, Ramqvist T, Klein G. Mutant p53 detected in a majority of Burkitt lymphoma cell lines by monoclonal antibody PAb240. Oncogene 1991; 6:1633–1639.

100. Michael D, Oren M. The p53-Mdm2 module and the ubiquitin system. Sem Cancer Biol 2003; 13(1):49–58.

101. Klangby U, Okan I, Magnusson KP, Wendland M, Lind P, Wiman KG. p16/INK4a and p15/INK4b gene methylation and absence of p16/INK4a mRNA and protein expression in Burkitt's lymphoma. Blood 1998; 91(5):1680–1687.

102. Stranks G, Height SE, Mitchell P, et al. Deletions and rearrangement of CDKN2 in lymphoid malignancy. Blood 1995; 85:893–901.

103. Wilda M, Bruch J, Harder L, et al. Inactivation of the ARF-MDM-2-p53 pathway in sporadic Burkitt's lymphoma in children. Leukemia 2003.

104. Sanchez-Beato M, Sanchez-Aguilera A, Piris MA. Cell cycle deregulation in B-cell lymphomas. Blood 2003; 101(4):1220–1235.

105. Capello D, Vitolo U, Pasqualucci L, et al. Distribution and pattern of BCL-6 mutations throughout the spectrum of B-cell neoplasia. Blood 2000; 95(2):651–659.

106. Capello D, Carbone A, Pastore C, Gloghini A, Saglio G, Gaidano G. Point mutations of the BCL-6 gene in Burkitt's lymphoma. Br J Haematol 1997; 99:168–170.

107. Artiga MJ, Saez AI, Romero C, et al. A short mutational hot spot in the first intron of BCL-6 is associated with increased BCL-6 expression and with longer overall survival in large B-cell lymphomas. Am J Pathol 2002; 160(4):1371–1380.

108. Cohen O, Feinstein E, Kimchi A. DAP-kinase is a Ca2+/calmodulin-dependent, cytoskeletal-associated protein kinase, with cell death-inducing functions that depend on its catalytic activity. EMBO J 1997; 16:998–1008.

109. Raveh T, Kimchi A. DAP kinase—a proapoptotic gene that functions as a tumor suppressor. Exp Cell Res 2001; 264(1):185–192.

110. Raveh T, Droguett G, Horwitz MS, DePinho RA, Kimchi A. DAP kinase activates a p19ARF/p53-mediated apoptotic checkpoint to suppress oncogenic transformation. Nat Cell Biol 2001; 3(1):1–7.

111. Katzenellenbogen RA, Baylin SB, Herman JG. Hypermethylation of the DAP-kinase CpG island is a common alteration in B-cell malignancies. Blood 1999; 93(12):4347–4353.

112. Ng MH. Death associated protein kinase: from regulation of apoptosis to tumor suppressive functions and B cell malignancies. Apoptosis 2002; 7(3):261–270.

113. Zhu J, Jiang J, Zhou W, Chen X. The potential tumor suppressor p73 differentially regulates cellular p53 target genes. Cancer Res 1998; 58:5061–5065.

114. Corn G, Kuerbitz SJ, Noesel Mv, et al. Transcriptional silencing of the p73 gene in acute lymphoblastic leukemia and Burkitt's lymphoma is associated with 5' CpG island methylation. Cancer Res 1999; 59(14):3352–3356.

115. Bartek J, Bartkova J, Lukas J. The retinoblastoma protein pathway and the restriction point. Curr Opin Cell Biol 1996; 8(6):805–814.

116. Ortega S, Malumbres M, Barbacid M. Cyclin D-dependent kinases, INK4 inhibitors and cancer. Biochim Biophys Acta—Rev Cancer 2002; 1602(1):73–87.

117. Sherr CJ. Cancer cell cycles. Science 1996; 274:1672–1677.

118. Sherr CJ, Weber JD. The ARF/p53 pathway. Curr Opin Genet Dev 2000; 10(1):94–99.

119. Herman JG, Civin CI, Issa JP, Collector MI, Sharkis SJ, Baylin SB. Distinct patterns of inactivation of p15INK4B and p16INK4A characterize the major types of hematological malignancies. Cancer Res 1997; 57:837–841.
120. Fredersdorf S, Burns J, Milne AM, et al. High level expression of p27(kip1) and cyclin D1 in some human breast cancer cells: inverse correlation between the expression of p27(kip1) and degree of malignancy in human breast and colorectal cancers. Proc Natl Acad Sci USA 1997; 94:6380–6385.
121. Barnouin K, Fredersdorf S, Eddaoudi A, et al. Antiproliferative function of p27kip1 is frequently inhibited in highly malignant Burkitt's lymphoma cells. Oncogene 1999; 18(46):6388–6397.
122. Sanchez-Beato M, Camacho FI, Martinez-Montero JC, et al. Anomalous high p27/KIP1 expression in a subset of aggressive B-cell lymphomas is associated with cyclin D3 overexpression. p27/KIP1—cyclin D3 colocalization in tumor cells. Blood 1999; 94(2):765–772.
123. Cinti C, Leoncini L, Nyongo A, et al. Genetic alterations of the retinoblastoma-related gene RB2/p130 identify different pathogenetic mechanisms in and among Burkitt's lymphoma subtypes. Am J Pathol 2000; 156(3):751–760.
124. Cinti C, Claudio PP, Howard CM, et al. Genetic alterations disrupting the nuclear localization of the retinoblastoma-related gene RB2/p130 in human tumor cell lines and primary tumors. Cancer Res 2000; 60(2):383–389.
125. Lazzi S, Bellan C, De Falco G, et al. Expression of RB2/p130 tumor-suppressor gene in AIDS-related non-Hodgkin's lymphomas: implications for disease pathogenesis. Hum Pathol 2002; 33(7):723–731.
126. Rubartelli A, Poggi A, Sitia R, Zocchi MR. HIV-I Tat: a polypeptide for all seasons. Immunol Today 1998; 19:543–545.
127. Babcock GJ, Decker LL, Volk M, Thorley-Lawson DA. EBV persistence in memory B-cells in vivo. Immunity 1998; 9(3):395–404.
128. Babcock GJ, Decker LL, Freeman RB, Thorley-Lawson DA. Epstein–Barr virus-infected resting memory B cells, not proliferating lymphoblasts, accumulate in the peripheral blood of immunosuppressed patients. J Exp Med 1999; 190(4):567–576.
129. Babcock GJ, Hochberg D, Thorley-Lawson AD. The expression pattern of Epstein–Barr virus latent genes in vivo is dependent upon the differentiation stage of the infected B cell. Immunity 2000; 13(4):497–506.
130. Kuppers R, Klein U, Hansmann ML, Rajewsky K. Cellular origin of human B-cell lymphomas. N Engl J Med 1999; 341:1520–1529.
131. Harris RS, Croom-Carter DSG, Rickinson AB, Neuberger MS. Epstein–Barr virus and the somatic hypermutation of immunoglobulin genes in Burkitt's lymphoma cells. J Virol 2001; 75(21):10,488–10,492.
132. Hochberg D, Middeldorp JM, Catalina M, Sullivan JL, Luzuriaga K, Thorley-Lawson DA. Demonstration of the Burkitt's lymphoma Epstein–Barr virus phenotype in dividing latently infected memory cells in vivo. Proc Natl Acad Sci USA 2004; 101(1):239–244.
133. Miyashita EM, Yang B, Babcock GJ, Thorley-Lawson DA. Identification of the site of Epstein–Barr virus persistence in vivo as a resting B cell [published erratum appears in J Virol 1998; 72(11):9419]. J Virol 1997; 71(7):4882–4891.
134. Rooney CM, Rowe M, Wallace LE, Rickinson AB. Epstein–Barr virus-positive Burkitt's lymphoma cells not recognized by virus-specific T-cell surveillance. Nature JID-0410462 1985; 317(6038):629–631.
135. Wang D, Liebowitz D, Wang F, et al. Epstein–Barr virus latent infection membrane protein alters the human B-lymphocyte phenotype: deletion of the amino terminus abolishes activity. J Virol 1988; 62(11):4173–4184.
136. Rowe DT, Rowe M, Evan GI, Wallace LE, Farrell PJ, Rickinson AB. Restricted expression of EBV latent genes and T lymphocyte-detected membrane antigen in Burkitt's lymphoma cells. EMBO J 1986; 5(10):2599–2607.

137. Rowe M, Rowe DT, Gregory CD, et al. Differences in B cell growth phenotype reflect novel patterns of Epstein–Barr virus latent gene expression in Burkitt's lymphoma cells. EMBO J 1987; 6(9):2743–2751.

138. Gregory CD, Rowe M, Rickinson AB. Different Epstein–Barr virus-B-cell interactions in phenotypically distinct clones of a Burkitt's lymphoma cell line. J Gen Virol 1990; 71(Pt 7):1481–1495.

139. Brooks LA, Lear AL, Young LS, Rickinson AB. Transcripts from the Epstein–Barr virus BamHI A fragment are detectable in all three forms of virus latency. J Virol 1993; 67(6):3182–3190.

140. Brooks L, Yao QY, Rickinson AB, Young LS. Epstein–Barr virus latent gene transcription in nasopharyngeal carcinoma cells: coexpression of EBNA1, LMP1, and LMP2 transcripts. J Virol 1992; 66(5):2689–2697.

141. Deacon EM, Pallesen G, Niedobitek G, et al. Epstein–Barr virus and Hodgkin's disease: transcriptional analysis of virus latency in the malignant cells. J Exp Med 1993; 177(2):339–349.

142. Fahraeus R, Fu HL, Ernberg I, et al. Expression of Epstein–Barr virus-encoded proteins in nasopharyngeal carcinoma. Int J Cancer 1988; 42(3):329–338.

143. Herbst H, Lymphomas F, Hummel M, et al. Epstein–Barr virus latent membrane protein expression in Hodgkin and Reed-Sternberg cells. Proc Natl Acad Sci USA 1991; 88(11):4766–4770.

144. Pallesen G, Hamilton-Dutoit SJ, Rowe M, Young LS. Expression of Epstein–Barr virus latent gene products in tumour cells of Hodgkin's disease [see comments]. Lancet 1991; 337(8737):320–322.

145. Smith PR, Griffin BE. Differential expression of Epstein–Barr viral transcripts for two proteins (TP1 and LMP) in lymphocyte and epithelial cells. Nucleic Acids Res 1991; 19(9):2435–2440.

146. Young LS, Dawson CW, Clark D, et al. Epstein–Barr virus gene expression in nasopharyngeal carcinoma. J Gen Virol 1988; 69(Pt 5):1051–1065.

147. Swaminathan S, Tomkinson B, Kieff E. Recombinant Epstein–Barr virus with small RNA (EBER) genes deleted transforms lymphocytes and replicates in vitro. Proc Natl Acad Sci USA 1991; 88(4):1546–1550.

148. Robertson ES, Tomkinson B, Kieff E. An Epstein–Barr virus with a 58-kilobase-pair deletion that includes BARF0 transforms B lymphocytes in vitro. J Virol 1994; 68(3):1449–1458.

149. Lee MA, Diamond ME, Yates JL. Genetic evidence that EBNA-1 is needed for efficient, stable latent infection by Epstein–Barr virus. J Virol 1999; 73(4):2974–2982.

150. Humme S, Reisbach G, Feederle R, et al. The EBV nuclear antigen 1 (EBNA1) enhances B cell immortalization several thousandfold. Proc Natl Acad Sci USA 2003;1832776100.

151. Kuppers R. B cells under influence: transformation of B cells by Epstein–Barr virus. Nat Rev Immunol 2003; 3(10):801–812.

152. Muller JR, Janz S, Goedert JJ, Potter M, Rabkin CS. Persistence of immunoglobulin heavy chain/c-myc recombination-positive lymphocyte clones in the blood of human immunodeficiency virus-infected homosexual men. Proc Natl Acad Sci USA 1995; 92:6577–6581.

153. Roschke V, Kopantzev E, Dertzbaugh M, Rudikoff S. Chromosomal translocations deregulating c-myc are associated with normal immune responses. Oncogene 1997; 14:3011–3016.

154. Uchida J, Yasui T, Takaoka-Shichijo Y, et al. Mimicry of CD40 signals by Epstein–Barr virus LMP1 in B lymphocyte responses. Science 1999; 286(5438):300–303.

155. Laichalk LL, Hochberg D, Babcock GJ, Freeman RB, Thorley-Lawson DA. The dispersal of mucosal memory B cells: evidence from persistent EBV infection. Immunity 2002; 16(5):745–754.

156. Kurth J, Hansmann ML, Rajewsky K, Kuppers R. Epstein–Barr virus-infected B cells expanding in germinal centers of infectious mononucleosis patients do not participate in the germinal center reaction. Proc Natl Acad Sci USA 2003; 100(8):4730–4735.
157. Kurth J, Spieker T, Wustrow J, et al. EBV-infected B cells in infectious mononucleosis. Viral strategies for spreading in the B cell compartment and establishing latency. Immunity 2000; 13(4):485–495.
158. Babcock GJ, Hochberg DDA. The expression pattern of Epstein–Barr virus latent genes in vivo is dependent upon the differentiation stage of the infected B cell. Immunity 2000; 13(4):497–506.
159. Thorley-Lawson DA. Epstein–Barr virus: exploiting the immune system. Nat Rev Immunol 2001; 1(1):75–82.
160. Shimizu N, Tanabe-Tochikura A, Kuroiwa Y, Takada K. Isolation of Epstein–Barr virus (EBV)-negative cell clones from the EBV-positive Burkitt's lymphoma (BL) line Akata: malignant phenotypes of BL cells are dependent on EBV. J Virol 1994; 68(9):6069–6073.
161. Komano J, Takada K. Role of bcl-2 in Epstein–Barr virus-induced malignant conversion of Burkitt's lymphoma cell line Akata. J Virol 2001; 75(3):1561–1564.
162. Rawlins DR, Milman G, Hayward SD, Hayward GS. Sequence-specific DNA binding of the Epstein–Barr virus nuclear antigen (EBNA-1) to clustered sites in the plasmid maintenance region. Cell 1985; 42(3):859–868.
163. Gahn TA, Sugden B. An EBNA-1-dependent enhancer acts from a distance of 10 kilobase pairs to increase expression of the Epstein–Barr virus LMP gene. J Virol 1995; 69(4):2633–2636.
164. Reisman D, Sugden B. Trans activation of an Epstein–Barr viral transcriptional enhancer by the Epstein–Barr viral nuclear antigen 1. Mol Cell Biol 1986; 6(11): 3838–3846.
165. Sugden B, Warren N. A promoter of Epstein–Barr virus that can function during latent infection can be transactivated by EBNA-1, a viral protein required for viral DNA replication during latent infection. J Virol 1989; 63(6):2644–2649.
166. Sample J, Henson EB, Sample C. The Epstein–Barr virus nuclear protein 1 promoter active in type I latency is autoregulated. J Virol 1992; 66(8):4654–4661.
167. Sung NS, Wilson J, Davenport M, Sista ND, Pagano JS. Reciprocal regulation of the Epstein–Barr virus BamHI-F promoter by EBNA-1 and an E2F transcription factor. Mol Cell Biol 1994; 14(11):7144–7152.
168. Schaefer BC, Strominger JL, Speck SH. Host-cell-determined methylation of specific Epstein–Barr virus promoters regulates the choice between distinct viral latency programs. Mol Cell Biol 1997; 17(1):364–377.
169. Kennedy G, Sugden B. EBNA-1, a bifunctional transcriptional activator. Mol Cell Biol 2003; 23(19):6901–6908.
170. Kang MS, Hung SC, Kieff E. Epstein–Barr virus nuclear antigen 1 activates transcription from episomal but not integrated DNA and does not alter lymphocyte growth. Proc Natl Acad Sci USA 2001; 98(26):15,233–15,238.
171. Kube D, Vockerodt M, Weber O, et al. Expression of Epstein–Barr virus nuclear antigen 1 is associated with enhanced expression of CD25 in the Hodgkin cell line L428. J Virol 1999; 73(2):1630–1636.
172. Kennedy G, Komano J, Sugden B. Epstein–Barr virus provides a survival factor to Burkitt's lymphomas. Proc Natl Acad Sci USA 2003; 100(24):14,269–14,274.
173. Drotar ME, Silva S, Barone E, et al. Epstein–Barr virus nuclear antigen-1 and Myc cooperate in lymphomagenesis. Int J Cancer 2003; 106(3):388–395.
174. Wilson JB, Bell JL, Levine AJ. Expression of Epstein–Barr virus nuclear-antigen-1 induces B cell neoplasia in transgenic mice. EMBO J 1996; 15:3117–3126.
175. Glickman JN, Howe JG, Steitz JA. Structural analyses of EBER1 and EBER2 ribonucleoprotein particles present in Epstein–Barr virus-infected cells. J Virol 1988; 62(3): 902–911.

176. Howe JG, Shu MD. Epstein–Barr virus small RNA (EBER) genes: unique transcription units that combine RNA polymerase II and III promoter elements. Cell 1989; 57: 825–834.

177. Howe JG, Shu MD. Upstream basal promoter element important for exclusive RNA polymerase III transcription of the EBER 2 gene. Mol Cell Biol 1993; 13(5): 2655–2665.

178. Lerner MR, Andrews NC, Miller G, Steitz JA. Two small RNAs encoded by Epstein–Barr virus and complexed with protein are precipitated by antibodies from patients with systemic lupus erythematosus. Proc Natl Acad Sci USA 1981; 78(2):805–809.

179. Arrand JR, Rymo L. Characterization of the major Epstein–Barr virus-specific RNA in Burkitt lymphoma-derived cells. J Virol 1982; 41(2):376–389.

180. Komano J, Maruo S, Kurozumi K, Oda T, Takada K. Oncogenic role of Epstein–Barr virus-encoded RNA in Burkitt's lymphoma cell line Akata. J Virol 1999; 73(12): 9827–9831.

181. Ruf IK, Rhyne PW, Yang C, Cleveland JL, Sample JT. Epstein–Barr virus small RNAs potentiate tumorigenicity of Burkitt lymphoma cells independently of an effect on apoptosis. J Virol 2000; 74(21):10,223–10,228.

182. Yamamoto N, Takizawa T, Iwanaga Y, Shimizu N, Yamamoto N. Malignant transformation of B lymphoma cell line BJAB by Epstein–Barr virus-encoded small RNAs. FEBS Lett 2000; 484(2):153–158.

183. Toczyski DP, Steitz JA. EAP, a highly conserved cellular protein associated with Epstein–Barr virus small RNAs (EBERs). EMBO J 1991; 10(2):459–466.

184. Toczyski DP, Steitz JA. The cellular RNA-binding protein EAP recognizes a conserved stem-loop in the Epstein–Barr virus small RNA EBER 1. Mol Cell Biol 1993; 13(1):703–710.

185. Toczyski DP, Matera AG, Ward DC, Steitz JA. The Epstein–Barr virus (EBV) small RNA EBER1 binds and relocalizes ribosomal protein L22 in EBV-infected human B lymphocytes. Proc Natl Acad Sci USA 1994; 91(8):3463–3467.

186. Clarke PA, Schwemmle M, Schickinger J, Hilses K, Clemens MJ. Binding of the Epstein–Barr virus small RNA EBER-1 to the double-stranded RNA-activated protein kinase DAI. Nucleic Acids Res 1991; 19:243–248.

187. Vuyisich M, Spanggord RJ, Beal PA. The binding site of the RNA-dependent protein kinase (PKR) on EBER1 RNA from Epstein–Barr virus. EMBO Rep 2002; 3(7): 622–627.

188. Maraia RJ, Intine RVA. Recognition of nascent RNA by the human La antigen: conserved and divergent features of structure and function. Mol Cell Biol 2001; 21(2): 367–379.

189. Intine RV, Dundr M, Misteli T, Maraia RJ. Aberrant nuclear trafficking of La protein leads to disordered processing of associated precursor tRNAs. Mol Cell 2002; 9(5):1113–1123.

190. Intine RV, Tenenbaum SA, Sakulich AL, Keene JD, Maraia RJ. Differential phosphorylation and subcellular localization of La RNPs associated with precursor tRNAs and translation-related mRNAs. Mol Cell 2003; 12(5):1301–1307.

191. Howe JG, Steitz JA. Localization of Epstein–Barr virus-encoded small RNAs by in situ hybridization. Proc Natl Acad Sci USA 1986; 83(23):9006–9010.

192. Trotta R, Vignudelli T, Candini O, et al. BCR/ABL activates mdm2 mRNA translation via the La antigen. Cancer Cell 2003; 3(2):145–160.

193. Holcik M, Korneluk RG. Functional characterization of the X-linked inhibitor of apoptosis (XIAP) internal ribosome entry site element: role of La autoantigen in XIAP translation. Mol Cell Biol 2000; 20(13):4648–4657.

194. Crosio C, Boyl PP, Loreni F, Pierandrei-Amaldi P, Amaldi F. La protein has a positive effect on the translation of TOP mRNAs in vivo. Nucl Acids Res 2000; 28(15):2927–2934.

195. Clarke PA, Sharp NA, Clemens MJ. Translational control by the Epstein–Barr virus small RNA EBER-1. Reversal of the double-stranded RNA-induced inhibition of protein synthesis in reticulocyte lysates. Eur J Biochem 1990; 193(3):635–641.

196. Clemens MJ, Laing KG, Jeffrey IW, et al. Regulation of the interferon-inducible eIF-2 alpha protein kinase by small RNAs. Biochimie 1994; 76(8):770–778.
197. Nanbo A, Inoue K, Adachi-Takasawa K, Takada K. Epstein–Barr virus RNA confers resistance to interferon-{alpha}-induced apoptosis in Burkitt's lymphoma. EMBO J 2002; 21(5):954–965.
198. Koromilas AE, Roy S, Barber GN, Katze MG, Sonenberg N. Malignant transformation by a mutant of the IFN-inducible dsRNA-dependent protein kinase. Science 1992; 257(5077):1685–1689.
199. Meurs EF, Galabru J, Barber GN, Katze MG, Hovanessian AG. Tumor suppressor function of the interferon-induced double-stranded RNA-activated protein kinase. Proc Natl Acad Sci USA 1993; 90(1):232–236.
200. Williams BRG. PKR: a sentinel kinase for cellular stress. Oncogene 1999; 18(45): 6112–6120.
201. Galabru J, Hovanessian A. Autophosphorylation of the protein kinase dependent on double-stranded RNA. J Biol Chem 1987; 262(32):15,538–15,544.
202. Swaminathan S, Huneycutt BS, Reiss CS, Kieff E. Epstein–Barr virus-encoded small RNAs (EBERs) do not modulate interferon effects in infected lymphocytes. J Virol 1992; 66(8):5133–5136.
203. Dobbelstein M, Shenk T. In vitro selection of RNA ligands for the ribosomal L22 protein associated with Epstein–Barr virus-expressed RNA by using randomized and cDNA-derived RNA libraries. J Virol 1995; 69(12):8027–8034.
204. Nakatogawa H, Ito K. The ribosomal exit tunnel functions as a discriminating gate. Cell 2002; 108(5):629–636.
205. Berisio R, Schluenzen F, Harms J, et al. Structural insight into the role of the ribosomal tunnel in cellular regulation. Nat Struct Biol 2003; 10(5):366–370.
206. Leopardi R, Ward PL, Ogle WO, Roizman B. Association of herpes simplex virus regulatory protein ICP22 with transcriptional complexes containing EAP, ICP4, RNA polymerase II, and viral DNA requires posttranslational modification by the U(L)13 proteinkinase. J Virol 1997; 71:1133–1139.
207. Leopardi R, Roizman B. Functional interaction and colocalization of the herpes simplex virus 1 major regulatory protein ICP4 with EAP, a nucleolar-ribosomal protein. Proc Natl Acad Sci USA 1996; 93:4572–4576.
208. Kim SK, Buczynski KA, Caughman GB, O'Callaghan DJ. The equine herpesvirus 1 immediate-early protein interacts with EAP, a nucleolar-ribosomal protein. Virology 2001; 279(1):173–184.
209. Hitt MM, Allday MJ, Hara T, et al. EBV gene expression in an NPC-related tumour. EMBO J 1989; 8(9):2639–2651.
210. Gilligan K, Sato H, Rajadurai P, et al. Novel transcription from the Epstein–Barr virus terminal EcoRI fragment, DIJhet, in a nasopharyngeal carcinoma. J Virol 1990; 64(10):4948–4956.
211. Chen HL, Lung MM, Sham JS, Choy DT, Griffin BE, Ng MH. Transcription of BamHI-A region of the EBV genome in NPC tissues and B cells. Virology 1992; 191(1):193–201.
212. Zhang CX, Ooka T. Expression of the complementary-strand transcripts from BamHI-A region of the Epstein–Barr virus genome in various induced virus-carrying B cell lines. Virology 1995; 208:180–188.
213. Chen H, Smith P, Ambinder RF, Hayward SD. Expression of Epstein–Barr virus BamHI-A rightward transcripts in latently infected B cells from peripheral blood. Blood 1999; 93(9):3026–3032.
214. Robertson E, Kieff E. Reducing the complexity of the transforming Epstein–Barr virus genome to 64 kilobase pairs. J Virol 1995; 69(2):983–993.
215. Gilligan KJ, Rajadurai P, Lin JC, et al. Expression of the Epstein–Barr virus BamHI A fragment in nasopharyngeal carcinoma: evidence for a viral protein expressed in vivo. J Virol 1991; 65(11):6252–6259.

216. Smith PR, de Jesus O, Turner D, et al. Structure and coding content of CST (BART) family RNAs of Epstein–Barr virus. J Virol 2000; 74(7):3082–3092.

217. Zhang J, Chen H, Weinmaster G, Hayward SD. Epstein–Barr virus BamHI-A rightward transcript-encoded RPMS protein interacts with the CBF1-associated corepressor CIR to negatively regulate the activity of EBNA2 and NotchIC. J Virol 2001; 75(6):2946–2956.

218. Kusano S, Raab-Traub N. An Epstein–Barr virus protein interacts with Notch. J Virol 2001; 75(1):384–395.

219. Henkel T, Ling PD, Hayward SD, Peterson MG. Mediation of Epstein–Barr virus EBNA2 transactivation by recombination signal-binding protein J kappa. Science 1994; 265(5168):92–95.

220. Zhao B, Marshall DR, Sample CE. A conserved domain of the Epstein–Barr virus nuclear antigens 3A and 3C binds to a discrete domain of J kappa. J Virol 1996; 70(7):4228–4236.

221. Robertson ES, Grossman S, Johannsen E, et al. Epstein–Barr virus nuclear protein 3C modulates transcription through interaction with the sequence-specific DNA-binding protein J kappa. J Virol 1995; 69(5):3108–3116.

222. Robertson ES, Lin J, Kieff E. The amino-terminal domains of Epstein–Barr virus nuclear proteins 3A, 3B, and 3C interact with RBPJ(kappa). J Virol 1996; 70(5):3068–3074.

223. Marshall D, Sample C. Epstein–Barr virus nuclear antigen 3C is a transcriptional regulator. J Virol 1995; 69:3624–3630.

224. Radkov SA, Bain M, Farrell PJ, West M, Rowe M, Allday MJ. Epstein–Barr virus EBNA3C represses Cp, the major promoter for EBNA expression, but has no effect on the promoter of the cell gene CD21. J Virol 1997; 71(11):8552–8562.

225. Ling PD, Hsieh JJ, Ruf IK, Rawlins DR, Hayward SD. EBNA-2 upregulation of Epstein–Barr virus latency promoters and the cellular CD23 promoter utilizes a common targeting intermediate, CBF1. J Virol 1994; 68(9):5375–5383.

226. Zimber-Strobl U, Strobl LJ, Meitinger C, et al. Epstein–Barr virus nuclear antigen 2 exerts its transactivating function through interaction with recombination signal binding protein RBP-J kappa, the homologue of Drosophila suppressor of hairless. EMBO J 1994; 13(20):4973–4982.

227. Waltzer L, Logeat F, Brou C, Israel A, Sergeant A, Manet E. The human J kappa recombination signal sequence binding protein (RBP-J kappa) targets the Epstein–Barr virus EBNA2 protein to its DNA responsive elements. EMBO J 1994; 13:5633–5638.

228. Sakai T, Taniguchi Y, Tamura K, et al. Functional replacement of the intracellular region of the Notch1 receptor by Epstein–Barr virus nuclear antigen 2. J Virol 1998; 72(7):6034–6039.

229. Maillard I, Adler SH, Pear WS. Notch and the immune system. Immunity 2003; 19(6):781–791.

230. Maillard I, Pear WS. Notch and cancer: best to avoid the ups and downs. Cancer Cell 2003; 3(3):203–205.

231. Chang BY, Conroy KB, Machleder EM, Cartwright CA. RACK1, a receptor for activated C kinase and a homolog of the beta subunit of G proteins, inhibits activity of Src tyrosine kinases and growth of NIH 3T3 cells. Mol Cell Biol 1998; 18(6):3245–3256.

232. Karran L, Gao Y, Smith PR, Griffin BE. Expression of a family of complementary-strand transcripts in Epstein–Barr virus-infected cells. Proc Natl Acad Sci USA 1992; 89(17):8058–8062.

233. Moghaddam A, Rosenzweig M, Lee-Parritz D, Annis B, Johnson RP, Wang F. An animal model for acute and persistent Epstein–Barr virus infection. Science 1997; 276(5321):2030–2033.

234. Collins WE, Warren M, Sullivan JS, Galland GG. Plasmodium coatneyi: observations on periodicity, mosquito infection, and transmission to Macaca mulatta monkeys. Am J Trop Med Hyg 2001; 64(3):101–110.

11
Epstein–Barr Virus Infection in Hodgkin Lymphomas

Hermann Herbst
Gerhard-Domagk-Institut für Pathologie, Westfälische Wilhelms-Universität, Münster, Germany

Gerald Niedobitek
Institut für Pathologie, Friedrich-Alexander-Universität, Erlangen, Germany

INTRODUCTION

Prior to the demonstration in situ of Epstein–Barr virus (EBV) genomes and antigens in Hodgkin's lymphomas (HLs), several lines of evidence already pointed to the involvement of EBV in its pathogenesis. In particular, seroepidemiological investigations showed an increased risk of HL following infectious mononucleosis (IM) (1,2). Until the late 1980s, however, attempts had failed to unequivocally demonstrate EBV particles or gene products in HL tissues. Methodological advancements and development of EBV-specific probes and monoclonal antibodies made it possible to establish a firm association of EBV with HL. In 1997, a working group of the International Agency for Research on Cancer categorized the EBV as a group I carcinogen and concluded that there was sufficient evidence to consider the association between EBV and HL as causal (3).

An association of HL with EBV was originally suggested on the basis of serological findings and because of a threefold increase in the risk of developing HL in young adults following acute IM (1,2). Unexpectedly, Sleckman et al. reported that a history of IM was not predictive of EBV-positivity in the Hodgkin and Reed–Sternberg (HRS) cells (4). In contrast, two subsequent studies investigating larger numbers of patients have indicated that IM increased the risk of developing EBV-associated HL in young adults (5,6). On the basis of these findings, Jarrett has proposed that HL cases fall into four different categories, including EBV-associated pediatric HL, EBV-positive HL in young adults, EBV-positive HL in older individuals, and EBV-negative HL, the latter representing most cases occurring in young adults (7).

HISTOLOGY OF HL

According to the recent World Health Organization (WHO) classification, malignant neoplasms of lymphoid tissues are divided into two large groups, HL and non-HL (NHL) (8). HL, previously designated Hodgkin's disease or lymphogranulomatosis, a term now obsolete, is considered a lymphoma because of growing evidence that the atypical cells are truly lymphoid in nature. HL is divided into two major entities: nodular lymphocyte-predominant HL (NLPHL) and classical HL (cHL). These forms differ in their clinical and histopathologic features and other characteristics. Lymphoid tissues of NLPHL display small numbers of atypical tumor cells known as "popcorn" or "L&H" (lymphocytic and/or histiocytic) Reed–Sternberg (RS) cell variants on a background of numerous non-neoplastic small lymphocytes arranged in a nodular, or nodular and diffuse, growth pattern, and associated with meshworks of follicular dendritic cells. cHL is characterized by the presence of characteristic atypical cells, Hodgkin cells and RS cells, which are collectively designated as HRS cells. These large cells display one (Hodgkin cells) or several to numerous (RS cells) atypical large nuclei with large eosinophilic nucleoli. They are embedded in an abundance of reactive cells without cytological atypia comprising lymphocytes, plasma cells, macrophages, and neutrophilic and eosinophilic granulocytes, as well as fibroblasts. RS cells arise from Hodgkin cells by endomitosis. The evidence for their derivation from the same cell population stems from their virtually identical phenotypic and genotypic features. Based on the composition of the nonmalignant cell admixture and the presence or absence of annular fibrosis, four histological types, or histotypes, of cHL are distinguished: (*i*) lymphocyte-rich HL (LRHL), (*ii*) nodular sclerosing HL (NSHL), (*iii*) mixed cellularity HL (MCHL), and (*iv*) lymphocyte-depleted HL (LDHL) (8, Table 1). Most cases comprise the histotypes of NSHL with encirclement of cellular nodules by a fibrosing mesenchymal response, or MCHL that displays typical HRS cells in a reactive cellular admixture of variable composition.

BIOLOGY OF HRS CELLS

The variant RS cells of NLPHL are recognized as B-cells by virtue of their display of B-lymphocyte antigens such as CD19, CD20, and CD22. Moreover, they often express immunoglobulin (Ig) transcripts with a monotypic pattern of light chain expression. In fact, rearrangement analysis of Ig genes at the single-cell level showed rearrangements and signs of somatic hypermutation characteristic for germinal center and postgerminal center B-cells, in some cases even with intraclonal V gene diversity due to continuing somatic mutations in the tumor cell clones (9,10). In agreement with this, the lymphocytic and histiocytic cells frequently express the activation-induced cytidine deaminase (AID),

Table 1 Hodgkin's Lymphoma

Nodular lymphocyte-predominant Hodgkin's lymphoma (NLPHL)

Classical Hodgkin's lymphoma (cHL)
  • Lymphocyte-rich HL (LRHL)
  • Nodular sclerosing HL (NSHL)
  • Mixed cellularity HL (MCHL)
  • Lymphocyte-depleted HL (LDHL)

---

a protein structurally related to RNA-editing enzymes, which is required for somatic hypermutation and Ig class switching (11).

HRS cells of cHL share a number of phenotypic characteristics with antigen- or mitogen-activated lymphocytes, such as expression of interleukin (IL)-2 receptor CD25, CD70, and members of the nerve-growth factor receptor family [CD30, CD40, tumor necrosis factor (TNF)-receptor], in addition to downregulation of CD45 antigens. A similar phenotype can also be found in EBV- or human T-lymphotropic virus type I–transformed cells (12). However, typical B-cell markers such as CD19, CD20, and CD22 are expressed in only a minority of cases, and then in only a small proportion of tumor cells. In HRS cells of some cHL cases, most often of NSHL histotype, expression of T-cell markers such as CD3, T-cell receptor (TCR)β chains, or CD4 was observed and considered evidence for a T lymphoid origin of such tumor cells (13). The lymphoid origin of HRS cell in cHL was obscured by inappropriate lineage marker expression, characteristic of macrophages and dendritic cells such as CD15, CD83, fascin, restin, and thymus and activation-regulated chemokine (TARC), leaving room for continued speculation about the exact origin of HRS cells (14–16). More recently, the lymphoid nature of HRS cells became clear when individual cells were isolated and analyzed for their Ig and TCR gene rearrangements (9). Most of these cases, the number of which is still limited, displayed clonal Ig gene rearrangements with evidence of somatic hypermutation. However, HRS cells of cHL lack signs of ongoing somatic hypermutation and generally do not express AID, pointing to a post-germinal center B-cell origin of HRS cells (11,17). In some cases, the mutations are "crippling," i.e., leading to mutations abolishing the binding potential of the Ig heavy or light chain (17). This however, does not seem to be biologically relevant because HRS cells of cHL typically do not express Ig. This is most likely due to the relative lack or absence of transcription factors that regulate Ig gene expression, such as Oct-2, Bob-1, or Pu-1 (18,19), or epigenetic mechanisms such as promoter methylation (20). The B-cell nature of HRS cells in most cHL cases is further confirmed by the expression of Pax-5, a transcription factor required for establishment and maintenance of B-cell identity (21). However, paradoxically, most B-cell–specific genes upregulated by Pax-5 are not expressed in HRS cells (21). The basis of this phenomenon is currently unclear. In a smaller number of cases, clonal TCR gene rearrangements were discovered, supporting previously published patterns of TCR β and CD3 expression by HRS cells and providing unequivocal evidence for a T-cell nature of HRS cells in some cases (22,23). Expression of various cytokine, chemokine, and other growth factor genes by HRS and the reactive cellular admixture is held to explain many of the characteristics of the different histotypes of cHL, systemic symptoms such as fever, and immune evasion of HRS cells expressing neo-antigens (24).

EBV DNA AND RNA IN HLs

After EBV gene probes became available in the late 1980s, EBV DNA was detected in HL tissue extracts by the application of direct filter hybridization techniques using probes for the internal repeat sequences (25–29). Southern blots probed for the EBV terminal repeats most frequently displayed viral episomal genomes in monoclonal composition (27,28,30). Application of this technique to metachronous (i.e., detected more than one month apart) HL manifestations also supported these conclusions (31). In concert with the visualization of EBV DNA in HRS cells, these findings provided evidence for the monoclonal nature of the atypical cells: EBV DNA was found in HRS cells of up to 40% of HL cases when in situ hybridization was used with radioactive (27,28) or biotinylated probes specific for the internal repeat sequences (32,33).

In HL involving several anatomic localizations, HRS cells at all sites were virus infected (31,34). Similarly, EBV persisted in the HRS cell population of EBV-positive HL cases in virtually all cases of relapsed disease, with maintenance of the clonal episomal and strain characteristics (35). Disappearance of EBV during relapse seems to be a very rare event (36). Moreover, EBV-encoded RNA (EBER)–specific in situ hybridization revealed EBV infection of virtually all HRS cells (37). All of these observations imply that EBV infection occurs before clonal expansion of the HRS cell population and suggest that HRS cells represent monoclonal proliferations, at least in EBV-positive HL cases. Thus, these findings are not easily reconciled with previous reports on the detection of polyclonal Ig gene rearrangements in HRS cells obtained by micromanipulation of frozen sections (38).

The application of the polymerase chain reaction (PCR) to amplify unique or repetitive EBV DNA sequences from HL tissue samples resulted in a considerably increased frequency of EBV detection ranging from 40% to 80% of the cases in different series (39–42). These findings led to the conclusion that EBV genomes may be present not only in HRS cells but in cells of the reactive admixture as well. These and many other problems regarding the cellular sources of EBV DNA could be resolved by in situ hybridization with EBER-specific probes. Because EBER transcripts are present in very high copy numbers within latently EBV-infected cells, they may be detected with high sensitivity and specificity by nonradioactive procedures in paraffin-embedded archival tissue samples, and even in autopsy materials. Thus, their detection has quickly become routine practice for the study of latent EBV infection, replacing PCR for the mere demonstration of the virus and producing a large body of data from different regions of the world.

By EBER-specific in situ hybridization, variable, but usually small numbers of nonmalignant small lymphocytes were found in the majority of the HL cases, regardless of the EBV status of the HRS cells. Increased numbers of small EBER-positive lymphocytes were observed in only a few cases, providing an explanation for the higher frequency of EBV-positive cases in most PCR studies and emphasizing the value of morphological analysis of EBV infection in HL (37,42). Double-labeling experiments revealed that the population of EBER-positive small, reactive cells was largely composed of B-lymphocytes (37). As opposed to the monoclonal nature of the neoplastic cells, reactive EBER-positive cells expressed Ig light chains in a polytypic, mosaic-like pattern, thus displaying the phenotype of mature B-cells of oligoclonal origin (37). This conclusion was substantiated by the analysis of the Ig gene rearrangement patterns of EBER-positive small lymphocytes in HL that showed functional rearrangements and a heterogeneous clonal composition strongly contrasting with the findings in neighboring HRS cells of monoclonal origin (43). The same conclusion was drawn from EBV strain analysis that showed the presence of different EBV strains in HRS cells and admixed lymphocytes (44). EBER-positive small B-cells with similar cytomorphologic and immunophenotypic characteristics were also found in lymph nodes from normal healthy controls and are likely to be part of the pool of circulating latent EBV-infected B-cells in virus carriers (45).

EBV infection of HRS cells is not evenly distributed among the different histotypes of HL. The largest proportion of EBV-positive cases, with up to 80% in Western series, was consistently found in MCHL, whereas the smallest proportions were seen in NLPHL and LDHL. HL arising in HIV-infected patients was exclusively of MCHL histotype and in virtually all cases associated with latent EBV infection of HRS cells (46). The literature is not yet informative as to LRHL, because this entity has only recently been defined.

More importantly, the frequency of HL cases with EBER-positive HRS cells showed considerable geographic variability: overall, EBER is present in 47% in North American cases of cHL (42), 50% (37) and 45% (47) in European cases, 57% in China (48), 60% and 85% in Korea (49), 72% in Algeria (50), 54% in Argentina (51), 64% in Brazil, 70% in Mexico (52), 96% in Peru (53), and even 100% in cases of pediatric HL in Honduras (54). In all of these studies, EBV was most prevalent in MCHL, less commonly associated with NSHL, and only rarely found in NLPHL and LDHL. Although rare in some developing countries, on a worldwide scale, the majority of HL cases are associated with EBV because of the larger populations in the developing compared to Western countries. The association of MCHL and EBV is also reflected in the age distribution. The MCHL histotype is more frequent in HL arising in patients younger than 15 years as well as in those patients over 50 years old, as opposed to NSHL, which predominates in young adults and is less frequently associated with EBV (55–57). HL originating in neck lymph nodes, i.e., close to the putative site of primary infection with EBV, is more frequently associated with the virus (58).

The prevalence of HL in immunosuppressed and HIV-infected individuals is increased compared to appropriate control populations. Virtually all of these cases are associated with EBV and are of the MCHL histotype (59). Interestingly, HL tissues of patients with AIDS displayed monoclonal EBV episomes by Southern blot analysis, which points to the fact that even in situations where expansion of EBV-positive clones may be expected, the EBV genomes of HRS cells remain dominant (59). This implies that even in a situation where immunodeficiency would be expected to allow the development of a multiclonal EBV-infected population, HL remains a clonal disease. HLs arising in the background of ulcerative colitis are EBV positive, indicating that the immunological disturbance underlying this form of inflammatory bowel disease may be relevant for the development of HL, which again were of the MCHL histotype in all reported cases (60). The close association of EBV with virtually all HL cases arising in states of immunocompromise contrasts with the situation in immunocompetent individuals and raises the possibility that all or most HL cases are initially EBV-positive, and selection against the virus in immunocompetent individuals results in the appearance of EBV-negative HL. This scenario would favor a "hit-and-run" mechanism, attributing a role to EBV even for EBV-negative HL. However, in at least some of such secondarily EBV-negative cases, the virus would have left traces in the host genome. A recent PCR and PCR in situ hybridization study on detection of heterogeneous EBV DNA in EBER-negative HL cases seemed to support this idea (61). However, a different group using fluorescence in situ hybridization with probes spanning the entire EBV genome on latent membrane protein (LMP) 1–negative HL found no hybridization to HRS cells, indicating that remnants of EBV genomes were not present (62).

PCR was also used to distinguish EBV strains present within HL lesions, in most cases revealing type A EBV (40). However, type B EBV sequences were also found in a proportion of cases, most of which were related to a clinical setting of immunodeficiency (63). In addition, by PCR, polymorphisms were detected within the LMP1 open reading frame. Some cases characterized by particularly bizarre tumor cells presented with LMP1 sequences identical to those previously detected in cases of nasopharyngeal carcinoma (64). These LMP1 variants are characterized by a 30 base pair (bp) deletion at the $3'$ end of the gene resulting in the loss of amino acids 343 to 352 from the carboxy terminus of the LMP1 protein (65,66). Transfectants expressing this LMP1 deletion variant displayed an increased tumorigenicity and proved less immunogenic than the wild-type protein (65,67,68). The finding of two HL cases with wild-type, full length LMP1 at diagnosis and the presence of additional deletion variants of LMP1 at relapse suggested that progressive accumulation of mutations during the course of the disease might have occurred (34). However, the relevance of the LMP1 deletion variant for the pathogenesis of HL remains uncertain. In studies comparing virus isolates from tumors and from the corresponding background population, full length and deleted forms of LMP1 were similarly prevalent in normal healthy carriers in European studies (69,70), suggesting that LMP1 deletions do not confer an increased risk of developing EBV-positive HL. Analysis of Danish Hodgkin's disease cases for mutations within the LMP1 promoter indicated a selection pressure against EBV strains with weak promoter activity (71).

EBV ANTIGEN EXPRESSION IN HLs

Application of polyclonal and monoclonal antibodies on tissue sections revealed EB nuclear antigen (EBNA)-1 and LMP1 in the absence of EBNA2 in EBV-positive HRS cells, a pattern previously established for undifferentiated nasopharyngeal carcinoma, i.e., latency type II (72–74). Whereas EBNA1 may also be found in occasional cells of the lymphoid cell admixture, LMP1 is exclusive to HRS cells (72–74). As predicted from studies at the transcriptional level, HRS cells express the LMP2 (terminal protein) gene in addition to LMP1 in a proportion of cases (75,76). Furthermore, it was established that EBNA1 transcripts initiate at the Op promoter, but not at the Cp and Wp promoters, indicating the absence of EBNA2-6 open reading frame transcripts in HL (75).

This pattern of latent viral antigen expression is strictly maintained in the vast majority of HRS cells. Expression of lytic cycle antigens such as the membrane glycoprotein, gp350/250 (72,77), viral capsid antigen (32,77), and early antigen (77) was not detected in most studies. Latency is disrupted by expression of the BZLF1 transactivator protein, which precedes expression of all other late EBV proteins. BZLF1 immunoreactivity was found in the nuclei of a very small proportion of neoplastic cells in few EBV-positive cases in two studies, which is consistent with an abortive lytic infection in only occasional HRS cells (77,78). In only one of the cases was BZLF1 reactivity accompanied by the expression of late EBV proteins, although BZLF1-specific antibodies were detected frequently in sera from HL patients (78,79).

EBV INFECTION AND THE PHENOTYPE OF HRS CELLS

LMP1 is a 63 kDa transmembrane protein with a short amino terminus and a long carboxy terminus, both cytoplasmic, and six membrane-spanning domains (80). Following oligomerization at the membrane to produce characteristic patches, LMP1 activates signaling through two distinct domains in its cytoplasmic terminus, carboxyl-terminal activating region 1(CTAR1) and CTAR2, both of which interact with TNF-associated factors (TRAF) (81). Ultimately, signaling involves the nuclear factor (NF)-κB, Jun N-terminal kinase (JNK)/activator protein-1 (AP-1), and mitogen-activated protein kinase pathways (82,83). TRAF molecules are physiologically recruited by membrane receptors like TNF-R, and this binding leads to a rise in NF-κB levels (84). Thus, by molecular mimicry, LMP1 utilizes and potentiates signaling mechanisms common to the TNF receptor/CD40 family of receptors to elicit its pleiotropic effects (85).

LMP2A and LMP2B are encoded by the same viral gene, with the exception of the first exon, which is unique to LMP2A (86). LMP2B is considered a negative regulator of LMP2A function. Like LMP1, LMP2 is an integral membrane protein, with 12 transmembrane domains, that forms patches and interferes with cell signaling pathways (87). At variance with LMP1, LMP2A is present in healthy individuals and is apparently not required for transformation of B-lymphocytes. The LMP2A cytoplasmic tail contains an immunoreceptor tyrosine–based activation motif (ITAM) domain that can recruit the Src and Syk family of kinases, which are physiologically involved in signal transduction from the B-cell receptor (88,89). Binding of the tyrosine kinases to the phosphorylated LMP2A ITAM sequences suppresses the activating signal normally generated by the B-cell receptor (90). Alternatively, LMP2A can replace a functional pre–B-cell receptor in B-cell development in mice (91,92). Thus, LMP2A seems to interfere with Ig signal transduction.

EBV infection of lymphocytes and epithelial cells in vitro is associated with a variety of immunophenotypic changes, most notably, the induction of some lymphocyte activation antigens, e.g., CD23, CD25, CD30, and CD70, and adhesion molecules such as intercellular adhesion molecule 1 (ICAM-1), leukocyte function-antigen molecule 1 (LFA-1), and LFA-3 (93–95). In attempts to define the role of EBV in the pathogenesis of HL, several investigators have studied EBV-positive and EBV-negative cases for phenotypic differences. Although expressed in most HL cases, the CD30 molecule was significantly more frequently detectable in EBV-positive cases (96). At least one of the TRAF molecules, TRAF1, is induced by LMP1 in vitro in an NF-κB–dependent manner and might protect lymphoid cells from apoptosis. In HL and EBV-positive non-Hodgkin's lymphoma (NHL), TRAF1 is strongly expressed, indicating that interference with proapoptotic pathways may be a distinct function of LMP1 in HRS cells (97). However, NF-κB is constitutively active in HRS cells independent of EBV status and expression of TRAF1 has been observed in EBV-positive and EBV-negative HRS cells (98). Bcl-2 and A20, both of which are proteins with antiapoptotic function, are induced by LMP1 in vitro. LMP1 and A20 both protect epithelial cells from p53-mediated apoptosis induced by serum withdrawal (99). In B-cells, LMP1 has been shown to upregulate Bcl-2 protein expression, which prevents cells from undergoing programmed cell death (95). There are no data as to A20 expression in HL, but Bcl-2 and p53 expression have been studied in EBV-positive and -negative HL. No significant differences were seen distinguishing EBV-associated and EBV-negative HL with respect to p53 and Bcl-2 (100). Expression of CD99, a molecule with putative functions in cell–cell interactions, apoptosis, and T-cell activation, is downregulated in EBV-positive HRS cells. This downregulation was considered attributable to LMP1, specifically to its NF-κB activation domains (101).

A statistically significant effect related to the presence of EBV in HRS cells was also observed with respect to the CD20 B-cell antigen (96,102) and the CD3 T-cell antigen (102). However, CD20 and CD3 were less frequently detectable in EBV-positive than in EBV-negative cases. In contrast to the upregulation of CD30, this effect is not evidently related to LMP1 expression as a reduced CD20-specific staining has also been observed for LMP1-negative EBV-infected lymphocytes in chronic virus carriers (37). Another LMP1-mediated phenotypic change that may be relevant in HRS cell biology is the association of LMP1 with the intermediate filament, vimentin (103,104). Thus, EBV may modulate the expression of some leukocyte differentiation antigens and other gene products in HRS cells. Because some of these markers are often used for lineage assignment of HRS cells in paraffin sections, the presence or absence of EBV should be considered when evaluating immunostaining patterns in HL.

Several cytokines have been shown to be expressed in EBV-transformed lymphoblastoid cell lines and to act as autocrine growth factors in this cellular environment. For this reason, the expression of cytokines in HRS cells in the context of EBV infection is of interest. Although some cytokines, such as lymphotoxin and TNF, are expressed in most HL cases regardless of the EBV status (105), studies of large HL series have recently demonstrated some potentially important differences between EBV-negative and EBV-positive cases. IL-6 (106,107) and, in particular, IL-10 are significantly more often expressed in EBV-positive than in EBV-negative HRS cells (106–108). Interestingly, this feature is also shared by EBV-infected blasts in IM (106,109). Because IL-6 as well as IL-10 expression are upregulated in LMP1-transfected epithelial cells, it is likely that this effect is also LMP1-mediated in HRS cells (110). In support of this idea, LMP1 has been shown to activate NF-κB signaling pathways (111,112) and an NF-κB–binding site was located in the IL-6 promoter (113). The BCRF1 open reading frame of EBV, which codes for a cytokine with IL-10 homology ("viral IL-10") is not transcribed in latent infection. Accordingly, BCRF1 transcripts were not found in HRS cells either by in situ hybridization or by real time or reverse transcriptase (RT)-PCR (114,115). Thus, HRS cells express cellular IL-10 and not "viral IL-10."

IL-12, which has functions in Th1 cell differentiation, (116) was detected by immunohistology in reactive cells but not in HRS cells in 28 of 33 (85%) HL cases (117). IL-12–positive cells could be detected within the reactive infiltrate in all 22 EBV-positive cases, but in only 5 of 10 EBV-negative cHL cases of that study (117). However, these authors did not differentiate sufficiently between the subunits of the IL-12 system. In HL-derived cell lines, expression of the p35 subunit of IL-12 but not of the p40 subunit has been observed; thus, functional IL-12 should not be expressed (118). EBV-induced gene 3 (EBI3), an EBV-induced cytokine homologous to the IL-12 p40 subunit, was found to be strongly expressed by HRS cells in 32 of 33 cHL cases independent of the EBV status (118). It has been suggested that EBI3 may function to antagonize IL-12 and to inhibit the development of a Th1 immune response. On the other hand, EBI3 together with p28 form a novel cytokine—termed IL-27—that cooperates with IL-12 in the induction of Th1 reactions (119). Thus, interpretation of IL-12 subunit expression in HL requires detailed knowledge of the cellular context. The Th1-associated chemokines, inducible protein (IP)-10, Mig-1, and macrophage inflammatory protein (MIP)-1α, were expressed at higher levels in cHL compared to benign lymphoid tissues (120,121). Elevated expression of these chemokines was also associated with EBV-positive cHL (120). In particular, expression of IP-10, a putative Th1 chemokine, in HRS cells is associated with EBV infection (120,122). Finally, expression of the Th2 chemokine TARC is a unique and consistent feature of HRS cells regardless of the EBV status (107,123).

Thus, these studies suggest that the presence of EBV and, particularly, LMP1 expression may contribute to the phenotype of HRS cells. This notion has been further underlined by the demonstration that HRS-like cells arising in some EBV-negative–B-cell NHL of low malignancy are often EBV-infected, suggesting that superinfection of tumor cells may induce an HRS-like cytomorphology (124,125). Also, non-neoplastic HRS-like cells are frequently found in IM (126,127). Phenotypic similarities between these blasts and HRS cells include the expression of LMP1 and CD30 as well as cytokines such as TNF-α, lymphotoxin, IL-6, and IL-10 (109,114,126,127). Together with the observation that HL frequently arises in cervical lymph nodes close to the site of primary EBV infection, these findings have been taken as evidence to suggest that HRS-like blasts in IM may represent HRS cell precursors (58). This idea has been further supported by the fact that HL arising in the lymphoreticular tissue of the Waldeyer's ring is more frequently EBV-associated than HL arising at other sites (128). Although IM patients may be at increased risk of developing HL, the question as to whether HL arising in temporal relationship to IM is indeed EBV-associated is controversial (4,57). Furthermore, HRS-like IM blasts are CD15 negative, but may display EBNA2, and whereas chromosomal abnormalities are a consistent feature of HRS cells, no cytogenetic alterations seem to be associated with IM. Thus, phenotypic similarities between the malignant HRS cells in HL and morphologically similar cells in IM should not be overemphasized.

HL AND EBV-SPECIFIC IMMUNITY

The development of EBV-associated lymphoproliferations with expression of potential cytotoxic T-lymphocyte (CTL) targets in transplant patients is easily understood in view of the iatrogenic suppression of T-cell immunity in these patients. In the absence of an intact T-cell system, tumors expressing viral antigens such as LMP and EBNA are not eliminated by CTLs (129,130). Thus, viral antigen expression patterns of tumor cells may reflect not only cell type–specific gene expression, but also the host's immune status.

In contrast, it has been much more difficult to understand how EBV-positive tumors develop in the face of an apparently normal immune system. In Burkitt lymphoma, the downregulation of all virus-encoded latent proteins with the exception of EBNA1 seems to help lymphoma cells escape immunosurveillance (131). HL patients frequently suffer from an impaired immune system, although they are often able to mount high anti-LMP1 antibody titers indicating the presence of an intact humoral immune response against this antigen (132). In this context, it is of interest that cHL lesions are commonly infiltrated by numerous small T-cells, mainly of CD4 phenotype, frequently forming rosettes around HRS cells. CD8-positive T-cells make up a small proportion of the T-cell infiltrate and are typically not in close contact with HRS cells (133). They do not appear to be directed against a common antigen (134). The numbers of CD8-positive T-cells are higher in EBV-associated cases of cHL than in EBV-negative cases and, paradoxically, indicate a poorer prognosis (135–137).

Several authors studied EBV-specific CTL responses from peripheral blood and tumor infiltrating lymphocytes from both EBV-negative and EBV-positive HL patients. In general, as in healthy EBV carriers, LMP-specific CTL precursors occurred only at low frequencies in the blood of HL patients, and less frequently in the EBV-negative HL lesions, whereas no EBV-specific CTL could be reactivated in vitro from EBV-related HL lesions (138–140). These data indicate that EBV-specific CTL that could potentially target the HRS cells either fail to penetrate the tumor site or fail to function within the tumor microenvironment. Anti-inflammatory cytokines and immunosuppressive factors produced by the tumor cells and/or the reactive cellular admixture may be responsible for this effect.

The association between EBV-infection and IL-10 expression by HRS cells suggests one potential mechanism to explain this phenomenon. IL-10 is a pleiotropic Th2 cytokine with numerous inhibitory effects on cell-mediated immunity. IL-10 inhibits T-cell growth, blocks IL-2 and interferon-γ production by Th1 cells, and downregulates proinflammatory cytokine production by lipopolysaccharide-stimulated monocytes. In addition, IL-10 is a growth and differentiation factor for B-cells (141).

Conceivably, IL-10 secretion by EBV-positive HRS cells may not only provide another growth factor for EBV-infected B-cells (142), but may also contribute to suppression of EBV-specific immunity in the HRS cell microenvironment (143). Numerous other mechanisms that may not necessarily be restricted to EBV-related HL seem to contribute to this immunological scenario, such as secretion of proteinase inhibitors or chemokines. In addition to being sources of granzyme themselves (144), HRS cells of a small proportion of HL cases express the granzyme inhibitor, protein-ase inhibitor 9 (145). Tissue inhibitor of metalloproteinases (TIMP)-1 is expressed by varying numbers of HRS cells in a large proportion of HL cases (146). In the latter study, it was further shown that TIMP1 may efficiently block T-cell activation.

In addition to secretion of IL-10, LMP1-positive HRS cells seem to influence the local immune response by another, distinct mechanism. It was previously shown that EBV may have functions of a superantigen (147). This superantigen was recently iden-tified as a gene product of the human endogenous retrovirus (HERV)-K18, and it was shown that HERV-K18 expression is induced by LMP1 (148). Moreover, LMP1 shares distinct peptide sequences and immunosuppressive properties with a retroviral protein, p15E, which derives from the *env* gene of certain animal endogenous retro-viruses (149). Thus, EBV seems to utilize phylogenetically ancient mechanisms to manipulate the host immune response in its favor. In addition, LMP1 seems to induce regulatory T-cells that have the ability to inhibit effector T-cells, suggesting a mechan-ism by which EBV-positive HRS cells may escape EBV-specific T-cell immunity (150).

CONCLUSIONS

Application of molecular biological methods has substantiated the previous seroepi-demiological identification of EBV as a major candidate etiologic agent in the devel-opment of HL. The combined evidence from PCR, EBV DNA, and EBER in situ hybridization as well as LMP1 immunostaining studies clearly demonstrates that EBV is present in the tumor cell population of up to 50% of HL cases in Western countries. The bulk of viral genomes are found in monoclonal form in most of these cases, indicating that the virus had entered the tumor cells prior to their clonal expansion. Furthermore, altered EBV serology preceding the onset of the disease places the virus in the appropriate time frame to have a role in the pathogenesis of HL. All histological types of HL are represented among these EBV-positive cases, though in varying proportions. These findings support a monoclonal origin of the HRS cell population and, by implication and in conjunction with studies demon-strating monoclonal Ig gene rearrangements in HRS cells and clonal karyotypic abnormalities, suggest that HL represents a true neoplasm. These observations are reinforced by the detection of LMP1, the only EBV gene with established oncogenic potential, in HRS cells of EBV-positive HL cases. By interference with CD40/TNF receptor signaling pathways, LMP1 may confer an apoptosis-resistant phenotype to HRS cells and modulate expression of numerous gene products including lineage markers and certain cytokines. In addition, LMP2A may substitute for the lack of functional Igs in HRS cells. These proteins may jointly provide the necessary survival signals for germinal center B-cells with "crippling" Ig gene mutations. EBV infection of lymphoid cells may provide a growth advantage to these cells by circumventing mechanisms resulting in apoptosis of lymphoid cells without func-tional antigen receptors. Thus, present evidence strongly suggests that the virus is more than a "silent passenger," but rather supports the notion of an etiologic role for EBV in the pathogenesis of a significant proportion of HL cases. Today, many of the mechanisms by which EBV contributes to the development of EBV-associated tumors are known, but it is also evident that EBV alone is not sufficient for the induction of HL (nor of any other EBV-associated malignancy) but has to be complemented by genetic factors and an impairment of antiviral immunity.

The consistent expression of LMP1 and LMP2 in HRS cells has been difficult to understand in view of studies showing that these proteins may provide target epitopes for EBV-specific cytotoxicity. Analyses of EBV-specific cytotoxic T-cells from HL lesions and peripheral blood from patients with EBV-positive and -negative HL have indicated that HL patients do not suffer from a generalized deficiency of EBV-specific immunity. However, virus-specific cytotoxic T-cells do not seem to be active in HL lesions despite the local presence of sufficient numbers of CD8- and granzyme B–positive cells. These results would seem to suggest that a disturbed EBV-specific immunity in the microenvironment of HRS cells may contribute to the pathogenesis of virus-associated HL. The observation of an association between the detection of EBV and the expression of IL-10 in HRS cells may explain some aspects of this phenomenon. Further studies will be required to substantiate these observations and to elucidate the underlying mechanisms. In any case, these factors have to be taken into account when embarking on studies aimed at treating HL patients with EBV-specific CTLs.

REFERENCES

1. Gutensohn N, Cole P. Epidemiology of Hodgkin's disease. Semin Oncol 1980; 7:92–102.
2. Mueller N, Evans A, Harris NL, et al. Hodgkin's disease and Epstein-Barr virus. Altered antibody pattern before diagnosis. N Engl J Med 1989; 320:689–695.
3. IARC. Epstein-Barr virus and Kaposi's sarcoma herpesvirus/herpesvirus 8. Proceedings of the IARC Working Group on the Evaluation of Carcinogenic Risks to Humans, Lyon, France, June 17–24, 1997. IARC Monogr Eval Carcinog Risks Hum 1997; 70:1–492.
4. Sleckman BG, Mauch PM, Ambinder RF, et al. Epstein-Barr virus in Hodgkin's disease: correlation of risk factors and disease characteristics with molecular evidence of viral infection. Cancer Epidemiol Biomarkers Prev 1998; 7:1117–1121.
5. Hjalgrim H, Askling J, Rostgaard K, et al. Characteristics of Hodgkin's lymphoma after infectious mononucleosis. N Engl J Med 2003; 349:1324–1332.
6. Alexander FE, Lawrence DJ, Freeland J, et al. An epidemiological study of index and family infectious mononucleosis and adult Hodgkin's disease (HD): evidence of a specific association with EBV+ve HD in young adults. Int J Cancer 2003; 107: 298–302.
7. Jarrett RF. Viruses and Hodgkin's lymphoma. Ann Oncol 2002; 13(suppl 1):23–29.
8. Jaffe ES, Harris NL, Stein H, Jardiman JW. Pathology and Genetics of Tumours of Haematopoietic and Lymphoid Tissues. In: WHO Classification of Tumors. Lyon: IARC Press, 2001.
9. Küppers R. Molecular biology of Hodgkin's lymphoma. Adv Cancer Res 2002; 84:277–312.
10. Chan WC. The Reed–Sternberg cell in classical Hodgkin's lymphoma. Hematol Oncol 2001; 19:1–17.
11. Greiner A, Tobollik S, Buettner M, et al. Differential expression of AID in nodular lymphocyte predominant and classical Hodgkin lymphoma. J Pathol 2005; 205:541–547.
12. Herbst H, Stein H, Niedobitek G. Epstein–Barr virus in CD30+ malignant lymphomas. Crit Rev Oncogenesis 1993; 4:191–239.
13. Dallenbach FE, Stein H. Expression of T-cell-receptor ß-chain in Reed–Sternberg cells. Lancet 1989; 2:828–830.

14. Drexler HG. Recent results on the biology of Hodgkin and Reed–Sternberg cells. I. Biopsy material. Leuk Lymphoma 1992; 8:283–313.

15. Pinkus GS, Pinkus JL, Langhoff E, et al. Fascin, a sensitive new marker for Reed–Sternberg cells of Hodgkin's disease. Evidence for a dendritic or B-cell derivation? Am J Pathol 1997; 150:543–562.

16. Sorg UR, Morse TM, Patton WN, et al. Hodgkin's cells express CD83, a dendritic cell lineage associated antigen. Pathology 1997; 29:294–299.

17. Kanzler H, Küppers R, Hansmann ML, Rajewski K. Hodgkin and Reed–Sternberg cells in Hodgkin's disease represent the outgrowth of a dominant tumor clone derived from (crippled) germinal center B-cells. J Exp Med 1996; 184:1495–1505.

18. Re D, Müshen M, Ahmadi T, et al. Oct-2 and Bob-1 deficiency in Hodgkin and Reed–Sternberg cells. Cancer Res 2001; 61:2080–2084.

19. Stein H, Marafioti T, Foss HD, et al. Down-regulation of BOB.1/OBF.1 and Oct2 in classical Hodgkin disease but not in lymphocyte predominant Hodgkin disease correlates with immunoglobulin transcription. Blood 2001; 97:496–501.

20. Ushmorov A, Ritz O, Hummel M, et al. Epigenetic silencing of the immunoglobulin heavy-chain gene in classical Hodgkin lymphoma-derived cell lines contributes to the loss of immunoglobulin expression. Blood 2004; 104:3326–3334.

21. Schwering I, Bräuninger A, Klein U, et al. Loss of the B-lineage-specific gene expression program in Hodgkin and Reed–Sternberg cells of Hodgkin lymphoma. Blood 2003; 101:1505–1512.

22. Müschen M, Rajewsky K, Bräuninger A, et al. Rare occurrence of classical Hodgkin's disease as a T-cell lymphoma. J Exp Med 2000; 191:387–394.

23. Seitz V, Hummel M, Marafioti T, Anagnostopulos I, Assaf C, Stein H. Detection of clonal T-cell receptor g-chain rearrangement in Reed–Sternberg cells of Hodgkin's disease. Blood 2000; 95:3020–3024.

24. Skinnider BF, Mak TW. The role of cytokines in classical Hodgkin lymphoma. Blood 2002; 99:4283–4297.

25. Weiss LM, Strickler JG, Warnke RA, Purtillo DT, Sklar J. Epstein–Barr viral DNA in tissues of Hodgkin's disease. Am J Pathol 1987; 129:86–89.

26. Herbst H, Tippelmann G, Anagnostopoulos I, et al. Immunoglobulin and T-cell receptor gene rearrangements in Hodgkin's disease and Ki-1-positive anaplastic large cell lymphoma: dissociation between phenotype and genotype. Leuk Res 1989; 13:103–116.

27. Weiss LM, Movahed LA, Warnke RA, Sklar J. Detection of Epstein–Barr virus genomes in Reed–Sternberg cells of Hodgkin's disease. N Engl J Med 1989; 320:502–506.

28. Anagnostopoulos I, Herbst H, Niedobitek G, Stein H. Demonstration of monoclonal EBV genomes in Hodgkin's disease and Ki-1 positive anaplastic large cell lymphoma by combined Southern blot and in situ hybridization. Blood 1989; 74:810–816.

29. Staal SP, Ambinder RF, Beschorner WE, Hayward GS, Mann R. A survey of Epstein–Barr virus DNA in lymphoid tissue. Frequent detection in Hodgkin's disease. Am J Clin Pathol 1989; 91:1–5.

30. Gulley ML, Eagan PA, Quintanilla-Martinez L, et al. Epstein-Barr virus DNA is abundant and monoclonal in the Reed–Sternberg cells of Hodgkin's disease: association with mixed cellularity subtype and Hispanic American ethnicity. Blood 1994; 83:1595–1602.

31. Boiocchi M, Dolcetti R, De Re V, Gloghini A, Carbone A. Demonstration of a unique Epstein–Barr virus-positive cellular clone in metachronous multiple localizations of Hodgkin's disease. Am J Pathol 1993; 142:33–38.

32. Uccini S, Monardo F, Stoppacciaro A, et al. High frequency of Epstein-Barr virus-genome detection in Hodgkin's disease of HIV-positive patients. Int J Cancer 1990; 46:581–585.

33. Brousset P, Chittal S, Schlaifer D, et al. Detection of Epstein-Barr virus messenger RNA in Reed–Sternberg cells of Hodgkin's disease by in situ hybridization with biotinylated probes on specially processed modified acetone methyl benzoate xylene (Mod-AMeX) sections. Blood 1991; 77:1781–1786.

34. Vasef MA, Kamel OW, Chen YY, Medeiros LJ, Weiss LM. Detection of Epstein–Barr virus in multiple sites involved by Hodgkin's disease. Am J Pathol 1995; 147:1408–1415.

35. Brousset P, Schlaifer D, Meggetto F, et al. Persistence of the same viral strain in early and late relapses of Epstein-Barr virus-associated Hodgkin's disease. Blood 1994; 84:2447–2451.

36. Delecluse HJ, Marafioti T, Hummel M, Dallenbach F, Anagnostopoulos I, Stein H. Disappearance of the Epstein–Barr virus in a relapse of Hodgkin's disease. J Pathol 1997; 182:475–479.

37. Herbst H, Steinbrecher E, Niedobitek G, et al. Distribution and phenotype of Epstein-Barr virus-harboring cells in Hodgkin's disease. Blood 1992; 80:484–491.

38. Hummel M, Ziemann K, Lammert H, Pileri S, Sabattini E, Stein H. Hodgkin's disease with monoclonal and polyclonal populations of Reed–Sternberg cells. N Engl J Med 1995; 333:901–906.

39. Herbst H, Niedobitek G, Kneba M, et al. High incidence of Epstein-Barr virus genomes in Hodgkin's disease. Am J Pathol 1990; 137:13–18.

40. Gledhill S, Gallagher A, Jones DB, et al. Viral involvement in Hodgkin's disease: detection of clonal type A Epstein-Barr virus genomes in tumour samples. Br J Cancer 1991; 64:227–232.

41. Knecht H, Odermatt BF, Bachmann E, et al. Frequent detection of Epstein-Barr virus DNA by the polymerase chain reaction in lymph node biopsies from patients with Hodgkin's disease without genomic evidence of B- or T-cell clonality. Blood 1991; 78:760–767.

42. Weiss LM, Chen YY, Liu XF, Shibata D. Epstein–Barr virus and Hodgkin's disease: a correlative in situ hybridization and polymerase chain reaction study. Am J Pathol 1991; 139:1259–1265.

43. Spieker T, Kurth J, Küppers R, Rajewsky K, Bräuninger A, Hansmann ML. Molecular single-cell analysis of the clonal relationship of small Epstein–Barr virus-infected cells and Epstein–Barr virus-harboring Hodgkin and Reed/Sternberg cells in Hodgkin disease. Blood 2000; 96:3133–3138.

44. Faumont N, Al Saati T, Brousset P, Offer C, Delsol G, Meggetto F. Demonstration by single-cell PCR that Reed–Sternberg cells and bystander B lymphocytes are infected by different Epstein-Barr virus strains in Hodgkin's disease. J Gen Virol 2001; 82:1169–1174.

45. Niedobitek G, Herbst H, Young LS, et al. Patterns of Epstein-Barr virus infection in non-neoplastic lymphoid tissue. Blood 1992; 79:2520–2526.

46. Siebert JD, Ambinder RF, Napoli VM, Quintanilla-Martinez L, Banks PM, Gulley ML. Human immunodeficiency virus-associated Hodgkin's disease contains latent, not replicative, Epstein–Barr virus. Hum Pathol 1995; 26:1191–1195.

47. Hummel M, Anagnostopulos I, Dallenbach F, Korbjuhn P, Dimmler C, Stein H. EBV infection patterns in Hodgkin's disease and normal lymphoid tissue: expression and cellular localization of EBV gene products. Br J Haematol 1992; 82:689–694.

48. Zhu ZG, Hamilton-Dutoit S, Yan QH, Pallesen G. The association between Epstein–Barr virus and Chinese Hodgkin's disease. Int J Cancer 1993; 55:359–363.

49. Huh J, Park C, Juhng S, Kim CE, Poppema S, Kim C. A pathologic study of Hodgkin's disease in Korea and its association with the Epstein–Barr virus. Cancer 1996; 77:949–955.

50. Belkaid MI, Briere J, Djebbara Z, Beldjord K, Andrieu JM, Colonna P. Comparison of Epstein–Barr virus markers in Reed–Sternberg cells in adult Hodgkin's disease tissues from an industrialized and a developing country. Leuk Lymphoma 1995; 17: 163–168.

51. Preciado MV, De Matteo E, Diez B, Menarguez J, Grinstein S. Presence of Epstein–Barr virus and strain type assignment in Argentine childhood Hodgkin's disease. Blood 1995; 86:3922–3929.

52. Quintanilla-Martinez L, Gamboa-Dominquez A, Gamez-Ledesma I, Angeles-Angeles A, Mohar A. Association of Epstein–Barr virus latent membrane protein and Hodgkin's disease in Mexico. Mod Pathol 1995; 8:675–679.

53. Chang KL, Albujar PF, Chen YY, Johnson RM, Weiss LM. High prevalence of Epstein–Barr virus in the Reed–Sternberg cells of Hodgkin's disease occurring in Peru. Blood 1993; 81:496–501.

54. Ambinder R, Browning PJ, Lorenzana I, et al. Epstein-Barr virus and childhood Hodgkin's disease in Honduras and the United States. Blood 1993; 81:462–467.

55. Jarrett RF, Gallagher A, Jones DB, et al. Detection of Epstein-Barr virus genomes in Hodgkin's disease: relation to age. J Clin Pathol 1991; 44:844–848.

56. Armstrong AA, Alexander FE, Pinto Paes R, et al. Association of Epstein-Barr virus with pediatric Hodgkin's disease. Am J Pathol 1993; 142:1683–1688.

57. Jarrett RF, Armstrong AA, Alexander E. Epidemiology of EBV and Hodgkin's lymphoma. Ann Oncol 1996; 7(suppl 4):S5–S10.

58. O'Grady J, Stewart S, Elton RA, Krajewski AS. Epstein–Barr virus in Hodgkin's disease and site of origin of tumour. Lancet 1994; 343:265–266.

59. Dolcetti R, Boiocchi M, Gloghini A, Carbone A. Pathogenetic and histogenetic features of HIV-associated Hodgkin's disease. Eur J Cancer 2001; 37:1276–1287.

60. Palli D, Trallori G, Bagnoli S, et al. Hodgkin's disease risk is increased in patients with ulcerative colitis. Gastroenterology 2000; 119:647–653.

61. Gan YJ, Razzouk BI, Su T, Sixbey JW. A defective, rearranged Epstein–Barr virus genome in EBER-negative and EBER-positive Hodgkin's disease. Am J Pathol 2002; 160:781–786.

62. Staratschek-Jox A, Kotkowski S, Belge G, et al. Detection of Epstein-Barr virus in Hodgkin-Reed–Sternberg cells: no evidence for the persistence of integrated viral fragment in latent membrane protein-1 (LMP-1)-negative classical Hodgkin's disease. Am J Pathol 2000; 156:209–216.

63. Boyle MJ, Vasak E, Tschuchnigg M, et al. Subtypes of Epstein-Barr virus in Hodgkin's disease: association between B-type EBV and immunocompromise. Blood 1993; 81:468–474.

64. Knecht H, Bachmann E, Brousset P, et al. Deletions within the LMP1 oncogene of Epstein-Barr virus are clustered in Hodgkin's disease and identical to those observed in nasopharyngeal carcinoma. Blood 1993; 82:2937–2942.

65. Chen ML, Tsai CN, Liang CL, et al. Cloning and characterization of the latent membrane protein (LMP) of a specific Epstein-Barr virus variant derived from nasopharyngeal carcinoma in the Taiwanese population. Oncogene 1992; 7:2131–2140.

66. Hu LF, Zabarovsky ER, Chen F, et al. Isolation and sequencing of the Epstein-Barr virus BNLF-1 (LMP1) from a Chinese nasopharyngeal carcinoma. J Gen Virol 1991; 72:2399–2409.

67. Hu LF, Chen F, Zheng X, et al. Clonability and tumourigenicity of human epithelial cells expressing the EBV-encoded membrane protein LMP1. Oncogene 1993; 8:1575–1583.

68. Trivedi P, Hu LF, Chen F, et al. Epstein-Barr virus (EBV)-encoded membrane protein LMP1 from a nasopharyngeal carcinoma is non-immunogenic in a murine model system, in contrast to a B-cell-derived homologue. Eur J Cancer 1994; 30A:84–88.

69. Sandvej K, Peh SC, Andresen BS, Pallesen G. Identification of potential hot spots in the carboxy-terminal part of the Epstein–Barr virus (EBV) BNLF-1 gene in both malignant and benign EBV-associated diseases: high frequency of a 30-bp deletion in Malaysian and Danish peripheral T-cell lymphomas. Blood 1994; 84:4053–4060.

70. Dolcetti R, Zancai P, De Re V, et al. Epstein-Barr virus strains with latent membrane protein-1 deletion: prevalence in the Italian population and high association with human immunodeficiency virus-related Hodgkin's disease. Blood 1997; 89:1723–1731.

71. Sandvej K, Andresen BS, Zhou XG, Gregersen N, Hamilton-Dutoit S. Analysis of the Epstein–Barr virus (EBV) latent membrane protein 1 (LMP-1) gene and promoter in Hodgkin's disease isolates: selection against EBV variants with mutations in the LMP-1 promoter ATF-1/CREB-1 binding site. Acta Biochim Pol 2000; 53:280–288.

72. Herbst H, Dallenbach F, Hummel M, et al. Epstein-Barr virus latent membrane protein expression in Hodgkin and Reed–Sternberg cells. Proc Natl Acad Sci USA 1991; 88:4766–4770.

73. Pallesen G, Hamilton-Dutoit SJ, Rowe M, Young LS. Expression of Epstein–Barr virus latent gene products in tumour cells of Hodgkin's disease. Lancet 1991; 337: 320–322.

74. Grässer FA, Murray PG, Kremmer E, et al. Monoclonal antibodies directed against the Epstein-Barr virus-encoded nuclear antigen 1 (EBNA1): immunohistologic detection of EBNA1 in the malignant cells of Hodgkin's disease. Blood 1994; 84:3792–3798.

75. Deacon EM, Pallesen G, Niedobitek G, et al. Epstein-Barr virus and Hodgkin's disease: transcriptional analysis of virus latency in the malignant cells. J Exp Med 1993; 177:339–349.

76. Niedobitek G, Kremmer E, Herbst H, et al. Immunohistochemical detection of the Epstein-Barr virus-encoded latent membrane protein 2A (LMP2A) in Hodgkin's disease and infectious mononucleosis. Blood 1997; 90:1664–1672.

77. Pallesen G, Sandvej K, Hamilton-Dutoit SJ, Rowe M, Young LS. Activation of Epstein–Barr virus replication in Hodgkin and Reed–Sternberg cells. Blood 1991; 78:1162–1165.

78. Brousset P, Knecht H, Rubin B, et al. Demonstration of Epstein-Barr virus replication in Reed–Sternberg cells of Hodgkin' s disease. Blood 1993; 82:872–876.

79. Drouet E, Brousset P, Fares F, et al. High Epstein-Barr virus serum load and elevated titers of anti-ZEBRA antibodies in patients with EBV-harboring tumor cells of Hodgkin's disease. J Med Virol 1999; 57:383–389.

80. Hudson GS, Farrell PJ, Barrell BG. Two related but differentially expressed potential membrane proteins encoded by the *Eco* RI Dhet region of Epstein–Barr virus B95–8. J Virol 1985; 53:528–535.

81. Devergne O, Hatzivassiliou E, Izumi KM, et al. Association of TRAF1, TRAF2, and TRAF3 with an Epstein-Barr virus LMP1 domain important for B-lymphocyte transformation: role in NF-kB activation. Mol Cell Biol 1996; 16:7098–7108.

82. Kieser A, Kilger E, Gires O, Ueffing M, Kolch W, Hammerschmidt W. Epstein–Barr virus latent membrane protein-1 triggers AP-1 activity via the c-jun N-terminal kinase cascade. EMBO J 1997; 16:6478–6485.

83. Gires O, Kohlhuber F, Kilger E, et al. Latent membrane protein 1 of Epstein-Barr virus interacts with JAK3 and activates STAT proteins. EMBO J 1999; 18:3064–3073.

84. Izumi KM, Kieff ED. The Epstein–Barr virus oncogene product latent membrane protein 1 engages the tumor necrosis factor-associated death domain protein to mediate B lymphocyte growth transformation and activate NF-kB. Proc Natl Acad Sci USA 1997; 94:12,592–12,597.

85. Brown KD, Hostager BS, Bishop GA. Differential signaling and tumor necrosis factor receptor-associated factor (TRAF) degradation mediated by CD40 and the Epstein–Barr virus oncoprotein latent membrane protein 1 (LMP1). J Exp Med 2001; 193:943–954.

86. Longnecker R, Kieff E. A second Epstein–Barr virus membrane protein (LMP2) is expressed in latent infection and colocalizes with LMP1. J Virol 1990; 64:2319–2326.

87. Dykstra ML, Longnecker R, Pierce SK. Epstein–Barr virus coopts lipid rafts to block the signaling and antigen transport functions of the BCR. Immunity 2001; 14:57–67.

88. Fruehling S, Longnecker R. The immunoreceptor tyrosine-based activation motif of Epstein–Barr virus LMP2A is essential for blocking BCR-mediated signal transduction. Virology 1997; 235:241–251.

89. Fruehling S, Swart R, Dolwick KM, Kremmer E, Longnecker R. Tyrosine 112 of latent membrane protein 2A is essential for protein tyrosine kinase loading and regulation of Epstein–Barr virus latency. J Virol 1998; 72:7796–7806.

90. Miller CL, Lee JH, Kieff E, Longnecker R. An integral membrane protein (LMP2) blocks reactivation of Epstein–Barr virus from latency following surface immunoglobulin crosslinking. Proc Natl Acad Sci USA 1994; 91:772–776.

91. Caldwell RG, Wilson JB, Anderson SJ, Longnecker R. Epstein–Barr virus LMP2A drives B-cell development and survival in the absence of normal B-cell receptor signals. Immunity 1998; 9:405–411.

92. Caldwell RG, Brown RC, Longnecker R. Epstein–Barr virus LMP2A-induced B-cell survival in two unique classes of EmuLMP2A transgenic mice. J Virol 2000; 74:1101–1113.

93. Calender A, Billaud M, Aubry J, Banchereau J, Vuillaume M, Lenoir G. EBV induces expression of B-cell activation markers on in vitro infection of EBV negative B lymphoma cells. Proc Natl Acad Sci USA 1987; 84:8060–8064.

94. Wang D, Leibowitz D, Wang F, et al. Epstein-Barr virus latent infection membrane protein alters the human B-lymphocyte phenotype: deletion of the amino terminus abolishes activity. J Virol 1988; 62:4173–4184.

95. Henderson S, Rowe M, Gregory C, et al. Induction of bcl-2 expression by Epstein-Barr virus latent membrane protein 1 protects infected B-cells from programmed cell death. Cell 1991; 65:1107–1115.

96. Herbst H, Raff T, Stein H. Phenotypic modulation of Hodgkin and Reed–Sternberg cells by Epstein–Barr virus. J Pathol 1996; 179:54–59.

97. Dürkop H, Foss HD, Demel G, Klotzbach H, Hahn C, Stein H. Tumor necrosis factor receptor-associated factor 1 is overexpressed in Reed–Sternberg cells of Hodgkin's disease and Epstein–Barr virus transformed lymphoid cells. Blood 1999; 93:617–623.

98. Siegler G, Kremmer E, Gonella R, Niedobitek G. Epstein–Barr Virus-encoded latent membrane protein (LMP) 1 and TNF receptor-associated factors (TRAF): co-localisation of LMP1 and TRAF1 in EBV-associated lymphoproliferations in vivo. J Clin Pathol: Mol Pathol 2003; 56:156–161.

99. Fries KL, Miller WE, Raab-Traub N. Epstein–Barr virus latent membrane protein-1 blocks p53-mediated apoptosis through the induction of the A20 gene. J Virol 1996:8653–8659.

100. Niedobitek G, Rowlands DC, Young LS, et al. Overexpression of p53 in Hodgkin's disease: lack of correlation with Epstein-Barr virus infection. J Pathol 1993; 169:207–212.

101. Lee I, Kim MK, Choi EY, et al. CD99 expression is positively regulated by Sp1 and is negatively regulated by Epstein–Barr virus latent membrane protein 1 through nuclear factor-kappaB. Blood 2001:3596–3604.

102. Bai MC, Jiwa NM, Horstman A, et al. Decreased expression of cellular markers in Eptein-Barr virus-positive Hodgkin's disease. J Pathol 1994; 174:49–55.

103. Birkenbach M, Liebowitz D, Wang F, Sample J, Kieff E. Epstein–Barr virus latent infection membrane protein increases vimentin expression in human B-cell lines. J Virol 1989; 63:4079–4084.

104. Liebowitz D, Kopan R, Fuchs E, Sample J, Kieff E. An Epstein–Barr virus transforming protein associates with vimentin in lymphocytes. Mol Cell Biol 1987; 7:2299–2308.

105. Foss HD, Herbst H, Oelmann E, et al. Lymphotoxin, tumour necrosis factor and interleukin-6 gene transcripts are present in Hodgkin and Reed–Sternberg cells of most Hodgkin's disease cases. Br J Haematol 1993; 84:627–635.

106. Herbst H, Samol J, Foss HD, Raff T, Niedobitek G. Modulation of interleukin-6 expression in Hodgkin and Reed–Sternberg cells by Epstein–Barr virus. J Pathol 1997; 182:299–306.

107. Beck A, Päzolt D, Grabenbauer GG, et al. Expression of cytokine and chemokine genes in Epstein-Barr virus-associated nasopharyngeal carcinoma and Hodgkin's disease. J Pathol 2001; 194:145–151.

108. Dukers DF, Jaspars LH, Vos W, et al. Quantitative immunohistochemical analysis of cytokine profiles in Epstein-Barr virus-positive and -negative cases of Hodgkin's disease. J Pathol 2000; 190:143–149.

109. Foss HD, Herbst H, Hummel M, et al. Patterns of cytokine gene expression in infectious mononucleosis. Blood 1994; 83:707–712.

110. Eliopoulos AG, Stack M, Dawson CW, et al. Epstein-Barr virus-encoded LMP1 and CD40 mediate IL-6 production in epithelial cells via an NF-kB pathway involving TNF receptor-associated factors. Oncogene 1997; 14:2899–2916.

111. Rowe M, Peng-Pilon M, Huen DS, et al. Upregulation of bcl-2 by the Epstein-Barr virus latent membrane protein LMP1: a B-cell specific response that is delayed relative to NF-kB activation and to induction of cell surface markers. J Virol 1994; 68:122–131.

112. Eliopoulos AG, Gallagher NJ, Blake SMS, Dawson CW, Young LS. Activation of the p38 mitogen-activated protein kinase pathway by Epstein–Barr virus-encoded latent membrane protein 1 coregulates interleukin-6 and interleukin-8 production. J Biol Chem 1999; 274:16,085–16,096.

113. Mori N, Shirakawa F, Shimizu F, et al. Transcriptional regulation of the human interleukin-6 gene promoter in human T-cell leukemia virus type I-infected T-cell lines: evidence for the involvement of NF-kB. Blood 1994; 84:2904–2911.

114. Herbst H, Foss HD, Samol J, et al. Frequent expression of interleukin-10 by Epstein–Barr virus-harboring tumor cells of Hodgkin's disease. Blood 1996; 87:2918–2929.

115. Hayes DP, Brink AA, Vervoort MB, Middeldorp JM, Meijer CJ, van den Brule AJ. Expression of Epstein–Barr virus (EBV) transcripts encoding homologues to important human proteins in diverse EBV associated diseases. Mol Pathol 1999; 52:97–103.

116. Gartely MK, Renzetti LM, Magram J, et al. The interleukin-12/interleukin-12-receptor system: role in normal and pathologic immune responses. Ann Rev Immunol 1998; 16:495–521.

117. Schwaller J, Tobler A, Niklaus G, et al. Interleukin-12 expression in human lymphomas and nonneoplastic lymphoid disorders. Blood 1995; 85:2182–2188.

118. Niedobitek G, Päzolt D, Teichmann M, Devergne O. Frequent expression of the Epstein–Barr virus (EBV)-induced gene, EBI3, an IL-12 p40-related cytokine, in Hodgkin and Reed–Sternberg cells. J Pathol 2002; 198:310–316.

119. Pflanz S, Timans JC, Cheung J, et al. IL-27, a heterodimeric cytokine composed of EBI3 and p28 protein, induces proliferation of naive CD4+ T-cells. Immunity 2002; 16:779–790.

120. Teruya-Feldstein J, Jaffe ES, Burd PR, Kingma DW, Setsuda JE, Tosato G. Differential chemokine expression in tissues involved by Hodgkin's disease: direct correlation of eotaxin expression and tissue eosinophilia. Blood 1999; 93:2463–2470.

121. Buri C, Körner M, Schärlii P, et al. CC chemokines and the receptors CCR3 and CCR5 are differentially expressed in the nonneoplastic leukocytic infiltrates of Hodgkin's disease. Blood 2001; 97:1543–1548.

122. Teichmann M, Meyer B, Beck A, Niedobitek G. Expression of the interferon-inducible chemokine IP-10 (CXCL10), a chemokine with proposed anti-neoplastic functions, in Hodgkin lymphoma and nasopharyngeal carcinoma. J Pathol 2005; 206:68–75.

123. van den Berg A, Visser L, Poppema S. High expression of the CC chemokine TARC in Reed–Sternberg cells. Am J Pathol 1999; 154:1685–1691.

124. Momose H, Chen YY, Benezra J, Weiss LM. Chronic lymphocytic leukemia small lymphocytic lymphoma with Reed–Sternberg like cells and possible transformation to Hodgkin's disease. Mediation by Epstein–Barr virus. Am J Surg Pathol 1992; 16:859–867.

125. Khan G, Coates PJ, Gupta RK, Kangro HO, Slavin G. Presence of Epstein–Barr virus in Hodgkin's disease is not exclusive to Reed–Sternberg cells. Am J Pathol 1992; 140:757–762.

126. Isaacson PG, Schmid C, Pan L, Wotherspoon AC, Wright DH. Epstein–Barr virus latent membrane protein expression by Hodgkin and Reed–Sternberg-like cells in acute infectious mononucleosis. J Pathol 1992; 167:267–271.

127. Reynolds DJ, Banks PM, Gulley ML. New characterisation of infectious mononucleosis and a phenotypic comparison with Hodgkin's disease. Am J Pathol 1995; 146:379–388.

128. Kapadia SB, Roman LN, Kingma DW, Jaffe ES, Frizzera G. Hodgkin's disease of Waldeyer's ring. Clinical and histoimmunophenotypic findings and association with Epstein–Barr virus in 16 cases. Am J Surg Pathol 1995; 19:1431–1439.

129. Murray RJ, Wang D, Young LS, et al. Epstein-Barr virus-specific cytotoxic T cell recognition of transfectants expressing the virus-coded latent membrane protein LMP. J Virol 1988; 62:3747–3755.

130. Thorley-Lawson DA, Israelsohn ES. Generation of specific cytotoxic T-cells with a fragment of the Epstein–Barr virus-encoded p63/latent membrane protein. Proc Natl Acad Sci USA 1987; 84:5384–5388.

131. Klein G. Viral latency and transformation: the strategy of Epstein–Barr virus. Cell 1989; 58:5–8.
132. Chen HF, Kevan-Jah S, Suentzenich KO, Grasser FA, Mueller-Lantzsch N. Expression of the Epstein–Barr virus latent membrane protein (LMP) in insect cells and detection of antibodies in human sera against this protein. Virology 1992; 190:106–115.
133. Poppema S, Bhan AK, Reinherz EL, Posner MR, Schlossman SF. In situ immunologic characterization of cellular constituents in lymph nodes and spleens involved by Hodgkin's disease. Blood 1982; 59:226–232.
134. Willenbrock K, Roers A, Blohbaum B, Rajewsky K, Hansmann ML. CD8(+) T-cells in Hodgkin's disease tumor tissue are a polyclonal population with limited clonal expansion but little evidence of selection by antigen. Am J Pathol 2000; 157:171–175.
135. Oudejans JJ, Jiwa NM, Kummer JA, et al. Analysis of major histocompatibility complex class I expression on Reed–Sternberg cells in relation to the cytotxic T-cell response in Epstein-Barr virus-positive and -negative Hodgkin's disease. Blood 1996; 87:3844–3851.
136. Oudejans JJ, Jiwa NM, Kummer JA, et al. Activated cytotoxic T-cells as prognostic marker in Hodgkin's disease. Blood 1997; 89:1376–1382.
137. Kandil A, Bazarbashi S, Mourad WA. The correlation of Epstein–Barr virus expression and lymphocyte subsets with the clinical presentation of nodular sclerosing Hodgkin's disease. Cancer 2001; 91:1957–1963.
138. Frisan T, Sjoberg J, Dolcetti R, et al. Local suppression of Epstein-Barr virus (EBV)-specific cytotoxicity in biopsies of EBV-positive Hodgkin's disease. Blood 1995; 86:1493–1501.
139. Dolcetti R, Frisan T, Sjoberg J, et al. Identification and characterization of an Epstein-Barr virus-specific T-cell response in the pathologic tissue of a patient with Hodgkin's disease. Cancer Res 1995; 54:3675–3681.
140. Chapman ALN, Rickinson AB, Thomas WA, Jarrett RF, Crocker J, Lee SP. Epstein–Barr virus-specific cytotoxic T lymphocyte responses in the blood and tumor site of Hodgkin's disease patients: implications for a T-cell-based therapy. Cancer Res 2001; 61:6219–6226.
141. Moore KW, de Waal Malefyt R, Coffman RL. Interleukin-10 and the interleukin-10 receptor. Ann Rev Immunol 2001; 19:683–765.
142. Beatty PR, Krams SM, Martinez OM. Involvement of IL-10 in the autonomouos growth of EBV-transformed B-cell lines. J Immunol 1997; 158:4045–4051.
143. Salazar-Onfray F. Interleukin-10: a cytokine used by tumors to escape immunosurveillance. Med Oncol 1999; 16:86–94.
144. Oudejans JJ, Kummer JA, Jiwa M, et al. Granzyme B expression in Reed–Sternberg cells of Hodgkin's disease. Am J Pathol 1996; 148:233–240.
145. Bladergroen BA, Meijerm CJLM, ten Berge RL, et al. Expression of the granzyme B inhibitor, protease inhibitor 9, by tumor cells in patients with non-Hodgkin and Hodgkin lymphoma: a novel protective mechanism for tumor cells to circumvent the immune system? Blood 2002; 99:232–237.
146. Oelmann E, Herbst H, Zühlsdorf M, et al. Tissue inhibitor of metalloproteinases 1 is an autocrine and paracrine survival factor, with additional immune-regulatory functions, expressed by Hodgkin/Reed–Sternberg cells. Blood 2002; 99:258–267.
147. Sutkowski N, Palkama T, Ciurli C, Sekaly RP, Thorley-Lawson DA, Huber BT. An Epstein–Barr virus-associated superantigen. J Exp Med 1996; 184:971–980.
148. Sutkowski N, Conrad B, Thorley-Lawson DA, Huber BT. Epstein–Barr virus transactivates the human endogenous retrovirus HERV-K18 that encodes a superantigen. Immunity 2001; 15:579–589.
149. Dukers DF, Meij P, Vervoort MBHJ, et al. Direct immunosuppressive effects of EBV-encoded latent membrane protein 1. J Immunol 2000; 165:663–670.
150. Marshall NA, Vickers MA, Barker RN. Regulatory T-cells secreting IL-10 dominate the immune response to EBV latent membrane protein 1. J Immunol 2003; 170:6183–6189.

12

Posttransplant Lymphoproliferative Disorder

Lode J. Swinnen

*Department of Oncology, Division of Hematologic Malignancies,
Johns Hopkins School of Medicine, Baltimore, Maryland, U.S.A.*

INTRODUCTION

Epstein–Barr virus (EBV)–associated lymphoproliferative disorders were first identified as a complication of immunodeficiency in the setting of organ transplantation. Similar lymphoproliferations have since been recognized in a variety of acquired and congenital immunodeficiency states. The clinical, pathologic, and molecular features of these disorders differ significantly from those of non-Hodgkin's lymphomas (HLs) encountered in immunocompetent individuals. Initially, these EBV-associated lymphoproliferations were viewed as EBV-associated B-cell tumors, but proliferations of T-cell origin and EBV-negative tumors have become increasingly common in such patients after survival for many years with immunodeficiency. The high prevalence in pediatric organ transplant recipients and following the use of intensive immunosuppressive regimens has also contributed to growing concerns about these disorders. Despite the curability of a proportion of patients, mortality from the disease has typically been high. Newer diagnostic and screening techniques and therapeutic advances such as monoclonal antibodies and adoptive T-cell therapy are likely to result in a lower prevalence and better treatment outcome.

EPIDEMIOLOGY

Transplant Type

Although several factors independently influence the risk for posttransplant lymphoproliferative disorder (PTLD), the type of transplant is clearly significant. The reason for the differences is unknown and may relate to the intensity of immunosuppression, factors specific to the graft, or to both (Table 1). An incidence of 3.4% following heart transplantation and 7.9% following lung transplantation was reported from the University of Pittsburgh (3). Large-scale registry data indicate a cumulative incidence of 5% by seven years in heart recipients, and of 1% by 10 years in renal recipients (2,4). The incidence of PTLD following allogeneic bone

Table 1   Incidence of PTLD by Type of Organ Transplant

Type of transplant (Ref.)	Incidence (%)
Bone marrow (1)	1
Kidney (2)	1
Liver (3)	2.2
Heart (2)	5
Lung (3)	7.9

Abbreviation: PTLD, posttransplant lymphoproliferative disorder.

marrow transplantation is generally low, of the order of 1%, unless the graft is mismatched or T-cell depleted. An analysis of data reported to the International Bone Marrow Transplant Registry (IBMTR) indicates a cumulative PTLD incidence of $1.0\% \pm 0.3\%$ at 10 years (1). However, one year following allogeneic bone marrow transplantation, a stable drop to a very low incidence rate of 120 cases per 10,000 patient-years was evident. That observation sharply contrasts with the unbroken rise in cumulative incidence seen after solid organ transplantation, and is likely due to the fact that immunosuppressive therapies are discontinued by the end of the first year following bone marrow transplantation, while they usually must be maintained indefinitely in solid organ recipients.

Immunosuppressive Drugs

Significant increases in PTLD incidence have repeatedly been linked with specific immunosuppressive drugs or regimens. A risk as high as 12% was associated with the use of cyclosporin prior to the advent of blood level monitoring (5). Agents specifically targeting or depleting T-cells result in the highest risk, with the effect at least partially dependent on the intensity and duration of T-cell suppression. The immunosuppressive antibody OKT3, a potent anti–T-cell agent, resulted in a ninefold higher incidence of PTLD in cardiac transplant recipients receiving induction immunotherapy, with an incidence of 35.7% in patients who had received two courses of the drug (6). In a recent analysis of the United Network for Organ Sharing (UNOS) registry data for 2713 renal transplant recipients, the use of various immunotherapy induction agents was compared with no induction therapy. The use of monoclonal antilymphocyte antibodies resulted in a 72% increase in risk, from an incidence of 0.51% to an incidence of 0.85%. The use of polyclonal antilymphocyte antibodies or of anti–interleukin-2 receptor antibody resulted in nonsignificant increases of 29% and 14%, respectively (7). Many other observations are consistent with the conclusion that the intensity of immunosuppression and, particularly, the use of selective anti–T-cell agents highly correlates with the risk for PTLD (8,9).

Analysis of the IBMTR data showed that the risk of PTLD following allogeneic bone marrow transplant (BMT) was strongly associated with donor–recipient mismatch ($RR = 4.1$), T-cell depletion of the allograft ($RR = 12.7$), prophylactic use of polyclonal antithymocyte globulin ($RR = 6.4$), and particularly administration of monoclonal antilymphocyte antibodies ($RR = 43.2$). The presence of two of these risk factors correlated with a PTLD incidence of 8%, and three or more risk factors with a 22% incidence. Selective depletion of T-cells was associated with a much higher risk than were approaches that removed both T- and B-cells, such as

Campath-1 monoclonal antibody or elutriation (1). The effect of the composition of the long-term maintenance immunosuppressive regimen on the risk of PTLD has been studied less extensively than that of induction regimens, other than observing that calcineurin inhibitors such as cyclosporin and tacrolimus require blood-level monitoring, and that the PTLD incidence with tacrolimus is comparable to that with cyclosporin (10,11). Interestingly, the UNOS database analysis showed that the use of mycophenolate mofetil maintenance immunosuppression correlated with a statistically significant 36% reduction in PTLD risk relative to azathioprine (7).

Although most common after solid organ transplantation, identical or very similar lymphoproliferations have been described in many other immunodeficiency settings and following the use of drugs other than the immunosuppressive therapies typically used in organ transplantation. These include methotrexate used in patients with rheumatoid arthritis (12), and fludarabine for non-HL (13) and following non-myeloablative allogeneic bone marrow transplantation.

Age and EBV Seropositivity

Pretransplant EBV seronegativity is perhaps the single greatest risk factor for PTLD (Table 2). Seronegative recipients almost universally seroconvert within one year of transplantation (19). Over 90% of adults in the general population are seropositive for EBV with children comprising the majority of seronegative persons. The likelihood of seronegativity is determined by age and by social and geographic factors (14,15). The incidence of PTLD in the pediatric age group is not as well defined as among adults, but is clearly appreciably higher with up to 15% incidence after heart transplantation; a series from the University of Pittsburgh identified a four times higher risk of PTLD for pediatric transplant recipients than for adult transplant recipients (14,20). The exact level of risk for pretransplant EBV seronegative patients is difficult to determine. Several single-institution data sets exist (14,16,17). A Mayo Clinic study found the risk of PTLD in EBV-seronegative recipients to be 76 times higher than in seropositive recipients (15). Among a cohort of adult heart recipients, a much higher proportion of patients who went on to develop PTLD were EBV seronegative prior to transplantation than were patients who did not develop the disease (30% versus 5%) (6), comparable to findings that have been reported in pediatric liver recipients (17). A retrospective study identifying a ninefold greater incidence of PTLD in pretransplant EBV seronegative renal recipients is of particular interest in that the risk appeared to extend to late onset PTLD as well as to PTLD occurring early after transplantation. The median interval from transplant for these late cases was more than five years, and many occurred at around 10 years (21).

Table 2 Populations at High Risk for PTLD and References

Pretransplant EBV seronegative/pediatric age group (14–17)
Administration of monoclonal anti-CD3 antibodies (1,7,18)
Mismatched BMT (1)
T-cell depleted BMT (1)

Abbreviations: BMT, bone marrow transplant; EBV, Epstein–Barr virus; PTLD, posttransplant lymphoproliferative disorder.

Association with EBV

Disease Model Based on T-Cell Function

Although EBV-negative PTLD is increasingly seen as a very late complication of solid organ transplantation, the majority of cases are EBV associated. The virus plays a central role in the pathogenesis of this disease. The role, if any, of EBV in EBV-negative tumors is unknown.

One of the earliest observations was that clinical or serologic indications of primary or reactivated EBV infection were frequently observed around the time of clinical appearance of the disorder (22). Tumor tissue was subsequently found to contain EBV DNA in much larger quantities than normal tissue, and to actively express viral proteins (23–25). Suppression of T-cell function or numbers, to prevent graft rejection, is believed to result in uncontrolled EBV-driven proliferation of B-cells (22,26). Continued proliferation would then result in clones with a growth advantage, giving rise to one or more clonal populations. Although the specific mechanisms that produce all the clinico-pathologic entities constituting the PTLD spectrum remain unclear, the model is consistent with many of the unusual clinical and pathologic features of the disease.

Tumor-associated EBV is clonal, further supporting an etiologic role for the virus, rather than incidental subsequent infection of an already expanded neoplastic B-cell proliferation. The virus is usually of type A (type 1) (27). Clonality of the virus can be determined on the basis of the specific number of terminal repeat sequences formed when the linear EBV genome circularizes upon infection of a B-cell. Viral clonality corresponds to B-cell clonality as determined by immunoglobulin gene rearrangement analysis. In addition, lesions consisting of polyclonal or multiclonal B-cell proliferations contain multiple EBV clones, whereas monoclonal proliferations show evidence of a single infectious event (28,29).

Subclinical EBV-related changes can be identified prior to the appearance of clinical disease. Analysis of prior archived liver biopsy specimens in liver transplant recipients has shown the presence of EBV, as determined by polymerase chain reaction (PCR) or by in situ immunohistochemical staining for EBV-encoded RNA (EBER), in 70% of cases who subsequently developed PTLD. Of the cases that did not go on to develop the disease, only 10% had such findings (25). A preclinical phase for PTLD is also suggested by observations that viral load as determined in peripheral blood mononuclear cells increases prior to the appearance of clinically detectable disease (30,31). It is not clear whether such rises in EBV load necessarily indicate EBV-driven neoplasia, or are reflective of severe immunodeficiency at that point in time. The clinical observations of increased PTLD risk following primary EBV infection and in association with progressively more potent anti–T-cell drugs are very consistent with a disease model based on insufficient or inadequate T-cell surveillance of EBV-driven lymphoproliferation. This model is less informative in cases of PTLD that occur late after transplantation and in cases of T-cell or EBV-negative PTLD.

EBV Latency in PTLD

EBV infection of resting B-cells in vitro results in immortalized lymphoblastoid cell lines that express the full range of latent viral cycle proteins [six nuclear antigens: Epstein–Barr nuclear antigen (EBNA)-1, EBNA-2, EBNA-3A, EBNA-3B, EBNA-3C, and EBNA-LP, and three membrane proteins: latent membrane protein (LMP)-1, LMP-2A, and LMP-2B]—the so-called latency III pattern. In the presence of adequate EBV-specific immunity in vivo, only the nonimmunogenic EBNA-1 is expressed in tumors (latency I) as exemplified in endemic Burkitt lymphoma (BL).

It is often stated that expression of viral latency proteins in PTLD is essentially the same as that seen in lymphoblastoid cell lines, consistent with severely diminished EBV-specific T-cell function. Unlike oral hairy leukoplakia in immunodeficiency, PTLD has not been associated with a fully productive viral lytic cycle (32–34). Restoration of T-cell surveillance by withdrawal or reduction in immunosuppressive therapy can in fact result in permanent regression of PTLD, particularly those presenting early after transplantation.

However, in many instances PTLD will not regress with such measures despite expression of immunodominant EBNA proteins in the tumor. Varying degrees of restriction of antigenic expression have been identified in tumor tissue, possibly reflecting varying degrees of immune control or evolution over time to proliferations with structural genetic alterations (32,35). A recent study identified some correlation between the pattern of viral latency antigen expression, the cell of origin of the tumor, and both the time since transplant and tumor responsiveness to reduced immunosuppression. PTLD of postgerminal center origin expressing the latency pattern seen in Hodgkin's disease (HD) (EBNA1, LMP-1, and LMP-2) was identified (36). Such cells may have been rescued from apoptosis by EBV, with chromosomal or structural gene alterations sustaining growth in the face of T-cell surveillance.

LMP-1 is the viral protein of greatest importance for EBV-induced transformation of B-cells, and it has been considered equivalent to an oncogene in that respect. In vitro, LMP-1 mimics the effects of ligand-induced aggregation of CD40, activating the transcriptional activators nuclear factor-kappa B and activator protein 1 (37,38). This activation is mediated by tumor necrosis factor-receptor associated factor (TRAF) signaling molecules that interact directly with a portion of LMP-1 (39). These observations have been extended to PTLD in vivo by showing physical localization of LMP-1 and TRAF1 and TRAF3 (40). Much more frequent TRAF1 protein expression was found in LMP-1 positive than in LMP-1 negative tumors in one series of PTLD cases (41), while in another study no correlation could be found between TRAF1, TRAF2, or TRAF3 expression and either LMP-1 or EBER (42). Overexpression of bcl-2 might confer resistance to apoptosis, and bcl-2 overexpression was in fact identified in all PTLD tumors expressing LMP-1 in one series, while absence of LMP-1 expression was always associated with a lack of bcl-2 expression. Interestingly, the viral homologue of bcl-2, BHRF1, was not overexpressed in these tumors. Viral induction of human bcl-2 therefore appears to be the case (34).

PATHOLOGY OF PTLD

Marked variability is characteristic of the pathology and molecular features of PTLD. A spectrum appears to exist, with polymorphic, polyclonal proliferations at one end, and monomorphic, predominantly monoclonal tumors closely resembling aggressive non-HLs at the other. Whether transition along this spectrum occurs in vivo, or whether the different entities are reflective of an individual pathogenesis in each case, remains an open question. PTLD following solid organ transplantation is most often of recipient origin, while it is typically of donor origin following allogeneic bone marrow transplantation (43–46). The disease is typically extranodal or involves visceral rather than superficial nodes.

Tissue biopsies are usually necessary for a diagnosis of PTLD, because of the challenging histology and the frequent need for additional studies such as immunohistochemical stains for EBV and immunoglobulin gene rearrangement

Table 3 WHO Classification of PTLD

Early lesions
  Plasmacytic hyperplasia
  IM-like PTLD
Polymorphic PTLD
Monomorphic PTLD
  Diffuse large B-cell lymphoma
  BL or Burkitt-like lymphoma
  Plasma cell myeloma
  Plasmacytoma
  Peripheral T-cell lymphoma
  Other types
HL and Hodgkin-like PTLD

Abbreviations: BL, Burkitt lymphoma; HL, Hodgkin's lymphoma; IM, infectious mononucleosis; PTLD, posttransplant lymphoproliferative disorder; WHO, World Health Organization.
Source: From Ref. 56.

analysis to determine clonality (47). Multiple clones may exist within a lesion, and lesions at separate anatomic sites may have a different histologic appearance and clonal composition (48–50). Several pathologic classifications have been used, the most recent being that of the World Health Organization (Table 3) (51–56).

PTLD Presenting Early After Transplantation

Although considerable overlap exists between the clinicopathologic entities most often seen early after transplantation and those presenting at later time points, the concept of early versus late PTLD does appear to be valid and is of some clinical utility. The terms early and late refer to the time following transplantation rather than to an evolution of the disease over time, which has not been described with any frequency. The early pattern of disease is most likely to occur in the first one to perhaps two years following transplantation.

Histologically, the lesions are polymorphic and are classified as plasmacytic hyperplasia and infectious mononucleosis (IM)-like PTLD (IM-PTLD). The proliferations are typically polyclonal or show only small clonal components. IM-PTLD closely resembles IM, and may simply be IM in an immunocompromised host. Whether this represents a true PTLD with the same potential for morbidity is controversial. With the exception of bcl-6 mutations seen in somewhat less than half of the cases, additional genotypic abnormalities are not expected. The vast majority of PTLD presenting early after transplantation are EBV associated. PTLD characteristically contains an admixture of reactive T-cells. Polymorphic PTLD especially can have greater than 50% T-cells with some monomorphic PTLD, also reported to be T-cell rich (57,58). The nature of these T-cells is variable and has not been extensively studied, with some cases showing a predominance of CD8+ cells and others predominantly CD4+ cells (58,59). Cytokine profiles have been investigated and appear to be consistent with a Th2 cytokine environment that promotes B-cell growth (60).

PTLD Presenting Late After Transplantation

The histology of lesions presenting late after transplantation tends to be monomorphic and may closely resemble non-HL, multiple myeloma, or HD. This need not mean that the biology or clinical behavior of such lesions is the same as that of the histologically equivalent lesions seen in the general population. There is considerable heterogeneity in immunophenotype, with some cases having a phenotype like follicular center cells (CD10+, bcl-6+, melanoma associated antigen (mutated) (MUM)-1−, CD138−), and others being clearly postfollicular (CD10−, bcl-6−, MUM-1+, CD138+). Lesions are predominantly clonal, and most will have bcl-6 mutations; various genotypic abnormalities have been described, including c-myc rearrangements, neuroblastones RAS (N-RAS) mutations, and p53 mutations (52,61,62). Plasmacytoid differentiation can be very pronounced, resembling multiple myeloma or, more frequently, an extramedullary plasmacytoma. Data regarding cytogenetic abnormalities in PTLD are limited. Abnormalities have been identified, usually in tumors with monomorphic histology, but no characteristic abnormality has been found. In a series of 28 patients, no clonal cytogenetic abnormalities were identified among 10 polymorphic tumors, all of which were either polyclonal or oligoclonal. Analysis of 12 monomorphic cases revealed a variety of abnormalities in 10 cases: chromosome 8 translocations involving the *myc* gene, trisomy 9, trisomy 11, and 11q27 (61). Occasional extranodal marginal zone B-cell lymphomas have also been described in the posttransplant setting (63,64).

Overall, 15% to 30% of PTLD show no evidence of EBV even with EBER in situ hybridization. The LMP-1 immunostain is less sensitive than the EBER stain, but is less likely to be positive in lesions other than PTLD. EBV-negative PTLD is mostly found among monomorphic lesions presenting late, often very late, after transplantation (65–67).

T-Cell and Hodgkin-Like PTLD

T-cell PTLD frequently resembles peripheral T-cell lymphoma (68,69). Hepatosplenic lymphomas have been reported (70), as have been cases of anaplastic large-cell lymphoma or extranodal natural killer cell/T-cell lymphoma of nasal type (68,71). Posttransplant lesions that meet the criteria for classic HD occur. In the clearest cases, the Reed–Sternberg cells should be CD45−, CD15+, and CD30+ with either negative or variable CD20 expression. With less typical phenotypes, the term "Hodgkin-like PTLD" is sometimes used. Interestingly, as many as one third of T-cell PTLDs are EBV associated. HD in the posttransplant setting is usually EBV positive (68,72).

CLINICAL FEATURES AND MANAGEMENT

It is not only the pathology of PTLD that is heterogeneous. The variability in clinical behavior manifested by this disease is striking. This, coupled with the retrospective nature and small size of most published series, makes it difficult to generalize. Certain clinical patterns and associations have nevertheless been recognized, and can be of clinical utility. The literature does, however, remain very variable and on certain issues, even contradictory.

Disease Early After Transplantation

Certain clinical features are seen most often early after transplantation, usually at less than one year. A clinical presentation with marked constitutional symptoms and rapid enlargement of the tonsils and/or extranodal lesions is frequent (73,74).

Highly immunosuppressed patients may present with rapidly progressive, wide-spread disease, diffusely infiltrative multiorgan involvement, and a systemic sepsis-like syndrome, sometimes within weeks of transplantation (75). The diagnosis can be difficult to distinguish from sepsis alone, because fever is frequent, the disease is typically extranodal, and mass lesions may not be evident. Multiorgan failure is often the outcome, and the diagnosis may not be evident until autopsy (76,77). The disease is usually polyclonal or oligoclonal with polymorphic histology and is EBV associated. The histologic category of polymorphic hyperplasia appears to be the one most likely to regress with decreased immunosuppression (78).

Disease Late After Transplantation

PTLD presenting later than about a year after transplantation is likely to be more circumscribed anatomically, manifest few or no systemic symptoms, and progress less rapidly. The disease is usually extranodal, or involves visceral nodes. Gastroin-testinal involvement is frequent; about 25% of patients in one series presented with gastrointestinal disease manifesting as acute abdominal pain, obstruction, or hemor-rhage (76). The transplanted organ itself may be affected in up to 20% of cases, in either the early or the late setting, and may be the only site of disease. Central ner-vous system (CNS) involvement is mainly seen as part of very extensive disease, but may occur in isolation. Unlike classic systemic non-HLs, parenchymal CNS involve-ment is not rare. Multiple pulmonary nodules have been commonly described, and must be differentiated from infectious etiologies in an immunocompromised host (77,79). Although multiple studies have indicated that polymorphic or reactive-appearing PTLD is more likely to respond to reduction in immunosuppression than are the monomorphic histologic categories (78,80–83), this distinction can be very difficult to make on clinical or histologic grounds and in some series, no correlation between histology and clinical behavior could be found (84,85). Mutations of bcl-6 have been found to correlate with refractoriness to decreased immunosuppression and with a poor outcome in general in one study (61). The number of patients in this series was small, and the clinical data were retrospective and subject to many vari-ables. The finding of a c-myc rearrangement or other genotypic abnormality has also been found to correspond with clinical behavior that more closely resembles that of malignancies seen in immunocompetent patients, although the numbers studied are again small (52,62).

Prognostic Categories

The prognosis for PTLD is again highly variable, determined in part by clinical vari-ables in the individual patient and by response to the treatment modality used. Attempts at identifying factors predictive of outcome have been made; one large ret-rospective series of 61 patients identified EBV-negativity in the tumor or T-cell phe-notype as a negative tumor-related prognostic factor. The International Prognostic Index as used in immunocompetent patients was less predictive in PTLD than was a specific index using two risk factors: performance status 0 or 1 versus ≥ 2, and number of involved sites (1 versus >1) (86). A similar retrospective review of 54 cases with analysis for prognostic variables revealed advanced stage, involvement of the allograft, poor performance status, and CD20 negativity to be statistically sig-nificant negative prognostic factors (87). In view of the therapeutic value of the anti-CD20 antibody rituximab, it is important not to underestimate CD20 positivity because many of the cells in a PTLD may be infiltrating benign T-cells. Only a minority of the cells present in a biopsy specimen may actually be neoplastic CD20+ B-cells, with only a few scattered CD20+ cells that are observed pathologically (88).

Treatment Approach

Initial Therapy

There is no clear or generally accepted approach to the treatment of PTLD other than a widely held view that a reduction in immunosuppressive agent therapy should be the initial treatment (Table 4). It is worth noting that unlike non-HL, PTLD can be permanently resolved in some cases by surgical resection or by irradiation of unresectable but strictly localized lesions (3,76). Reduction in immunosuppression can clearly result in regression of PTLD in some cases, with permanent resolution in a proportion of them (3,76).

The probability of a response to reduction in immunosuppression appears to correlate with the interval since transplantation, perhaps because the interval also shows a degree of correlation with the morphology and clonality of lymphoproliferations. As many as 80% of patients presenting at less than one year following transplantation were found to respond to reduction in immunosuppression (though not all durably), while none presenting at more than one year did so (3). Differing results have been reported in other series, namely, lower response rates and greater variability in terms of the interval since transplantation (89,90). A detailed study of 11 renal recipients with PTLD reported an 82% durable complete response (CR) rate with reduced immunosuppression and simultaneous acyclovir. Peripheral CD8+ T-cell numbers increased significantly in responding patients, and CD8+ cells from two such patients were found to specifically recognize an immunodominant peptide from the EBV lytic gene BZLF-1 (91). When studied prospectively in a cooperative group trial for adult organ transplant recipients with PTLD, complete remission was achieved in none out of 20 patients despite an aggressive immunosuppressive reduction algorithm. Moreover, 38% of patients experienced rejection and 50% progressive disease during the period of reduced immunosuppression (92). Rapid disease progression, rejection of a vital organ, or the loss of a renal allograft complicating subsequent management are all valid concerns. The extent and duration of a reduction in immunosuppression is furthermore subjective and poorly defined in most reports. The efficacy and toxicity profile of rituximab are such that a strong case can be made for combining rituximab therapy with some reduction in immunosuppressive agents as the initial management of PTLD in all adult cases. Experience with rituximab in the pediatric setting is more limited.

Table 4 Therapies in Use for PTLD

Reduction in immunosuppressive therapies
Rituximab
Surgical resection or limited field irradiation
Cytotoxic chemotherapy
INF-α
Donor leukocyte infusion (for PTLD after T-cell depleted allogeneic BMT)
EBV-specific adoptive T-cell therapy (primarily for PTLD after allogeneic BMT)

Abbreviations: BMT, bone marrow transplant; EBV, Epstein–Barr virus; INF, interferon; PTLD, posttransplant lymphoproliferative disorders.

Regression of lymphoproliferations has been attributed anecdotally to the use of high-dose acyclovir, but the therapeutic value of antiviral drugs remains unproven (79,93). Acyclovir and ganciclovir are of unproven value as prophylaxes for PTLD, with anecdotal observations suggesting a lack of efficacy (94–96). Regression of PTLD following foscarnet therapy has been reported in three cases (97). The role of antivirals in the management of PTLD remains very unclear, although a course of acyclovir has often been included in the initial treatment of PTLD.

Anti–B-Cell Monoclonal Antibodies

The large-scale availability of rituximab, with its significant activity and, to date, minimal toxicity, has changed the management of PTLD. In fact, two anti–B-cell monoclonal antibody preparations have been studied and have been shown to be effective. The first was a mixture of anti-CD21 and anti-CD24 anti–B-cell monoclonal antibodies found to be effective in patients with polyclonal or oligoclonal disease in a European multicenter trial reported in 1991 involving both organ transplant and BMT recipients with PTLD (98). Long-term follow-up on this study was reported seven years later (99). Fifty-eight patients with PTLD (27 following bone marrow and 31 following organ transplantation) had been treated. The overall CR rate was 61%. The relapse rate was low at 8%. The long-term overall survival was 46% (BMT 35%, organ transplant 55%) at a median follow-up of 61 months. Complete remission was achieved in 46% of monoclonal and 80% of oligoclonal cases ($p = 0.05$). Multivisceral disease, CNS involvement, and late onset PTLD (>1 year posttransplant) were identified as predictive of poorer response on multivariate analysis. Only 29% of patients with CNS involvement and 22% of patients presenting later than one year posttransplant achieved complete remission. Toxicity was mild, consisting of transient fever, hypotension, and neutropenia. The antibodies used are unfortunately not clinically available. This is an important study because it not only first demonstrated the efficacy of anti–B-cell monoclonal antibody therapy against PTLD, but also showed that the remissions were durable. PTLD is currently the only malignancy known to be curable with anti–B-cell monoclonal antibody monotherapy.

The commercially available anti-CD20 antibody rituximab has shown definite efficacy in PTLD, and has come to be widely used as treatment for the disease. Initial data consisted of anecdotes and information obtained from a retrospective study of 32 patients (100,101). Immunosuppressive therapies had been modified in a variable fashion; among 26 evaluable patients, 54% CR and 15% partial response (PR) was reported. A prospective multicenter study of rituximab for PTLD following solid organ or bone marrow transplantation has been reported in preliminary fashion. Fifty-five patients (19 renal, 11 cardiac, 7 lung or heart-lung, 7 liver, and 11 hematopoietic stem cell transplant recipients) were recruited from 19 centers. Rituximab was given as four weekly doses of $375 \, \text{mg/m}^2$; solid organ transplant recipients had not responded to prior tapering of immunosuppressive therapies. The median interval from transplant was 25 months (0.4 months to 17 years). Twenty-five patients (45.5%) had responded, and of these, 18 (33%) had a CR or an unconfirmed CR by 80 days; on reassessment at 360 days, the CR rate remained 33%, and overall survival 63%. Median survival was 454 days (102,103). Toxicity as reported to date has usually been minor and does not appear to differ from that seen with the use of this drug in the immunocompetent population. The long-term follow-up data from the earlier study using anti-CD21/CD24 antibodies suggest that CRs following antibody therapy can be durable in many patients. Rituximab therefore has significant efficacy against B-cell PTLD at the cost of minimal toxicity. However, a significant proportion of patients do not achieve complete remission and require other therapy.

Cytotoxic Chemotherapy

Cytotoxic agents have traditionally been viewed as a last resort in the treatment of PTLD because of early reports of very high mortality with such treatments (3,79). Sepsis and other complications of chemotherapy have been the major problems in some centers, while others have found refractory disease to be common (3,79,89). A number of regimens have been used.

The regimen most commonly used for aggressive lymphomas in the immuno-competent population, CHOP (cyclophosphamide, doxorubicin, vincristine, and prednisone), has not been studied very extensively in the treatment of PTLD. Early small series suggested poor results. A multicenter retrospective series of CHOP for 25 patients with PTLD refractory to reduced immunosuppression showed a 48% CR rate. Median survival was one year for the group as a whole; 50% of patients achiev-ing CR relapsed, with a median time to progression of less than one year. A 36% mortality from treatment toxicity was seen (104). The combination of rituximab and CHOP (R–CHOP) may be more efficacious, but remains to be studied.

An aggressive multiagent regimen, prednisone, doxorubicin cyclophosphamide, etoposide, cytarabine blcomycin, vincristine, methotrexate, leucovorin (ProMACE-CytaBOM), has been studied retrospectively, and in a prospective trial. Initially, a 75% durable complete remission rate was achieved with a median follow-up of 64 months (77). In a prospective multicenter trial conducted prior to the advent of ritu-ximab in patients refractory to reduced immunosuppression, this regimen resulted in a CR rate of 67% and 57% durable CR at more than two years follow-up (92). The advent of better supportive care measures, granulocyte colony-stimulating factor, and preventive antibiotics has likely reduced the toxicity of intensive chemotherapy in this patient population.

Exceptionally good results have been reported in a study of pediatric organ transplant recipients treated with low-dose chemotherapy. Thirty-six patients (17 liver, 6 liver/bowel/pancreas, 5 renal, 3 heart, 3 bowel, and 2 lung recipients) were treated with cyclophosphamide 600 mg/m^2 IV on day 1 and prednisone 2 mg/kg on days 1 to 5, repeated every three weeks for a total of six cycles. All patients had failed prior modification of immunosuppressive therapies; immunosuppressive agents were not re-escalated during chemotherapy. Median age was 4.9 years, and median time from transplant was 5.3 months. The overall response rate was 86% (77% CR, 9% PR). Four (11%) patients experienced progressive disease, while two died of treat-ment-related causes. Median follow-up was 32 months, and only 5 patients have relapsed (105). Preliminary data on six pediatric patients treated with this regimen in combination with rituximab indicate no additional toxicity and complete remis-sion in five of the six patients.

These pediatric studies show better results than what has been seen in the adult studies, and this was achieved with considerably less therapy. A large proportion of patients in the pediatric study are likely to have had PTLD following primary EBV infection early after transplant; polymorphic, polyclonal, or oligoclonal proliferations, with few structural genetic abnormalities, would be expected in that setting. The treat-ment may have controlled EBV-driven lymphoproliferation during the time required for EBV-specific immunocompetence to develop. Although this study represents an excellent result in a pediatric population, it is unclear how well low-dose therapy would work in adult patients, against tumors presenting later after transplant and in the face of established EBV-specific immunity, or against tumors with more malignant histologic and biochemical features.

Other Therapies for PTLD

INF-α. Durable CRs have been achieved with low-dose interferon (INF)-α 2b, usually a dose of 3 million units/m^2 given daily or three times a week. Toxicity has generally been low, and rejection has not emerged as a major problem with this drug in patients suffering from PTLD. Neither the response rate nor the mechanism of action is well defined at this point. The drug might exert an antiviral and/or an antitumor effect; both early polyclonal proliferations and late-presenting monoclonal lesions have been reported to respond (94,106). In a series of 18 pediatric liver recipients treated with INF and concurrent discontinuation of immunosuppressive agents, a 77% CR rate was achieved. The extent to which these responses were attributable to the immunosuppressive reduction, to the INF, or to both, is unknown. Median survival was poor at only six months, primarily because of infectious complications (107). A study of INF in 16 adult PTLD patients refractory to reduced immunosuppression resulted in 50% CRs, the durability of which was unclear (108). On the other hand, 12 adult PTLD patients who were treated in a prospective study and had disease refractory to reduced immunosuppression showed only a 17% CR rate, with 17% PRs also (92). INF-α clearly has activity in PTLD, but the response rate may be lower than that of rituximab. Whether INF might be useful in cases refractory to rituximab is unknown.

T-cell therapy. In a disease model where PTLD is the result of inadequate T-cell control over EBV-driven lymphoproliferation, infusion of EBV-specific T-cells would be expected to cause regression or resolution of the proliferation. EBV-specific immunocompetence can rapidly be restored in T-cell–depleted allogeneic bone marrow recipients by the infusion of a limited number of peripheral blood leukocytes from the donor. PTLD could be controlled in these cases without incurring a more general and nonspecific graft-versus-host disease, probably because of the high frequency of EBV-specific effector cells in the relatively small number of leukocytes transfused (109). Adoptive transfer of more selective T-cell immunity has been achieved using in vitro expanded EBV-specific T-cells as treatment and prophylaxis for PTLD in BMT recipients (110,111). Polyclonal T-cell lines containing both CD4+ and CD8+ cells were used because it is not presently clear which antigens expressed by EBV-infected cells are important in generating an effector response. Adoptive transfer of EBV-specific T-cell immunity in solid organ recipients is constrained by the major histocompatibility complex–restricted nature of the T-cell response, and the fact that the majority of cases of PTLD arise from recipient rather than donor lymphocytes in the organ transplant setting. Encouraging preliminary data obtained from the use of autologous EBV-specific T-cells expanded in vitro have been reported in pediatric liver recipients (112). In a different approach, eight patients were treated with infusions of partly human leukocyte antigen–matched allogeneic EBV-specific cytotoxic T-cells derived from normal blood donors. Three complete remissions occurred. Responses were predominantly seen in patients with localized, polyclonal disease presenting early after transplantation. Graft-versus-host disease did not occur (113).

Several challenges remain: most notably the elaboration of suitable cytotoxic T-cells for patients experiencing primary EBV infection posttransplant, a particular problem in pediatric recipients, and demonstration of efficacy in patients with malignant tumors having a monomorphic histology that usually does not respond to reduction in immunosuppressive therapies and may or may not be amenable to EBV-specific immune control.

EARLY DIAGNOSIS AND SCREENING

PTLD can be subtle and easily overlooked or misdiagnosed as infection or rejection. A definitive diagnostic test for clinically evident disease would clearly be desirable, in view of the poor prognosis attached to extensive disease or declining performance status. Of even greater value would be a reliable test for subclinical lymphoprolifera-tion, which might allow identification of a state of overimmunosuppression, or per-mit early preemptive treatment for PTLD. There are extensive data supporting the existence of a detectable subclinical phase to the disease. Analysis of prior liver biopsy specimens in liver transplant recipients has shown that the presence of EBV, as determined by PCR or by in situ immunohistochemical staining for EBER expressing cells, could be detected in 70% of cases who subsequently developed PTLD. Only 10% of cases who did not go on to develop PTLD had such findings (25). More accessible indications of a preclinical phase of the disease are evident from observations that circulating viral load, as determined in peripheral blood mononuclear cells or in serum, increases prior to the appearance of clinically detected disease. These increases in viral load resolve following eradication of the PTLD. Some transplant centers already perform routine EBV viral load determina-tions and attempt to integrate that information into the clinical management of patients. However, many uncertainties exist. It is not clear when such rises in EBV load are indicative of EBV-driven neoplasia, and when they might only reflect the degree of immunodeficiency at the time. Pediatric cases are particularly challenging because viral load may be chronically high in patients who develop a posttransplant primary EBV infection (114). Multiple questions still need to be resolved before an effective test for routine posttransplant screening is achieved, including determina-tion of the best compartment (peripheral blood mononuclear cells, serum, or whole blood) to sample, the most suitable probes and methodologies for detection, and the establishment of stringent parameters of sensitivity and specificity in specific patient populations. Existing data are generally from small series with, at times, conflicting results (30,31,90,115–122).

REFERENCES

1. Curtis RE, Travis LB, Rowlings PA, et al. Risk of lymphoproliferative disorders after bone marrow transplantation: a multiinstitutional study. Blood 1999; 94:2208–2216.
2. Opelz G, Henderson R. Incidence of non-Hodgkin lymphoma in kidney and heart transplant recipients. Lancet 1993; 342:1514–1516.
3. Armitage JM, Kormos RL, Stuart RS, et al. Posttransplant lymphoproliferative disease in thoracic organ transplant patients: ten years of cyclosporine-based immunosuppres-sion. J Heart Lung Transplant 1991; 10:877–886.
4. Opelz G. Are post-transplant lymphomas inevitable? [editorial]. Nephrol Dial Trans-plant 1996; 11:1952–1955.
5. Starzl TE, Nalesnik MA, Porter KA, et al. Reversibility of lymphomas and lymphopro-liferative lesions developing under cyclosporin-steroid therapy. Lancet 1984; 1:583–587.

6. Swinnen LJ, Costanzo-Nordin MR, Fisher SG, et al. Increased incidence of lymphopro-
    liferative disorder after immunosuppression with the monoclonal antibody OKT3 in
    cardiac-transplant recipients. N Engl J Med 1990; 323:1723–1728.
7. Cherikh WS, Kauffman HM, McBride MA, Maghirang J, Swinnen LJ, Hanto DW.
    Association of the type of induction immunosuppression with posttransplant lympho-
    proliferative disorder, graft survival, and patient survival after primary kidney trans-
    plantation. Transplantation 2003; 76(9):1289–1293.
8. Penn I. The changing pattern of posttransplant malignancies. Transplant Proc 1991;
    23:1101–1103.
9. Witherspoon RP, Fisher LD, Schoch G, et al. Secondary cancers after bone marrow
    transplantation for leukemia or aplastic anemia. N Engl J Med 1989; 321:784–789.
10. Armitage JM, Fricker FJ, del Nido P, Starzl TE, Hardesty RL, Griffith BP. A decade
    (1982 to 1992) of pediatric cardiac transplantation and the impact of FK 506 immuno-
    suppression. J Thorac Cardiovasc Surg 1993; 105:464–472.
11. Cacciarelli TV, Reyes J, Jaffe R, et al. Primary tacrolimus (FK506) therapy and the
    long-term risk of post-transplant lymphoproliferative disease in pediatric liver trans-
    plant recipients. Pediatr Transplant 2001; 5(5):359–364.
12. Harris NL, Swerdlow SH. Methotrexate-associated lymphoproliferative disorders. In:
    Jaffe ES, Harris NL, Stein H, Vardiman JW, eds. Pathology and Genetics of Tumours
    of Haematopoietic and Lymphoid Tissues World Health Organization Classification of
    Tumours. Lyon: IARC Press, 2001:270–271.
13. Abruzzo LV, Rosales CM, Medeiros LJ, et al. Epstein–Barr virus-positive B-cell lym-
    phoproliferative disorders arising in immunodeficient patients previously treated with
    fludarabine for low-grade B-cell neoplasms. Am J Surg Pathol 2002; 26(5):630–636.
14. Ho M, Jaffe R, Miller G, et al. The frequency of Epstein–Barr virus infection and asso-
    ciated lymphoproliferative syndrome after transplantation and its manifestations in
    children. Transplantation 1988; 45:719–727.
15. Walker RC, Paya CV, Marshall WF, et al. Pretransplantation seronegative Epstein–
    Barr virus status is the primary risk factor for posttransplantation lymphoproliferative
    disorder in adult heart, lung, and other solid organ transplantations. J Heart Lung
    Transplant 1995; 14:214–221.
16. Cacciarelli TV, Esquivel CO, Moore DH, et al. Factors affecting survival after orthoto-
    pic liver transplantation in infants. Transplantation 1997; 64:242–248.
17. Newell KA, Alonso EM, Whitington PF, et al. Posttransplant lymphoproliferative dis-
    ease in pediatric liver transplantation. Interplay between primary Epstein–Barr virus
    infection and immunosuppression. Transplantation 1996; 62(3):370–375.
18. Paredes J, Krown SE. Interferon-alpha therapy in patients with Kaposi's sarcoma and the
    acquired immunodeficiency syndrome. Int J Immunopharmacol 1991; 13(suppl 1):77–81.
19. Ho M, Miller G, Atchison RW, et al. Epstein–Barr virus infections and DNA hybridiza-
    tion studies in posttransplantation lymphoma and lymphoproliferative lesions: the role
    of primary infection. J Infect Dis 1985; 152:876–886.
20. Holmes RD, Sokol RJ. Epstein–Barr virus and post-transplant lymphoproliferative dis-
    ease. Pediatr Transplant 2002; 6(6):456–464.
21. Shahinian VB, Muirhead N, Jevnikar AM, et al. Epstein–Barr virus seronegativity is
    a risk factor for late-onset posttransplant lymphoproliferative disorder in adult renal
    allograft recipients. Transplantation 2003; 75(6):851–856.
22. Purtilo DT. Epstein–Barr-virus-induced oncogenesis in immune-deficient individuals.
    Lancet 1980; 1:300–303.
23. Hanto DW, Frizzera G, Purtilo DT, et al. Clinical spectrum of lymphoproliferative dis-
    orders in renal transplant recipients and evidence for the role of Epstein–Barr virus.
    Cancer Res 1981; 41:4253–4261.
24. Young L, Alfieri C, Hennessy K, et al. Expression of Epstein–Barr virus transforma-
    tion-associated genes in tissues of patients with EBV lymphoproliferative disease.
    N Engl J Med 1989; 321:1080–1085.

25. Randhawa PS, Jaffe R, Demetris AJ, et al. Expression of Epstein–Barr virus-encoded small RNA (by the EBER-1 gene) in liver specimens from transplant recipients with post-transplantation lymphoproliferative disease. N Engl J Med 1992; 327:1710–1714.

26. Klein G. Lymphoma development in mice and humans: diversity of initiation is followed by convergent cytogenetic evolution. Proc Natl Acad Sci USA 1979; 76:2442–2446.

27. Frank D, Cesarman E, Liu YF, Michler RE, Knowles DM. Posttransplantation lymphoproliferative disorders frequently contain type A and not type B Epstein–Barr virus. Blood 1995; 85:1396–1403.

28. Cleary ML, Nalesnik MA, Shearer WT, Sklar J. Clonal analysis of transplant-associated lymphoproliferations based on the structure of the genomic termini of the Epstein–Barr virus. Blood 1988; 72:349–352.

29. Kaplan MA, Ferry JA, Harris NL, Jacobson JO. Clonal analysis of posttransplant lymphoproliferative disorders, using both episomal Epstein–Barr virus and immunoglobulin genes as markers. Am J Clin Pathol 1994; 101:590–596.

30. Riddler SA, Breinig MC, McKnight JL. Increased levels of circulating Epstein–Barr virus (EBV)-infected lymphocytes and decreased EBV nuclear antigen antibody responses are associated with the development of posttransplant lymphoproliferative disease in solid-organ transplant recipients. Blood 1994; 84:972–984.

31. Rooney CM, Loftin SK, Holladay MS, Brenner MK, Krance RA, Heslop HE. Early identification of Epstein–Barr virus-associated post-transplantation lymphoproliferative disease. Br J Haematol 1995; 89:98–103.

32. Cen H, Williams PA, McWilliams HP, Breinig MC, Ho M, McKnight JLC. Evidence for restricted Epstein–Barr virus latent gene expression and anti-EBNA antibody response in solid organ transplant recipients with post-transplant lymphoproliferative disorders. Blood 1993; 81:1393–1403.

33. Rea D, Fourcade C, Leblond V, et al. Patterns of Epstein–Barr virus latent and replicative gene expression in Epstein–Barr virus B-cell lymphoproliferative disorders after organ transplantation. Transplantation 1994; 58:317–324.

34. Murray PG, Swinnen LJ, Constandinou CM, et al. BCL-2 but not its Epstein–Barr virus-encoded homologue, BHRF1, is commonly expressed in posttransplantation lymphoproliferative disorders. Blood 1996; 87:706–711.

35. Delecluse HJ, Kremmer E, Rouault JP, Cour C, Bornkamm G, Berger F. The expression of Epstein–Barr virus latent proteins is related to the pathological features of post-transplant lymphoproliferative disorders. Am J Pathol 1995; 146:1113–1120.

36. Timms JM, Bell A, Flavell JR, et al. Target cells of Epstein–Barr-virus (EBV)-positive post-transplant lymphoproliferative disease: similarities to EBV-positive Hodgkin's lymphoma. Lancet 2003; 361(9353):217–223.

37. Izumi KM, Kieff ED. The Epstein–Barr virus oncogene product latent membrane protein 1 engages the tumor necrosis factor receptor-associated death domain protein to mediate B lymphocyte growth transformation and activate NF-kappaB. Proc Natl Acad Sci USA 1997; 94:12592–12597.

38. Kieser A, Kilger E, Gires O, Ueffing M, Kolch W, Hammerschmidt W. Epstein–Barr virus latent membrane protein-1 triggers AP-1 activity via the c-Jun N-terminal kinase cascade. EMBO J 1997; 16:6478–6485.

39. Devergne O, Hatzivassiliou E, Izumi KM, et al. Association of TRAF1, TRAF2, and TRAF3 with an Epstein–Barr virus LMP1 domain important for B-lymphocyte transformation: role in NF-kappaB activation. Mol Cell Biol 1996; 16:7098–7108.

40. Liebowitz D. Epstein–Barr virus and a cellular signaling pathway in lymphomas from immunosuppressed patients. N Engl J Med 1998; 338:1413–1421.

41. Murray PG, Swinnen LJ, Flavell JR, et al. Frequent expression of the tumor necrosis factor receptor-associated factor 1 in latent membrane protein 1-positive posttransplant lymphoproliferative disease and HIV-associated lymphomas. Hum Pathol 2001; 32(9):963–969.

42. Ramalingam P, Chu WS, Tubbs R, Rybicki L, Pettay J, Hsi ED. Latent membrane protein 1, tumor necrosis factor receptor-associated factor (TRAF)-1, TRAF-2, TRAF-3, and nuclear factor kappa B expression in posttransplantation lymphoproliferative disorders. Arch Pathol Lab Med 2003; 127(10):1335–1339.
43. Shapiro RS, McClain K, Frizzera G, et al. Epstein–Barr virus associated B-cell lymphoproliferative disorders following bone marrow transplantation. Blood 1988; 71: 1234–1243.
44. Larson RS, Scott MA, McCurley TL, Vnencak-Jones CL. Microsatellite analysis of posttransplant lymphoproliferative disorders: determination of donor/recipient origin and identification of putative lymphomagenic mechanism. Cancer Res 1996; 56 (19):4378–4381.
45. Weissmann DJ, Ferry JA, Harris NL, Louis DN, Delmonico F, Spiro I. Posttransplantation lymphoproliferative disorders in solid organ recipients are predominantly aggressive tumors of host origin. Am J Clin Pathol 1995; 103:748–755.
46. Chadburn A, Suciu-Foca N, Cesarman E, Reed E, Michler RE, Knowles DM. Posttransplantation lymphoproliferative disorders arising in solid organ transplant recipients are usually of recipient origin. Am J Pathol 1995; 147:1862–1870.
47. Paya CV, Fung JJ, Nalesnik MA, et al. Epstein–Barr virus-induced posttransplant lymphoproliferative disorders. ASTS/ASTP EBV-PTLD Task Force and The Mayo Clinic Organized International Consensus Development Meeting. Transplantation 1999; 68 (10):1517–1525.
48. Nelson BP, Locker J, Nalesnik MA, Fung JJ, Swerdlow SH. Clonal and morphological variation in a posttransplant lymphoproliferative disorder: evolution from clonal T-cell to clonal B-cell predominance. Hum Pathol 1998; 29:416–421.
49. Swerdlow SH. Post-transplant lymphoproliferative disorders: a morphologic, phenotypic and genotypic spectrum of disease. Histopathology 1992; 20(5):373–385.
50. Chadburn A, Cesarman E, Liu YF, et al. Molecular genetic analysis demonstrates that multiple posttransplantation lymphoproliferative disorders occurring in one anatomic site in a single patient represent distinct primary lymphoid neoplasms. Cancer 1995; 75:2747–2756.
51. Frizzera G, Hanto DW, Gajl-Peczalska KJ, et al. Polymorphic diffuse B-cell hyperplasias and lymphomas in renal transplant recipients. Cancer Res 1981; 41:4262–4279.
52. Knowles DM, Cesarman E, Chadburn A, et al. Correlative morphologic and molecular genetic analysis demonstrates three distinct categories of posttransplantation lymphoproliferative disorders. Blood 1995; 85:552–565.
53. Nalesnik MA, Jaffe R, Starzl TE, et al. The pathology of posttransplant lymphoproliferative disorders occurring in the setting of cyclosporine A-prednisone immunosuppression. Am J Pathol 1988; 133:173–192.
54. Swerdlow SH. Classification of the posttransplant lymphoproliferative disorders: from the past to the present. Semin Diagn Pathol 1997; 14(1):2–7.
55. Harris NL, Ferry JA, Swerdlow SH. Posttransplant lymphoproliferative disorders: summary of Society for Hematopathology Workshop. Semin Diagn Pathol 1997; 14:8–14.
56. Harris NL, Swerdlow SH, Frizzera G, Knowles DM. Post-transplant lymphoproliferative disorders. In: Jaffe ES, Harris NL, Stein H, Vardiman JW, eds. Pathology and Genetics of Tumours of Haematopoietic and Lymphoid Tissues World Health Organization Classification of Tumours. Lyon: IARC Press, 2001:264–269.
57. Minervini MI, Swerdlow SH, Nalesnik MA. Polymorphism and T-cell infiltration in posttransplant lymphoproliferative disorders. Transplant Proc 1999; 31(1–2):1270.
58. Kowal-Vern A, Swinnen L, Pyle J, et al. Characterization of postcardiac transplant lymphomas. Histology, immunophenotyping, immunohistochemistry, and gene rearrangement. Arch Pathol Lab Med 1996; 120(1):41–48.
59. Perera SM, Thomas JA, Burke M, Crawford DH. Analysis of the T-cell micro-environment in Epstein–Barr virus-related post-transplantation B lymphoproliferative disease. J Pathol 1998; 184(2):177–184.

60. Nalesnik MA, Zeevi A, Randhawa PS, et al. Cytokine mRNA profiles in Epstein–Barr virus-associated post-transplant lymphoproliferative disorders. Clin Transplant 1999; 13(1 Pt 1):39–44.

61. Cesarman E, Chadburn A, Liu YF, Migliazza A, Dalla-Favera R, Knowles DM. BCL-6 gene mutations in posttransplantation lymphoproliferative disorders predict response to therapy and clinical outcome. Blood 1998; 92:2294–2302.

62. Locker J, Nalesnik M. Molecular genetic analysis of lymphoid tumors arising after organ transplantation. Am J Pathol 1989; 135:977–987.

63. Hsi ED, Singleton TP, Swinnen L, Dunphy CH, Alkan S. Mucosa-associated lymphoid tissue-type lymphomas occurring in post-transplantation patients. Am J Surg Pathol 2000; 24(1):100–106.

64. Wotherspoon AC, Diss TC, Pan L, Singh N, Whelan J, Isaacson PG. Low grade gastric B-cell lymphoma of mucosa associated lymphoid tissue in immunocompromised patients. Histopathology 1996; 28(2):129–134.

65. Muti G, De Gasperi A, Cantoni S, et al. Incidence and clinical characteristics of post-transplant lymphoproliferative disorders: report from a single center. Transpl Int 2000; 13(suppl 1):382–387.

66. Leblond V, Davi F, Charlotte F, et al. Posttransplant lymphoproliferative disorders not associated with Epstein–Barr virus: a distinct entity? J Clin Oncol 1998; 16(6):2052–2059.

67. Nelson BP, Nalesnik MA, Locker JD. EBV negative post-transplant lymphoproliferative disorders: a distinct entity? Lab Invest 1996; 74:118A.

68. Van Gorp J, Doornewaard H, Verdonck LF, Klopping C, Vos PF, van den Tweel JG. Posttransplant T-cell lymphoma. Report of three cases and a review of the literature. Cancer 1994; 73:3064–3072.

69. Kluin PM, Feller A, Gaulard P, et al. Peripheral T/NK-cell lymphoma: a report of the IXth Workshop of the European Association for Haematopathology. Histopathology 2001; 38(3):250–270.

70. Steurer M, Stauder R, Grunewald K, et al. Hepatosplenic gammadelta-T-cell lymphoma with leukemic course after renal transplantation. Hum Pathol 2002; 33(2):253–258.

71. Mukai HY, Kojima H, Suzukawa K, et al. Nasal natural killer cell lymphoma in a post-renal transplant patient. Transplantation 2000; 69(7):1501–1503.

72. Dockrell DH, Strickler JG, Paya CV. Epstein–Barr virus-induced T-cell lymphoma in solid organ transplant recipients. Clin Infect Dis 1998; 26(1):180–182.

73. Hanto DW, Birkenbach M, Frizzera G, Gajl-Peczalska KJ, Simmons RL, Schubach WH. Confirmation of the heterogeneity of posttransplant Epstein–Barr virus-associated B-cell proliferations by immunoglobulin gene rearrangement analyses. Transplantation 1989; 47:458–464.

74. Hanto DW, Gajl-Peczalska KJ, Frizzera G, et al. Epstein–Barr virus (EBV) induced polyclonal and monoclonal B-cell lymphoproliferative diseases occurring after renal transplantation. Clinical, pathologic, and virologic findings and implications for therapy. Ann Surg 1983; 198:356–369.

75. Swinnen LJ. Durable remission after aggressive chemotherapy for post-cardiac transplant lymphoproliferation. Leuk Lymphoma 1997; 28(1–2):89–101.

76. Nalesnik MA, Makowka L, Starzl TE. The diagnosis and treatment of posttransplant lymphoproliferative disorders. Curr Probl Surg 1988; 25:367–472.

77. Swinnen LJ, Mullen GM, Carr TJ, Costanzo MR, Fisher RI. Aggressive treatment for postcardiac transplant lymphoproliferation. Blood 1995; 86:3333–3340.

78. Chadburn A, Chen JM, Hsu DT, et al. The morphologic and molecular genetic categories of posttransplantation lymphoproliferative disorders are clinically relevant. Cancer 1998; 82(10):1978–1987.

79. Morrison VA, Dunn DL, Manivel JC, Gajlpeczalska KJ, Peterson BA. Clinical characteristics of post-transplant lymphoproliferative disorders. Am J Med 1994; 97:14–24.

80. Miller WT Jr, Siegel SG, Montone KT. Posttransplantation lymphoproliferative disorder: changing manifestations of disease in a renal transplant population. Crit Rev Diagn Imaging 1997; 38(6):569–585.
81. Hanto DW. Classification of Epstein–Barr virus-associated posttransplant lymphoproliferative diseases: implications for understanding their pathogenesis and developing rational treatment strategies. Annu Rev Med 1995; 46:381–394.
82. Hayashi RJ, Kraus MD, Patel AL, et al. Posttransplant lymphoproliferative disease in children: correlation of histology to clinical behavior. J Pediatr Hematol Oncol 2001; 23(1):14–18.
83. Cohen JI. Epstein–Barr virus lymphoproliferative disease associated with acquired immunodeficiency. Medicine (Baltimore) 1991; 70(2):137–160.
84. Green M, Michaels M, Weber S. Predicting outcome from post-transplant lymphoproliferative disease: a risky business. Pediatr Transplant 2001; 5(4):235–238.
85. Nalesnik MA. Involvement of the gastrointestinal tract by Epstein–Barr virus-associated posttransplant lymphoproliferative disorders. Am J Surg Pathol 1990; 14(suppl 1):92–100.
86. Leblond V, Dhedin N, Mamzer Bruneel MF, et al. Identification of prognostic factors in 61 patients with posttransplantation lymphoproliferative disorders. J Clin Oncol 2001; 19(3):772–778.
87. Ghobrial IM, Habermann TM, Maurer MJ, et al. Proposed prognostic model for survival in solid organ transplant recipients with post transplant lymphoproliferative disorders (PTLD) [abstr 1423]. Blood 2003; 102(11):392a.
88. Gulley ML, Swinnen LJ, Plaisance KT Jr, Schnell C, Grogan TM, Schneider BG. Tumor origin and CD20 expression in posttransplant lymphoproliferative disorder occurring in solid organ transplant recipients: implications for immune-based therapy. Transplantation 2003; 76(6):959–964.
89. Leblond V, Sutton L, Dorent R, et al. Lymphoproliferative disorders after organ transplantation: a report of 24 cases observed in a single center. J Clin Oncol 1995; 13:961–968.
90. Tsai DE, Hardy CL, Tomaszewski JE, et al. Reduction in immunosuppression as initial therapy for posttransplant lymphoproliferative disorder: analysis of prognostic variables and long-term follow-up of 42 adult patients. Transplantation 2001; 71(8):1076–1088.
91. Porcu P, Eisenbeis CF, Pelletier RP, et al. Successful treatment of posttransplantation lymphoproliferative disorder (PTLD) following renal allografting is associated with sustained CD8(+) T-cell restoration. Blood 2002; 100(7):2341–2348.
92. Swinnen LJ, LeBlanc M, Kasamon Y, et al. Phase II study of sequential reduction in immunosuppression, interferon alpha-2b, and ProMACE-CytaBOM chemotherapy for post-transplant lymphoproliferative disorder (PTLD) (SWOG/ECOG S9239) [abstr 1463]. Blood 2003; 102(11):403a.
93. Hanto DW, Frizzera G, Gajl-Peczalska KJ, et al. Epstein–Barr virus-induced B-cell lymphoma after renal transplantation: acyclovir therapy and transition from polyclonal to monoclonal B-cell proliferation. N Engl J Med 1982; 306:913–918.
94. Filipovich AH, Mathur A, Kamat D, Kersey JH, Shapiro RS. Lymphoproliferative disorders and other tumors complicating immunodeficiencies. Immunodeficiency 1994; 5:91–112.
95. McDiarmid SV, Jordan S, Lee GS, et al. Prevention and preemptive therapy of post-transplant lymphoproliferative disease in pediatric liver recipients. Transplantation 1998; 66:1604–1611.
96. Green M, Kaufmann M, Wilson J, Reyes J. Comparison of intravenous ganciclovir followed by oral acyclovir with intravenous ganciclovir alone for prevention of cytomegalovirus and Epstein–Barr virus disease after liver transplantation in children. Clin Infect Dis 1997; 25(6):1344–1349.
97. Oertel SH, Anagnostopoulos I, Hummel MW, Jonas S, Riess HB. Identification of early antigen BZLF1/ZEBRA protein of Epstein–Barr virus can predict the effectiveness of antiviral treatment in patients with post-transplant lymphoproliferative disease. Br J Haematol 2002; 118(4):1120–1123.

98. Fischer A, Blanche S, Le Bidois J, et al. Anti-B-cell monoclonal antibodies in the treatment of severe B-cell lymphoproliferative syndrome following bone marrow and organ transplantation. N Engl J Med 1991; 324:1451–1456.

99. Benkerrou M, Jais JP, Leblond V, et al. Anti-B-cell monoclonal antibody treatment of severe posttransplant B-lymphoproliferative disorder: prognostic factors and long-term outcome. Blood 1998; 92:3137–3147.

100. Grillo-Lopez AJ, Lynch J, Coiffier B, et al. Rituximab therapy of lymphoproliferative disorders in immunosuppressed patients [abstr]. Ann Oncol 1999; 10(3):179.

101. Milpied N, Vasseur B, Parquet N, et al. Humanized anti-CD20 monoclonal antibody (Rituximab) in post transplant B-lymphoproliferative disorder: a retrospective analysis on 32 patients. Ann Oncol 2000; 11(suppl 1):113–116.

102. Choquet S, Herbrecht R, Socie G, et al. Efficacy and safety of rituximab in B-cell post-transplantation lymphoproliferative disorders (B-PTLD): preliminary results of a multi-center, open label, phase II trial (M9037 Trial) [abstr 1811]. Blood 2002; 100(11):11–16.

103. Choquet S, Leblond V, Herbrecht R, et al. Efficacy and safety of rituximab in B-Cell post transplantation lymphoproliferative disorders (B-PTLD): final results of a multicenter, open label, phase II trial (M 39037 TRIAL) [abstr 986]. Blood 2003; 102(11):277a.

104. Choquet S, Leblond V, Jager U, et al. Efficacy of CHOP regimen as first line therapy in posttransplantation lymphoproliferative disorders (PTLD) [abstr 3897]. Blood 2003; 102(11):49b.

105. Gross TG, Park J, Bucuvalas J, et al. Low-dose chemotherapy for refractory EBV associated post transplant lymphoproliferative disease (PTLD) following solid organ transplant in children [abstr 598]. Blood 2002; 100(11):11–16.

106. Shapiro RS, Chauvenet A, McGuire W, et al. Treatment of B-cell lymphoproliferative disorders with interferon alfa and intravenous gamma globulin [letter]. N Engl J Med 1988; 318:1334.

107. Liebowitz D, Anastasi J, Hagos F, LeBeau MM, Olopade OI. Post-transplant lymphoproliferative disorders (PTLD): clinicopathologic characterization and response to immunomodulatory therapy with interferon-alpha [abstr]. Ann Oncol 1996; 7:28.

108. Davis CL, Wood BL, Sabath DE, Joseph JS, Stehman-Breen C, Broudy VC. Interferon-alpha treatment of posttransplant lymphoproliferative disorder in recipients of solid organ transplants. Transplantation 1998; 66:1770–1779.

109. Papadopoulos EB, Ladanyi M, Emanuel D, et al. Infusions of donor leukocytes to treat Epstein–Barr virus-associated lymphoproliferative disorders after allogeneic bone marrow transplantation. N Engl J Med 1994; 330:1185–1191.

110. Rooney CM, Smith CA, Ng CY, et al. Use of gene-modified virus-specific T lymphocytes to control Epstein–Barr-virus-related lymphoproliferation. Lancet 1995; 345:9–13.

111. O'Reilly RJ, Small TN, Papadopoulos E, Lucas K, Lacerda J, Koulova L. Biology and adoptive cell therapy of Epstein–Barr virus-associated lymphoproliferative disorders in recipients of marrow allografts. Immunol Rev 1997; 157:195–216.

112. Loren AW, Porter DL, Stadtmauer EA, Tsai DE. Post-transplant lymphoproliferative disorder: a review. Bone Marrow Transplant 2003; 31(3):145–155.

113. Haque T, Wilkie GM, Taylor C, et al. Treatment of Epstein–Barr-virus-positive post-transplantation lymphoproliferative disease with partly HLA-matched allogeneic cytotoxic T-cells. Lancet 2002; 360(9331):436–442.

114. Boyle GJ, Michaels MG, Webber SA, et al. Posttransplantation lymphoproliferative disorders in pediatric thoracic organ recipients. J Pediatr 1997; 131:309–313.

115. Tsai DE, Nearey M, Hardy CL, et al. Use of EBV PCR for the diagnosis and monitoring of post-transplant lymphoproliferative disorder in adult solid organ transplant patients. Am J Transplant 2002; 2(10):946–954.

116. Lucas KG, Burton RL, Zimmerman SE, et al. Semiquantitative Epstein–Barr Virus (EBV) polymerase chain reaction for the determination of patients at risk for EBV-induced lymphoproliferative disease after stem cell transplantation. Blood 1998; 91:3654–3661.

117. Rose C, Green M, Webber S, et al. Detection of Epstein–Barr virus genomes in peripheral blood B-cells from solid-organ transplant recipients by fluorescence in situ hybridization. J Clin Microbiol 2002; 40(7):2533–2544.

118. Rowe DT, Qu L, Reyes J, et al. Use of quantitative competitive PCR to measure Epstein–Barr virus genome load in the peripheral blood of pediatric transplant patients with lymphoproliferative disorders. J Clin Microbiol 1997; 35:1612–1615.

119. Wagner HJ, Wessel M, Jabs W, et al. Patients at risk for development of posttransplant lymphoproliferative disorder: plasma versus peripheral blood mononuclear cells as material for quantification of Epstein–Barr viral load by using real-time quantitative polymerase chain reaction. Transplantation 2001; 72(6):1012–1019.

120. Smets F, Latinne D, Bazin H, et al. Ratio between Epstein–Barr viral load and anti-Epstein–Barr virus specific T-cell response as a predictive marker of posttransplant lymphoproliferative disease. Transplantation 2002; 73(10):1603–1610.

121. George D, Barnett L, Boulad F, et al. Semi-quantitative PCR analysis of genomic EBV DNA post BMT allows close surveillance of patients at risk for development of EBV-lymphoproliferative disorders (EBV-LPD) allowing prompt intervention [abstr]. Blood 1998; 92(10 suppl 1):437a.

122. Swinnen LJ, Gulley ML, Hamilton E, Schichman SA. EBV DNA quantitation in serum is highly correlated with the development and regression of post-transplant lymphoproliferative disorder (PTLD) in solid organ transplant recipients [abstr]. Blood 1998; 92 (10 suppl 1):314–315.

13

T-Cell Lymphomas Associated with Epstein–Barr Virus

James F. Jones

Viral Exanthems and Herpesvirus Branch, Centers for Disease Control and Prevention, Atlanta, Georgia, and Department of Pediatrics, National Jewish Medical and Research Center, Denver, Colorado, U.S.A.

INTRODUCTION

In 1988, three patients undergoing evaluation for severe, chronic, active Epstein–Barr virus (EBV) infection developed peripheral T-cell lymphomas, which were subsequently shown by in situ hybridization to contain the EBV genome. The T-cells were $CD4^+$ and had undergone clonal T-cell receptor gene rearrangements. The clinical course was fatal in each case despite aggressive chemotherapy. Each of the patients had markedly elevated immunoglobulin G (IgG) antiviral capsid antigen (>1:10,000) and anti-early antigen (EA) titers (>1:640), but low (<1:40) to zero anti-EBV nuclear antigen (EBNA) titers by the immunofluorescent technique (1).

The tropism of EBV has long been recognized for B-cells and epithelial cells. The attempts to detect EBV in these T-cell neoplasms were stimulated by the cluster of a rare tumor type in the context of a rare disease known to be driven by EBV. Furthermore, the cellular receptor for the complement component, C3d [now known as complement receptor 2 (CR2)], which is known to subserve binding of EBV by B-cells, was also identified on T-cells (2). An early study identified the presence of this receptor on human thymic cells using complement-coated erythrocytes (3). More recently, direct EBV binding and entry into thymic cells have been demonstrated (4), with subsequent activation of the infected cells (5).

Following this initial observation, archived specimens of T-cell lymphomas as well as newly acquired tumors from around the world have been examined for the presence of EBV DNA, RNA, and protein expression. In the many studies performed so far, EBV has been found in a wide variety of T-cell tumors. However, the nomenclature of the tumor types and the methods used to query the presence of EBV have created a somewhat confusing picture.

Table 1 The WHO T-Cell Tumor Classification Scheme

WHO classification (2001)	Presentation	EBV
Leukemic/disseminated		
T-cell prolymphocytic leukemia	Hepatosplenomegaly, lymphadenopathy	−
T-cell large granular lymphocytic leukemia	Neutropenia, lymphocytosis, hepatosplenomegaly	−
Aggressive NK cell leukemia	Fever, B-symptoms[a], leukemic blood[b]	+
Adult T-cell leukemia/lymphoma	HTLV-1	−
Cutaneous		
Mycosis fungoides	Truncal patches/plaques	+
Sézary syndrome	Erythroderma, lymphadenopathy	+
Primary cutaneous anaplastic large cell lymphoma	Localized skin lesions	+
Lymphomatoid papulomatosis	Recurrent papules or nodules	−
Other extranodal		
Extranodal NK/T-cell lymphoma, nasaltype	Nasal/midface mass or destructive lesion	+
Enteropathy-type–T-cell lymphoma	Celiac disease, abdominal pain, intestinal perforation	+
Hepatosplenic T-cell lymphoma	Hepatosplenomegaly, thrombocytopenia, anemia, leukocytosis	+
Subcutaneous panniculitis-like–T-cell lymphoma	Subcutaneous nodules over the trunk, extremities and B-symptoms[a]	+
Nodal		
Angioimmunoblastic T-cell lymphoma	Systemic symptoms, polyclonal gammopathy	+
Peripheral T-cell lymphoma, unspecified	Lymphadenopathy, B-symptoms[a]	+
Anaplastic large cell lymphoma	B-symptoms[a], advanced lymphadenopathy	+
Neoplasm of uncertain lineage and stage of differentiation		
Blastic NK cell lymphoma	Skin tumors, disseminated lymphadenopathy	−
Precursor T-cell lymphoma		
Precursor T lymphoblastic leukemia/ lymphoblastic lymphoma (precursor T-cell acute lymphoblastic leukemia)	High leukocyte count, mediastinal/other mass	+

[a]B-symptoms—B refers to the presence of systemic symptoms (significant fever, night sweats, and/or unexplained weight loss of greater than 10% of normal body weight) in a clinical staging system in which A represents clinical illness without systemic symptoms, and B represents presence of these systemic symptoms.
[b]Leukemic blood–circulating leukemic cells; larger than normal large granular lymphocytes with irregular, hyperchromatic nuclei, and/or increased azurophilic granules.
Abbreviations: EBV, Epstein–Barr virus; WHO, World Health Organization; NK, natural killer; HTLV-1, human T-cell lymphotropic virus-1.
Source: Modified from Ref. 6.

CLASSIFICATION OF T-CELL LYMPHOMAS ASSOCIATED WITH EBV

A new, detailed classification scheme of lymphomas (Table 1) delineated by the World Health Organization (WHO) in 2001 (6) attempted to rectify some of the previous overlapping classifications such as Lukes, Kiel, Working Group, and Revised European-American Classification of Lymphoid Neoplasms (REAL). The WHO classification scheme is based on morphologic, genetic, immunophenotypic, and clinical parameters. Key points of the WHO classification include distinctions between precursor T-cell tumors and peripheral tumors, differentiation among anatomical sites, cytotoxic versus noncytotoxic cells by phenotype, and comparisons of names to those in previous classifications. Peripheral T-cells are post-thymic (or mature) T-cells, whereas precursor T-cells are pre-thymic (or developing) T-cells.

There is considerable overlap in the classification scheme. For example, tumors classified as "extranodal" are frequently associated with nodal tumors. Cutaneous tumors may be of several types. Thus, the anatomical site is only one consideration in identification of tumor behavior.

The interpretation of the presence of EBV in tumor cells is still evolving. As with other diseases, identification of EBV within cells should have a purpose, and the methods used for identification must be sensitive and specific. The significance of the detection of EBV is illustrated by the different tabulations of the association of EBV with T-cell lymphomas. A useful summary of T-cell lymphomas published in 2001 based on morphology, cell surface phenotypes, and genotypic characteristics (7) that was prepared prior to the availability of the WHO classification identified 12 types of T-cell lymphomas and three types of natural killer (NK) cell tumors (Table 2). The modifications included a numerical identifier of the existing WHO name for T-cell lymphomas for the sake of comparison. Of these 15 tumor types, EBV was noted as being present in only three types: nasal/nasal-type ("angiocentric lymphoma") T-cell lymphoma, aggressive NK lymphoma, and nasal/nasal-type NK lymphoma. None of the cutaneous tumors were characterized as containing EBV.

The classification published in 2001 by the WHO, however, lists five T-cell tumors as carrying EBV DNA: aggressive NK cell leukemia, extranodal NK/T-cell lymphoma nasal type, enteropathy-type T-cell lymphoma, angioblastic T-cell lymphoma, and peripheral T-cell lymphoma, unspecified (Table 1).

The sensitivity for detection of EBV in these tumors is dependent on the target used for detection [e.g., DNA, EBV encoded RNAs (EBERs), antigens] and the technique used [e.g., polymerase chain reaction (PCR), in situ hybridization]. For example, a closer examination of cutaneous T-cell tumors in which EBV is normally not considered to be present is instructive. Reports by Iwatsuki et al. (8) from Japan, Jumbou et al. (9), and Dreno et al. (10) from France, and others using both RNA and DNA PCR techniques describe the presence of EBV in several cutaneous tumor types including mycosis fungoides and Sézary syndrome. Several of the studies that failed to identify EBV in these lesions used only probes for EBERs, which is a potential methodological limitation. EBERs are small, untranslated RNA molecules expressed only during latent EBV infection. Therefore, if the neoplastic cells harbor EBV in the replicative state, EBERs will not be detected, and the neoplasm will be misclassified as being EBV-negative. Foulc et al. (11) provide support for this scenario by showing the presence of the *EBV* gene BHLF1 by in situ hybridization in Sézary syndrome specimens that were EBER-negative. They went on to show a poorer prognosis for patients with EBV-positive tumors. Another possible reason for the apparent inability to identify EBV in other tumors is a lack of uniformity in classification systems at the time of publication of many of these reports. Thus, it is likely that additional EBV-positive T-cell lymphomas may be identified in the future, which will need to be reclassified.

TYPES OF T-CELL LYMPHOMAS AND THEIR ASSOCIATION WITH EBV

Among the leukemic or disseminated T-cell lymphomas, EBV has not been found in T-cell prolymphocytic leukemia and T-cell large granular lymphocytic leukemia.

Table 2 A Modified T-Cell Tumor Classification

Lymphocyte neoplasm	Morphology	Phenotype	Genotype
Lymphomas			
T-cell lymphoma, nasal and nasal-type ("angiocentric lymphoma") **3a**	Angiocentric and angiodestructive growth	CD2, CD3$^{+/-}$, CD5$^{+/-}$, CD56, cytoplasmic CD3	TCR rearrangements variable
Cutaneous T-cell lymphoma	Small to large cells with cerebriform nuclei	TdT$^-$, CD2, CD3, CD4, CD5, CD7$^{+/-}$, CD30	α/β TCR rearrangement
Mycosis fungoides **2a**	Same as above	Same as above	Same as above
Sézary syndrome **2b**	Same as above	Same as above	Same as above
Angioimmunoblastic T-cell lymphoma **4a**	Small immunoblasts with pale staining or clear cells		α/β TCR rearrangement with rare incomplete IgR, trisomy 3 or 5 noted
Peripheral T-cell lymphoma (unspecified) **4b**	Highly variable	CD2, CD3, CD5, CD7$^-$, CD4 > CD8 > CD4/CD8	α/β TCR rearrangement often with incomplete IgR
Subcutaneous panniculitic–T-cell lymphoma **3d**	Medium-sized atypical cells with irregular nuclei and hyperchromasia	CD2, CD3, CD5, CD7$^-$, CD4$^-$/CD8	α/β TCR rearrangement
Intestinal T-cell lymphoma **3b**	Small to large atypical lymphocytes	CD2, CD3, CD5, CD7$^-$, CD4$^-$/CD8$^-$ or CD4$^-$/CD8$^+$, CD103	β TCR rearrangement

	Morphology	Immunophenotype	Genetics
Hepatosplenic γ;δ T-cell lymphoma **3c**	Small to medium-size cells with condensed chromatin and round nuclei	CD2, CD3, CD4−, CD5, CD7−, CD8+/−	γ/δ TCR, isochromosome 7q
Adult T-cell lymphoma **1d**	Highly variable with multilobed nuclei	CD2, CD3, CD5, CD7−, CD25, CD4 ≫ CD8	α/β TCR rearrangement and integrated HTLV-1
Anaplastic large cell lymphoma **4c**	Large blastic pleomorphic cells with "horseshoe"-shaped nuclei, prominent nucleoli, and abundant basophilic cytoplasm	TdT−, CD2, CD3, CD5, CD7+/−, CD25+/−, CD30, CD45+/−	TCR rearrangement, t(2;5) (p23;q35) resulting in nucleophosmin-anaplastic lymphoma kinase fusion protein
Primary cutaneous CD30-positive lymphoma **2c**	Anaplastic large cells as above in cutaneous nodules	TdT−, CD2, CD3, CD8+/−, CD57+/−, CD30	TCR rearrangement, without (2;5) (p23;q35)
NK cell neoplasms			
Large granular lymphocytic leukemia **1b**	Abundant cytoplasm and azurophilic granules	TdT−, CD2, CD3−, CD8+/−, CD16, CD56, CD57+/−	No TCR rearrangement
Aggressive NK cell leukemia **1c**	Same as above	Same as above	No TCR rearragement
NK cell lymphoma, nasal and nasal-type ("angiocentric lymphoma") **3a**	Angiocentric and angiodestructive growth	CD2, CD5+/−, CD56, cytoplasmic CD3	No TCR rearrangement

Abbreviations: HTLV, human T-cell lymphotropic virus; NK, natural killer; TCR, T-cell receptor.
Source: Modified from Ref. 7.

However, previous studies that used different nomenclature continue to confound the question of the presence or absence of EBV in these cells. Matsuo and Drexler (12) observed EBV in cell lines established from NK and NK/T leukemia–lymphomas that share morphological characteristics with T-cell large granular lymphocytic leukemia.

Cutaneous T-cell lymphomas include mycosis fungoides and a subtype known as Sézary syndrome; angiocentric lymphomas, currently known as extranodal NK/T-cell lymphomas, nasal type; and angiolymphoblastic lymphomas (13,14). Angiocentric tumors may occur in other sites, including the bowel, in association with ischemia and subsequent perforation. Angiolymphoblastic lymphomas are more serious and are associated with fever and generalized lymphadenopathy. This grouping also includes primary cutaneous anaplastic large cell lymphomas, in which the tumor cells express a protein recognized by the CD30 antibody Ki-1. Most attempts to identify EBV in these tumors have used EBER or latent membrane protein 1 (LMP1) detection methods and have been negative. de Bruin et al. (15) found EBV by DNA PCR in one tumor sample, but assumed that because in situ hybridization for EBERs was negative, the PCR result was a false-positive. This issue is clouded by the presence of EBV in these tumors that arise in sites other than the skin.

Peripheral T-cell lymphomas may occur in virtually any organ system including the gastrointestinal tract, skin, nasal passages, and in blood vessels and aortic aneurysms (16,17). These tumors continue to be associated with severe, chronic, active EBV disease with expression of viral genes associated with active replication, while in some instances the tumor cells express type II latency (EBNA1, LMP1, and LMP2A) (18). These tumors also appear in patients following transplantation (19). It is likely that some of these tumors would be classified under different names using the current WHO classification.

In Lennert's (lymphoepithelial) lymphoma (currently classified as peripheral T-cell lymphoma, unspecified), the malignant cells may be either helper or cytotoxic T-cells. The tumor is likely to occur in lymphoid organs of older patients, associated with systemic symptoms, and contains infiltrating histiocytes. The disease course may be aggressive or indolent. In one study, EBV was found in one case out of a series of 10, but only in situ testing using EBER probes was used (20).

T/NK-cell lymphomas are associated with midline lymphomas. Skin involvement is associated with a poor prognosis, whereas coexpression of CD30 is associated with a better prognosis (21). In one series, 69% of upper respiratory tract lymphomas (NK/T) were of T-cell origin, with 53% being EBV-positive (22). American patients are less likely to have EBV-positive tumor cells when compared to Chinese patients, but the more frequent association of EBV with tumors in Southeast Asia is not universally accepted as different methodologies may influence the results. T/NK tumors are one type of several non-Hodgkin's lymphomas (NHLs) found to have free viral DNA by PCR in serum or plasma, suggesting that virus replication may be present. This observation is in contrast to their observation of likely being EBER-positive because free viral DNA is thought to be a consequence of ongoing, productive viral replication. Type A EBV was found to be dominant in these tumors in China (23). This form expresses the same latency pattern (type II) as nasopharyngeal carcinoma and Hodgkin's disease (EBNA1 with QUK splice, LMP1 and LMP2 proteins, BamHI A reading frame, and absence of EBNA2 message) (24). The distribution of type A EBV is worldwide. Chan et al. (25) identified an unusual patient in whom the disease presented as a testicular tumor.

Two-thirds of immunosuppression-related NHL are T-cell in origin in some series (26). However, tumors containing EBV occurred among healthy persons as frequently as among immunosuppressed individuals in Japan (27). Therefore, immunosuppression does not appear to be a prerequisite for the development of T-cell lymphomas in general or of those containing EBV.

Enteropathy caused by celiac disease with an human leukocyte antigen (HLA) DQA1*0501, DQB1*0201 phenotype may be associated with virus-positive T-cell lymphomas (28). The frequency of intestinal NHL appeared to be particularly high in Mexico, as well as among post-transplant tumors (29).

Intravascular lymphomatosis, a proliferation of tumor cells in vascular space without tissue involvement, was found to contain EBER-positive cells (30). This disease is rare, and the clinical consequences depend on the anatomic site of the infiltrate in the vessel lumen.

γ/δ T-cell tumors are peripheral T-cell lymphomas with cytopenia that are $CD2^+$, $CD3^+$, T-cell receptor δ-1^+, β F^-, and EBER-positive, which are frequently found in the liver and spleen (31). These lymphomas were also described in fatal cases, occurring in subcutaneous tissue, vocal cords, gastric mucosa, and the central nervous system (32). Apparent primary γ/δ tumors of the larynx (33), intestinal tract (34), and the lung need to be added to this list (35). Familial cases have also been described (36). Gaulard et al. (37) reviewed these tumors in 2003.

The hemophagocytic syndrome is characterized by fever, malaise, myalgia, lethargy, and hepatosplenomegaly, and may be familial or sporadic. The sporadic form is associated with infections, particularly EBV, and is found in hepatosplenic γ/δ tumors, peripheral T-cell lymphomas, and NK cell peripheral–T-cell lymphomas, all of which may carry the EBV genome (35,37). Anaplastic large cell lymphomas, which were not included in the WHO classification as containing the EBV genome, were subsequently described as being EBV-positive in the presence of the hemophagocytosis syndrome (38,39).

Richter syndrome is the conversion of chronic lymphocytic leukemia to a diffuse large cell lymphoma of either B- or T-cell origin. The lymphoma cells of both cell types have been found to be EBV-positive (40).

Patients undergoing immunosuppressive therapy for rheumatoid arthritis and other inflammatory diseases with low dose methotrexate and other drugs have been reported to develop EBV-positive, large T-cell lymphomas (41). Other immunosuppressive conditions, such as human immunodeficiency virus infection and the acquired immunodeficiency syndrome (AIDS), predispose to central nervous system T-cell lymphomas that frequently contain EBV (42). Usually, primary central nervous system lymphomas in patients with AIDS are B-cell lymphomas.

Discordant lymphomas occur when B-cell tumors change to T-cell tumors, T-cell tumors become B-cell tumors, and B-cell and T-cell tumors coexist. EBV was found in coexisting B-cell and T-cell tumors and in the B-cell to T-cell tumor transitions (43).

Several T-cell lymphomas have been misidentified as malignant histiocytosis. These cases had a fulminant course associated with pancytopenia, liver dysfunction, and disseminated intravascular coagulopathy. The pathology has included extranodal, histiocytic infiltrates in multiple tumor types (38,44).

FUTURE CONSIDERATIONS

Methods used for identification of EBV in T-cell lymphomas include probes that detect EBNA1, EBNA2, *Bam*HI H, *Bam*HI W, *Bam*HI Z, and antibodies that identify specific EBV proteins. Both in situ and PCR molecular techniques, along with histochemistry, have been used in the study of T-cell lymphomas, and the percentages of positive T-cells in the varying studies are somewhat different. For example, one study identified EBV DNA in 59% of archived T-cell lymphomas using EBNA1 probes versus 47% positive using EBER probes by in situ hybridization, while another showed similar differences using primers for the glycoprotein gp220 as compared to presence of EBER (45).

Other markers have been used to characterize the EBV-positive tumor cells. Peripheral T-cell lymphomas contain anaplastic large cells in 73% of cases. Pleomorphic cells were present in 18% of these cases. Interleukin-10 was expressed in 43% of nasal NK tumors, but in none of angioimmunoblastic and γ/δ tumors. Nodal T-cell lymphomas with EBNA1-expressing tumor cells were associated with an aggressive course and hepatosplenomegaly (15). Fulminant CD8$^+$ extranodal T-cell lymphomas (NK and cytotoxic T-cell types) were identified using TIA-1 and granzyme B as markers (46).

Epidemiologic studies show ethnic differences between the West and the East, as well as within the two regions. Peh and Quen (47) identified the incidence of T-cell lymphomas, in general, with decreasing incidence from Indian > Chinese > Malay backgrounds, with the overall incidence higher in Asia than in the West. In one study from Japan in 1996, it was recognized that T-cell lymphomas were more frequently EBV-positive than were B-cell tumors, even though B-cell lymphomas were more common (48). The same phenomenon was observed in Denmark (49). Differential diagnoses have not been studied in depth, but include EBV-positive T-cells in viral lymphadenitis occurring with infectious mononucleosis and other multicentric lymphadenopathy syndromes (50). It was also noted in these reports that T-cell tumors with EBV were associated with a poorer prognosis and significant constitutional symptoms (B-symptoms of night sweats, fever, metabolic wasting, and 10% loss of body weight within six months).

The discussion of the role of EBV in the development of T-cell tumors varies from none at all to hypothesized infiltration of tumor with cytotoxic T-cells that then become infected and contribute to additional tumor development (51). Enteropathy-associated T-cell lymphomas demonstrate decreased HLA expression on tumor cells (52). The unsatisfactory status and incomplete explanations of the role of EBV in the pathogenesis of B-cell and epithelial tumors extends to T-cell lymphomas.

Because some overlap in phenotypic and genotypic characteristics of mature T-cell leukemias on using the new WHO classification were reported by Herling et al. (53), it is not surprising that the EBV status of these and other T-cell tumors is unclear. The role of EBV in T-cell lymphomas in the assignment of causality, understanding of tumor biology, need for specific therapy, and clinical prognosis continues to evolve (31), but as observed in 1996 (54), the distribution of EBV in T-cell tumors is quite variable.

This statement continues to describe the field and is exemplified by a need for additional studies of the incidence and causal role of EBV in T-cell lymphomas. These tumors as a group account for almost 15% of NHL throughout the world (6), but accurate percentages of T-cell tumors that carry the EBV genome are not available for various reasons. In particular, viral genome detection methods must include analysis of viral DNA and RNA and not use of only selected methods. The most common association of EBV is with NK/T-cell tumors, where a majority of tumors carry the viral genome even though the NK cell is not thought of as a primary cell target for EBV infection. Thus, understanding of EBV in T-cell lymphomas requires a broad, perhaps new approach to evaluate EBV and its relationships to humans.

REFERENCES

1. Jones JF, Shurin S, Abramowsky C, et al. T-cell lymphomas containing Epstein–Barr viral DNA in patients with Epstein–Barr virus infections. N Engl J Med 1988; 318:733–741.
2. Fingeroth JD, Clabby ML, Strominger JD. Characterization of a T-lymphocyte Epstein–Barr virus/C3d receptor (CD21). J Virol 1988; 62:1442–1447.
3. Shore A, Dosch HM, Gelfand EW. Expression and modulation of C3 receptors during early T-cell ontogeny. Cell Immunol 1979; 45:157–166.
4. Paterson RL, Kelleher C, Amankonah TD, et al. Model of Epstein–Barr virus infection of human thymocytes: expression of viral genomes and impact on cellular receptor expression in the T-lymphoblastic cell line, HPB-ALL. Blood 1995; 85:456–464.
5. Paterson RL, Kelleher CA, Streib JE, et al. Activation of human thymocytes after infection by EBV. J Immunol 1995; 154:1440–1449.
6. Jaffe ES, Harris NL, Stein H, Vardiman J. World Health Organization Classification of Tumours/Pathology and Genetics of Tumours of Haematopoietic and Lymphoid Tissues. Lyon, France: International Agency for Research on Cancer, 2001.
7. Kipps TJ. Classification of malignant lymphoid disorders. In: Beutler E, Lichtman MA, Coller BS, Kipps TJ, Seligsohn U, eds. Williams Hematology. 6th ed. New York: McGraw-Hill, 2001.
8. Iwatsuki K, Xu Z, Ohtsukia M, Kaneko F. Cutaneous lymphoproliferative disorders associated with Epstein–Barr virus: a clinical overview. J Dermatol Sci 2000; 22:181–195.
9. Jumbou O, Huet S, Bureau B, et al. Epstein–Barr virus research by in situ hybridization in 65 cutaneous T-cell epidermotropic lymphomas. Ann Dermatol Venereol 1998; 125:90–93.
10. Dreno B, Celerier P, Fleischmannn M, et al. Presence of Epstein–Barr virus in cutaneous lesions of mycosis fungoides and Sezary syndrome. Acta Derm Venereol 1994; 74: 355–357.
11. Foulc P, Guyen JMN, Dreno B. Clinical and laboratory investigations; prognostic factors in Sezary syndrome: a study of 28 patients. Br J Dermatol 2003; 149:1152–1158.
12. Matsuo Y, Drexler HG. Immunoprofiling of cell lines derived from natural killer-cell and natural killer-like T-cell leukemia-lymphoma. Leuk Res 2003; 27:935–945.
13. Wechsler J, Willemze R, van der Brule A, et al. Differences in Epstein–Barr virus expression between primary and secondary cutaneous angiocentric lymphomas. French Study Group of Cutaneous lymphomas. Arch Dermatol 1998; 134:479–484.
14. Sugaya M, Nakaura K, Asahina A, Tamaki K. Leukocystic vasculitis with IgA deposits in angioimmunoblastic T-cell lymphoma. J Dermatol 2001; 28:32–37.
15. de Bruin PC, Jiwa M, Oudejans JJ, et al. Presence of Epstein–Barr virus in extranodal T-cell lymphomas: differences in relation to site. Blood 1994; 83:1612–1618.
16. Luo CY, Ko WC, Tsao CJ, et al. Epstein–Barr virus-containing T-cell lymphoma and atherosclerotic abdominal aortic aneurysm in a young adult. Hum Pathol 1999; 30:1114–1117.
17. Huh J, Hong SM, Kim SS, et al. Angiocentric lymphoma masquerading as acute appendicitis. Histopathology 1999; 334:378–380.
18. Kanegane H, Bhatia K, Gutierrez M, et al. A syndrome of peripheral blood T-cell infection with Epstein–Barr virus (EBV) followed by EBV-positive T-cell lymphoma. Blood 1998; 91:2085–2091.
19. Frias C, Lauzurica R, Vauero M, Ribera JM. Detection of Epstein–Barr virus in post-transplantation T-cell lymphoma in a kidney transplant recipient: case report and review. Clin Infect Dis 2000; 30:576–578.

20. Yamashita Y, Nakamura S, Kagami Y, et al. Lennert's lymphoma: a variant of cytotoxic T-cell lymphoma? Am J Surg Pathol 2000; 24:1627–1633.
21. Mraz-Gernhard S, Natkunam Y, Hoppe RT, et al. Natural killer/natural killer-like T-cell lymphoma, CD56$^+$, presenting in the skin: an increasingly recognized entity with an aggressive course. J Clin Oncol 2001; 19:2179–2188.
22. Gao Z, Wang H, Pan Z. Investigation of the clinicopathologic features, immunophenotype and Epstein–Barr infection of the upper respiratory tract lymphomas in patients. Zhonghua Bing Li Xu Za Zhi 1998; 27:251–254.
23. Chiang AK, Tao Q, Srivastava G, Ho FC. Nasal NK- and T-cell lymphomas share the same type of Epstein–Barr virus latency as nasopharyngeal carcinoma and Hodgkin's disease. Int J Cancer 1996; 68:285–290.
24. Chiang AK, Wong KY, Liang AC, Srivastava G. Comparative analysis of Epstein–Barr virus gene polymorphisms in nasal T/NK cell lymphomas and nasal tissues: implications on virus strain selection in malignancy. Int J Cancer 1999; 80:356–364.
25. Chan JK, Tsang WY, Lau WH, et al. Aggressive T/natural killer cell lymphoma presenting as testicular tumor. Cancer 1996; 77:1198–1205.
26. Leong IT, Fernandes BJ, Mock D. Epstein–Barr virus detection in non-Hodgkin's lymphoma of the oral cavity: an immunocytochemical and in situ hybridization study. Oral Surg Oral Med Oral Pathol Oral Radiol Endod 2001; 92:184–193.
27. Sidigas J, Ueno K, Tokunaga M, et al. Molecular epidemiology of Epstein–Barr virus (EBV) in EBV-related malignancies. Int J Cancer 1997; 72:72–76.
28. Wright DH. Enteropathy associated T-cell lymphoma. Cancer Surv 1997; 30:249–261.
29. Quintanilla-Martinez L, Lome-Maldonado C, Ott g, et al. Primary intestinal non-Hodgkin's lymphoma and Epstein–Barr virus: high frequency of EBV-infection in T-cell lymphomas of Mexican origin. Leuk Lymphoma 1998; 30:111–121.
30. Au WY, Shek TW, Kwong YL. Epstein–Barr virus-related intravascular lymphomatosis. Am J Surg Pathol 2000; 24:309–310.
31. Oshima K, Liu Q, Koga T, et al. Classification of cell lineage and anatomical site, and prognosis of extranodal T-cell lymphoma—natural killer cell, cytotoxic T-lymphocyte, and non-NK/CTL types. Virchows Arch 2002; 440:425–435.
32. Shapira MY, Caspi O, Amir G, et al. Gastric-mucocutaneous gammadelta T-cell lymphoma: possible association with Epstein–Barr virus? Leuk Lymphoma 1999; 35:397–401.
33. Marianowski R, Wassef M, Amanou L, et al. Primary T-cell non-Hodgkin lymphoma of the larynx with subsequent cutaneous involvement. Arch Otolaryngol Head Neck Surg 1998; 124:1037–1040.
34. Lavergne A, Brocheriou I, Delfau MH, et al. Primary intestinal gamma-delta T-cell lymphoma with evidence of Epstein–Barr virus. Histopathology 1998; 32:271–276.
35. Arnulf B, Copie-Bergman C, Delfau-Larue MH, et al. Non hepatosplenic gammadelta T-cell lymphoma: a subset of cytotoxic lymphomas with mucosal or skin localization. Blood 1998; 91:1723–1731.
36. Donadieu J, Canioni D, Cuenod B, et al. A familial T-cell lymphoma with gamma delta phenotype and an original location. Possible role of chronic Epstein–Barr virus infection. Cancer 1996; 77:1571–1577.
37. Gaulard P, Balhadj K, Reyes F. $\gamma\delta$ T-cell lymphomas. Semin Hematol 2003; 40:233–243.
38. Takahashi N, Miura I, Chubachi A, et al. A clinicopathological study of 20 patients with T/natural killer (NK)-cell lymphoma-associated hemophagocytic syndrome with special reference to nasal and nasal-type NK/T-cell lymphoma. Int J Hematol 2001; 74:303–308.
39. Kikukawa M, Shin K, Iwamoto T, et al. A case of anaplastic large cell lymphoma associated with Epstein–Barr virus infection, representing clinicopathological features of malignant histiocytosis. Nippon Ronen Igakkai Zasshi 2003; 40:515–519.
40. Ansell SM, Li C-Y, Lloyd RV, Phyliky RL. Epstein–Barr virus in Richter's transformation. Am J Hematol 1999; 60:99–104.

41. Le Goff P, Chicault P, Saraux A, et al. Lymphoma with regression after methotrexate withdrawal in a patient with rheumatoid arthritis. Role for the Epstein–Barr virus. Rev Rheum Engl Ed 1998; 65:283–286.
42. Aydin F, Bartholomew PM, Vinson DG. Primary T-cell lymphoma of the brain in a patient at advanced stage of acquired immunodeficiency syndrome. Arch Pathol Lab Med 1998; 122:361–365.
43. Abruzzo LV, Griffith LM, Nandedkar M, et al. Histologically discordant lymphomas with B-cell and T-cell components. Am J Clin Pathol 1997; 108:316–323.
44. Oshima K, Suzumiya J, Kanda M, et al. Genotypic and phenotypic alterations in Epstein–Barr virus associated lymphoma. Histopathology 199; 35:539–550.
45. Noorali S, Pervez S, Moatter T, et al. Characterization of T-cell non-Hodgkin's lymphoma and its association with Epstein–Barr virus in Pakistani patients. Leuk Lymphoma 2003; 44:807–813.
46. Kagami Y, Nakamura S, Suzuki R, et al. A nodal gamma/delta T-cell lymphoma with an association of Epstein–Barr virus. Am J Surg Pathol 1997; 21:729–736.
47. Peh SC, Quen QW. Nasal and nasal-type natural killer (NK)/T-cell lymphoma: immunophenotype and Epstein–Barr virus (EBV) association. Med J Malaysia 2003; 58:196–204.
48. Teramoto N, Sarker AB, Tonoyama Y, et al. Epstein–Barr virus infection in the neoplastic and nonneoplastic cells of lymphoid malignancies. Cancer 1996; 77:2339–2347.
49. d'Amore F, Johansen P, Houmand A, et al. Epstein–Barr virus genome in non-Hodgkin's lymphomas occurring in immunocompetent patients: highest prevalence in nonlymphoblastic T-cell lymphoma and correlation with a poor prognosis with a poor prognosis. Danish Lymphoma Study Group, LYFO. Blood 1996; 87:1045–1055.
50. Kojima M, Nakamura S, Itoh H, et al. Acute viral lymphadenitis mimicking low-grade peripheral T-cell lymphoma. A clinicopathological study of nine cases. APMIS 2001; 109:419–427.
51. Chiang AK, Chan AC, Srivastiva G, Ho FC. Nasal T/natural killer (NK)-cell lymphomas are derived from Epstein–Barr virus-infected cytotoxic lymphocytes of both NK- and T-cell lineage. Int J Cancer 1997; 73:332–338.
52. Ashton-Key M, Singh N, Pan LX, Smith ME. HLA antigen expression in enteropathy associated T-cell lymphoma. J Clin Pathol 1996; 49:545–548.
53. Herling M, Khoury JD, LaBaron T, et al. A systematic approach to diagnosis of mature T-cell leukemias reveals heterogeneity among WHO categories. Blood 2004; 104:328–335.
54. Meijer CJ, Jiwa NM, Dukers DF, et al. Epstein–Barr virus and human T-cell lymphomas. Semin Cancer Biol 1996; 7:191–196.

14

Nasopharyngeal Carcinoma[a]

Sai Wah Tsao
*Department of Anatomy, The University of Hong Kong, Pokfulam, Hong Kong Special
Administration Region, P.R. China*

Kwok Wai Lo
*Department of Anatomical and Cellular Pathology, The Chinese University of Hong
Kong, Shatin, N.T., Hong Kong Special Administration Region, P.R. China*

Dolly P. Huang[†]
*Sir Y. K. Pao Centre for Cancer, The Chinese University of Hong Kong, Prince of Wales
Hospital, Shatin, N.T., Hong Kong Special Administration Region, P.R. China*

INTRODUCTION

Epstein–Barr virus (EBV) is a highly successful human pathogen, with greater than 95% of the world's population harboring latent EBV in their B-cells. This remarkable infection rate is achieved by the highly efficient transmission route of the virus from persistently infected persons to naïve individuals, most likely through saliva. Infection with EBV most frequently occurs in early childhood and is usually asymptomatic. Infection during early adulthood is frequently associated with infectious mononucleosis which is a benign and self-limiting lymphoproliferative disease. Seroepidemiological evidence suggests that EBV infection is widespread in China and that practically all Chinese children in Hong Kong are EBV positive before 15 years of age (1).

In most individuals, EBV establishes a harmonious relationship with the host with no major pathology. However, in immunocompromised patients including those who underwent transplantation and among patients with AIDS, this intricate balance is tipped, resulting in posttransplant lymphoproliferative disease (PTLD) and oral hairy leukoplakia (OHL), a benign replicative disorder of oral tongue mucosa in AIDS patients (2).

The transformation potential of EBV is demonstrated by the efficient transformation of B-cells to generate lymphoblastoid cell lines in the laboratory. EBV has been implicated in the pathogenesis of lymphoproliferative tumors, including Burkitt

---

[†] Deceased.

[a] In fond memory of our teacher, friend and colleague, Prof. Dolly P. Huang, who passed away before the publishing of this work.

lymphoma (BL) and Hodgkin's lymphoma, as well as epithelial tumors including nasopharyngeal carcinoma (NPC) and gastric carcinoma (3). The highest association of cancer with EBV is observed in NPC where the EBV genome can be detected in practically every NPC cell (4). Furthermore, EBV infection is closely related to the differentiation status of epithelial cancers (5). EBV infection is present mainly in the undifferentiated type carcinoma of the nasopharynx and stomach. EBV is not commonly detected in other head and neck cancers that are predominantly squamous cell carcinoma with various degrees of differentiation. EBV infection is absent in normal nasopharyngeal epithelium but can be detected in premalignant lesions, particularly in high-grade precancerous lesions and carcinoma in situ (6–8). A role of EBV in transforming premalignant nasopharyngeal epithelial cells into invasive cancer cells has been proposed (9). EBV infection has also been reported in breast (10) and liver cancers (11), but there is controversy about the involvement of EBV in the development of these cancers (12). Notably, the EBV genome copy numbers detected in breast and liver cancers are low, and the characteristic expression of EBV-encoded RNAs (EBERs) and Epstein–Barr nuclear antigen (EBNA)1, which are commonly detected in all EBV latent infections, is absent (3,13).

EBV GENE EXPRESSION DURING LATENT INFECTION

Latent EBV infection is associated with several human malignancies. Expression of the EBV proteins during latent infection triggers a host immune response, and thus only a restricted number of EBV proteins are expressed (14). In BL, only the EBNA1 protein is expressed in addition to EBERs and BamHI A RNAs (type I latency). In NPC, the EBV genes expressed include EBNA1, LMP1, LMP2A, and LMP2B in addition to EBERs and BamHI A RNAs (type II latency). Interestingly, BamHI fragment, right forward open reading frame 1 (BARF1) which was previously classified as an early EBV gene, was detected in about 85% of North African NPC biopsies (15). BARF1 is able to transform rodent fibroblasts and immortalize simian epithelial cells (16,17). In EBV-mediated transformation of B-cells in vitro and lymphoproliferative diseases in immunocompromised patients, the full range of latent genes that includes EBNA1, EBNA2, EBNA3A, EBNA3B, LMP1, LMP2A, and LMP2B in addition to EBERs and BamHI A RNAs (type III latency) are expressed. The precise regulatory mechanism of gene expression in different types of EBV latent infection is not fully understood and likely involves feedback regulatory mechanisms of EBV proteins on the usage of various promoters in the EBV genome, as well as specific promoter methylation (14,18). The functions of EBV genes expressed in latent infection and their involvement in human cancers have been recently reviewed (3).

GENETIC SUSCEPTIBILITY OF NPC

NPC is commonly observed in Hong Kong and the Southern provinces of China. The worldwide incidence of NPC is low in most countries (approximately 1/100,000 per year) (19), but in Hong Kong and Southern China the incidence rate of NPC is 25 to 50 per 100,000 per year (20). The male-to-female ratio is 2–3 to 1. The histopathology is mainly of the undifferentiated type (5). Multiple etiological factors are believed to be involved in NPC development including EBV infection, genetic susceptibility, and diet.

The ethnic clustering of NPC in Southern Chinese strongly suggests the involvement of genetic susceptibility and environmental factors in its development. Migrant and association studies of genetic markers and familial aggregation of the disease strongly indicated that genetic predisposition plays an important role in NPC development (21–23). Cellular susceptibility to the transformative action of EBV oncogenes may be one of the genetic predisposition factors to NPC in Southern Chinese. An earlier study identified a genetic risk factor for NPC and mapped it to the human leukocyte antigen (HLA) locus (24). An association of NPC with HLA alleles, A2, B14, and B46, was observed among Chinese patients. The candidate gene closely linked to HLA for increased risk of NPC has not yet been identified. The involvement of HLA in NPC may be related to the activity of cytotoxic T-cell recognition and host immune response to EBV infection.

Genetic polymorphisms for genes involved in metabolism of carcinogens may also play a role in the increased risk of NPC among Southern Chinese. For example, one genetic predisposition factor may be related to the metabolism of nitrosamine, a known carcinogen that is present in salt fish, a common part of the diet of Southern Chinese (Cantonese) living in Hong Kong in earlier days (25,26). The CYP2E1, one of the cytochrome P450 genes, is responsible for the metabolic activation of nitrosamines and the related carcinogens. Case–control studies have shown a strong association of the C2 allele of CYP2E1 with increased risk of NPC in Chinese (27). Salt fish is no longer a major component in the daily diet in present-day Hong Kong, which might alter the incidence rate of NPC in the population of Hong Kong. Indeed, there is a decreasing trend of incidence rate of NPC in Hong Kong over the past 20 years (28). The incidence rates of NPC for males and females in Hong Kong decreased by 29% and 30%, respectively. The glutathione S-transferase M1 (GSTM1) gene is involved in the detoxification of several carcinogens in tobacco smoke. A twofold increase in risk for NPC was also observed to be associated with the GSTM1 null genotype (29).

The close community and sharing of microenvironment and similar diet among Chinese living in Hong Kong and Southern China present immense difficulties in distinguishing the influence of environmental factors from the bonafide predisposing genetic factors involved in the development of NPC. Nevertheless, an recent study using a genome-wide linkage analysis approach was able to map an NPC susceptibility locus to chromosome 4 (D4S405 and D4S3002 loci) in 20 familial NPCs in the Cantonese population (30). The cloning and identification of the NPC susceptibility gene will help in the understanding of the pathogenic mechanisms of NPC.

ASSOCIATION OF EBV INFECTION WITH NPC

Detection of EBV in NPC

The indication that EBV infection is linked with NPC was first suggested by the serological detection of antibodies in NPC patients against the EBV antigen (31). In situ hybridization also demonstrated the presence of EBV DNA in NPC biopsies (32). The complete EBV genome is maintained in the NPC cells. There are 1 to approximately 30 copies of EBV genome per NPC cell, most of which are episomes and not integrated into the chromosomes. Analysis of the number of terminal repeat elements in the circularized EBV DNA in NPC showed that the EBV episomes within an NPC tumor are all derived from one copy of EBV, strongly indicating that NPC is derived from clonal expansion of a singly EBV-infected cell (see Chapter 7) (9). In situ hybridization of EBERs, which are present at high copy in EBV-infected cells, is a reliable marker of EBV infection. EBER can be detected in most high-grade pre-cancerous nasopharyngeal lesions but not in low-grade lesions or histologically normal nasopharyngeal epithelium (6–8). This suggests that other changes or genetic events in the precancerous lesions might be present in nasopharyngeal epithelium prior to EBV infection.

Serology of EBV in Patients with NPC

EBV infection in NPC induces an immunological response. The typical serological profile of NPC patients consists of an increase in both immunoglobulin G (IgG) and IgA antibodies against the viral capsid antigen (VCA) and early antigen (EA) and IgG antibodies against EBNA (33,34). Antibodies against ZEBRA (replication activator of EBV) can also be detected (35). The presence of antibodies against both latent and replication (lytic) antigens of EBV suggests that both latent and lytic EBV infections are present in NPC patients. The infiltrating lymphocytes in NPC may contribute significantly to the elevation of antibodies to the lytic antigens of EBV. The serological titers of antibodies against various EBV antigens have been used clinically to monitor tumor burden, remission, and recurrence in NPC (36).

Serum EBV DNA in Patients with NPC

The EBV genome is present in serum and can be easily detected by polymerase chain reaction (PCR) amplification. With the advance of real-time (RT) and quantitative PCR, it is possible to accurately quantitate the levels of circulating EBV DNA in the serum of NPC patients. The quantitation of EBV DNA as a tumor marker for NPC has a lower false positive rate compared to the antibody-based serological markers (37). EBV DNA can be detected in the plasma of 96% of NPC patients but only in 7% of healthy individuals (38). Furthermore, the EBV DNA concentrations are positively correlated with the clinical staging of the NPC patients (39). The median plasma levels of EBV DNA in advanced-stage NPC (stages III and IV) were approximately eight times higher than those with early-stage NPC (stages I and II), suggesting that the plasma concentration of EBV DNA in NPC patients reflects tumor load. In addition, the persistence of EBV DNA after radiotherapy is associated with poor prognosis. Furthermore, plasma levels of EBV DNA is higher in NPC patients with recurrence than in those remaining in clinical remission.

GENETIC ALTERATIONS IN NPC

Early Genetic Events in the Development of NPC

EBV latent infection, Bcl-2 overexpression, and telomerase activation are early events in NPC development (9,40,41). We have examined the relationship of EBV infection and genetic alterations in early stages of NPC development. By microdissection and microsatellite analysis, we have examined EBER expression with genetic changes in the histological normal epithelia, low- and high-grade dysplastic lesions, and invasive carcinoma of the nasopharynx (Fig. 1). The nasopharyngeal epithelium in Southern Chinese appears to be prone to allelic deletion of chromosomes 3p and 9p, which can be detected by a loss of heterozygosity (LOH) study (7,8).

LOH study involves the detection of loss of one of the two heterozygous alleles at a specific chromosomal locus, indicating inactivation of one functional copy of a gene(s) mapped to that specific locus. LOH at a specific locus is a hallmark for the

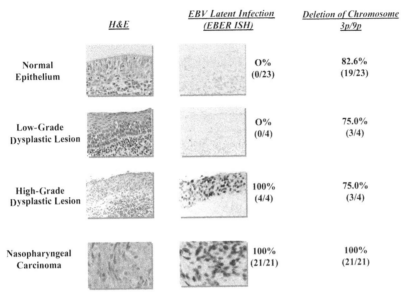

	H&E	*EBV Latent Infection (EBER ISH)*	*Deletion of Chromosome 3p/9p*
Normal Epithelium		0% (0/23)	82.6% (19/23)
Low-Grade Dysplastic Lesion		0% (0/4)	75.0% (3/4)
High-Grade Dysplastic Lesion		100% (4/4)	75.0% (3/4)
Nasopharyngeal Carcinoma		100% (21/21)	100% (21/21)

Figure 1 (*See color insert.*) Expression of EBER in premalignant nasopharyngeal epithelium carrying allelic deletion of chromosomes 3p and 9p. Note the expression of EBER in the high-grade precancerous lesion but its absence in the low-grade precancerous lesion. Allelic deletion of chromosomes 3p (at locus D3S1076) and 9p (at loci IFNA and DS9161) could be detected in both high- and low-grade precancerous lesions of nasopharyngeal epithelium, suggesting that the deletions occur before EBV infection. *Abbreviations*: EBER, Epstein–Barr virus encoded ribonucleic acids; EBV, Epstein–Barr virus.

presence of a tumor suppressor gene mapped to that locus. High frequencies of LOH on chromosomes 3p and 9p (80% and 45%, respectively) were detected in both low- and high-grade dysplastic lesions and even in histologically normal epithelia of the nasopharynx from Southern Chinese living in an area known to be endemic for NPC (7,8). A much lower LOH rate was observed in normal nasopharyngeal epithelium in low-risk Northern Chinese. Moreover, we have also detected the aberrant methylation of the tumor suppressor gene located at 3p21.3, *RASSF1A*, in some dysplastic lesions and adjacent epithelia (unpublished observation). These findings imply that losses of 3p and 9p are earlier events in NPC development. Inactivation of the target tumor suppressor genes on these regions may confer a growth advantage on the initiated cells. Interestingly, EBV infection was not detected in low-grade lesions harboring LOH of 3p and 9p, suggesting that these genetic alterations are early events in NPC development and precede EBV infection. The postulate is that the latent EBV infection and expression of viral oncogene, such as LMP1 and other EBV viral gene products, in the high-grade dysplastic nasopharyngeal epithelium may transform the genetically altered cells into invasive cancer cells (9).

Global Genetic Changes in NPC

Knowledge of the genetic and epigenetic changes in NPC and their interaction with EBV oncogenes is crucial for the understanding of the molecular basis of development of NPC. EBV-infected cells may drive the clonal expansion of premalignant nasopharyngeal epithelial cells, resulting in further genetic alterations detected in NPC. Multiple genomic-wide studies have defined important tumor suppressor loci and amplicons of NPC (42–45). High-resolution allelotyping and comparative genome hybridization (CGH) studies have identified, in addition to the losses on 3p and 9p, losses on chromosomes 9q, 11q, 13q, 14q, and 16q, and gains on 1q, 3q, 12p, and 12q. Common regions of loss were 3p14–21, 14q24-qter, and 11q21-qter, while common regions of gain were 3q21–26 and 12q13–15 (42–45). Recent array-based CGH analyses have further identified cryptic amplification at the chromosomal region 3q26 (46,47). The highest frequencies of allelic losses were found in chromosomes 3p (96.3%), 9p (85.2%), and 14q (85.2%). Multiple minimally deleted regions including 3p14–24.2, 11q21–23, 13q12–14, 13q31–32, 14q24–32, and 16q22–23 have been identified, which may harbor multiple tumor suppressor genes (42). Monochromosome transfer studies have provided functional evidence for the involvement of tumor suppressors at chromosomes 3p, 9p, 11q, and 14q in NPC (48–50).

Candidate Tumor Suppressors and Oncogenes Identified in NPC

Dysfunction of Rb and p53 antioncogene regulatory pathways plays a major role in human carcinogenesis. However, mutational inactivation of the Rb and *p53* genes are rare events in NPC (51,52). Disruption of the Rb and p53 functions in NPC may be achieved by indirect mechanisms. The *p16* gene, a cyclin-dependent kinase (CDK) inhibitor located within 9p21 region, has been reported to be a target tumor suppressor in NPC. Inactivation of *p16* genes disrupts the cell cycle entry regulated by Rb (53,54). The *p16* gene was inactivated in about 80% of primary tumors by either homozygous deletions or promoter methylation. NPC cells transfected with wild-type p16 showed in vitro growth inhibition, fewer colonies in soft agar, shifting of G2 phase to G1 phase in cell cycle, and suppressed tumorigenicity in athymic nude mice (55). The *p14/ARF* gene, which is also located in 9p21 region, was inactivated in about 54% of primary tumors of NPC (53,56,57). The p14/ARF binds to the Mdm2 and inhibits the ubiquitination and degradation of p53 protein. Mutation of *p53* is rare in NPC (52). The *p14/ARF* loss may facilitate p53 degradation in NPC cells. Recent study in transgenic animals showed that the loss of the p16INKA/p14ARF locus facilitates the transformative action of LMP1 in epithelial cells (58). Another study has shown that overexpression of the *deltaN-p63*, which has dominant negative function to p53, may disrupt p53 function in NPC cells (59). The *deltaN-p63* transcript as well as protein is consistently overexpressed in NPC and may be one of the target oncogenes on the 3q26 amplicon. These findings suggest that inactivation of both Rb and p53 pathways are critical genetic events in NPC tumorigenesis.

The chromosome 3p region is commonly lost in NPC. The *RASSF1A* gene at 3p21.3 is a target tumor suppressor of NPC. A high frequency of *RASSF1A* inactivation was found in the NPC cell lines and primary tumors (75% to 100%) (60). Exogenous expression of *RASSF1A* in a *RASSF1A*-deficient NPC cell line C666-1 inhibited tumor cell growth. Reduced colony formation of the *RASSF1A*-expressing clones was noted in both anchorage-dependent and -independent assays while tumor formation in nude mice was remarkably suppressed (61). The RASSF1A protein might function as an effector of the Ras signaling pathway (62). Recent study has demonstrated that RASSF1A is a microtubule-binding protein that can stabilize microtubules and prevent their depolymerization in vivo (63). Another report suggests that RASSF1A may be involved in cell cycle regulation in lung cancer cells through the inhibition of cyclin D1 accumulation (64); neither significant change in expression of cyclin D1 nor G1 arrest was found in the *RASSF1A*-transfected NPC cells (61). Our microarray study revealed multiple candidate *RASSF1A* target genes suggesting that RASSF1A may be involved in multiple cellular pathways, including the transforming growth factor (TGF)-beta superfamily and G-protein signaling in NPC (unpublished observations).

In addition to potential tumor suppressor genes and oncogenes on chromosome 3p and 9p, mutations of the *RB2/p130* gene, overexpression of the bcl-2, and c-met oncoproteins and reduced expression of p27 and MAD2 cell cycle regulatory proteins have also been reported in NPC (65–69). Furthermore, epigenetic studies on NPC have also identified multiple gene targets transcriptionally silenced by promoter hypermethylation (56). Widespread hypermethylation of CpG islands over the entire genome implies a methylator phenotype in NPC. Epigenetic inactivation of these genes may cause disruption of retinoid signaling pathway [e.g., retinoic acid receptor beta (RARB)] (56), endothelin-1 pathway [e.g., endothelin B receptor (ENDRB)] (70), cell cycle and apoptosis control [e.g., death associated protein (DAP)-kinase, retinomablastoma interacting zinc-finger protein 1 (RIZ1)] (71), cell adhesion [e.g., E-cadherin, tumor suppressor in lung cancer-1 (TSLC-1)] (72,73), and other novel pathways [e.g., harpin-induced (HIN), BLU] (74,75). The functional interaction of these genetic alterations and EBV oncogenes remains to be determined.

EBV INFECTION IN EPITHELIAL CELLS AND B LYMPHOCYTES

Cell Types Involved in Primary and Persistent EBV Infection

The spread of EBV in humans is efficiently achieved through salivary transmission, with B-lymphocytes in the oropharyngeal mucosa believed to be the cell type involved in the spread of primary EBV infection (76). The presence of mature B-cells is required to establish persistent EBV infection. This is indicated by the absence of EBV infection in patients with X-linked agammaglobulinemia, a rare disease affecting B-cell development (77). The pharyngeal epithelium covering the lymphoid tissue is loose and disrupted in places where the underlying B-cells can be exposed to EBV transmitted by saliva (76). Infection of the pharyngeal epithelial cells may be a secondary event that involves migration of EBV-infected B-cells into the pharyngeal epithelium. The expression of CD48 on the surfaces of B-cells is dramatically upregulated after EBV infection (78). The CD48 can bind to a heparan sulfate proteoglycan on the surfaces of epithelial cells, which facilitates the homing-in of EBV-infected B-cells to the epithelial cells in the pharynx. In patients with AIDS, epithelial cells at the lateral borders of the tongue can be infected with EBV, resulting in OHL, a benign lesion with EBV undergoing lytic replication in proliferative epithelial cells (79). Another important observation is that persistent EBV infection is not maintained in bone marrow transplantation patients whose bone marrow cells but not the epithelial cells have been eradicated, hence suggesting that latently infected memory B-cells in the bone marrow, instead of epithelial cells, are the pool for persistent EBV infection (80).

Switches in Receptors for EBV Infection and Tropism

EBV infection of B-lymphocytes is facilitated by the presence of complement receptor 2 (CR2) or CD21, which interacts with the glycoprotein gp350/220 protein of viral envelope of EBV and mediates viral entry (81). EBV infection of B-lymphocytes readily gives rise to lymphoblastoid cell lines that can be propagated in vitro. Infection of normal nasopharyngeal epithelial cells is rare in vivo and difficult to accomplish in vitro.

Different viral receptors are believed to be involved in the infection of B-lymphocytes and human epithelial cells (82). In addition to the gp350/220 protein of EBV envelope, entry of the virus into the B-lymphocytes requires three additional viral envelope glycoproteins: gH, gL, and gp42. EBV infection in B-lymphocytes involves interaction of gp42 with the HLA class II complex on infected cells. In epithelial cells, which do not express HLA class II complex, EBV infection involves only gH and gL, and not gp42. EBV virus which does not express gp42 can only infect epithelial cells but not B-cells. Addition of the gp42 to the gH and gL complex produces a virus that can only infect B-cells. This provides a molecular switch in EBV to change its tropism. Interestingly, the presence of the HLA class II in the virus-producing cells can alter the ratio of the three-part envelope protein complex (gH, gL, and gp42) to a two-part (gH and gL) complex and hence will alter the tropism of the virus (82). As a consequence, virus originating from the infected epithelial cells and B-cell–derived EBV efficiently infect B-cells and epithelial cells, respectively. This suggests a cycle of infection and reinfection of EBV when they switch host cell type from epithelial cells to B-cells and cause reinfection of pharyngeal epithelial cells.

EBV INFECTION IN NASOPHARYNGEAL EPITHELIAL CELLS

Routes of Entry

EBV infection is commonly detected in NPC but not in healthy nasopharyngeal epithelium (83). The route of EBV entry and maintenance of EBV infection in nasopharyngeal epithelial cells are poorly understood. The high rate of LOH of 3p and 9p in nasopharyngeal epithelium of Southern Chinese may be a predisposing factor for EBV infection. Several routes of entry of EBV into nasopharyngeal epithelial cells have been implicated.

An early study demonstrated that EBV could enter human epithelial cells via IgA-mediated endocytosis (84). Polymeric IgA (pIgA) specific for EBV, isolated from acute infectious mononucleosis, was shown to promote EBV infection in a human epithelial cell line, HT-29. Presumably, the plasma cells at the mucosa secrete pIgA that binds by means of the J (joining) chain to the secretory component (SC), a transmembrane protein expressed on the basolateral surface of epithelial cells. IgA against EBV-VCA and gp350 can be detected at high titers in patients with NPC (33,85). Expression of SC could be detected in the pseudostratified columnar epithelium and intermediate epithelium covering the lateral nasopharyngeal walls including the fossa of Rosenmüller, where NPC commonly develops. Binding of EBV to the pIgA/SC receptor complex and endocytosis of the EBV/IgA/SC complex may facilitate the entry of EBV into nasopharyngeal epithelial cells. This route of EBV infection has been demonstrated in vitro using NPC cells (86). It is well known that NPC cells established in culture commonly lose the EBV genome on prolonged propagation (87,88). Treatment of two of these EBV-negative NPC cell lines (TW01 and TW06) with serum of NPC patients containing high titers of IgA against EBV-VCA facilitated their reinfection by EBV. The expression of EBV-encoded proteins, including LMP1 and EBNA1, in EBV-reinfected NPC cells could be detected 10 days after EBV infection. Increased expression of epithelial growth factor receptor, TGF-α, interleukin (IL)-1β, IL-6, and granulocyte–macrophage colony–stimulating factors were observed in NPC cells within one to two weeks after reinfection with EBV. However, the EBV genome was not retained in the EBV-reinfected NPC cells. The EBV genomes in the infected NPC cells were eventually lost by exocytosis after three to four weeks. This is reminiscent of the continuous loss of EBV in cell lines established from NPC biopsies. The switch of growth condition from in vivo to in vitro environment may trigger lytic replication and exocytosis of EBV. Propagation of NPC biopsies in athymic nude mice, however, allows retention of the EBV genome, resulting in the establishment of an EBV-positive NPC cell line, C666–1 (89), and several EBV-positive NPC xenografts (90), suggesting the importance of cellular factors in supporting latent infection of EBV.

Direct cell-to-cell contact between the EBV-producing B-cells (Akata) and target cells was recently shown to be highly efficient in transmission of EBV into a variety of human epithelial cells. The introduction of a G418-resistant (neomycin resistance) gene into the EBV genome allows selective growth of EBV-infected epithelial cells. EBV transmission by cell-to-cell contact occurs independently of the CR2 receptor that mediates EBV entry in B-cells. EBV infection of NPC cells was achieved by cell-to-cell contact in the NPC cell lines TW03 (91), TW01, and HONE1 (92) and CNE1, CNE2, HK1, and TW04 in our laboratories with different degrees of infection efficiency.

Polarization of the epithelial cells was shown to be a major determining factor for EBV infection by cell-to-cell contact (93). A recent study examined the binding and entry of EBV into tongue and oropharyngeal epithelial cells that do not express the CR2 receptor. The epithelial cells were cultured on microporous membranes to form polarized monolayers with tight junctions at the apical regions. Incubation of these polarized monolayers of cells with EBV-producing B-cell lines results in high efficiency of EBV infection (7% to 16% infection rate) suggesting that primary EBV infection in polarized cells occurs at the apical surface by direct cell-to-cell contact with EBV-infected B-cells. EBV infection of these polarized pharyngeal epithelial cells could also be achieved by attachment of cell-free EBV virions to the lateral and basal surfaces of the polarized epithelium. The attachment of virus to cell is mediated by the interaction of the arginine-glycine-aspartate (RGD) motif of the EBV BMRF-2 glycoprotein and the $\beta 1$ or $\alpha 5 \beta 1$ integrins of the cell membrane at the lateral and basal surfaces of the polarized epithelial cells. Antibodies against both BMRF-2 and $\beta 1$ integrins neutralize binding and entry of EBV into pharyngeal epithelial cells but not in CR2 positive BJAB cells. In addition, the polarized epithelial cells that were previously infected with EBV by cell-to-cell contact at the apical surface could release EBV virions from the apical as well as the basolateral surfaces to achieve spreading of EBV infection to adjacent cells. This study clearly demonstrated the route of CR2-independent infection of EBV into pharyngeal epithelial cells and its subsequent spread to adjacent epithelial cells.

Maintenance of the EBV Genome in Nasopharyngeal Epithelial Cells

While the EBV genome can readily be detected in NPC in vivo, maintenance of the EBV genome in NPC, generally, is not supported in vitro. It is well known that NPC cell lines established from NPC commonly lose their EBV genomes on prolonged culture. This is distinct from human papillomavirus (HPV) infection in cervical carcinoma cells where HPV16 and HPV18 genomes are retained as integrated forms in established cervical carcinoma cell lines such as HeLa and CaSki. In contrast, the EBV genome could be maintained in NPC xenograft maintained in nude mice. The C666–1 cell line, which retains the EBV genome in culture, was derived from a xenografted NPC that has been passed for a long time. It would be interesting to examine the cellular factors important for the maintenance of the EBV genome in C666–1 cells.

Several factors have been proposed to be involved in the maintenance of the EBV genome. The contribution of cellular signal transducers and activators of transcription (STAT) signaling activity has been implicated in the maintenance of EBV infection in NPC cells. The STAT proteins are latent in the cytoplasm and are critical in mediating cytokine-driven signaling. In response to the binding of ligand to the cytokine receptors, the tyrosine residues on the STAT proteins are phosphorylated by Janus activated kinase (JAK) family kinases. The STAT3 and STAT5 proteins are associated with cell proliferation and prevention of apoptosis through upregulation of the antiapoptotic proteins Bcl-xL, Bcl-2, and Mcl-1, and cell cycle regulators such as cyclin D1, cyclin D2, and c-Myc (94). Maintenance of the EBV episome is dependent on the expression of EBNA1, which involves the usage of BamHI-Q promoter (Qp). The observation that STAT can regulate Qp activity suggests that STAT activation may play a role in maintaining the EBV genome in cells (95). Expression of BZLF1, which codes for Zta expression, induces lytic EBV infection that is associated with downregulation of Qp activity. Interestingly, increased tyrosine phosphorylation of STAT3 and STAT5 were observed in EBV-infected HeLa cells. Increased phosphorylation of STAT3 and STAT5 could be observed in NPC cell lines expressing LMP1. Activation of STAT3 by LMP1 is mostly mediated by IL6 secretion that forms an autocrine loop to maintain the EBV genome in cells (96). The STAT3 and STAT5 proteins are commonly activated in human cancers, including NPC (97), which would support the Qp activity and contribute to the maintenance of EBV genome in NPC cells in vivo.

A recent study showed that high levels of nuclear factor κB (NF-κB) inhibit lytic replication of gamma-herpesviruses, including EBV (98). The inhibition of virus replication protects the cell from the cytopathic effects of viral protein synthesis and promotes the establishment of latent infection. Inhibition of NF-κB in latently infected cells leads to lytic protein synthesis. The EBV-encoded LMP1 is a potent activator of NF-κB. The expression of LMP1 upregulates intracellular NF-κB activity and further inhibits lytic gene expression which stabilizes the latent infection. Details of the mechanism by which NF-κB inhibits lytic promoters of gamma-herpesvirus are unknown but involves both the N-terminal DNA-binding/dimerization domain and the C-terminal activation domain of p65.

Biological Properties of EBV-Infected Nasopharyngeal Epithelial Cells

EBV infection of human epithelial cells was achieved in an earlier study by first expressing the CR2 receptor in an SV40-immortalized keratinocyte cell line (SVK) followed by infection with EBV containing supernatant harvested from Akata cells, an EBV-producing cell line (99). About 50% to 90% of CR2-expressing SVK (SVK-CR2) cells could be infected by EBV via this method. The EBV-infected SVK-CR2 cells expressed the EBV gene characteristic of latency type II infection that includes EBNA1, LMP1, LMP2A, and LMP2B, in addition to EBERs and BamHI A RNAs. The EBNA1 transcripts in SVK-CR2 infected with EBV mainly used the Qp instead of the C promoter/W promoter (Cp/Wp). The expression level of LMP1 was low and could only be detected by RT-PCR. This is reminiscent of LMP1 expression in NPC in vivo, which is often heterogeneous and low in expression. EBV infection in the SVK-CR2 cells was unstable. At 24 days postinfection, only 10% of the EBV-infected SVK-CR2 cells retained the EBV genome (100). The lytic cycle proteins of EBV infection, such as BZLF1 and EA-D, can be detected in EBV-infected SVK-CR2 cells. Lytic infection of EBV is enhanced by stimulating the EBV-infected SVK-CR2 cells to undergo epithelial differentiation using 12-O-tetradecanoyl-phorbol-13-acetate. Cloning of SVK-CR2 cells stably infected with EBV showed that they become refractory to differentiation-inducing agents. EBV lytic proteins are not detectable in these EBV stably infected clones. These findings suggest that stable latent infection of EBV can only be established in undifferentiated epithelial cells. This is reminiscent of the common detection of EBV genome in undifferentiated NPC and less frequent detection in other head and neck carcinomas, which are largely squamous cell carcinomas with more differentiated histology.

While the earlier studies using SVK have been highly informative about EBV infection in human epithelial cells, the presence of SV40 gene products in the SVK cells may interact with the actions of EBV genes. Recent studies have employed the genetically recombinant EBV carrying G418-resistant (neomycin resistance) drug selection marker that allows selective growth of EBV-infected epithelial cells for long-term functional analysis (101). EBV infection was achieved by direct cell-to-cell contact of EBV-producing cells and target epithelial cells without the involvement of the CR2 receptor. This clearly indicates that EBV infects epithelial cells via an entry route distinct from that of B-cells, which is dependent on the CR2 receptor. As mentioned earlier, most of the NPC cell lines established in culture eventually lost their EBV genome upon prolonged propagation. These resulting EBV-negative NPC cell lines can be reinfected with EBV using the cell-to-cell contact method. Functional studies of EBV reinfection of NPC cells have been reported in TW01, HONE1 (92), and TW03 cells (91). In our laboratories, we have also successfully infected HONE1, CNE1, CNE2, HK1, and TW04 cells with EBV using supernatants from the Akata cells (unpublished results). In addition, two immortalized but nonmalignant nasopharyngeal epithelial cell lines (NP69 and NP39) immortalized by SV40T and HPV16E6E6 were also successfully infected with EBV. There are variations in the efficiency of EBV infection among the NPC and immortalized NP cell lines. EBV infection was highly efficient in HONE1 cells and less efficient in HK1 and immortalized NP cells. The ease of EBV infection may be related to the stage of differentiation of the epithelial cells. The HK1 was established from a well-differentiated NPC (102) while the immortalized nasopharyngeal epithelial cells retain many differentiation properties of normal nasopharyngeal epithelial cells (103). These observations are in line with the earlier studies that showed that latent EBV infection is better supported in undifferentiated cells. The presence of EBV in these reinfected NPC and immortalized nasopharyngeal epithelial cell lines was confirmed by in situ hybridization of EBER. Examination of EBV latent gene expression in these EBV-infected NPC cells revealed latency type II gene expression with EBNA1, LMP1, LMP2A, and LMP2B, in addition to EBERs and *Bam*HI A RNAs in all the EBV-infected cells. The transcription of EBNA1 was predominantly from the Qp. We also detected expression of BARF1 in all EBV-infected NPC and immortalized NP cells (unpublished observations). Interestingly, EBV reinfection of NPC cells did not appear to result in growth stimulation in cultured NPC cells (unpublished observations); this was also reported by others (91). This is not surprising as the EBV genome in SVK-CR2 cells as well as primary NPC cells is continuously lost upon prolonged culture, suggesting the lack of selective growth advantage for EBV-infected NPC cells in culture (100). One explanation is that the established NPC cell lines are highly adapted to growth in culture conditions and may not be responsive to stimulation of cell growth by EBV infection. The in vitro culture environment may also trigger lytic infection of EBV. However, enhancement in invasive properties and tumorigenicity in nude mice was reported in EBV-infected NPC cells

(100). These observations suggest that EBV infection may play a more important role in induction of invasive property in premalignant nasopharyngeal epithelial cells in vivo. It should be noted that all the studies reported involved the use of recombinant EBV generated from Akata cells that are originated from B-lymphocytes and may not fully represent the biological properties of EBV isolated from NPC. Nonetheless, they have provided insights into the role of EBV infection in NPC.

The transformation ability of EBV in epithelial cells was demonstrated in EBV-infected simian kidney epithelial cells (104). EBV infection could lead to immortalization of nonmalignant gastric epithelial cell lines (GT38 and FT 39) (105,106). EBV infection of a nonmalignant gastric epithelial cell line (PGE-5) resulted in enhanced population doubling, higher saturation density, anchorage-independent growth in soft agar, and tumorigenicity in SCID mice (107). All these observations support a role of EBV infection in human epithelial malignancies.

TRANSFORMATION PROPERTIES OF GENE PRODUCTS ENCODED BY EBV

The transformation properties and intracellular signaling activity have been examined in several gene products encoded by EBV during latent infection.

LMP1

Transformation and Cell Signaling

The signaling pathways and transformation properties of LMP1 have been intensively investigated. LMP1 is essential for EBV-induced immortalization of B-lymphocytes. The significance of LMP1 in NPC has been recently reviewed (108). Expression of LMP1 transforms Rat-1 fibroblasts (109) and induces various phenotypic changes in epithelial cells (110), including loss of contact inhibition, anchorage-independent growth in soft agar, and the ability to grow in reduced serum concentration. LMP1 expression is common in EBV-positive NPC, although the level of expression is generally low and heterogeneous. Expression of LMP1 in immortalized nasopharyngeal epithelial cells induces an array of genes involved in growth stimulation, enhanced survival, and increased invasive potentials (111). LMP1 is an integral membrane protein consisting of a short N-terminal cytoplasmic domain, a six-transmembrane-spanning domain, and a 200-residue-long C-terminal cytoplasmic domain (112). Aggregation or oligomerization of LMP1 in the membrane is essential for activation of cell signaling. LMP1 functions as a constitutively active tumor necrosis factor receptor, activating a number of signaling pathways in a ligand-independent manner (113). Two distinct functional domains have been identified within the C-terminal regions: C-terminal activation regions 1 and 2 (CTAR1 and CTAR2). The CTAR1 region (residue 194–231) has been shown to initiate cell proliferation, and the CTAR2 region (residue 351–386) is essential for permanent lymphoblastoid cell line outgrowth. Several major signaling pathways from the C-terminal regions of LMP1 including NF-κB, the mitogen-activated protein kinase (MAPK) family (extracellular signal–regulated kinases, p38, and c-Jun N-terminal kinases), the JAK/STAT protein, and recently the phosphatidylinositol 3-kinase have been identified (114).

LMP1 is a potent activator of NF-κB activation in cells, which mediates many downstream events of LMP1 expression (112,115). Both the CTAR1 and CTAR2 domains of LMP1 are responsible for activation of NF-κB (115). LMP1 activates expression of myriads of cellular genes involved in cell growth [e.g., epidermal growth factor receptor (EGFR)], antiapoptosis [e.g., Bcl-2, Bfl-1, A20, and cellular inhibitor of apoptosis proteins (cIAPs)], proinflammatory cytokines (e.g., IL6 and IL8), cell surface antigens (e.g., CD40, CD54, and CD95), angiogenesis factors [e.g., vascular endothelial cell growth factor (VEGF) and cyclo-oxygenase (COX) 2], and invasion [matrix metalloproteinases (MMPs)].

LMP1 Variants

There are controversies over the association of LMP1 variants with specific types of human diseases (116). The predominant LMP1 strain in China (China 1) (117) is characterized by 13 nucleotide changes with respect to the prototypic B95–8 LMP1, including a point mutation resulting in the loss of an *Xho*1 restriction site. The China 1 strain is also distinguished by changes in the C-terminal region of LMP1, notably the deletion of amino acids 343 to 352. It has been postulated that the LMP1 variant isolated from Chinese NPC may have distinct functional and possibly transformation properties (118). The LMP1 from NPC is shown to be more potent in activation of NF-κB, a major cell-signaling pathway activated by LMP1 (119,120). Activation of NF-κB induces an array of downstream events facilitating cell survival and invasion. There is a great deal of interest in whether specific sequence variations of LMP1 may be associated with different EBV-associated diseases, including NPC. A comprehensive study on the sequences of LMP1 variants from 92 EBV-positive NPC specimens collected from different geographical regions of China was analyzed using a phylogenetic analysis method (121). Seven strains of LMP1—B95–8, Med, China 1, China 2, China 3, Alaskan, and North Carolina strains—could be identified. China 1 LMP1 is the prevalent strain that makes up 85% of the LMP1 variants surveyed in published literature. The China 1 strain carries a 30-base pair (bp) deletion at the C-cytoplasmic region at codon 346 to 355, and other specific amino acid sequence differences.

The biological properties of the CAO-LMP1 have been compared with the prototype B95–8 LMP1 by stable expression in SCC12F human squamous epithelial cells, which revealed distinct biological properties (122). The CAO-LMP1 is less toxic than the B95–8-LMP1. Significant functional differences between these two variants with respect to cellular toxicity, production of IL6 and IL8, and expression of CD40, CD44, and CD54 were observed. An enhancement of signaling activity of NF-κB and activator protein (AP) was mapped to the transmembrane domain of the CAO-LMP1 but not to the region of C-cytoplasmic domain where a 30-bp deletion is present (119). This agrees with other studies indicating that the 30-bp deletion may not be the major effector of functional differences between variant LMP1 genes in human lymphocytes (123). Apart from the 30-bp deletion at the C-cytoplasmic terminal, there are also multiple sequence variations in the transmembrane domain of the CAO-LMP1 variant, which are not present in the prototype B95–8-LMP1. The sequence variations in the transmembrane domain of CAO-LMP1 may account for the enhanced ability to activate cell signaling by enabling a long intracellular half-life of CAO-LMP1.

We have also examined the sequence variations of LMP1 isolated from NPC patients and healthy subjects in Hong Kong (89). More than 80% of NPC patients in Hong Kong harbor a specific variant of LMP1 (2117-LMP1). The sequence of 2117-LMP1 is similar to that of CAO-LMP1, including a 30-bp deletion at the C-terminal cytoplasmic domain. There are amino acid variations between the

2117-LMP1 in Hong Kong NPC (HK NPC) and CAO-LMP1. The 2117-LMP1 carries a unique substitution at codon 335 (replacing a glycine with an aspartic acid) that is absent in the prototypic B95–8-LMP1 and in the two LMP1 variants isolated from Chinese NPC patients (CAO-LMP1 and C1510-LMP1). The codon 355 is located outside the known functional domains involved in cell signaling. The 2117-LMP1 is more efficient in stimulating NF-κB activation and displays a distinct functional difference from the prototypic B95–8 LMP1 (120).

LMP2

The LMP2 gene encodes two structurally similar proteins, LMP2A and LMP2B. Neither protein is essential for B-cell transformation in vitro (124). The LMP2A has been shown to block the B-cell receptor–stimulated lytic cycle of EBV in B-cells (125). Expression of LMP2 abrogates normal B-cell development in a transgenic mouse model and drives the proliferation and survival of B-cells (126). LMP2A may function in maintenance of EBV latency in B-cells. Recent studies showed that LMP2 could augment many transformation properties of LMP1, including activation of NK-κB (127). Oncogenic effects of LMP2A have also been demonstrated in HaCaT-cells (128). Activation of the phosphoinositide 3 (PI3) kinase–Akt pathway and the MAPK pathway resulting in the phosphorylation of c-Jun are believed to be involved in the transformation process.

BARF1

The BARF1 gene is transcribed early after the EBV infection from the *Bam*HI A fragment of the EBV genome and encodes a 33-kDa protein homologous to the human colony-stimulating factor-1 (hCSF-1) receptor (129). The BARF1 protein is functional and can neutralize the activity of hCSF-1 in vitro, suggesting a role in the support of cell growth in EBV-infected cells. The BARF1 protein inhibits alpha interferon secretion from mononuclear cells and may modulate the innate host response to the virus. The transformation properties of BARF1 have been demonstrated in rodent fibroblast (130), monkey salivary epithelial cells (131), and EBV-negative Akata cells (132). Expression of BARF1 is detected in greater than 85% of nasopharyngeal biopsies (15) and in greater than 80% of EBV-positive gastric carcinoma (131). Expression of BARF1 appears to be epithelial specific, and it is rarely expressed in lymphoid neoplasias such as Hodgkin's disease and T-cell lymphoma (132,133).

The transformation mechanism of BARF1 is poorly understood. Transfection of primate tissue explants with a specific subfragment (p31) of EBV DNA results in immortalization of primate epithelial cells (134). The gene for BARF1 is encoded within the p31 fragment. BARF1 expression was detected in early as well as late passages of p31-immortalized primate epithelial cells. Expression of BARF1 in the p31-immortalized primate epithelial cells results in enhanced growth rate and clonal expansion of cells with multiple double minutes (amplified chromosomal sequences). All of these studies support a role of BARF1 in EBV-induced epithelial cancers.

EBERs

The EBERs are small, unpolyadenylated RNAs encoded by EBV upon infection of a cell (135). The expression of EBERs is detected at a high level in most EBV-associated human malignancies and is used as a reliable marker for latent EBV infection. Expression level of EBER is the highest among the viral genes expressed in latently EBV-infected cells. The EBERs are localized to the cell nucleus and in the cytoplasm, where they form complexes with cellular proteins La (136), EBER-associated protein (EAP)/L22 (137), and the double-stranded RNA–dependent protein kinase (PKR) (138). Activation of PKR is a cell defense mechanism against viral infection (139). PKR is an interferon-induced protein kinase that can be activated by double-stranded RNA and other cytokines, including IL-2 and TNFα. Activation of PKR involves autophosphorylation of the PKR protein which then induces phosphorylation of eukaryotic initiation factor 2α (eIF2α) (a translation initiation factor). The phosphorylation of eIF2α inhibits protein synthesis in cells and induces apoptosis. EBERs can bind to PKR and block its activity and may thereby prevent apoptosis in EBV-infected cells (140). In BL, EBERs were shown to play a key role in the maintenance of malignant phenotype (see Chapter 10) (141). Expression of EBERs confers clonability on soft agarose, tumorigenicity on nude mice, and resistance to apoptotic stimuli in BL. EBERs induce transcription of IL-10, which may function as an autocrine growth factor of BL.

Very little is known about the functions of EBER expression in nasopharyngeal epithelial cells. EBER expression could be detected at high level in dysplastic nasopharyngeal epithelium (9). It remains to be determined if EBERs may inactivate PKR activation in premalignant nasopharyngeal epithelial cells and inhibit apoptosis in cells during EBV infection. EBER-1 expression in rodent fibroblasts slightly increased their ability to form colonies in soft agar (142). However, clones containing a high concentration of EBER-1 were not invariably tumorigenic in nude mice. A recent study showed that EBERs may induce autocrine growth of EBV-positive gastric carcinoma by induction of insulin-like growth factor-1 (IGF-1) (143). The functional role of EBER in EBV-positive NPC remains to be explored.

PROPOSED SEQUENCE OF EVENTS FOR NPC DEVELOPMENT

In summary, a sequence of events involved in the development of NPC is proposed (Fig. 2). The development of NPC is the result of a unique interaction of environmental factors, predisposing genetic factors, and latent EBV infection, which drive the progression of a clonal cell population to evolve from normal nasopharyngeal epithelium, eventually progressing to preinvasive lesions and invasive cancer. Some of the genetic and epigenetic changes involved in this transformation process have been identified. Early genetic events include allelic loss on chromosomes 3p and 9p, involving the inactivation of *RASSF1A* and *p16/INK4* on the respective chromosomes, facilitating the expansion of multiple clonal cell populations in nasopharyngeal epithelium. EBV infection in these genetically altered nasopharyngeal epithelial cell clones appears to be critical in NPC development. EBV entry into nasopharyngeal epithelial cells may be achieved through pIgA-mediated mechanisms or direct cell-to-cell contact with infiltrating EBV-bearing lymphocytes in nasopharyngeal epithelium. Alteration of cellular environments in premalignant nasopharyngeal epithelial cells, including STAT3 activation, may support the establishment of latent infection of EBV. Expression of the latent gene products of EBV drives the clonal expansion of EBV-infected nasopharyngeal cells. Activation of telomerase protects the telomere ends of continuously dividing cells and sustains the clonal expansion of EBV-infected precancerous clones. Accumulation of further genetic and epigenetic alterations

Nasopharyngeal Carcinoma Tumorigenesis

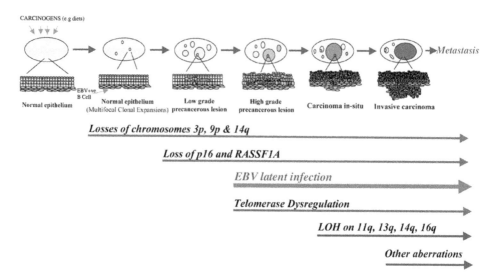

Figure 2 Proposed sequence of events in the development of NPC. *Abbreviations*: EBV, Epstein–Barr virus; LOH, loss of heterozygosity; NPC, nasopharyngeal carcinoma.

eventually converts these EBV-infected premalignant epithelial cells into invasive cancer cells. These later genetic changes may involve deletion of 11q, 13q, 14q, and 16q, inactivation of the *TSLC1* and *ENDRB* genes, downregulation of E-cadherin, and other perturbations.

ACKNOWLEDGMENTS

The authors acknowledge the funding support received from the Research Grant Council, Hong Kong (Grant numbers: HKU7356/02M, HKU7475/03M, HKU7457/04), Joint National Science Foundation, PRC and Research Grant Council, Hong Kong (NSF/HKU 728/04), Kadoorie Charitable Foundations and the CRCG grant from the University of Hong Kong

REFERENCES

1. Chan CW, Chiang AK, Chan KH, Lau AS. Epstein–Barr virus-associated infectious mononucleosis in Chinese children. Pediatr Infect Dis J 2003; 22:974–978.
2. De Souza YG, Greenspan D, Felton JR, Hartzog GA, Hammer M, Greenspan JS. Localization of Epstein–Barr virus DNA in the epithelial cells of oral hairy leukoplakia by in situ hybridization of tissue sections. N Engl J Med 1989; 320:1559–1560.
3. Young LS, Murray PG. Epstein–Barr virus and oncogenesis: from latent genes to tumours. Oncogene 2003; 22:5108–5121.
4. Wolf H, Zur HH, Becker V. EB viral genomes in epithelial nasopharyngeal carcinoma cells. Nat New Biol 1973; 244:245–247.
5. Spano JP, Busson P, Atlan D, et al. Nasopharyngeal carcinomas: an update. Eur J Cancer 2003; 39:2121–2135.

6. Pathmanathan R, Prasad U, Chandrika G, Sadler R, Flynn K, Raab-Traub N. Undifferentiated, nonkeratinizing, and squamous cell carcinoma of the nasopharynx. Variants of Epstein–Barr virus-infected neoplasia. Am J Pathol 1995; 146:1355–1367.

7. Chan AS, To KF, Lo KW, et al. Frequent chromosome 9p losses in histologically normal nasopharyngeal epithelia from southern Chinese. Int J Cancer 2002; 102:300–303.

8. Chan AS, To KF, Lo KW, et al. High frequency of chromosome 3p deletion in histologically normal nasopharyngeal epithelia from southern Chinese. Cancer Res 2000; 60:5365–5370.

9. Pathmanathan R, Prasad U, Sadler R, Flynn K, Raab-Traub N. Clonal proliferations of cells infected with Epstein–Barr virus in preinvasive lesions related to nasopharyngeal carcinoma. N Engl J Med 1995; 333:693–698.

10. Bonnet M, Guinebretiere JM, Kremmer E, et al. Detection of Epstein–Barr virus in invasive breast cancers. J Natl Cancer Inst 1999; 91:1376–1381.

11. Sugawara Y, Mizugaki Y, Uchida T, et al. Detection of Epstein–Barr virus (EBV) in hepatocellular carcinoma tissue: a novel EBV latency characterized by the absence of EBV-encoded small RNA expression. Virology 1999; 256:196–202.

12. Herrmann K, Niedobitek G. Epstein–Barr virus-associated carcinomas: facts and fiction. J Pathol 2003; 199:140–145.

13. Junying J, Herrmann K, Davies G, et al. Absence of Epstein–Barr virus DNA in the tumor cells of European hepatocellular carcinoma. Virology 2003; 306:236–243.

14. Kieff E, Rickinson AB. Epstein–Barr virus. In: Knipe DM, Howley PM, eds. Field's Virology. Philadelphia: Lippincott/Williams & Wilkins, 2001:2575–2627.

15. Decaussin G, Sbih-Lammali F, Turenne-Tessier M, Bouguermouh A, Ooka T. Expression of BARF1 gene encoded by Epstein–Barr virus in nasopharyngeal carcinoma biopsies. Cancer Res 2000; 60:5584–5588.

16. Wei MX, Turenne-Tessier M, Decaussin G, Benet G, Ooka T. Establishment of a monkey kidney epithelial cell line with the BARF1 open reading frame from Epstein–Barr virus. Oncogene 1997; 14:3073–3081.

17. Wei MX, Ooka T. A transforming function of the BARF1 gene encoded by Epstein–Barr virus. EMBO J 1989; 8:2897–2903.

18. Li H, Minarovits J. Host cell-dependent expression of latent Epstein–Barr virus genomes: regulation by DNA methylation. Adv Cancer Res 2003; 89:133–156.

19. Muirs CS, Waterhous J, Mack T. Cancer incidence in five continents. IARC Sci Publ 1987; 5(88):463–469.

20. Huang DP. Epidemiology of nasopharyngeal carcinoma. Ear Nose Throat J 1990; 69:222–225.

21. Jeannel D, Ghnassia M, Hubert A, et al. Increased risk of nasopharyngeal carcinoma among males of French origin born in Maghreb (north Africa). Int J Cancer 1993; 54:536–539.

22. Hildesheim A, Apple RJ, Chen CJ, et al. Association of HLA class I and II alleles and extended haplotypes with nasopharyngeal carcinoma in Taiwan. J Natl Cancer Inst 2002; 94:1780–1789.

23. Kirk RL, Blake NM, Serjeantson S, Simons MJ, Chan SH. Genetic components in susceptibility to nasopharyngeal carcinoma. IARC Sci Publ 1978:283–297.

24. Lu SJ, Day NE, Degos L, et al. Linkage of a nasopharyngeal carcinoma susceptibility locus to the HLA region. Nature 1990; 346:470–471.

25. Ho JH, Huang DP, Fong YY. Salted fish and nasopharyngeal carcinoma in southern Chinese. Lancet 1978; 2:626.

26. Yu MC, Henderson BE. Intake of Cantonese-style salted fish as a cause of nasopharyngeal carcinoma. IARC Sci Publ 1987:547–549.

27. Hildesheim A, Chen CJ, Caporaso NE, et al. Cytochrome P4502E1 genetic polymorphisms and risk of nasopharyngeal carcinoma: results from a case-control study conducted in Taiwan. Cancer Epidemiol Biomarkers Prev 1995; 4:607–610.

28. Lee AW, Foo W, Mang O, et al. Changing epidemiology of nasopharyngeal carcinoma in Hong Kong over a 20-year period (1980–99): an encouraging reduction in both incidence and mortality. Int J Cancer 2003; 103:680–685.
29. Nazar-Stewart V, Vaughan TL, Burt RD, Chen C, Berwick M, Swanson GM. Glutathione S-transferase M1 and susceptibility to nasopharyngeal carcinoma. Cancer Epidemiol Biomarkers Prev 1999; 8:547–551.
30. Feng BJ, Huang W, Shugart YY, et al. Genome-wide scan for familial nasopharyngeal carcinoma reveals evidence of linkage to chromosome 4. Nat Genet 2002; 31:395–399.
31. Klein G, Geering G, Old LJ, Henle G, Henle W, Clifford P. Comparison of the anti-EBV titer and the EBV-associated membrane reactive and precipitating antibody levels in the sera of Burkitt lymphoma and nasopharyngeal carcinoma patients and controls. Int J Cancer 1970; 5:185–194.
32. Zur HH, Schulte-Holthausen H, Klein G, et al. EBV DNA in biopsies of Burkitt tumours and anaplastic carcinomas of the nasopharynx. Nature 1970; 228:1056–1058.
33. Henle G, Henle W. Epstein–Barr virus-specific IgA serum antibodies as an outstanding feature of nasopharyngeal carcinoma. Int J Cancer 1976; 17:1–7.
34. Klein G. The biology and serology of Epstein–Barr virus (EBV) infections. Bull Cancer 1976; 63:399–410.
35. Joab I, Nicolas JC, Schwaab G, et al. Detection of anti-Epstein–Barr-virus transactivator (ZEBRA) antibodies in sera from patients with nasopharyngeal carcinoma. Int J Cancer 1991; 48:647–649.
36. Dolcetti R, Menezes J. Epstein–Barr virus and undifferentiated nasopharyngeal carcinoma: new immunobiological and molecular insights on a long-standing etiopathogenic association. Adv Cancer Res 2003; 87:127–157.
37. Chan KC, Lo YM. Circulating EBV DNA as a tumor marker for nasopharyngeal carcinoma. Semin Cancer Biol 2002; 12:489–496.
38. Lo YM, Chan LY, Lo KW, et al. Quantitative analysis of cell-free Epstein–Barr virus DNA in plasma of patients with nasopharyngeal carcinoma. Cancer Res 1999; 59:1188–1191.
39. Lo YM, Chan LY, Chan AT, et al. Quantitative and temporal correlation between circulating cell-free Epstein–Barr virus DNA and tumor recurrence in nasopharyngeal carcinoma. Cancer Res 1999; 59:5452–5455.
40. Sheu LF, Chen A, Meng CL, Ho KC, Lin FG, Lee WH. Analysis of bcl-2 expression in normal, inflamed, dysplastic nasopharyngeal epithelia, and nasopharyngeal carcinoma: association with p53 expression. Hum Pathol 1997; 28:556–562.
41. Chang JT, Liao CT, Jung SM, Wang TC, See LC, Cheng AJ. Telomerase activity is frequently found in metaplastic and malignant human nasopharyngeal tissues. Br J Cancer 2000; 82:1946–1951.
42. Lo KW, Teo PM, Hui AB, et al. High resolution allelotype of microdissected primary nasopharyngeal carcinoma. Cancer Res 2000; 60:3348–3353.
43. Hui AB, Lo KW, Leung SF, et al. Detection of recurrent chromosomal gains and losses in primary nasopharyngeal carcinoma by comparative genomic hybridisation. Int J Cancer 1999; 82:498–503.
44. Chen YJ, Ko JY, Chen PJ, et al. Chromosomal aberrations in nasopharyngeal carcinoma analyzed by comparative genomic hybridization. Genes Chromosomes Cancer 1999; 25:169–175.
45. Fang Y, Guan X, Guo Y, et al. Analysis of genetic alterations in primary nasopharyngeal carcinoma by comparative genomic hybridization. Genes Chromosomes Cancer 2001; 30:254–260.
46. Hui AB, Lo KW, Teo PM, To KF, Huang DP. Genome wide detection of oncogene amplifications in nasopharyngeal carcinoma by array based comparative genomic hybridization. Int J Oncol 2002; 20:467–473.
47. Guo X, Lui WO, Qian CN, et al. Identifying cancer-related genes in nasopharyngeal carcinoma cell lines using DNA and mRNA expression profiling analyses. Int J Oncol 2002; 21:1197–1204.

48. Cheng Y, Ko JM, Lung HL, Lo PH, Stanbridge EJ, Lung ML. Monochromosome transfer provides functional evidence for growth-suppressive genes on chromosome 14 in nasopharyngeal carcinoma. Genes Chromosomes Cancer 2003; 37:359–368.
49. Cheng Y, Chakrabarti R, Garcia-Barcelo M, et al. Mapping of nasopharyngeal carcinoma tumor-suppressive activity to a 1.8-megabase region of chromosome band 11q13. Genes Chromosomes Cancer 2002; 34:97–103.
50. Cheng Y, Stanbridge EJ, Kong H, Bengtsson U, Lerman MI, Lung ML. A functional investigation of tumor suppressor gene activities in a nasopharyngeal carcinoma cell line HONE1 using a monochromosome transfer approach. Genes Chromosomes Cancer 2000; 28:82–91.
51. Sun Y, Hegamyer G, Colburn NH. Nasopharyngeal carcinoma shows no detectable retinoblastoma susceptibility gene alterations. Oncogene 1993; 8:791–795.
52. Spruck CH III, Tsai YC, Huang DP, et al. Absence of p53 gene mutations in primary nasopharyngeal carcinomas. Cancer Res 1992; 52:4787–4790.
53. Lo KW, Huang DP, Lau KM. p16 gene alterations in nasopharyngeal carcinoma. Cancer Res 1995; 55:2039–2043.
54. Lo KW, Cheung ST, Leung SF, et al. Hypermethylation of the p16 gene in nasopharyngeal carcinoma. Cancer Res 1996; 56:2721–2725.
55. Wang GL, Lo KW, Tsang KS, et al. Inhibiting tumorigenic potential by restoration of p16 in nasopharyngeal carcinoma. Br J Cancer 1999; 81:1122–1126.
56. Kwong J, Lo KW, To KF, Teo PM, Johnson PJ, Huang DP. Promoter hypermethylation of multiple genes in nasopharyngeal carcinoma. Clin Cancer Res 2002; 8:131–137.
57. Huang DP, Lo KW, van Hasselt CA, et al. A region of homozygous deletion on chromosome 9p21-22 in primary nasopharyngeal carcinoma. Cancer Res 1994; 54: 4003–4006.
58. Macdiarmid J, Stevenson D, Campbell DH, Wilson JB. The latent membrane protein 1 of Epstein–Barr virus and loss of the INK4a locus: paradoxes resolve to cooperation in carcinogenesis in vivo. Carcinogenesis 2003; 24:1209–1218.
59. Crook T, Nicholls JM, Brooks L, O'Nions J, Allday MJ. High level expression of deltaN-p63: a mechanism for the inactivation of p53 in undifferentiated nasopharyngeal carcinoma (NPC)? Oncogene 2000; 19:3439–3444.
60. Lo KW, Kwong J, Hui AB, et al. High frequency of promoter hypermethylation of RASSF1A in nasopharyngeal carcinoma. Cancer Res 2001; 61:3877–3881.
61. Chow LS, Lo KW, Kwong J, et al. RASSF1A is a target tumor suppressor from 3p21.3 in nasopharyngeal carcinoma. Int J Cancer 2004; 109(6):839–847.
62. Dammann R, Li C, Yoon JH, Chin PL, Bates S, Pfeifer GP. Epigenetic inactivation of a RAS association domain family protein from the lung tumor suppressor locus 3p21.3. Nat Genet 2000; 25:315–319.
63. Liu L, Tommasi S, Lee DH, Dammann R, Pfeifer GP. Control of microtubule stability by the RASSF1A tumor suppressor. Oncogene 2003; 22:8125–8136.
64. Shivakumar L, Minna J, Sakamaki T, Pestell R, White MA. The RASSF1A tumor suppressor blocks cell cycle progression and inhibits cyclin D1 accumulation. Mol Cell Biol 2002; 22:4309–4318.
65. Claudio PP, Howard CM, Fu Y, et al. Mutations in the retinoblastoma-related gene RB2/p130 in primary nasopharyngeal carcinoma. Cancer Res 2000; 60:8–12.
66. Lu QL, Elia G, Lucas S, Thomas JA. Bcl-2 proto-oncogene expression in Epstein–Barr-virus-associated nasopharyngeal carcinoma. Int J Cancer 1993; 53:29–35.
67. Qian CN, Guo X, Cao B, et al. Met protein expression level correlates with survival in patients with late-stage nasopharyngeal carcinoma. Cancer Res 2002; 62:589–596.
68. Wang X, Jin DY, Wong YC, et al. Correlation of defective mitotic checkpoint with aberrantly reduced expression of MAD2 protein in nasopharyngeal carcinoma cells. Carcinogenesis 2000; 21:2293–2297.
69. Baba Y, Tsukuda M, Mochimatsu I, et al. Reduced expression of p16 and p27 proteins in nasopharyngeal carcinoma. Cancer Detect Prev 2001; 25:414–419.

70. Lo KW, Tsang YS, Kwong J, To KF, Teo PM, Huang DP. Promoter hypermethylation of the EDNRB gene in nasopharyngeal carcinoma. Int J Cancer 2002; 98:651–655.

71. Chang HW, Chan A, Kwong DL, Wei WI, Sham JS, Yuen AP. Detection of hyper-methylated RIZ1 gene in primary tumor, mouth, and throat rinsing fluid, nasopharyn-geal swab, and peripheral blood of nasopharyngeal carcinoma patient. Clin Cancer Res 2003; 9:1033–1038.

72. Tsao SW, Liu Y, Wang X, et al. The association of E-cadherin expression and the methylation status of the E-cadherin gene in nasopharyngeal carcinoma cells. Eur J Cancer 2003; 39:524–531.

73. Hui AB, Lo KW, Kwong J, et al. Epigenetic inactivation of TSLC1 gene in nasophar-yngeal carcinoma. Mol Carcinog 2003; 38:170–178.

74. Wong TS, Kwong DL, Sham JS, et al. Promoter hypermethylation of high-in-normal 1 gene in primary nasopharyngeal carcinoma. Clin Cancer Res 2003; 9:3042–3046.

75. Liu XQ, Chen HK, Zhang XS, et al. Alterations of BLU, a candidate tumor suppressor gene on chromosome 3p21.3, in human nasopharyngeal carcinoma. Int J Cancer 2003; 106:60–65.

76. Faulkner GC, Krajewski AS, Crawford DH. The ins and outs of EBV infection. Trends Microbiol 2000; 8:185–189.

77. Faulkner GC, Burrows SR, Khanna R, Moss DJ, Bird AG, Crawford DH. X-Linked agammaglobulinemia patients are not infected with Epstein–Barr virus: implications for the biology of the virus. J Virol 1999; 73:1555–1564.

78. Ianelli CJ, DeLellis R, Thorley-Lawson DA. CD48 binds to heparan sulfate on the sur-face of epithelial cells. J Biol Chem 1998; 273:23,367–23,375.

79. Greenspan JS, Greenspan D, Lennette ET, et al. Replication of Epstein-Barr virus within the epithelial cells of oral "hairy" leukoplakia, an AIDS-associated lesion. N Engl J Med 1985; 313:1564–1571.

80. Gratama JW, Oosterveer MA, Zwaan FE, Lepoutre J, Klein G, Ernberg I. Eradication of Epstein–Barr virus by allogeneic bone marrow transplantation: implications for sites of viral latency. Proc Natl Acad Sci USA 1988; 85:8693–8696.

81. Hutt-Fletcher LM, Lake CM. Two Epstein–Barr virus glycoprotein complexes. Curr Top Microbiol Immunol 2001; 258:51–64.

82. Borza CM, Hutt-Fletcher LM. Alternate replication in B-cells and epithelial cells switches tropism of Epstein–Barr virus. Nat Med 2002; 8:594–599.

83. Tao Q, Srivastava G, Chan AC, Chung LP, Loke SL, Ho FC. Evidence for lytic infec-tion by Epstein–Barr virus in mucosal lymphocytes instead of nasopharyngeal epithelial cells in normal individuals. J Med Virol 1995; 45:71–77.

84. Sixbey JW, Yao QY. Immunoglobulin A-induced shift of Epstein–Barr virus tissue tropism. Science 1992; 255:1578–1580.

85. Xu J, Ahmad A, Blagdon M, et al. The Epstein–Barr virus (EBV) major envelope glycoprotein gp350/220-specific antibody reactivities in the sera of patients with differ-ent EBV-associated diseases. Int J Cancer 1998; 79:481–486.

86. Lin CT, Kao HJ, Lin JL, Chan WY, Wu HC, Liang ST. Response of nasopharyngeal carcinoma cells to Epstein–Barr virus infection in vitro. Lab Invest 2000; 80:1149–1160.

87. Lin CT, Chan WY, Chen W, et al. Characterization of seven newly established naso-pharyngeal carcinoma cell lines. Lab Invest 1993; 68:716–727.

88. Lin CT, Wong CI, Chan WY, et al. Establishment and characterization of two naso-pharyngeal carcinoma cell lines. Lab Invest 1990; 62:713–724.

89. Cheung ST, Leung SF, Lo KW, et al. Specific latent membrane protein 1 gene sequences in type 1 and type 2 Epstein–Barr virus from nasopharyngeal carcinoma in Hong Kong. Int J Cancer 1998; 76:399–406.

90. Huang DP, Ho JH, Chan WK, Lau WH, Lui M. Cytogenetics of undifferentiated nasopharyngeal carcinoma xenografts from southern Chinese. Int J Cancer 1989; 43:936–939.

91. Teramoto N, Maeda A, Kobayashi K, et al. Epstein–Barr virus infection to Epstein–Barr virus-negative nasopharyngeal carcinoma cell line TW03 enhances its tumorigenicity. Lab Invest 2000; 80:303–312.

92. Chang Y, Tung CH, Huang YT, Lu J, Chen JY, Tsai CH. Requirement for cell-to-cell contact in Epstein–Barr virus infection of nasopharyngeal carcinoma cells and keratinocytes. J Virol 1999; 73:8857–8866.

93. Gan YJ, Chodosh J, Morgan A, Sixbey JW. Epithelial cell polarization is a determinant in the infectious outcome of immunoglobulin A-mediated entry by Epstein–Barr virus. J Virol 1997; 71:519–526.

94. Kisseleva T, Bhattacharya S, Braunstein J, Schindler CW. Signaling through the JAK/STAT pathway, recent advances and future challenges. Gene 2002; 285:1–24.

95. Chen H, Lee JM, Wang Y, Huang DP, Ambinder RF, Hayward SD. The Epstein–Barr virus latency BamHI-Q promoter is positively regulated by STATs and Zta interference with JAK/STAT activation leads to loss of BamHI-Q promoter activity. Proc Natl Acad Sci USA 1999; 96:9339–9344.

96. Chen H, Hutt-Fletcher L, Cao L, Hayward SD. A positive autoregulatory loop of LMP1 expression and STAT activation in epithelial cells latently infected with Epstein–Barr virus. J Virol 2003; 77:4139–4148.

97. Hsiao JR, Jin YT, Tsai ST, Shiau AL, Wu CL, Su WC. Constitutive activation of STAT3 and STAT5 is present in the majority of nasopharyngeal carcinoma and correlates with better prognosis. Br J Cancer 2003; 89:344–349.

98. Brown HJ, Song MJ, Deng H, Wu TT, Cheng G, Sun R. NF-kappaB inhibits gamma-herpesvirus lytic replication. J Virol 2003; 77:8532–8540.

99. Li QX, Young LS, Niedobitek G, et al. Epstein–Barr virus infection and replication in a human epithelial cell system. Nature 1992; 356:347–350.

100. Knox PG, Li QX, Rickinson AB, Young LS. In vitro production of stable Epstein–Barr virus-positive epithelial cell clones which resemble the virus: cell interaction observed in nasopharyngeal carcinoma. Virology 1996; 215:40–50.

101. Imai S, Nishikawa J, Takada K. Cell-to-cell contact as an efficient mode of Epstein–Barr virus infection of diverse human epithelial cells. J Virol 1998; 72:4371–4378.

102. Huang DP, Ho JH, Poon YF, et al. Establishment of a cell line (NPC/HK1) from a differentiated squamous carcinoma of the nasopharynx. Int J Cancer 1980; 26:127–132.

103. Tsao SW, Wang X, Liu Y, et al. Establishment of two immortalized nasopharyngeal epithelial cell lines using SV40 large T and HPV16E6/E7 viral oncogenes. Biochim Biophys Acta 2002; 1590:150–158.

104. Danve C, Decaussin G, Busson P, Ooka T. Growth transformation of primary epithelial cells with a NPC-derived Epstein–Barr virus strain. Virology 2001; 288:223–235.

105. Tajima M, Komuro M, Okinaga K. Establishment of Epstein–Barr virus-positive human gastric epithelial cell lines. Jpn J Cancer Res 1998; 89(3):262–268.

106. Takasaka N, Tajima M, Okinaga K, et al. Productive infection of Epstein–Barr virus (EBV) in EBV-genome-positive epithelial cell lines (GT38 and GT39) derived from gastric tissues. Virology 1998; 247(2):152–159.

107. Nishikawa J, Imai S, Oda T, Kojima T, Okita K, Takada K. Epstein–Barr virus promotes epithelial cell growth in the absence of EBNA2 and LMP1 expression. J Virol 1999; 73(2):1286–1292.

108. Tsao SW, Tramoutanis G, Dawson CW, Lo AK, Huang DP. The significance of LMP1 expression in nasopharyngeal carcinoma. Semin Cancer Biol 2002; 12:473–487.

109. Wang D, Liebowitz D, Kieff E. An EBV membrane protein expressed in immortalized lymphocytes transforms established rodent cells. Cell 1985; 43:831–840.

110. Dawson CW, Rickinson AB, Young LS. Epstein–Barr virus latent membrane protein inhibits human epithelial cell differentiation. Nature 1990; 344:777–780.

111. Lo AK, Liu Y, Wang XH, et al. Alterations of biologic properties and gene expression in nasopharyngeal epithelial cells by the Epstein–Barr virus-encoded latent membrane protein 1. Lab Invest 2003; 83:697–709.

112. Eliopoulos AG, Young LS. LMP1 structure and signal transduction. Semin Cancer Biol 2001; 11:435–444.

113. Mosialos G, Birkenbach M, Yalamanchili R, VanArsdale T, Ware C, Kieff E. The Epstein–Barr virus transforming protein LMP1 engages signaling proteins for the tumor necrosis factor receptor family. Cell 1995; 80:389–399.

114. Dawson CW, Tramountanis G, Eliopoulos AG, Young LS. Epstein–Barr virus latent membrane protein 1 (LMP1) activates the phosphatidylinositol 3-kinase/Akt pathway to promote cell survival and induce actin filament remodeling. J Biol Chem 2003; 278:3694–3704.

115. Mosialos G. Cytokine signaling and Epstein–Barr virus-mediated cell transformation. Cytokine Growth Factor Rev 2001; 12:259–270.

116. Jenkins PJ, Farrell PJ. Are particular Epstein–Barr virus strains linked to disease? Semin Cancer Biol 1996; 7:209–215.

117. Sung NS, Edwards RH, Seillier-Moiseiwitsch F, Perkins AG, Zeng Y, Raab-Traub N. Epstein–Barr virus strain variation in nasopharyngeal carcinoma from the endemic and non-endemic regions of China. Int J Cancer 1998; 76:207–215.

118. Hu LF, Chen F, Zheng X, et al. Clonability and tumorigenicity of human epithelial cells expressing the EBV encoded membrane protein LMP1. Oncogene 1993; 8:1575–1583.

119. Blake SM, Eliopoulos AG, Dawson CW, Young LS. The transmembrane domains of the EBV-encoded latent membrane protein 1 (LMP1) variant CAO regulate enhanced signalling activity. Virology 2001; 282:278–287.

120. Lo AKF, Huang DP, Lo KW, Pang JC, Li HM, Tsao SW. Phenotypic alterations induced by the Hong Kong-prevalent Epstein–Barr virus-encoded LMP1 variant (2117-LMP1) in nasopharyngeal epithelial cells. Int J Cancer 2004; 109(6):919–925.

121. Edwards RH, Seillier-Moiseiwitsch F, Raab-Traub N. Signature amino acid changes in latent membrane protein 1 distinguish Epstein–Barr virus strains. Virology 1999; 261:79–95.

122. Dawson CW, Eliopoulos AG, Blake SM, Barker R, Young LS. Identification of functional differences between prototype Epstein–Barr virus-encoded LMP1 and a nasopharyngeal carcinoma-derived LMP1 in human epithelial cells. Virology 2000; 272:204–217.

123. Johnson RJ, Stack M, Hazlewood SA, et al. The 30-base-pair deletion in Chinese variants of the Epstein–Barr virus LMP1 gene is not the major effector of functional differences between variant LMP1 genes in human lymphocytes. J Virol 1998; 72:4038–4048.

124. Lon gn ecker R. Epstein–Barr virus latency: LMP2, a regulator or means for Epstein–Barr virus persistence? Adv Cancer Res 2000; 79:175–200.

125. Miller CL, Lee JH, Kieff E, Longnecker R. An integral membrane protein (LMP2) blocks reactivation of Epstein–Barr virus from latency following surface immunoglobulin crosslinking. Proc Natl Acad Sci USA 1994; 91:772–776.

126. Caldwell RG, Wilson JB, Anderson SJ, Longnecker R. Epstein–Barr virus LMP2A drives B cell development and survival in the absence of normal B-cell receptor signals. Immunity 1998; 9:405–411.

127. Dawson CW, George JH, Blake SM, Longnecker R, Young LS. The Epstein–Barr virus encoded latent membrane protein 2A augments signaling from latent membrane protein 1. Virology 2001; 289:192–207.

128. Scholle F, Bendt KM, Raab-Traub N. Epstein–Barr virus LMP2A transforms epithelial cells, inhibits cell differentiation, and activates Akt. J Virol 2000; 74:10,681–10,689.

129. Strockbine LD, Cohen JI, Farrah T, et al. The Epstein–Barr virus BARF1 gene encodes a novel, soluble colony-stimulating factor-1 receptor. J Virol 1998; 72:4015–4021.

130. Sheng W, Decaussin G, Ligout A, Takada K, Ooka T. Malignant transformation of Epstein–Barr virus-negative Akata cells by introduction of the BARF1 gene carried by Epstein–Barr virus. J Virol 2003; 77:3859–3865.

131. Zur HA, Brink AA, Craanen ME, Middeldorp JM, Meijer CJ, van den Brule AJ. Unique transcription pattern of Epstein–Barr virus (EBV) in EBV-carrying gastric adenocarcinomas: expression of the transforming BARF1 gene. Cancer Res 2000; 60:2745–2748.

132. Brink AA, Vervoort MB, Middeldorp JM, Meijer CJ, van den Brule AJ. Nucleic acid sequence-based amplification, a new method for analysis of spliced and unspliced

Epstein–Barr virus latent transcripts, and its comparison with reverse transcriptase PCR. J Clin Microbiol 1998; 36:3164–3169.

133. Hayes DP, Brink AA, Vervoort MB, Middeldorp JM, Meijer CJ, van den Brule AJ. Expression of Epstein–Barr virus (EBV) transcripts encoding homologues to important human proteins in diverse EBV associated diseases. Mol Pathol 1999; 52:97–103.

134. Gao Y, Lu YJ, Xue SA, Chen H, Wedderburn N, Griffin BE. Hypothesis: a novel route for immortalization of epithelial cells by Epstein–Barr virus. Oncogene 2002; 21:825–835.

135. Nanbo A, Takada K. The role of Epstein–Barr virus-encoded small RNAs (EBERs) in oncogenesis. Rev Med Virol 2002; 12:321–326.

136. Lerner MR, Andrews NC, Miller G, Steitz JA. Two small RNAs encoded by Epstein–Barr virus and complexed with protein are precipitated by antibodies from patients with systemic lupus erythematosus. Proc Natl Acad Sci USA 1981; 78:805–809.

137. Toczyski DP, Steitz JA. EAP: a highly conserved cellular protein associated with Epstein–Barr virus small RNAs (EBERs). EMBO J 1991; 10:459–466.

138. Clarke PA, Schwemmle M, Schickinger J, Hilse K, Clemens MJ. Binding of Epstein–Barr virus small RNA EBER-1 to the double-stranded RNA-activated protein kinase DAI. Nucleic Acids Res 1991; 19:243–248.

139. Williams BR. PKR: a sentinel kinase for cellular stress. Oncogene 1999; 18:6112–6120.

140. Elia A, Laing KG, Schofield A, Tilleray VJ, Clemens MJ. Regulation of the double-stranded RNA-dependent protein kinase PKR by RNAs encoded by a repeated sequence in the Epstein–Barr virus genome. Nucleic Acids Res 1996; 24:4471–4478.

141. Nanbo A, Inoue K, Adachi-Takasawa K, Takada K. Epstein–Barr virus RNA confers resistance to interferon-alpha-induced apoptosis in Burkitt's lymphoma. EMBO J 2002; 21:954–965.

142. Laing KG, Elia A, Jeffrey I, et al. In vivo effects of the Epstein–Barr virus small RNA EBER-1 on protein synthesis and cell growth regulation. Virology 2002; 297:253–269.

143. Iwakiri D, Eizuru Y, Tokunaga M, Takada K. Autocrine growth of Epstein–Barr virus-positive gastric carcinoma cells mediated by an Epstein–Barr virus-encoded small RNA. Cancer Res 2003; 63:7062–7067.

15
Leiomyosarcoma

Hal B. Jenson
Baystate Health, Springfield, and Tufts University School of Medicine, Boston, Massachusetts, U.S.A.

INTRODUCTION

The emergence of the epidemic of the acquired immunodeficiency syndrome (AIDS) resulting from infection with human immunodeficiency virus (HIV) brought the consequences of many uncommon or previously unrecognized secondary infections to the forefront of clinical infectious diseases. This included an expansion of the recognized role of Epstein–Barr virus (EBV) in human disease (see Chapter 9). In addition to its role in oral hairy leukoplakia and lymphoid interstitial pneumonitis, EBV was linked with an increased risk of lymphoma, especially of the central nervous system.

The experience of AIDS patients with EBV infection also led to the most recent identification of an EBV-associated human cancer, and simultaneously led to an extraordinary new finding about the biology of EBV. In the mid-1990s, investigators identified the causal association of EBV with leiomyosarcomas, or smooth muscle tumors, and the role of host immune status as the primary determinant for this rare cancer. These findings also showed the ability of EBV to infect smooth muscle cells, expanding the range of cell types that have been shown to be infected with EBV.

Immunocompromised persons, whether the underlying cause of immunocompromise is congenital or acquired, have an approximately 10- to 100-fold higher incidence of malignancies than immunocompetent persons, with higher frequency of unusual tumor types (1). Because of their sentinel role, some cancers, including the rare Kaposi's sarcoma and the more common non-Hodgkin's lymphoma (HL) and cervical carcinoma, are included as AIDS-defining conditions (2). Several other types of cancers, including Hodgkin's disease, squamous cell carcinoma, testicular neoplasms (seminoma and nonseminoma), and, as recently demonstrated, leiomyosarcoma, are seen with increased frequency but are not AIDS defining.

Many of the cancers associated with immunosuppression are also associated with viral infections. These include non-HL, which is also associated with EBV; Kaposi's sarcoma, which is causally linked to Kaposi's sarcoma–associated herpesvirus (KSHV), also known as human herpesvirus type 8 (HHV8); hepatocellular carcinoma, which is linked to hepatitis B and C viruses; cervical cancer, which is linked to human papillomaviruses types 16 and 18; and squamous cell carcinoma of the skin, which is linked to human papillomaviruses types 5 and 8 (3,4). Leiomyosarcoma associated with EBV is the most recent addition to the list of tumors associated with immuno-suppression that are also linked to a specific viral etiology.

EPIDEMIOLOGY

Leiomyosarcomas are rare. They present in a wide spectrum of anatomic locations, and are reflected in a wide variety of clinical presentations. Despite the number of individual cases of leiomyosarcomas reported in the medical literature, the rarity and isolated occurrence has impeded the advancement in understanding their basic biology and pathogenesis.

The overall incidence of leiomyosarcomas in the general population is one to two cases per million (5). They occur most frequently in the uterus of adult women, and also in the gastrointestinal and hepatobiliary tracts of both sexes. Smooth muscle tumors have been reported in every organ and appendage, reflecting the ubiquitous distribution of smooth muscle in blood vessels. Clinical classification of leiomyosarcomas based on anatomic location (i.e., superficial soft tissue, deep soft tissue, and visceral) are arbitrary and have not been shown to provide prognostic significance.

Leiomyosarcomas account for approximately 2% to 9% of all soft tissue sarcomas in adults, and are among the more common sarcomas of adults (6–10). The peak incidence is from 40 to 50 years of age (11–13). There is no racial or sexual difference, except for the obvious limitation of uterine leiomyosarcoma to women (5,6,14). Leiomyosarcomas are rarely reported in children, accounting for only 2% of soft tissue sarcomas, which as a group are fifth in order of the most common types of tumors in children (15,16). The three largest series of smooth muscle tumors in children reported only 10 original cases each (16–18).

Epidemiology in Immunocompromised Persons

Before 1985, rare leiomyosarcomas were reported in immunocompromised persons, including renal transplant recipients (19,20) and patients who received gastric irradiation as therapy for peptic ulcer disease (21), and in association with Alport's syndrome (22). From 1985 to 1990, five cases of leiomyosarcoma associated with HIV-1 infection, all of which occurred in children, were reported (23–25). Eleven additional cases of leiomyomas and leiomyosarcomas in HIV-1–infected persons were subsequently reported by others (26–34), including nine children (26,27,29–34), one adolescent (28), and one adult (32) from 1991 through 1994. [One case reported in the series by Chadwick et al. (25) was also reported separately (35,36); the imaging studies of the case reported by Sabatino et al. (26) were reported by Balsam and Segal (37)].

During this period, leiomyoma and leiomyosarcoma were also being reported with increasing frequency in patients following kidney or liver organ transplantation (1,38,39). Similar to leiomyosarcomas associated with HIV-1 infection, there was a surprisingly high proportion of cases in children, despite the fewer number of organ transplants in children. In a review of 8724 malignancies that developed in 8191 organ allograft recipients, 5 of 15 (33%) leiomyosarcomas that were reported occurred in children (1). In all the 15 transplant recipients with leiomyosarcoma, the allograft or the surrounding tissues was the major site of tumor involvement.

PATHOGENESIS

Histopathology

Tumors of smooth muscle may be benign, as hamartomas and leiomyomas, or malignant, as leiomyosarcomas (40,41). Hamartomas are the disorganized over-growth of mature cells. Leiomyomas are well-differentiated neoplasms of histologically normal cells without cytologic atypia. They are composed primarily of smooth muscle cells and occasionally of some myofibroblasts, fibroblasts, and incompletely differentiated mesenchymal cells. Leiomyomas are well circumscribed and have little or no predilection for malignant transformation. Soft tissue leiomyomas typically occur in women in the pelvic retroperitoneum, and bear histologic similarity to uterine leiomyomas, and they occur in both sexes in deep somatic soft tissues (41).

Smooth muscle cells have an elongated, fusiform, or spindle-shaped appearance with centrally placed nuclei and a fibrillary, deeply eosinophilic cytoplasm. Myofilaments are well developed throughout the cytoplasm, with continuous basal lamina, which differentiate smooth muscle cells from myofibroblasts, which have an appearance between smooth muscle cells and fibroblasts. Smooth muscle tumors are sometimes identified as spindle-cell tumors based on the characteristic cell morphology. Individual cells align in bundles or fascicles that intersect at right angles or align in palisades (Fig. 1, panel B). Smooth muscle cells, including leiomyomas and leiomyosarcomas, express characteristic cell markers. The smooth muscle cell form of calponin is restricted to smooth muscle cells in the adult but is also expressed in the early cardiac tube in embryos (42). Smooth muscle α-actin is also detected in skeletal and, to a lesser degree, in cardiac muscles (43). Smooth muscle cells also express desmin. They do not express skeletal muscle myosin heavy chain—a skeletal muscle marker.

The histopathologic identification of smooth muscle is straightforward based on the typical cellular morphology, with confirmation by identification of smooth muscle elements by immunohistochemical staining. However, the distinction between leiomyoma and leiomyosarcoma, and, occasionally, among other spindle-cell tumors, can be obscure (6,40). Poorly differentiated smooth muscle tumors may be difficult to distinguish from fibrosarcoma, neurogenic sarcoma, malignant fibrous histiocytoma, or undifferentiated sarcoma. Definitive histopathologic criteria defining benign (leiomyoma) and malignant (leiomyosarcoma) smooth muscle tumors are not well established. Increased tumor size, poorly differentiated cellularity, cytologic atypia, infiltration, necrosis, hemorrhage, and multifocal lesions roughly correlate with smooth muscle cell malignancy. The mitotic index has been frequently used to define leiomyosarcoma, but this has not been standardized. Proposed criteria include a mitotic index of ≥ 5 mitoses per 10 high-power microscope fields for uterine tumors (44), ≥ 2 mitoses per 50 high-power fields for gastrointestinal tract tumors (14,45), and ≥ 5 mitoses per 50 high-power fields for pulmonary tumors (46). However, malignant behavior of smooth muscle tumors does not correlate well even with the degree of mitotic activity (14,47,48). Some smooth muscle tumors with a benign histology, and even devoid of mitoses, have been reported to behave as malignant leiomyosarcoma (14,48,49).

The uncertainty between benign and malignant smooth muscle tumors has resulted in many reported cases of "smooth muscle tumors" that are not further classified. Capricious and unpredictable biological and clinical behavior characterize leiomyosarcomas. Metastatic spread may be the only certain indicator of malignancy.

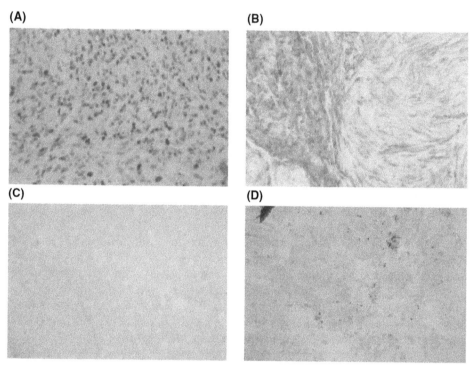

Figure 1 (*See color insert.*) Photomicrographs of tumor specimens studied to detect EBV. Panel (**A**) (×630) shows in situ hybridization of a leiomyosarcoma specimen from an HIV-positive patient (Patient 1). When tested with the EBER probe, the sample shows bright-red nuclear staining, indicating prominent hybridization of the biotinylated probe. Panel (**B**) (×250) shows immunoperoxidase staining of the tissue from Patient 1 with antibody to the EBV receptor (CD21). The golden-brown precipitate observed on staining with DAB peroxidase reveals masses of tumor cells that bound the CD21 antibody. Under identical conditions, a pan-B cell antibody, CD20, did not react with the tissue. Panel (**C**) (×630) shows in situ hybridization of a leiomyoma specimen from an HIV-negative patient (Patient 10). When this sample was tested with the EBER probe as in Panel A, there was no detectable hybridization of the probe. Panel (**D**) (×250) shows immunoperoxidase staining of the tissue from Patient 10 with antibody to CD21. There are moderate numbers of golden-brown precipitates in the muscle fibers on staining with DAB peroxidase. *Abbreviations*: DAB, 3,3′-diaminobenzidine; EBV, Epstein–Barr virus; EBER, EBV-encoded ribonucleic acid; HIV, human immunodeficiency virus. *Source*: From Ref. 51.

Association of EBV with Leiomyosarcoma

The identification of EBV infection of smooth muscle cells of leiomyosarcoma was first reported in a single case of an adult with HIV-1 infection, by Prévot et al. (50) in 1994, and, in two subsequent series published together in early 1995, of six HIV-1–infected persons (51), and three organ transplant recipients (52). These initial reports have been substantiated by many additional reports of cases of EBV-associated leiomyosarcomas in immunocompromised persons, including 11 adults and six children with HIV-1 infection (49,53–64), and nine patients following organ transplants (65–72), including four children (65,69,71), one adolescent, and four adults (66–68,72,73). A peculiar aspect is the development of large cysts associated with hepatic leiomyosarcomas in the two adult patients following kidney transplant (66–68).

In addition to HIV-1 infection and posttransplant immunosuppression, other forms of immunosuppression also facilitate development of EBV-associated leiomyosarcoma. A leiomyosarcoma originally reported in 1976 (74), in a five-year-old boy, three years after remission of acute lymphocytic leukemia that was treated with chemotherapy and radiation, was subsequently tested and found to contain EBV (75). EBV-associated leiomyosarcomas have also been reported in a 14-year-old girl with common variable immunodeficiency syndrome (49,76) and in a 10-year-old girl with ataxia-telangiectasia (77).

One of the sentinel findings of EBV-associated leiomyosarcomas is that all of the smooth muscle cells harbor EBV (Fig. 1). Using in situ hybridization for EBV-encoded ribonucleic acid (EBER), reports consistently document the EBV EBER in all or greater than 90% of the smooth muscle cells of the tumor, but not in adjacent normal tissues. A series of seven smooth muscle cell tumors from four patients with AIDS near or at the time of tumor diagnosis by semiquantitative polymerase chain reaction (PCR) amplification, showed EBV levels from 170,442 to 659,668 EBV copies per 100,000 cells, with an average of 451,140 copies per 100,000 cells. If all cells are uniformly infected with EBV, as indicated by the uniform staining for EBER by in situ hybridization, this equates to an average of 4.5 EBV genome copies per cell (55), consistent with the amounts of EBV in lymphoblastoid cell lines, which characteristically have 10 or fewer episomes per cell (78). These results are also consistent with the semiquantitation of EBV reported in smooth muscle cell tumors from patients with organ transplant (52). There are no lymphocytic infiltrates in, or surrounding, leiomyosarcomas that might account for the high levels of EBV detected by PCR (59,79). The extraordinarily high copy numbers of EBV in the tumor cells, as determined by semiquantitative PCR, are consistent with and supportive of the in situ hybridization results for the presence of EBV in all tumor cells. High levels of cell-free EBV present in plasma of three patients tested (16,740, 12,440, and 3973 genome copies/mL) also support the hypothesis of high levels of EBV replication in immunosuppressed patients with EBV-associated leiomyosarcoma (57). The presence of HIV-1 has been tested by in situ hybridization and by semiquantitative PCR, and has not been found in the smooth muscle cells of HIV-1–associated leiomyosarcomas (30,51,57).

Leiomyosarcomas in one adult heart transplant recipient and three adult renal transplant recipients, and a laryngeal leiomyosarcoma (80), that have been studied for the presence of EBV have been reported as EBV-negative (80–83). One leiomyosarcoma in a child with HIV-1 infection was tested for EBV in 1992 and reported as being EBV-negative (30). The absence of centralized testing for EBV and adequate controls in all cases leaves open the possibility that these are false-negative results. Another leiomyosarcoma in a child with HIV-1 infection was reported after the association with EBV was identified, but the tumor was not tested for EBV infection (84).

The results of the EBV serologic testing are consistent with remote EBV infection in all patients with smooth muscle cell tumors that have been reported. There is not a characteristic serologic profile such as that often found in nasopharyngeal carcinoma and Burkitt lymphoma, which are also associated with EBV but which occur primarily in immunocompetent persons (85).

The growing number of these cases that consistently show uniform EBV infection of leiomyosarcoma cells provides clear evidence of the ability of EBV to infect smooth muscle cells. This recent discovery is a remarkable new finding. The contribution of EBV to the development of leiomyosarcomas appears to be limited to the milieu of immunodeficiency, which may be congenital (e.g., common variable immunodeficiency, ataxia-telangiectasia) or acquired (e.g., HIV-1 infection, immunosuppressive therapy following organ transplant). EBV has not been found in smooth muscle cells from healthy individuals, in leiomyomas, or in leiomyosarcomas in the absence of HIV-1 infection or other immunocompromising conditions (49,51,56,79,86). The absence of EBV in the leiomyosarcomas of immunocompetent persons, coupled with its consistent presence in leiomyosarcomas of immunocompromised persons lends support to the hypothesis that EBV has an etiologic role in the increased incidence of soft tissue tumors in immunocompromised persons but that other mechanisms of smooth muscle tumorigenicity exist.

Pathogenesis of EBV-Associated Leiomyosarcoma

The sequence of events in the transformation from normal smooth muscle cells to EBV-infected leiomyosarcomatous cells has been studied. A critical finding of evidence of EBV infection of the muscle cells prior to malignant transformation is the finding of EBV monoclonality of leiomyosarcomas (51,52,66), even in individuals with multiple tumor nodules, which are common in immunocompromised persons who develop leiomyosarcoma. In the tumors that have been tested, only monoclonal episomal EBV has been found, confirming that EBV infection precedes malignant transformation. Viral integration into the cell genome, which might account for malignant transformation, has not been found. The most striking case is that of a five-year-old female with two separate tumors taken at different times and from different sites, with each tumor demonstrating different EBV monoclonality, demonstrating that these two tumors developed independently (51). A 15-year-old male with multiple leiomyosarcomas following heart–lung transplant, was found to have pulmonary tumors of donor origin and hepatic tumors of host origin (70). A 24-year-old male had equimolar biclonality of EBV in a leiomyosarcoma, consistent with dual EBV infection of tumor cells or a uniformly mixed cell population derived from two independent EBV infection events (51). Either scenario is strong evidence of causal linkage of EBV to the tumor. It appears that the principal factor that predisposes to leiomyosarcoma—impaired host immunity—facilitates the simultaneous development of multiple primary tumors. The critical role of the immune system is underscored by a recent case report, which suggests that posttransplant EBV-associated leiomyosarcoma can be controlled by surgical intervention and reduction of immunosuppression (73).

The presence of EBV in both a leiomyoma and leiomyosarcoma occurring in an eight-year-old girl (51) suggests that EBV infects the smooth muscle cells before they undergo malignant transformation, and thus plays a pivotal role in the progression to malignancy. High levels of EBV, as shown in the leiomyoma by in situ hybridization and semiquantitative PCR, is supportive of such an scenario. Taken as a whole, the evidence of multiple discrete EBV cell infection events associated with the tumors of these patients demonstrates that EBV infection of smooth muscle cells and proliferation is probably not an infrequent occurrence under circumstances of impaired immunity.

The increased numbers of cases of leiomyosarcomas in children compared to adults is even more remarkable considering the much greater number of adults compared to children with HIV-1 infection or organ transplant. After non-HL, leiomyosarcoma is the second leading cancer in children with HIV-1 infection (87,88). Children may be more susceptible to developing EBV-associated tumors because primary EBV infection occurs in childhood (89–91). The host may be less well prepared to limit primary EBV infection and the contribution of EBV to malignant transformation than under the typical scenario that is present in adults, with development of impaired immunosurveillance in the setting of previously established but well-controlled, latent EBV infection.

EBV Receptor Studies in Leiomyosarcomas

The presence of the EBV receptor CD21 [also known as complement receptor 2 (CR2)], which is also the receptor for the C3d component of complement (92,93), on smooth muscle cells would appear to be a prerequisite for EBV infection of smooth muscle cells. The EBV receptor has been identified on a variety of nonlymphoid cells including smooth muscle cells, striated muscle cells, epithelial cells of the parotid gland and tonsil, skin, lung, esophagus, jejunum, colon, pancreas, kidney, and adrenal cortical cells and hepatocytes from healthy persons (57,94).

The EBV receptor has been found to be present at relatively higher levels on the cells of both leiomyomas and leiomyosarcomas of HIV-1–infected patients but at lower levels in tumors from HIV-1–uninfected patients (Fig. 1) (51,57). The CD21 receptor is detected best with biotin–streptavidin procedures using the OKB7 (95) monoclonal antibody, and is undetectable using the hepatitis B surface antigen antibody (HB5) (96) monoclonal antibody (97), which may account for reported differences in identification of the CD21 on smooth muscle cells (51,57,70). This also suggests that the CD21 antigen on smooth muscle cells (97) may not be identical to that found on epithelial cells or lymphocytes (98,99).

Alternatively, the presence of CD21 may not be required because the mechanism of EBV entry into different cell types may be by different routes (100,101). It is possible that the fusion of smooth muscle cells with EBV-infected lymphocytes could be the route of cell entry into nonlymphoid cells by EBV-induced formation of polykaryocytes of EBV-superinfected lymphoblastoid cells with cells devoid of EBV receptors (102).

The presence of EBV in the leiomyosarcomas of HIV-1–infected persons but not in those from immunocompetent persons suggests that the entry of EBV into muscle cells is directly or indirectly influenced by HIV-1 infection. In HIV-1–infected patients, EBV infection of smooth muscle cells may be facilitated by switching-on or increased expression of the EBV receptor, and by the much higher circulating levels of EBV. However, given the increased incidence of leiomyosarcomas in organ transplant recipients as well as persons with HIV-1 infection, it is likely that the contribution of HIV-1 to leiomyosarcoma is also the result of a common effect of decreased immunity rather than a direct gene effect of HIV-1 infection. Although the CD21 receptor is present in low amounts on leiomyomas and leiomyosarcomas from immunocompetent children (51,57), EBV infection of these cells is not found. This also emphasizes the important role of immunity, which normally controls circulating EBV levels and may target EBV-infected smooth muscle cells if such infection should occasionally occur. Under any scenario, previous EBV infection and impaired immunity are sufficient prerequisites for development of leiomyosarcoma.

In Vitro Cell Studies of EBV-Associated Leiomyosarcoma

The biology of EBV infection of smooth muscle cells has been studied best in explanted cells from a single leiomyosarcoma of a woman with HIV-1 infection (97).

The cells exhibited very slow growth in vitro with unusual elliptical and spindle-shaped morphology, and fragmentation of the cytoplasm into long, tapering cytoplasmic processes. Greater than 90% of cells expressed diffuse distribution of the smooth muscle isoform of actin by immunoperoxidase staining. Approximately 25% of cells expressed very bright fluorescence to the smooth muscle isoforms of calponin and actin by immunostaining. The majority of cells demonstrated a weak signal for CD21, and approximately 5% to 10% of cells showed a strong signal confined to cell surfaces. The cultured cells harbored EBV, and infectious EBV continued to be detected by PCR and virus culture through several passages in vitro. Several EBV antigens including latent antigen Epstein–Barr nuclear antigen-1, immediate early antigen BZLF1, early antigen EA-D, late antigens including viral capsid antigen p160, glycoprotein gp125, and membrane antigen gp350. Human umbilical cord lymphocytes, transformed with virus isolated from cultured cells, yielded immortalized cell lines that expressed EBV antigens similar to other EBV-transformed lymphocyte cell lines. These findings confirm that EBV is capable of lytic infection of smooth muscle cells with expression of a repertoire of latent and replicative viral products, and production of infectious virus, and may contribute to the oncogenesis of leiomyosarcomas.

The inability to derive immortalized, EBV-infected smooth muscle cell lines that are tumorigenic is, in many ways, similar to the inability to establish non-lymphoid cell lines from Kaposi sarcoma harboring KSHV. The biology of these two gamma herpesviruses in these two tumors may have many similarities.

CONCLUSIONS

Leiomyosarcomas expand the spectrum of EBV-associated malignancies, and also of malignancies associated with impaired immunity. Immune dysfunction appears to facilitate EBV infection of smooth muscle cells, which is followed by malignant transformation and proliferation.

REFERENCES

1. Penn I. Sarcomas in organ allograft recipients. Transplantation 1995; 60:1485–1491.
2. Centers for Disease Control and Prevention. 1993 revised classification system for HIV infection and expanded surveillance case definition for AIDS among adolescents and adults. Morb Mortal Wkly Rep 1992;41:1–19.
3. Beral V, Newton R. Overview of the epidemiology of immunodeficiency-associated cancers. J Natl Cancer Inst 1998; Monographs:1–6.
4. Remick SC. Non-AIDS-defining cancers. Hematol Oncol Clin North Am 1996; 10:1203–1213.
5. Polednak AP. Incidence of soft-tissue cancers in blacks and whites in New York State. Int J Cancer 1986; 38:21–26.
6. Cavazzana AO, Ninfo V, Tirabosco R, Montaldi A, Frunzio R. Leiomyosarcoma. Curr Top Pathol 1995; 89:313–332.
7. Myhre-Jensen O, Kaae S, Madsen EH, Sneppen O. Histopathological grading in soft-tissue tumours. Relation to survival in 261 surgically treated patients. Acta Pathol Microbiol Immunol Scand [A] 1983; 91:145–150.
8. Trojani M, Contesso G, Coindre JM, et al. Soft-tissue sarcomas of adults; study of pathological prognostic variables and definition of a histopathological grading system. Int J Cancer 1984; 33:37–42.

9. Enjoji M, Hashimoto H. Diagnosis of soft tissue sarcomas. Pathol Res Pract 1984; 178:215–226.

10. Markhede G, Angervall L, Stener B. A multivariate analysis of the prognosis after surgical treatment of malignant soft-tissue tumors. Cancer 1982; 49:1721–1733.

11. Hashimoto H, Daimaru Y, Tsuneyoshi M, Enjoji M. Leiomyosarcoma of the external soft tissues. A clinicopathologic, immunohistochemical, and electron microscopic study. Cancer 1986; 57:2077–2088.

12. Wile AG, Evans HL, Romsdahl MM. Leiomyosarcoma of soft tissue: a clinicopathologic study. Cancer 1981; 48:1022–1032.

13. Neugut AI, Sordillo PP. Leiomyosarcomas of the extremities. J Surg Oncol 1989; 40:65–67.

14. Evans HL. Smooth muscle tumors of the gastrointestinal tract. A study of 56 cases followed for a minimum of 10 years. Cancer 1985; 56:2242–2250.

15. Young JLJ, Miller RW. Incidence of malignant tumors in U.S. children. J Pediatr 1975; 86:254–258.

16. Lack EE. Leiomyosarcomas in childhood: a clinical and pathologic study of 10 cases. Pediatr Pathol 1986; 6:181–197.

17. Yannopoulos K, Stout AP. Smooth muscle tumors in children. Cancer 1962; 15:958–971.

18. Botting AJ, Soule EH, Brown AL Jr. Smooth muscle tumors in children. Cancer 1965; 18:711–720.

19. Walker D, Gill TJI, Corson JM. Leiomyosarcoma in a renal allograft recipient treated with immunosuppressive drugs. JAMA 1971; 215:2084–2086.

20. Pritzker KPH, Huang SN, Marshall KG. Malignant tumours following immunosuppressive therapy. Can Med Assoc J 1970; 103:1362–1365.

21. Lieber MR, Winans CS, Griem ML, Moossa R, Elner VM, Franklin WA. Sarcomas arising after radiotherapy for peptic ulcer disease. Dig Dis Sci 1985; 30:593–599.

22. Cohen SR, Thompson JW, Sherman NJ. Congenital stenosis of the lower esophagus associated with leiomyoma and leiomyosarcoma of the gastrointestinal tract. Ann Otol Rhinol Laryngol 1988; 97:454–459.

23. Case records of the Massachusetts General Hospital. Weekly clinicopathological exercises. Case 9–1986. A 40-month-old girl with the acquired immunodeficiency syndrome and spinal-cord compression [published erratum appears in N Engl J Med 1986 Jun 5; 314(23):1523]. N Engl J Med 1986; 314:629–640.

24. Ninane J, Moulin D, Latinne D, et al. AIDS in two African children–one with fibrosarcoma of the liver. Eur J Pediatr 1985; 144:385–390.

25. Chadwick EG, Connor EJ, Guerra Hanson IC, et al. Tumors of smooth-muscle origin in HIV-infected children. JAMA 1990; 263:3182–3184.

26. Sabatino D, Martinez S, Young R, Balbi H, Ciminera P, Frieri M. Simultaneous pulmonary leiomyosarcoma and leiomyoma in pediatric HIV infection. Pediatr Hematol Oncol 1991; 8:355–359.

27. Mueller BU, Butler KM, Higham MC, et al. Smooth muscle tumors in children with human immunodeficiency virus infection. Pediatrics 1992; 90:460–463.

28. Orlow SJ, Kamino H, Lawrence RL. Multiple subcutaneous leiomyosarcomas in an adolescent with AIDS. Am J Pediatr Hematol Oncol 1992; 14:365–368.

29. Radin R, Kiyabu M. Multiple smooth muscle tumors of the colon and adrenal gland in an adult with AIDS. Am J Radiol 1992; 159:545–546.

30. Ross JS, Del Rosario A, Bui HX, Sonbati H, Solis O. Primary hepatic leiomyosarcoma in a child with the acquired immunodeficiency syndrome. Hum Pathol 1992; 23:69–72.

31. Challapalli M. Leiomyomata and leiomyosarcomata in HIV-infected children. [letter]. Diagn Cytopathol 1993; 9:366.

32. Steel TR, Pell MF, Turner JJ, Lim GH. Spinal epidural leiomyoma occurring in an HIV-infected man. Case report. J Neurosurg 1993; 79:442–445.

33. van Hoeven KH, Factor SM, Kress Y, Woodruff JM. Visceral myogenic tumors. A manifestation of HIV infection in children. Am J Surg Pathol 1993; 17:1176–1181.

34. Levin TL, Adam HM, van Hoeven KH, Goldman HS. Hepatic spindle cell tumors in HIV positive children. Pediatr Radiol 1994; 24:78–79.

35. McLoughlin LC, Nord KS, Joshi VV, DiCarlo FJ, Kane MJ. Disseminated leiomyosarcoma in a child with acquired immune deficiency syndrome. Cancer 1991; 67:2618–2621.

36. Murphy SB, Chadwick EG. HIV and smooth muscle tumors [letter]. Pediatrics 1993; 91:1020–1021.

37. Balsam D, Segal S. Two smooth muscle tumors in the airway of an HIV-infected child. Pediatr Radiol 1992; 22:552–553.

38. Ha C, Haller JO, Rollins NK. Smooth muscle tumors in immunocompromised (HIV negative) children. Pediatr Radiol 1993; 23:413–414.

39. Danhaive O, Ninane J, Sokal E, et al. Hepatic localization of a fibrosarcoma in a child with a liver transplant. J Pediatr 1992; 120:434–437.

40. Spencer JM, Amonette RA. Tumors with smooth muscle differentiation. Dermatol Surg 1996; 22:761–768.

41. Weiss SW. Smooth muscle tumors of soft tissue. Adv Anat Pathol 2002; 9:351–359.

42. Miano JM, Olson EN. Expression of the smooth muscle cell calponin gene marks the early cardiac and smooth muscle cell lineages during mouse embryogenesis. J Biol Chem 1996; 271:7095–7103.

43. Ruzicka DL, Schwartz RJ. Sequential activation of alpha-actin genes during avian cardiogenesis: vascular smooth muscle alpha-actin gene transcripts mark the onset of cardiomyocyte differentiation. J Cell Biol 1988; 107:2575–2586.

44. Christopherson WM, Williamson EO, Gray LA. Leiomyosarcoma of the uterus. Cancer 1972; 29:1512–1517.

45. Morgan BK, Compton C, Talbert M, Gallagher WJ, Wood WC. Benign smooth muscle tumors of the gastrointestinal tract. A 24-year experience. Ann Surg 1990; 211:63–66.

46. Gal AA, Brooks JS, Pietra GG. Leiomyomatous neoplasms of the lung: a clinical, histologic, and immunohistochemical study. Mod Pathol 1989; 2:209–216.

47. Evans HL, Chawla SP, Simpson C, Finn KP. Smooth muscle neoplasms of the uterus other than ordinary leiomyoma. A study of 46 cases, with emphasis on diagnostic criteria and prognostic factors. Cancer 1988; 62:2239–2247.

48. Hashimoto H, Tsuneyoshi M, Enjoji M. Malignant smooth muscle tumors of the retroperitoneum and mesentery: a clinicopathologic analysis of 44 cases. J Surg Oncol 1985; 28:177–186.

49. Kleinschmidt-DeMasters BK, Mierau GW, Sze CI, et al. Unusual dural and skull-based mesenchymal neoplasms: a report of four cases. Hum Pathol 1998; 29:240–245.

50. Prévot S, Néris J, de Saint Maur PP. Detection of Epstein Barr virus in an hepatic leiomyomatous neoplasm in an adult human immunodeficiency virus 1-infected patient. Virchows Archiv 1994; 425:321–325.

51. McClain KL, Leach CT, Jenson HB, et al. Association of Epstein–Barr virus with leiomyosarcomas in young people with AIDS. N Engl J Med 1995; 332:12–18.

52. Lee ES, Locker J, Nalesnik M, et al. The association of Epstein–Barr virus with smooth-muscle tumors occurring after organ transplantation. N Engl J Med 1995; 332:19–25.

53. Jimenez-Heffernan JA, Hardisson D, Palacios J, Garcia-Viera M, Gamallo Nistal M. Adrenal gland leiomyoma in a child with acquired immunodeficiency syndrome. Pediatr Pathol Lab Med 1995; 15:923–929.

54. Zetler PJ, Filipenko D, Bilbey JH, Schmidt N. Primary adrenal leiomysarcoma in a man with acquired immunodeficiency syndrome (AIDS). Further evidence for an increase in smooth muscle tumors related to Epstein–Barr infection in AIDS. Arch Pathol Lab Med 1995; 119:1164–1167.

55. Bluhm JM, Yi ES, Diaz G, Colby TV, Colt HG. Multicentric endobronchial smooth muscle tumors associated with the Epstein–Barr virus in an adult patient with the acquired immunodeficiency syndrome. A case report. Cancer 1997; 80:1910–1913.

56. Boman F, Gultekin H, Dickman PS. Latent Epstein–Barr virus infection demonstrated in low-grade leiomyosarcomas of adults with acquired immunodeficiency syndrome, but

not in adjacent Kaposi's lesion or smooth muscle tumors in immunocompetent patients. Arch Pathol Lab Med 1997; 121:834–838.

57. Jenson HB, Leach CT, McClain KL, et al. Benign and malignant smooth muscle tumors containing Epstein–Barr virus in children with AIDS. Leuk Lymphoma 1997; 27: 303–314.

58. Morgello S, Kotsianti A, Gumprecht JP, Moore F. Epstein–Barr virus-associated dural leiomyosarcoma in a man infected with human immunodeficiency virus. Case report. J Neurosurg 1997; 86:883–887.

59. Creager AJ, Maia DM, Funkhouser WK. Epstein–Barr virus-associated renal smooth muscle neoplasm. Report of a case with review of the literature. Arch Pathol Lab Med 1998; 122:277–281.

60. Krishnan R, Freeman JA, Creager AJ. Epstein–Barr virus induced renal leiomyoma. J Urol 1999; 161:212.

61. Blumenthal DT, Raizer JJ, Rosenblum MK, Bilsky MH, Hariharan S, Abrey LE. Primary intracranial neoplasms in patients with HIV. Neurology 1999; 52:1648–1651.

62. Brown HG, Burger PC, Olivi A, Sills AK, Barditch-Crovo PA, Lee RR. Intracranial leiomyosarcoma in a patient with AIDS. Neuroradiology 1999; 41:35–39.

63. Barbashina V, Heller DS, Hameed M, et al. Splenic smooth-muscle tumors in children with acquired immunodeficiency syndrome: report of two cases of this unusual location with evidence of an association with Epstein–Barr virus. Virchows Arch 2000; 436:138–139.

64. Ritter AM, Amaker BH, Graham RS, Broaddus WC, Ward JD. Central nervous system leiomyosarcoma in patients with acquired immunodeficiency syndrome. Report of two cases. J Neurosurg 2000; 92:688–692.

65. Timmons CF, Dawson DB, Richards CS, Andrews WS, Katz JA. Epstein–Barr virus-associated leiomyosarcomas in liver transplantation recipients. Origin from either donor or recipient tissue. Cancer 1995; 76:1481–1489.

66. Le Bail B, Morel D, Merel P, et al. Cystic smooth-muscle tumor of the liver and spleen associated with Epstein–Barr virus after renal transplantation. Am J Surg Pathol 1996; 20:1418–1425.

67. Morel D, Merville P, Le Bail B, Berger F, Saric J, Potaux L. Epstein–Barr virus (EBV)-associated hepatic and splenic smooth muscle tumours after kidney transplantation. Nephrol Dial Transplant 1996; 11:1864–1866.

68. Sadahira Y, Moriya T, Shirabe T, Matsuno T, Manabe T. Epstein–Barr virus-associated post-transplant primary smooth muscle tumor of the liver: report of an autopsy case. Pathol Int 1996; 46:601–604.

69. Davidoff AM, Hebra A, Clark BJ III, et al. Epstein–Barr virus-associated hepatic smooth muscle neoplasm in a cardiac transplant recipient. Transplantation 1996; 61:515–517.

70. Somers GR, Tesoriero AA, Hartland E, et al. Multiple leiomyosarcomas of both donor and recipient origin arising in a heart-lung transplant patient. Am J Surg Pathol 1998; 22:1423–1428.

71. Brichard B, Smets F, Sokal E, et al. Unusual evolution of an Epstein–Barr virus—associated leiomyosarcoma occurring after liver transplantation. Pediatr Transplant 2001; 5:365–369.

72. Rogatsch H, Bonatti H, Menet A, Larcher C, Feichtinger H, Dirnhofer S. Epstein–Barr virus—associated multicentric leiomyosarcoma in an adult patient after heart transplantation: case report and review of the literature. Am J Surg Pathol 2000; 24: 614–621.

73. Bonatti H, Hoefer D, Rogatsch H, Margreiter R, Larcher C, Autretter H. Successful management of recurrent Epstein–Barr virus—associated multilocular leiomyosarcoma after cardiac transplantation. Transplant Proc 2005; 37:1839–1844.

74. Shen SC, Yunis EJ. Leiomyosarcoma developing in a child during remission of leukemia. J Pediatr 1976; 89:780–782.

75. Yunis EJ. Role of Epstein–Barr virus in tumor development. J Pediatr 1996; 128:438.

76. Mierau GW, Greffe BS, Weeks DA. Primary leiomyosarcoma of brain in an adolescent with common variable immunodeficiency syndrome. Ultrastruct Pathol 1997; 21:301–315.
77. Reyes C, Abuzaitoun O, de Jong A, Hanson C, Langston. Epstein–Barr virus—associated smooth muscle tumors in ataxia-telangiectasia: a case report and review. Hum Pathol 2002; 33:133–136.
78. Kaschka-Dierich C, Adams A, Lindahl T, et al. Intracellular forms of Epstein–Barr virus DNA in human tumour cells in vivo. Nature 1976; 260:302–306.
79. Hill MA, Araya JC, Eckert MW, Gillespie AT, Hunt JD, Levine EA. Tumor specific Epstein–Barr virus infection is not associated with leiomyosarcoma in human immunodeficiency virus negative individuals. Cancer 1997; 80:204–210.
80. Marioni G, Bertino G, Mariuzzi L, Bergamin-Bracale AM, Lombardo M, Beltrami CA. Laryngeal leiomyosarcoma. J Laryngol Otol 2000; 114:398–401.
81. van Gelder T, Vuzevski VD, Weimar W. Epstein–Barr virus in smooth-muscle tumors [letter]. N Engl J Med 1995; 332:1719.
82. van Gelder T, Jonkman FAM, Niesters HGM, et al. Absence of Epstein–Barr virus involvement in an adult heart transplant recipient with an epitheloid leiomyosarcoma [letter]. J Heart Lung Transplant 1996; 15:650–651.
83. Ashfaq A, Haller E, Mossey R, et al. Recurrent membranous nephropathy and leiomyosarcoma in the renal allograft of a lupus patient. J Nephrol 2004; 17:134–138.
84. Dugan MC. Primary adrenal leiomyosarcoma in acquired immunodeficiency syndrome [letter]. Arch Pathol Lab Med 1996; 120:797–798.
85. Jenson HB, Ench Y. Epstein–Barr virus. In: Rose NR, Hamilton RG, Detrick B, eds. Manual of Clinical Laboratory Immunology, 6th ed., Washington, D.C: American Society for Microbiology, 2002:615–626.
86. Lam KY. Oesophageal mesenchymal tumors: clinical features and absence of Epstein–Barr virus. J Clin Pathol 1999; 52:758–760.
87. Granovsky MO, Mueller BU, Nicholson HS, Rosenberg PS, Rabkin CS. Cancer in human immunodeficiency virus-infected children: a case series from the Children's Cancer Group and the National Cancer Institute. J Clin Oncol 1998; 16:1729–1735.
88. Pollock BH, Jenson HB, Leach CT, et al. Risk factors for pediatric human immunodeficiency virus (HIV)-related malignancy. JAMA 2003; 289:2393–2399.
89. Evans AS. New discoveries in infectious mononucleosis. Mod Med 1974; 1:18–24.
90. Evans AS, Niederman JC, McCollum RW. Seroepidemiologic studies of infectious mononucleosis with EB virus. N Engl J Med 1968; 279:1123–1127.
91. Wang PS, Evans AS. Prevalence of antibodies to Epstein–Barr virus and cytomegalovirus in sera from a group of children in the People's Republic of China. J Infect Dis 1986; 153:150–152.
92. Jondal M, Klein G, Oldstone MB, Bokish V, Yefenof E. Surface markers on human B and T lymphocytes. VIII. Association between complement and Epstein–Barr virus receptors on human lymphoid cells. Scand J Immunol 1976; 5:401–410.
93. Hutt-Fletcher LM, Fowler E, Lambris JD, Feighny RJ, Simmons JG, Ross GD. Studies of the Epstein Barr virus receptor found on Raji cells. II. A comparison of lymphocyte binding sites for Epstein Barr virus and C3d. J Immunol 1983; 130:1309–1312.
94. Timens W, Boes A, Vos H, Poppema S. Tissue distribution of the C3d/EBV-receptor: CD21 monoclonal antibodies reactive with a variety of epithelial cells, medullary thymocytes, and peripheral T-cells. Histochemistry 1991; 95:605–611.
95. Nemerow GR, McNaughton ME, Cooper NR. Binding of monoclonal antibody to the Epstein Barr virus (EBV)/CR2 receptor induces activation and differentiation of human B lymphocytes. J Immunol 1985; 135:3068–3073.
96. Fingeroth JD, Weis JJ, Tedder TF, Strominger JL, Biro PA, Fearon DT. Epstein–Barr virus receptor of human B lymphocytes is the C3d receptor CR2. Proc Natl Acad Sci USA 1984; 81:4510–4514.

97. Jenson HB, Montalvo EA, McClain KL, et al. Characterization of natural Epstein–Barr virus infection and replication in smooth muscle cells from a leiomyosarcoma. J Med Virol 1999; 57:36–46.

98. Sixbey JW, Davis DS, Young LS, Hutt-Fletcher L, Tedder TF, Rickinson AB. Human epithelial cell expression of an Epstein–Barr virus receptor. J Gen Virol 1987; 68:805–811.

99. Young L, Alfieri C, Hennessy K, et al. Expression of Epstein–Barr virus transformation-associated genes in tissues of patients with EBV lymphoproliferative disease. N Engl J Med 1989; 321:1080–1085.

100. Miller N, Hutt-Fletcher LM. Epstein–Barr virus enters B-cells and epithelial cells by different routes. J Virol 1992; 66:3409–3414.

101. Yoshizaki T, Takimoto T, Takeshita H, et al. Epstein–Barr virus lytic cycle spreads via cell fusion in a nasopharyngeal carcinoma hybrid cell line. Laryngoscope 1994; 104:91–94.

102. Bayliss GJ, Wolf H. Epstein–Barr virus-induced cell fusion. Nature 1980; 287:164–165.

16
X-Linked Lymphoproliferative Disease

Thomas A. Seemayer
Department of Pathology/Microbiology, University of Nebraska Medical Center, Nebraska Medical Center, Omaha, Nebraska, U.S.A.

Thomas G. Gross
Department of Pediatrics, Ohio State University, and Division of Hematology/ Oncology/BMT, Children's Hospital, Columbus, Ohio, U.S.A.

Arpad Lanyi
Department of Pathology/Microbiology and Center for Human Molecular Genetics, University of Nebraska Medical Center, Nebraska Medical Center, Omaha, Nebraska, U.S.A.

Janos Sumegi
Division of Hematology/Oncology, Children's Hospital Medical Center, Cincinnati, Ohio, U.S.A.

THE DISCOVERY OF THE DISEASE

The disease to be described was discovered neither by serendipity nor accident. Rather it was brought to light over the course of years by the persistence and unquenchable curiosity of David T. Purtilo, a young pathologist marked in his formative years by the brilliant and stimulating Robert A. Good at the University of Minnesota.

The story begins in 1969 in the autopsy suite of Children's Hospital, Boston. Under the supervision of Gordon Vawter, a premier pediatric pathologist, Purtilo, a pathology resident, performed an autopsy on an eight-year-old boy who died after a virulent (31 days duration) illness that produced symptoms one month following exposure to the child with infectious mononucleosis (IM). The deceased had clinical and laboratory features of IM: positive heterophile antibodies, atypical lymphocytosis, hypergammaglobulinemia, and massive hepatosplenomegaly. At necropsy, a disseminated lymphoid infiltrate permeated the spleen, liver, bone marrow, brain, kidney, pancreas, adrenals, and esophagus. The child was thought to have died from hepatic and medullary failure. In due course (see below), the findings were interpreted to represent fulminant IM (FIM). At the time, FIM was regarded as a very rare outcome of the natural disease (1).

Purtilo sought to determine whether other family members had incurred similar illnesses. He learned that a brother had died in 1961 (eight years earlier) at three years of age following a two-week history of sore throat, fever, and cervical lymphadenopathy, terminating with convulsions and death. The child was diagnosed to have had "acute lymphoblastic leukemia." The autopsy report delineated hepatosplenomegaly and a disseminated lymphoproliferative process affecting diverse viscera. No laboratory studies had been performed, as the child died two hours following hospitalization. Regrettably, the autopsy slides were not available for review.

In 1973, Dr. Vawter notified Purtilo that a third brother had developed a similar fulminant lymphoproliferative condition and died 30 days after the onset of symptoms. The necropsy findings were similar to that in the other two siblings. On the mother's side, Purtilo learned that three maternally related male cousins had died: a nine-year-old boy with aplastic anemia following IM and hypogammaglobulinemia; a three-year-old boy with lymphoma of the ileal-cecal region; and a 19-year-old boy with cerebral lymphoma. The central nervous system lymphoma was histopathologically identical to the intestinal lymphoma in his half-brother. Lastly, an 11-year-old maternally related male cousin was found to have hypo-immunoglobulin G (IgG) and hyper-IgM. This boy developed generalized vaccinia following a smallpox vaccination, but survived.

A preliminary communication on this kindred appeared in 1974 (2). In the same year, an abstract describing acquired agammaglobulinemia in three related males following IM was reported (3), as was a publication describing fatal IM in four related males (4).

The seminal paper describing this unique family, surname Duncan after the original kindred, was published in *The Lancet* in 1975 (5). Of 18 boys in the Duncan kindred, six died of a lymphoproliferative disease. At the time, the disease appeared to bridge the gap between IM and lymphoma. A common thread [Epstein–Barr virus (EBV) infection] in four of the six boys suggested that a viral infection had triggered the uncontrolled proliferation of lymphocytes, the latter stemming from "inadequate immunologic shut-off mechanisms."

Following *The Lancet* publication, Purtilo devoted his life to study this disease, which over the course of time came to be known as X-linked lymphoproliferative (XLP) disease. He relentlessly scoured the literature, contacted authors of reports which might be describing patients with XLP, and traveled extensively to interview physicians, patients, and family members. In these venues, he synthesized the clinical, laboratory, and pathologic data and, above all, obtained precious DNA to bank for the eventual quest of the gene.

THE XLP REGISTRY

Not long after the discovery of XLP, Purtilo recognized that it was important that an XLP Registry be established. The XLP Registry was established in 1980 (6), its *raison d'être* to serve as a referral center for clinical (family/physician) counseling relevant to the investigation, diagnosis, and treatment of XLP and, *above all, to orchestrate research to better understand the disease*. Initially based at the University of Massachusetts Medical Center in Worcester, the Registry was brought to Omaha in 1981 when Purtilo was appointed Chairperson in Pathology at the University of Nebraska Medical Center.

For years, the XLP Registry, while retained in assorted files, was stored in Purtilo's memory. He knew, in no small detail, each affected male and kindred.

Table 1 Summary of XLP Registry Data (as of 2002)

Total affected males	314
Alive	73 (23%)
Dead	241 (77%)

Abbreviation: XLP, X-linked lymphoproliferative.

Following his untimely sudden death (at age 53) in 1992, the XLP Registry data were entered into a computer database created and maintained by Jack R. Davis, M.T. American Society for Clinical Pathology (ASCP).

Over the past 22 years, well over 2500 individuals have been studied and entered in the XLP Registry. Ninety-one kindred have been defined with 314 affected males (Table 1). Over three-quarters of the affected males have died, many prior to the age of 10 years. The oldest living affected male is 49 years old. Initially, Registry studies were a reflection of the times and related to the patients' EBV status, heterophile serology, serum immunoglobulin (Ig) levels, white blood cell count, and differential and Monospot test. Later on, assessments for T/B-lymphocyte populations, natural killer (NK) cells, and cytokines were performed. Whenever possible, surgical and autopsy histological sections were reviewed to complement the clinical and laboratory data. As time passed, DNA analysis utilizing restriction fragment length polymorphisms was offered to attempt to delineate the genetic status of a putative XLP male or female carrier. Following the cloning of the XLP gene, the Registry has offered sequence analysis of the gene to identify affected males and female carriers. For many of these studies, the costs were absorbed by the William C. Havens Foundation and the Lymphoproliferative Research Foundation at the University of Nebraska.

THE DIAGNOSIS OF XLP

XLP is a rare disorder, affecting an estimated one out of every million male individuals (7). Prior to the isolation of the XLP gene, *SH2D1A*, it was difficult to make a diagnosis of XLP based solely on clinical and/or laboratory features. Laboratory studies of lymphocyte numbers, immunophenotype, and function were generally not helpful, because results were either normal or hard to interpret due to immune depletion resulting from primary EBV infection or lymphoma treatment (8–10). Evaluation of humoral responses led to inconsistent results with some patients displaying normal values and others demonstrating increases in IgA and/or IgM, as well as variable deficiencies in the levels of total IgG, or the IgG1 and IgG3 subclasses (11). Studies of EBV-specific immunity have been controversial, as well. Initial results suggested that XLP patients could not mount an effective anti-EBV immune response, as demonstrated by deficient production of EBV-specific antibodies, (12,13) and defective killing of EBV-infected B-cells by autologous T or NK cells (9,14–16). Other studies, however, demonstrated that some XLP patients can generate normal anti-EBV responses during both acute and latent infection (9,17). The only consistent findings are as follows: the lack of anti-EBNA response in EBV infected males many months (or several years) later and the inability to undergo isotype IgM → IgG switch following secondary challenge with MX174 bacteriophage. Regrettably, (18) both of these aberrations can be seen in other inherited T-cell deficiencies; hence they are not diagnostic of XLP.

Establishing a definitive XLP diagnosis until recently was based on the clinical identification of two or more maternally related males demonstrating an XLP phenotype following EBV infection (7,19). The definition was clinical, since no laboratory test was judged to be diagnostic.

Now the diagnosis can more easily be made based on the identification of an abnormal *SH2D1A* gene sequence (20) or protein expression (21). Based on clinical similarities, the differential diagnosis for XLP is broad and includes sporadic FIM, hemophagocytic lymphohistiocytosis that may or may not be EBV associated, X-linked hyper-IgM syndrome, X-linked agammaglobulinemia, autoimmune lymphoproliferative disease syndrome, common variable immunodeficiency, and chronic active EBV infection (22–24). Because distinguishing among these conditions can be difficult, we suggest that males suspected as having one of these disorders undergo genetic testing for the *SH2D1A* gene. Establishing the correct diagnosis of XLP is important, as it may heighten patient/family surveillance for early signs of the disease, but more importantly promote studies to explore the potential value of hematopoietic stem cell transplantation (HSCT) as curative therapy (25,26).

In female XLP carriers, only 50% of their lymphocytes express *SH2D1A* due to random X chromosome inactivation (27). Because carriers display no overt clinical manifestations, normal lymphocytes must compensate for those for which the gene is nonfunctional. Despite this observation, abnormalities in serum Ig and anti-EBV antibody titers have been reported in carriers (28,29). Molecular analysis should be pursued in females at risk of being a carrier to provide accurate genetic counseling. Recent genetic studies have also demonstrated that *SH2D1A* mutations can arise in affected boys whose mothers do not have a mutated gene (24).

CLINICAL MANIFESTATIONS OF XLP

Initially, three phenotypes were described in XLP patients, and these continue to characterize the majority of patients: FIM, malignant lymphoma [lymphoproliferative disease(LPD)], and dysgammaglobulinemia (DYS) (7). Less commonly reported manifestations include disorders such as vasculitis, pulmonary lymphomatoid granulomatosis, and hematologic cytopenias (HC), including aplastic anemia and pure red cell aplasia (7,30–32). The "disease state" is capricious, as it may feature a single phenotype (Table 2) or two or more phenotypes (Table 3) which may develop sequentially in susceptible individuals.

Table 2 Single Phenotype (as of 2002)

	#	# Alive	# Dead
FIM	141	3 (2.1%)	138 (97.9%)
DYS	34	27 (79%)	7 (21%)
Lymphoma/lymphoproliferative disease	53	12 (22%)	41 (78.1%)
HC	6	1 (16%)	5 (84%)
Total	234		

Abbreviations: FIM, fulminant infectious mononucleosis; DYS, dysgammaglobulinemia; HC, hematologic cytopenias.

Table 3 Multiple Phenotypes (as of 2002)

	#	# Alive	# Dead
FIM	41	10 (24%)	31 (76%)
DYS	58	20 (34%)	38 (66%)
Lymphoma/lymphoproliferative disease	35	11 (31%)	24 (69%)
HC	11	2 (18%)	9 (82%)
Vasculitis	4	0 (0%)	4 (100%)
Total	149		

Abbreviations: FIM, fulminant infectious mononucleosis; DYS, dysgammaglobulinemia; HC, hematologic cytopenias.

The clinical features affecting XLP patients can vary among kindreds, as well as among different members within the same family, suggesting that environmental or genetic factors influence the clinical expression of the disease (20). The cumulative data of XLP phenotypes and survival are presented in Table 4.

Fatal Infectious Mononucleosis

Reflecting the ubiquitous nature of EBV infection, FIM (usually with a concomitant virus-associated hemophagocytic syndrome) is the most common XLP phenotype affecting approximately 46% of patients in the XLP Registry (7,30,31). FIM is decisively the most lethal of the XLP phenotypes, as most of the boys die within one month and only 7% of FIM patients have survived. The median age of XLP-associated FIM onset is five years, but the condition has occurred up to 40 years of age. This contrasts with sporadic (non-XLP-associated) FIM which occurs in approximately 1:3000 IM cases (50 cases annually in the United States), at a median age of 13 years (30).

Table 4 Total XLP Phenotypes and Survival

	# Total	%	Median age at onset (yrs)	# Alive	%
FIM	182	46	5	13	7
DYS	92	23.3	9	47	51
Lymphoma/ lymphoproliferative disease	88	22.3	6	23	26
HC	17	4.3	8	3	18
Genetic diagnosis (asymptomatic children)	11	3		11	100
Vasculitis	4	1	7	0	0
Total	394				

Abbreviations: XLP, X-linked lymphoproliferative; FIM, fulminant infectious mononucleosis; DYS, dysgammaglobulinemia; HC, hematologic cytopenias.

In contrast to the well-orchestrated normal immune response (likened to a Mozart divertimento) to EBV, boys with XLP mount a dysregulated, exuberant response to the virus, with CD8+ T-cells, EBV-infected B-cells, and macrophages infiltrating body tissues. This results in extensive parenchymal damage, most vividly in the liver (as fulminant hepatitis) and bone marrow (as medullary destruction). Other tissues, and even vessels, are affected, as mononuclear cellular infiltrates and cell injury are manifest in the spleen (extensive necrosis of white pulp), brain (perivascular mononuclear cell infiltrates), heart (mild mononuclear cell myocarditis), and kidneys (mild interstitial nephritis) (7,32–37). The thymus incurs thymocyte depletion and necrosis of thymic epithelia, reminiscent of that observed in experimental and human graft-versus-host disease and AIDS (38–40). Excessive release of interleukin (IL)-2 and interferon (IFN)-gamma (γ) by activated T-lymphocytes contributes to uncontrolled macrophage activation, and culminates in the hemophagocytosis, tissue destruction, and cellular depletion of FIM (37,41,42). Interestingly, 39% of XLP patients with evidence of current or prior EBV infection never develop FIM (20). This latter observation remains unexplained.

Dysgammaglobulinemia

Affecting 23% of patients, DYS is the second most common XLP phenotype (7,20,30). Most boys developing this phenotype demonstrate global decreases of serum Ig levels. However, some feature increased levels of IgM and/or IgA, as well as variable deficiencies in IgG1 and IgG3 subclasses (11). The median age at the time of DYS diagnosis is nine years. The pathogenesis of DYS is not understood. Although hypogammaglobulinemia often occurs after EBV infection, some XLP patients develop hypogammaglobulinemia without prior evidence of EBV infection (20). *SH2D1A* knockout mice (the murine XLP model) can manifest progressive hypogammaglobulinemia (J. Sumegi, personal communication). These observations suggest that mutations of *SH2D1A* contribute to a defect in humoral memory responses and the maintenance of lifelong ability to produce appropriate humoral immunity.

Lymphoproliferative Disease

Lymphomas develop in 22% of XLP patients at a median age of six years, and half of them occur following EBV infection (7,20,30). Most lymphomas are of B-cell immunophenotype and are characterized by a small noncleaved (Burkitt lymphoma) or diffuse large cell histology (41,43). Karyotypic analysis has not been extensively performed; however, the t(8;14) associated with conventional African Burkitt lymphoma has been identified twice (44,45). Approximately 10% of LPD are not of B-cell phenotype. Small numbers of patients with Hodgkin's disease or T-cell lymphoproliferative disorders, including lymphoblastic lymphoma, lymphomatoid granulomatosis, or angiocentric immunoproliferative lesions have been reported to the XLP Registry (30,41). Relapses are common and may be of different clonal origins (46). Together, these observations suggest that the *SH2D1A* mutation affects immune function that provides immunosurveillance against LPD or lymphoma development.

Hematologic Cytopenia

Distinct from the marrow depletion seen with FIM, a limited number (4%) of boys have developed isolated HC (Table 1) (7,30). Most manifest with two or more hematologic cell lines suppressed or worse, with aplastic anemia. Curiously, pure red cell aplasia has also been observed (7,47). EBV infection is more often associated with aplastic anemia in patients without XLP, yet 40% of cases observed in XLP have occurred without evidence of prior EBV infection (20). Therefore, whether the mutations of *SH2D1A* contribute to the pathogenesis of this marrow suppression remains an unsettled issue.

GENOTYPE–PHENOTYPE CORRELATION

One might predict that mutations which delete the XLP gene or truncate the protein would be more likely to be associated with a severe phenotype, whereas missense mutations would occur preferentially in mildly affected patients. A study was performed to define the correlation between the mutations found in the *SH2D1A* gene and the clinical manifestations of XLP (20). The results were startling, namely, that it was not uncommon to observe different phenotypes with identical mutations, even within the same family. No significant differences were observed in the phenotypes or in severity of disease based on the type (missense, nonsense, and truncating) or in localization of *SH2D1A* mutations (Table 5). The age of onset of clinical manifestations of XLP varied considerably, from younger than 1 to 40 years, as did survival, but there was no correlation with the type of mutation. *The clinical significance of these results was clear: genetic analysis did not predict the phenotype or the severity of disease.*

THE ROLE OF EBV INFECTION IN XLP

Initially, it was thought that males affected with XLP manifest symptoms following primary EBV infection. While IM is, by definition, caused by EBV, other XLP phenotypes, including lymphoma and hypogammaglobulinemia, occasionally developed in EBV-seronegative patients (20,48). Hence, this early assumption was proved to be incorrect over time.

Data from the XLP Registry suggest that as many as 12.5% of affected boys will manifest symptoms of XLP prior to exposure to EBV (7). Although FIM is always associated with acute EBV infection, the frequencies of the other major XLP phenotypes are similar, regardless of EBV status (Table 5) (20).

The effect of EBV infection on outcome of XLP has been studied (Table 6) (20). There is no difference in the age of onset of clinical symptoms between males who have or have not been previously exposed to EBV. But in general, survival is slightly better in patients who manifest clinical symptoms of XLP prior to EBV infection. Therefore, prevention of EBV infection in boys with XLP may not avert clinical manifestations of the disease but may slightly prolong survival. These data suggest that other genetic and/or environmental factors influence host susceptibility to EBV and are important in the determination of the clinical phenotype of XLP.

TREATMENT AND PROGNOSIS

XLP is highly lethal, as most (75%) patients die by 10 years of age, though the oldest known survivor is 49 years old (7,30). Antiviral therapies, including acyclovir,

Table 5 Correlation of Mutation Type, EBV Status, Clinical Phenotype, and Outcome in XLP

Mutation type	Number of kindreds	Phenotype	% affected	EBV status at first manifestation	% affected	Median age of onset (yr)	Median survival (yr)
Deletion (no *SH2D1A*)	5	FIM	25	EBV positive	31	5 (0.5–26)	7 (1–41)
		DYS	44				
		Lymphoma/ lymphoproliferative disease	25	EBV negative	31		
		HC	0				
		Asymptomatic (diagnosed genetically)	6	EBV status indeterminable	38		
Deletion (truncated *SH2D1A*)	8	FIM	51	EBV positive	46	4 (0.5–34)	9 (1–41)
		DYS	26				
		Lymphoma/ lymphoproliferative disease	17	EBV negative	14		
		HC	6				
		Asymptomatic (diagnosed genetically)	0	EBV status indeterminable	40		
Splice defect	3	FIM	69	EBV positive	31	2 (0.1–5)	3 (1–20)
		DYS	6				

Mutation	n	Clinical phenotype	%	EBV status	%	Age	Age
		Lymphoma/lymphoproliferative disease	19	EBV negative	25		
		HC	0				
		Asymptomatic (diagnosed genetically)	6	EBV status indeterminable	44		
Nonsense	9	FIM	65	EBV positive	50	3 (0.5–23)	6 (0.5–38)
		DYS	8				
		Lymphoma/lymphoproliferative disease	23	EBV negative	17		
		HC	2				
		Asymptomatic (diagnosed genetically)	2	EBV status indeterminable	33		
Missense	9	FIM	36	EBV positive	25	4 (1–33)	7 (1–45)
		DYS	17				
		Lymphoma/lymphoproliferative disease	39	EBV negative	13		
		HC	4				
		Asymptomatic (diagnosed genetically)	4	EBV status indeterminable	62		

Abbreviations: DYS, dysgammaglobulinemia; EBV, Epstein-Barr virus; FIM, fulminant infectious mononucleosis; HC, hematologic cytopenias; XLP, X-linked lymphoproliferative.

Source: From Ref. 20.

Table 6 The Effect of EBV Infection on Clinical Outcome in XLP

	Median age of first manifestation (yrs)	Median survival age (yrs)
EBV positive		
Overall	4 (0.5–40)	6 (0.5–40)
FIM	3 (0.5–40)	4 (0.5–40)
DYS	6 (0.5–32)	14 (0.5–38)
Lymphoma/lymphoproliferative disease	5 (2–19)	6 (2–32)
HC	6 (2–24)	12 (2–27)
EBV negative		
Overall	6 (0–34)	16.5[a](1-41)
DYS	4.5 (0.1–34)	19 (4–41)
Lymphoma/lymphoproliferative disease	8 (3–33)	17 (4–39)
HC[b]	1, 11	7, 14

[a]P value < 0.05 comparing EBV-positive versus EBV-negative cohorts.
[b]Two cases of HC reported. Ages in each column represent age at the time of diagnosis and age at the time of death, respectively.
Abbreviations: XLP, X-linked lymphoproliferative; FIM, fulminant infectious mononucleosis; DYS, dysgammaglobulinemia; HC, hematologic cytopenias; EBV, Epstein–Barr virus.
Source: From Ref. 20.

ganciclovir, intravenous Ig, and IFN-α have been used to treat primary EBV infection; none have been particularly effective (7,49).

The only therapy that has been consistently beneficial for males with FIM includes etoposide, a topoisomerase II inhibitor that is cytotoxic against activated macrophages, complemented with glucocorticoids or cyclosporine to suppress reactive T-lymphocytes (7,50). Recently, a patient with FIM was successfully treated with corticosteroids and monoclonal anti–B-cell antibody (K. Nichols, personal communication). While symptoms may have initially resolved, relapses are invariable. Therefore, an allogeneic HSCT (umbilical cord blood, adult blood, or bone marrow) is recommended once the patient's condition is stabilized and a suitable donor has been identified (25,50).

Patients with XLP hypogammaglobulinemia require regular Ig supplementation to prevent bacterial and viral infections. However, Ig infusions do not offer the guarantee of protection from primary EBV infection in an EBV seronegative patient (20,30,51).

For patients with lymphoma or HC, standard therapeutic protocols suffice. Although treatment can induce disease remissions, relapses and other XLP phenotypes invariably occur.

For definitive treatment, a new immune system has to efface the old one. This involves the replacement of defective immune system with an allogeneic HSCT (25). In the literature, a total of 15 male XLP patients have undergone an allogeneic bone marrow transplant (BMT). Although usually successful, four died from infectious or therapy-related causes. All were over 15 years of age at the time of BMT, suggesting that treatment at a younger age may be beneficial for XLP. It is estimated that there have been over 50 males with XLP who have undergone BMT. However, the number of boys treated is too small to make specific recommendations regarding the optimal timing of the transplant, the source (umbilical cord blood, adult blood, or bone marrow) of the graft, and other specifics concerning the patient and the procedure.

Wiskott–Aldrich syndrome (WAS), another X-linked immunodeficiency, is similar to XLP in that the vast majority of affected males have clinical manifestations of the disease before age 10, and life expectancy is less than 20 years. Over 30 years of experience has demonstrated that BMT for treating WAS, as in the case of XLP, is best when performed before significant problems with infections or lymphoma develop. Even boys with WAS without symptoms, who receive BMT at an earlier age, i.e., less than five years, do better with BMT (52). These data lead us to recommend that BMT be performed as early as possible for XLP. BMT has been performed successfully in two XLP boys with a genetic diagnosis prior to the onset of EBV infection and clinical symptoms other than hypogammaglobulinemia (26). To conclude, given the dismal results in older XLP and WAS patients, i.e., greater than 20 years of age, BMT of older patients should be undertaken only in those who are in good physical condition and after extensive counseling regarding the involved risks.

An approach that may offer a better outcome for older patients is nonmyeloablative HSCT. Because lower doses of radiation and chemotherapy are used, nonmyeloablative BMT is anticipated to cause less transplant-related toxicity. To date, only one XLP patient has reportedly undergone nonmyeloablative transplantation (53). The patient succumbed to recurrent disease following transplantation. Clearly, although novel, additional studies of nonmyeloablative therapy in this clinical setting should be explored.

THE XLP GENE

The gene absent or mutated in XLP patients, *SH2D1A* (also known as DSHP or SAP), is located in the chromosomal Xq25 region between DXS1001 and DXS8057 in the vicinity of the Tenascin-M gene (54–56). The human gene, spanning 25 kb, consists of four exons and three introns which are transcribed into two messenger RNA (mRNA) species of 2.5 and 0.9 kb, respectively. These mRNAs code the same open reading frame (ORF), but their 3′ untranslated sequences are different. Homologues of the human *SH2D1A* have been identified in murines (*Mus musculus*), primates (*Macaca rhesus* and *Sanguineous oedipus*), and turkeys (*Gallus gallus*) (57). The murine gene has a similar exon/intron structure as the human counterpart but expresses only a single mRNA transcript of 790 nucleotides, shorter than the human mRNAs.

SH2D1A is expressed in the thymus in CD8+ and CD4+ cells. The expression is prevalent in Th1 cells, but Th2 cells also express the gene. *SH2D1A* expression is downregulated upon anti-CD3 stimulation of both CD4+ and CD8+ cells. The mouse gene, *Sh2d1a*, is expressed in low levels in resting NK cells, but increases upon infection with murine cytomegalovirus or lymphocytic choriomeningitis virus. IL-2 activates *Sh2d1a* expression in cultured NK cells. *Sh2d1a* is expressed in some B-cells (58).

The human *SH2D1A* has an ORF of 462 nucleotides flanked by untranslated 5′ and 3′ sequences. The protein translation initiation site (AUG for methionine) is 78 nucleotides downstream from the start of the ORF, and therefore the length of the protein encoding sequence is 384 nucleotides. The *SH2D1A* mRNA encodes a protein of 128 amino acid (aa) residues that consists of a SH2 domain and a 25 aa C-terminal tail. The murine gene *SH2D1A* expresses a transcript of 790 nucleotides, which encodes a protein of 127 aa, which we will denote as SAP [signaling lymphocyte activating protein (SLAM)–associated protein]. The conceptual translation of the *M. rhesus* and *Sanguineus oedipusSH2D1A* cDNA results in proteins of 127 and 137 aa, respectively. The *SH2D1A* protein, SAP, is conserved during evolution; there are but few positions in the protein with deviations in the aa sequence.

A close homolog of *SH2D1A EAT-2*, has been found in humans and mice (59). The human and mouse EAT-2 genes encode a protein of 132 aa consisting of a single SH2 domain and a short sequence at the C-terminal of the protein. The gene was first identified as a transcript induced by the EWS/FL11 fusion oncogenic protein (60). *SH2D1A* and *EAT-2* represent the first members of a family of genes that contain only a single SH2 domain and are expressed in various tissues.

THE XLP PROTEIN

The XLP protein SAP is a cytoplasmic protein, and it interacts with the cytoplasmic tail of cell surface proteins of two distinct classes: the CD2 family of proteins, such as SLAM, 2B4, and Ly-9 and the Dok family of cytosolic adaptor proteins (see below).

SAP is not detected in the nucleus, but rather physically and functionally links SLAM and other immune cell receptors to the Src-related protein kinase Fyn. The relevant domain of the protein is an SH2 domain (Src-homology region 2) that recognizes phosphotyrosine residues.

The single SH2 domain is unusual among SH2 domain–containing proteins (61). The SH2 domain is typically found in signaling and adapter proteins with multidomain architecture in association with SH1, SH3 (another type of phosphotyrosine recognition sequence which recognizes phosphotyrosine residues imbedded in aa sequences containing multiple proline residues, in contrast to SH2 domains), or phosphatase domains. The lack of these domains in *SH2D1A* and EAT-2 suggests that they function as signaling molecules blocking or regulating the binding of other SH2 domain–containing proteins to their particular docking sites.

SAP has a characteristic SH2 fold, which includes a central β-sheet with α-helices packed against either side (61). The classical SH2 domains bind phosphopeptides in a "two-pronged" fashion; the phosphorylated tyrosine binds in a pocket on one side of the central sheet, and the three to five residue C-terminal binds to the pocket or groove on the opposite side (61). The SH2D1A protein interacts via its SH2 domain with a motif (TIpYXXV/I) in the cytoplasmic tail of SLAM (CD150), 2B4 (CD244), Ly-9, and CD84, suggesting that the combinations of dysfunctional signaling pathways initiated by these four cell surface receptors may contribute to the complex phenotypes of the disease. The SH2 domain in SAP is unusual among SH2 domain–containing proteins for its ability to bind to nonphosphorylated proteins. All other SH2 domain–containing proteins bind with high affinity only to sequences containing phosphorylated tyrosine. Indeed, SAP has been shown to block recruitment of the SHP-2 phosphatase to the tail of SLAM (55,61). SHP-2 is responsible for maintaining the optimal level of tyrosine phosphorylation.

The CD2 Family of Cell Membrane Receptors

SAP binds to the cytoplasmic tails of all of the CD2 family of surface molecules. At present, the CD2 subfamily of membrane receptors includes CD2, CD48, CD583, SLAM, CD84, Ly-9, 2B4, (62–69) and two recent members, BLAME, (70) expressed in activated monocytes and dendritic cells, and CS-1 (71), a new receptor found on NK cells. CD48, SLAM, CD84, Ly-9, 2B4, BLAME, and CS-1 map to a gene cluster on the chromosome 1q21–24 region, suggesting that the CD2 receptor family developed from an ancestral gene via multiple gene duplications (72). CD2 and CD58 reside at chromosome 1p13. Interestingly, the ligands for these receptors are within the same receptor family; CD2 and CD58 (73) or 2B4 and CD48 (74). SLAM, CD84, and Ly-9 are homophilic receptors (55).

The extracellular region of these receptors consists of an N-terminal Ig-like variable (V) domain and two Ig-like constant domains (C2) stabilized by two intrachain disulfide bonds (75). In Ly-9, these domains are duplicated, and they adopt a V/C2/V/C2 structure (67,76). The cytoplasmic domains of 2B4, SLAM, CD84, and Ly-9 all contain multiple copies of the consensus binding site (TxYxxV/I) for SAP and the tyrosine phosphatase SHP-2. The cytoplasmic domain of CD2 is unique in that it lacks tyrosine residues that upon phosphorylation could make contact with SH2 domains (59).

SLAM is expressed in CD45RO^{high} peripheral blood memory T-cells, CD4+ and CD8+ immature thymocytes, in B-cells, in some EBV-transformed lymphoblastoid cell lines (LCLs), tonsillar B-cells, and in activated dendritic cells (65,77–82). Engagement of SLAM by a SLAM-specific antibody can potentiate antigen or anti-CD3–induced T-cell proliferation, or directly induce proliferation of preactivated T-cells or CD4-positive T-cell clones (70). In addition, the same stimuli can induce IFN-γ production in CD4 positive Th0 cells and in polarized Th1 and Th2 cells. Polarized Th2 cells can be reverted to the Th0 or Th1 phenotype by SLAM/SLAM ligation, indicating that SLAM is important in the maintenance of the Th1/Th2 balance. In activated B-lymphocytes, SLAM engagement by specific antibody or by soluble SLAM can induce proliferation and Ig synthesis. SLAM augments CD95-induced apoptosis in certain B-cell lines. These results indicate that SLAM can transmit CD28 or CD40 independent costimulatory as well as inhibitory signals in lymphoid cells.

The cytoplasmic domain of SLAM contains two copies of the T/SIYxxV/I consensus sequence for high affinity binding of SAP (83). Y281 can bind SAP in both its phosphorylated or nonphosphorylated forms, while Y327 can only engage in SAP binding upon phosphorylation. Phosphorylated Y281 and Y327 of SLAM motifs are essential in binding the phosphatase SHP-2, both in T and B-lymphocytes (84). The N-terminal SH2 domain of SHP-2 is instrumental in regulating the phosphatase activity of SHP-2 and in binding SHP-2 to its targets (85–89). The N-terminal SH2 domains of SHP-2 and SAP share significant homology with 30% identity at the protein level. Overexpression of SAP in COS-7 cells blocks SHP-2 binding to SLAM, indicating that SAP and SHP-2 compete for the same phosphotyrosine on SLAM.

In T-cells, two distinct signaling SLAM complexes may exist with fundamentally different functions: one complex in which SLAM is bound to SHP-2 and another which binds to SAP. The details of the molecular events following SAP binding to SLAM are unknown, but it is likely that preventing SHP-2 from binding to SLAM may facilitate the phosphorylation of the SLAM cytoplasmic domain by tyrosine kinases. Y281 can bind SAP in its nonphosphorylated form at relatively high affinity. On the other hand, Y327 needs to be phosphorylated to bind to SAP. SAP binding to Y281 may render Y327 available for phosphorylation by cytoplasmic protein–tyrosine kinases. Phosphorylation of Y327 renders the SLAM cytoplasmic domain accessible for SH2 domain–mediated protein interactions. Whether SAP is able to block SH2 domain proteins from binding to SLAM Y327 may depend on the actual concentration of SAP.

The kinetics of SLAM and SAP expression are regulated differently following T-cell activation, significantly changing the stoichiometry of SLAM and SAP in the cell. SLAM expression is quickly induced by T-cell activation, and its level gradually decreases with time. However, SAP levels first drop sharply following T-cell activation by α-CD3, and expression increases later. It is conceivable that during T-cell activation both forms of SLAM signal complex with or without SAP may exist. Alternatively, SAP binding to SLAM may be regulated by post-translational modifications of SAP.

In B-cells, SLAM has been found to associate with SH2 containing inositol phosphatase (SHIP), an SH2 domain containing inositol phosphate 5'-phosphatase. The binding of SHIP to SLAM seems to be regulated by SH2D1A/SAP. SLAM was found to be associated with SAP and SHIP in LCLs that expressed SAP, while in SAP-negative LCLs and SHP-2, SHIP was not associated with SLAM. SHIP binding was dependent on the presence of pY281 and pY327. It was proposed that SAP would act as a "switch" that regulates the association of SLAM with SHIP or SHP-2. Phosphorylation of SLAM in B-cells is controlled by Fgr and Lyn and the phosphotyrosine phosphatase CD45. Ligation of SLAM by a specific antibody resulted in rapid dephosphorylation of SHIP mediated by SLAM-associated CD45. Dephosphorylation of SHIP could affect its binding to the phosphotyrosine-binding domain of Shc and affect downstream signaling toward p21ras (90). It is important that the model we described for SLAM signal transduction in T-cells is consistent with experimental data obtained in B-cells. Because SLAM impacts on the regulation of IFN-γ production by CD4+ T-cells, on the induction of Th1 cytokines in polarized Th2 cells, and on the CD95-induced apoptosis in B-cells, the data suggest that the absence of the SLAM/SAP signal transduction could account for some of the immune defects seen in XLP. 2B4 is a receptor present on all NK cells and T-cells that mediate non–major histocompatibility comlex–restricted cytotoxicity (69). 2B4 is also expressed on the surface of γδ T-cells, monocytes, some CD8+ thymocytes, and a subset of peripheral CD8+ T-cells (75). Engagement of 2B4 via specific antibody or its high affinity ligand CD48 augments lysis of a variety of target cells by 2B4 bearing cells. Signals via 2B4 also induce increased cytokine release, Ca^{2+} influx, and degranulation in NK cells (74,91,92). In CD8+ T-cells, however, 2B4 seems to function as an adhesion molecule, as these cells are not directly activated by 2B4 engagement (92).

The extracellular region of 2B4 adopts the Ig-like structure characteristic of the SLAM family. Within the 120 aa cytoplasmic region, four tyrosines are part of a putative consensus binding site for SAP and SHP-2. In agreement with this, mutually exclusive binding of SAP or SHP-2 to 2B4 was demonstrated by immunoprecipitation in stable transfected, pervanadate treated pre-B (BAF3) cell lines (77). Unlike that of SLAM, 2B4 phosphorylation is essential for SAP binding. Induction of SAP in NK cells would result in SHP-2 displacement and increased signaling by 2B4. Recent observations suggest that in the absence of functional SAP, the 2B4/CD48 signaling pathway is altered, resulting in the failure of XLP patients to control EBV-infected B-cells in the early phase of the infection (93–95).

In polyclonal or clonal populations of XLP-derived NK cells, engagement of 2B4 by specific antibody or via CD48 failed to augment killing of a variety of cells. In addition to the lack of an activating 2B4-mediated signal in XLP-derived NK cells, in the absence of SAP, 2B4 engagement via CD48 mediated inhibitory signals rather than activating signals. Importantly, this suppressor effect was resolved by interrupting the 2B4/CD48 interaction by specific antibody. These data not only shed light on a previously unknown inhibitory function of 2B4, but also open a window on how EBV-infected B-cells may escape NK and CD8+ T-cell surveillance in XLP patients (95).

SAP, besides its interaction with the members of the CD2 family of receptors, can interact with the RasGAP adapter protein p62Dok. p62Dok [downstream of kinases-1 (Dok-1)] is a member of a new family of adapters that includes p62Dok (Dok-1), p56Dok (Dok-2), and Dok-3 (96–99). While Dok-1 and Dok-2 are expressed in T-cells at high levels, Dok-3 is expressed in B-cells, macrophages, and myeloid cells, but not in T-cells (99). Dok-1 is also expressed and was shown to function in B-lymphocytes, in vivo (100). SAP binds weakly to Dok-2 in transfected 293 T-cells. There are no data on the binding of SAP to Dok-3.

The Dok Family of Cytosolic Adapter Proteins

Dok-1 was first identified as a major phosphoprotein in cells transformed by the oncogenes v-src, v-fps, and v-abl (101–103). Besides viral oncogenes, it is also the target for a host of receptor tyrosine kinases as well as nonreceptor tyrosine kinases (99,100,104). Upon phosphorylation, Dok-1 binds the SH2 domains of RasGAP and recruits C-terminal Src kinase to the membrane (105,106). The function of Dok-1 in B-cells in FcR-γRIIB and BCR-mediated signals is well documented (99,100,107,108). In primary B lymphocytes, cross-linking the FcR-γRIIB fragment with the BCR induced Dok-1 phosphorylation by the Src kinase Lyn and was followed by a decrease in the MAP kinase activity and growth inhibition. B-lymphocytes from Doc-1 deficient mice, however, continue to proliferate under the same conditions, indicating that this strong inhibitory signal, presumably via the inhibition of the Ras pathway, is delivered by Doc-1. The function of Dok-1 in T-lymphocytes is not yet established. Recent reports have indicated that, in Jurkat T-lymphocytes, as in primary B-cells, Dok-1 may also transmit inhibitory signals (108,109). Overexpression of Dok-1 in Jurkat cell clones inhibited CD2-mediated signals, including increase in intracellular [Ca^{2+}], phospholipase C-g activation, and activation of MAP kinases. Similarly, pretreatment of Jurkat cells with CD3-specific antibody prior to activation via CD2 amplified the CD2-induced tyrosine phosphorylation.

SAP binds to one of the C-terminal phosphotyrosines (pY449) on Dok-1 (110). The process requires both the C-terminal 35 aa region and the pleckstrin homology domain of Dok-1. How SAP can regulate Dok-1 is yet to be defined. By inhibiting SHP-2 binding, SAP may prolong the phosphorylation of Dok-1 and promote inhibitory signals. Many alternative mechanisms can be envisioned, as Dok-1 has at least seven tyrosines that can potentially interact with SH2 domain proteins (111). The possibility that Dok-1 is recruited to SLAM-family receptors should also be investigated. Because Dok-1 transmits inhibitory signals in both T and B-lymphocytes, the lack of SAP-controlled Dok-1–mediated signals may contribute to the development of unchecked T-cell and B-cell proliferation in XLP.

In T-cells the SLAM receptor molecule is capable of triggering SH2D1-dependent protein tyrosine phosphorylation. SAP promotes the recruitment of Fyn into the SLAM/SAP complex, activating a signal transduction pathway that involves inositol phosphatase SHIP, the adaptor molecules Dok-2, Dok-1, Shc, and RasGAP. Because SAP facilitates the recruitment of T-cell–specific Fyn it is essential for this pathway (111).

In conclusion, interactions of SAP with the members of the SLAM family of receptors and Dok-1 may mediate signals that ensure proper surveillance of EBV-specific T-cell and B-cell proliferation or appropriate control of EBV-negative B-cell proliferation.

XLP MUTATIONS

Since the identification of the *SH2D1A* gene, several forms of functional mutations have been described in XLP families (112–117):

- macro- and micro-deletions;
- mutations interfering with transcription and splicing;
- mutations interfering with protein synthesis or affecting protein function;
- missense mutations

  - mutations that affect the stability of the SH2D1A protein,
  - mutations that disrupt the specific actions between SH2D1A and target proteins.

Macro- and micro deletions: The most common mutations are deletions ranging from several nucleotides to several megabase pairs of DNA leading to a complete or partial loss of the gene and truncation or absence of a functional SH2D1A protein. These deletions account for 40% to 50% of the SH2D1A mutations.

Mutations interfering with normal transcription and splicing: These mutations account for 10% to 15% of all SH2D1A mutations.

Mutations interfering with protein synthesis or affecting protein function: The replacement of methionine by isoleucine interferes with translation and precludes the initiation of translation. The consequence is an absence of the SH2D1A protein.

Missense mutations: Eleven missense mutations identified in XLP families were analyzed in vitro and in vivo. The missense mutations can be assigned to two categories: mutations which alter the stability of the protein by substantially decreasing its half-life and mutations which disrupt the specific interactions between SH2D1A and target proteins.

Examination of the missense mutations in XLP patients suggests that the full complement of binding interaction(s) is critical for SH2D1A function. These point mutations are distributed evenly along the SH2-domain structure, and mutations have been found in N-terminal seven aa sequences and the 25 aa long C-terminal tail sequence of the protein.

Mutations that affect the stability of the SH2D1A protein: The wild-type SH2D1A protein has a half-life of 18 hours. When the stability of the mutated SH2D1A proteins was analyzed it was found that missense mutations (Y7C, S28R, R32T, Q99P, P101L, V10G, and X128R) that affect the structure of the backbone of the SH2D1A SH2 domain and disrupt hydrophilic and hydrophobic bonding shorten the half-life of the protein. Interestingly, one of the mutations observed outside of the SH2 domain, X129R, dramatically shortened the half-life of the protein (118).

The R32T mutation affects the stability of the protein by introducing a change in the most conserved aa among various SH2 domains (118). This arginine located in betaB5 is required for phosphotyrosine recognition and binding. An identical mutation in the SH2 domain of Btk causes X-linked agammaglobulinemia (XLA) when mutated to glycine or threonine (119). There are no reports describing the stability of the Btk wild-type or mutant proteins. In vitro mutagenesis of the arginine has led to impaired function of SH2 domains.

The E67D and T68I mutations change the conformation of the loop connecting the beta 5 and beta 6 strands. The T68I mutation changes the half-life of the protein (118). Although the SH2D1A protein with an E67D mutation was not assayed for protein stability, the position of this aa relative to T68 may impart the same effect.

The aa residue in Btk corresponding to T68 of SH2D1A is also mutated, leading to XLA (120). E67 as well as T68 are located near amino acids involved in residue +3 binding.

P101 at the C-terminus of the SH2 domain is strongly conserved. This residue is located in the short loop connecting the last two beta strands. Substitution of the peptide backbone turning proline by isoleucine will most likely affect folding, because the tangle formed by proline is hardly preserved by the other residue.

Mutations that disrupt the specific interactions between SH2D1A and target proteins: The SH2D1A/R32Q mutant protein is unable to bind both phosphorylated and nonphosphorylated SLAM proteins and block the recruitment of SHP-2 to the cytoplasmic tail of SLAM. The R32Q mutation also affects the half-life of the protein. *Therefore, it is most likely that an inability of SH2D1A to bind to SLAM is central to both impairments.*

The cytosine at aa position 42 plays an important role in the interactions with tyrosines. The mutation at this position results in SH2D1A/C24W, a relatively stable protein which shows a reduced binding to both phosphorylated and unphosphorylated SLAM.

The SH2D1A protein/T68I maintains its ability to bind to phosphorylated tyrosine of SLAM but is unable to bind to nonphosphorylated SLAM. The threonine 68 is involved in the interaction with valine in the +3 position of the SLAM peptide. SH2D1A/T53I fails to bind to nonphosphorylated SLAM. Mutant SH2D1A/R32T was greatly compromised in its ability to bind to SLAM, whereas the SLAM-binding properties of mutants 2 (T68I, G93D, and Q99P) were less affected. Interestingly, the ability of mutant P101L to bind SLAM was actually enhanced. Mutants P101L, Q99P, and T68I are unable to displace SHP-1 or SHP-2 (118). This might be either due to an altered affinity for the competing site on the receptor or due to a reduced stability of the SAP protein, as has been previously postulated. Another possibility is that the mutations may disrupt interactions with other, as yet unknown, proteins.

CONCLUSIONS

Although the first XLP patient was encountered in 1969, it took six years to define and present the disease entity to the medical community. Fourteen more years passed until the chromosomal location of the disease gene was established. In 1998, the gene mutated in XLP was identified and cloned, and the various inactivating mutations responsible for the disease were subsequently described. A mouse model of the disease was created by targeted mutagenesis.

The crystal structure of the protein product has been defined, and interacting proteins have been identified. Based on the structure of the XLP protein, a single SH2 domain with a short C-terminal tail sequence, it may act as a natural blocker (inhibitor) or as a regulator (adaptor) in the critical events in T-cell and NK cell signal transduction. The role of the protein in B-cell signal transduction was also explored but requires further study.

The gene, the protein, and the identified disease-causing mutations have not only opened a window to the molecular etiology of the disease but will also teach us about fundamental events in the T-cell and B-cell immunoregulation during EBV infection. All of this illustrates that a very rare condition can lead to the acquisition of very fundamental knowledge. This, of course, is not new, as many rare genetically determined immune deficiencies have contributed greatly to our understanding of the immune system.

ACKNOWLEDGMENTS

The authors dedicate this chapter to the memory of our cherished friend and colleague, David T. Purtilo. The XLP Registry is supported by the William C. Havens Foundation, Omaha, Nebraska and the Lymphoproliferative Research Fund.

REFERENCES

1. Penman HG. Fatal infectious mononucleosis: a critical review. J Clin Pathol 1970; 23:765–771.
2. Purtilo DT, Cassels C, Yang JPS. Fatal infectious mononucleosis in familial lymphohistiocytosis. New Engl J Med 1974; 291:736.
3. Provisor J, Iacuone JJ, Chilcote RR, Neiburger RG, Baehner RL. Acquired agammaglobulinemia in three related male children following an illness with clinical and laboratory features of infectious mononucleosis. Pediatr Res 1974; 8:417.
4. Bar RS, DeLor CJ, Clausen KP, Hurtubise P, Henle W, Hewetson JF. Fatal infectious mononucleosis in a family. N Engl J Med 1974; 290:363–367.
5. Purtilo DT, Cassel CK, Yang JPS, et al. X-linked recessive progressive combined variable immunodeficiency (Duncan's disease). Lancet 1975; 1:935–941.
6. Hamilton JK, Paquin LA, Sullivan JL, et al. X-linked lymphoproliferative syndrome registry report. J Pediatr 1980; 96:669–673.
7. Seemayer TA, Gross TG, Egeler RM, et al. X-linked lymphoproliferative disease: twenty-five years after the discovery. Pediatr Res 1995; 38:471–478.
8. Lindsten T, Seeley JK, Ballow M, et al. Immune deficiency in the X-linked lymphoproliferative syndrome. II. Immunoregulatory T-cell defects. J Immunol 1982; 129:2536–2540.
9. Sullivan JL, Byron KS, Brewster FE, Baker SM, Ochs HD. X-linked lymphoproliferative syndrome—natural history of the immunodeficiency. J Clin Invest 1983; 71:1765–1778.
10. Sullivan JL, Woda BA. X-linked lymphoproliferative syndrome. Immunodef Rev 1989; 1:325–347.
11. Grierson HL, Skare J, Hawk J, Pauza M, Purtilo DT. Immunoglobulin class and subclass deficiencies prior to Epstein–Barr virus infection in males with X-linked lymphoproliferative disease. Am J Med Genet 1991; 40:294–297.
12. Harada S, Sakamoto K, Seeley JK, et al. Immune deficiency in the X-linked lymphoproliferative syndrome. I. Epstein–Barr virus-specific defects. J Immunol 1982; 129:2532–2535.
13. Sakamoto K, Freed HJ, Purtilo DT. Antibody responses to Epstein-Barr virus in families with the X-linked lymphoproliferative syndrome. J Immunol 1980; 125:921–925.
14. Sullivan JL, Byron KS, Brewster FE, Purtilo DT. Deficient natural killer cell activity in X-linked lymphoproliferative syndrome. Science 1980; 210:543–545.
15. Harada S, Bechtold T, Seeley JK, Purtilo DT. Cell-mediated immunity to Epstein–Barr virus (EBV) and natural killer (NK)-cell activity in the X-linked lymphoproliferative syndrome. Int J Cancer 1982; 30:739–744.
16. Argov S, Johnson DR, Collins M, Koren HS, Lipscomb H, Purtilo DT. Defective natural killing activity but retention of lymphocyte-mediated antibody-dependent cellular cytotoxicity in patients with the X-linked lymphoproliferative syndrome. Cell Immunol 1986; 100:1–9.
17. Rousset F, Souillet G, Roncarolo MG, Lamelin JP. Studies of EBV-lymphoid cell interactions in two patients with the X- linked lymphoproliferative syndrome: normal EBV-specific HLA-restricted cytotoxicity. Clin Exp Immunol 1986; 63:280–289.
18. Purtilo DT, Grierson HL, Ochs H. Detection of X-linked lymphoproliferative disease (XLP) using molecular and immunovirological markers. Am J Med 1989; 87:421–424.
19. Seemayer TA, Grierson H, Pirruccello SJ, et al. X-linked lymphoproliferative disease. Am J Dis Child 1993; 147:1242–1245.

20. Sumegi J, Huang D, Lanyi A, et al. Correlation of mutations of the SH2D1A gene and Epstein–Barr virus infection with clinical phenotype and outcome in X-linked lymphoproliferative disease. Blood 2000; 96:3118–3125.

21. Gilmour KC, Cranston T, Jones A, et al. Diagnosis of X-linked lymphoproliferative disease by analysis of SLAM-associated protein expression. Eur J Immunol 2000; 30:1691–1697.

22. Okano M, Gross TG. A review of Epstein–Barr virus infection in patients with immunodeficiency disorders. Am J Med Sci 2000; 319:392–396.

23. Morra M, Silander O, Calpe S, et al. Alterations of the X-linked lymphoproliferative disease gene SH2D1A in common variable immunodeficiency syndrome. Blood 2001; 98:1321–1325.

24. Arico M, Imashuku S, Clementi R, et al. Hemophagocytic lymphohistiocytosis due to germline mutations in SH2D1A, the X-linked lymphoproliferative disease gene. Blood 2001; 97:1131–1133.

25. Gross TG, Filipovich AH, Conley ME, et al. Cure of X-linked lymphoproliferative disease (XLP) with allogeneic hematopoietic stem cell transplantation (HSCT): report from the XLP registry. Bone Marrow Transplant 1996; 17:741–744.

26. Ziegner UH, Ochs HD, Schanen C, et al. Unrelated umbilical cord stem cell transplantation for X-linked immunodeficiencies. J Pediatr 2001; 138:570–573.

27. Conley ME, Sullivan JL, Neidich JA, Puck JM. X chromosome inactivation patterns in obligate carriers of X-linked lymphoproliferative syndrome. Clin Immunol Immunopathol 1990; 55:486–491.

28. Sakamoto K, Seeley JK, Lindsten T, et al. Abnormal anti-Epstein–Barr virus antibodies in carriers of the X-linked lymphoproliferative syndrome and in females at risk. J Immunol 1982; 128:904–907.

29. Grierson H, Purtilo DT. Epstein–Barr virus infections in males with X-linked lymphoproliferative syndrome. Ann Intern Med 1987; 106:538–545.

30. Seemayer TA, Greiner TG, Gross TG, Davis JR, Lanyi A, Sumegi J. X-linked lymphoproliferative disease. In: Goedert JJ, ed. Infectious Causes of Cancer, Targets for Intervention. Totowa, NJ: Humana Press, 2000:51–61.

31. Sumegi J, Gross TG, Seemayer TA. The molecular genetics of X-linked lymphoproliferative (Duncan's) disease. Cancer J Sci Am 1999; 5:57–62.

32. Dutz JP, Benoit L, Wang X, et al. Lymphocytic vasculitis in X-linked lymphoproliferative disease. Blood 2001; 97:95–100.

33. Mroczek EC, Weisenburger DD, Grierson HL, Markin R, Purtilo DT. Fatal infectious mononucleosis and virus-associated hemophagocytic syndrome. Arch Pathol Lab Med 1987; 111:530–535.

34. Mroczek EC, Seemayer TA, Grierson HL, et al. Thymic lesions in fatal infectious mononucleosis. Clin Immunol Immunopathol 1987; 43:243–255.

35. Harrington DS, Weisenburger DD, Purtilo DT. Epstein–Barr virus-associated lymphoproliferative lesions. Clin Lab Med 1988; 8:97–118.

36. Seemayer TA, Gross TG, Hinrichs SH, Egeler RM. Massive diffuse histiocytic myocardial infiltration in Epstein–Barr virus-associated hemophagocytic syndrome and fulminant infectious mononucleosis. Cell Vision 1994; 1:260–264.

37. Okano M, Gross TG. Epstein–Barr virus-associated hemophagocytic syndrome and fatal infectious mononucleosis. Am J Hematol 1996; 53:111–115.

38. Seemayer TA, Lapp WS, Bolande RP. Thymic involution in murine graft-*versus*-host reaction: epithelial injury mimicking human dysplasia. Am J Pathol 1977; 88:119–134.

39. Seemayer TA, Bolande RP. Thymic involution mimicking thymic dysplasia, a consequence of transfusion-induced graft-*versus*-host disease in a premature infant. Arch Pathol Lab Med 1980; 104:141–144.

40. Seemayer TA, Laroche AC, Russo P, et al. Precocious thymic involution manifest by epithelial injury in the acquired immune deficiency syndrome. Hum Pathol 1984; 15:469–474.

41. Greiner TC, Gross TG. Atypical immune lymphoproliferations. In: Hoffman R, Benz EJ Jr, Shantill SJ, eds. Hematology: Basic Principles and Practice. New York: Churchill Livingstone, 2000:1432–1443.

42. Gross TG, Goyo-Rivas JJ, Hinrichs SH, Kamani NR, Baker KS. T helper cell (Th) cell responses following Epstein–Barr virus (EBV) infections in X-linked lymphoproliferative disease (XLP) and Chediak-Higashi syndrome (CHS). J Allergy Clin Immunol 1997; 99:S6.

43. Harrington DS, Weisenburger DD, Purtilo DT. Malignant lymphoma in the X-linked lymphoproliferative syndrome. Cancer 1987; 59:1419–1429.

44. Egeler RM, de Kraker J, Slater R, Purtilo DT. Documentation of Burkitt lymphoma with t(8;14) (q24;q32) in X-linked lymphoproliferative disease. Cancer 1992; 70:683–687.

45. Williams LL, Rooney CM, Conley ME, Brenner MK, Krance RA, Heslop HE. Correction of Duncan's syndrome by allogeneic bone marrow transplantation. Lancet 1993; 2:587–588.

46. Hoffmann T, Heilmann C, Madsen HO, Vindeløv L, Schmiegelow K. Matched unrelated allogeneic bone marrow transplantation for recurrent malignant lymphoma in a patient with X-linked lymphoproliferative disease (XLP). Bone Marrow Transplant 1998; 22:603–604.

47. Filipovich AH, Blazar BR, Ramsay NK, et al. Allogeneic bone marrow transplantation for X-linked lymphoproliferative syndrome. Transplantation 1986; 42:222–224.

48. Brandau O, Schuster V, Weiss M, et al. Epstein–Barr virus-negative boys with non-Hodgkin lymphoma are mutated in the SH2D1A gene, as are patients with X-linked lymphoproliferative disease (XLP). Hum Mol Genet 1999; 8:2407–2413.

49. Okano M, Pirruccello SJ, Grierson HL, Johnson DR, Thiele GM, Purtilo DT. Immunovirological studies of fatal infectious mononucleosis in a patient with X-linked lymphoproliferative syndrome treated with intravenous immunoglobulin and interferon-alpha. Clin Immunol Immunopathol 1990; 54:410–418.

50. Pracher E, Grumayer-Panzer ER, Zoubek A, Peters C, Gadner H. Bone marrow transplantation in a boy with X-linked lymphoproliferative syndrome and acute severe infectious mononucleosis. Bone Marrow Transplant 1994; 13:655–658.

51. Okano M, Bashir RM, Davis JR, Purtilo DT. Detection of primary Epstein–Barr virus infection in a patient with X-linked lymphoproliferative disease receiving immunoglobulin prophylaxis. Am J Hematol 1991; 36:294–296.

52. Filipovich AH, Stone JV, Tomany SC, et al. Impact of donor type on outcome of bone marrow transplantation for Wiskott-Aldrich syndrome: collaborative study of the International Bone Marrow Transplant Registry and the National Marrow Donor Program. Blood 2001; 97:1598–1603.

53. Amrolia P, Gaspar HB, Hassan A, et al. Nonmyeloablative stem cell transplantation for congenital immunodeficiencies. Blood 2000; 96:1239–1246.

54. Coffey AJ, Brooksbank RA, Brandau O, et al. The aberrant host response to EBV infection in X-linked lymphoproliferative disease results from mutations in a novel SH2-domain encoding gene, SH2D1A. Nat Genet 1998; 20:129–135.

55. Sayos J, Wu C, Morra M, et al. The X-linked lymphoproliferative-disease gene product SAP regulates signals induced through the co-receptor SLAM. Nature 1998; 395:462–469.

56. Nichols KE, Harkin DP, Levitz S, et al. Inactivating mutations in an SH2 domain-encoding gene in X-linked lymphoproliferative syndrome. Proc Natl Acad Sci USA 1998; 95:13,765–13,770.

57. Wu C, Sayos J, Wang N, Howie D, Coyle A, Terhorst C. Genomic organization and characterization of mouse SH2D1A, the gene that is altered in X-linked lymphoproliferative disease. Immunogenet 2000; 51:805–815.

58. Nagy N, Cerboni C, Mattsson K, et al. SH2D1A and SLAM protein expression in human lymphocytes and derived cell lines. Int J Cancer 2000; 88:439–447.

59. Morra M, Howie D, Grande MS, et al. X-linked lymphoproliferative disease: a progressive immunodeficiency. Ann Rev Immunol 2001; 19:657–682.

60. Thompson AD, Braun BS, Arvand A, et al. Eat-2 is a novel SH2 domain containing protein that is up-regulated by Ewing's sarcoma EWS/FLI1 fusion gene. Oncogene 1996; 13:2649–2658.

61. Poy F, Yaffe B, Sayos J, et al. Crystal structures of the XLP protein SAP reveal a class of SH2 domains with extended, phosphotyrosine-independent sequence recognition. Mol Cell 1999; 4:555–559.

62. Seed B, Aruffo A. Molecular cloning of the CD2 antigen, the T-cell erythrocyte receptor, by a rapid immunoselection procedure. Proc Natl Acad Sci USA 1987; 84:3365.

63. Staunton DE, Thorley-Lawson DA. Molecular cloning of the lymphocyte activation marker Blast-1. EMBO 1987; 6:3695.

64. Seed B. An LFA-3 cDNA encodes a phospholipid-linked membrane protein homologous to its receptor CD2. Nature 1987; 329:840–842.

65. Cocks BG, Chang C-CJ, Carballido JM, Yssel H, de Vries JE, Aversa G. A novel receptor involved in T-cell activation. Nature 1995; 376:260–263.

66. De la Fuente MA, Pizcueta P, Nadal M, Bosch J, Engel P. CD84 leukocyte antigen is a new member of the Ig superfamily. Blood 1997; 90:2398–2405.

67. Sandrin MS, Gumley TP, Henning HM, et al. Isolation and characterization of cDNA clones for mouse Ly-9. J Immunol 1992; 149:1636–1641.

68. Valiante NM, Trinchieri G. Identification of a novel signal transduction surface molecule on human cytotoxic lymphocytes. J Exp Med 1993; 178:1397–1406.

69. Garni-Wagner BA, Purohit A, Matthew PA, Bennett M, Kumar V. A novel function-associated molecule related to non-MHC-restricted cytotoxicity mediated by activated natural killer cells and T-cells. J Immunol 1993; 151:60–70.

70. Kingsbury GA, Feeney LA, Nong Y, et al. Cloning, expression, and function of blame, a novel member of the cd2 family. J Immunol 2001; 166:5675–5680.

71. Boles KS, Matthew PA. Molecular cloning of CS1, a novel human natural killer cell receptor belonging to the CD2 subset of the immunoglobulin superfamily. Immunogenetics 2001; 52:302–307.

72. Williams AF, Barclay AN. The immunoglobulin superfamily-domains for cell surface recognition. Ann Rev Immunol 1988; 6:381–405.

73. Davis SJ, Ikemizu S, Wild MK, Van der Merwe PA. CD2 and the nature of protein interactions mediating cell-cell recognition. Immunol Rev 1998; 163:217–236.

74. Brown MH, Boles K, van der Merwe PA, Kumar V, Mathew PA, Barclay AN. 2B4, the natural killer and T-cell immunoglobulin superfamily surface protein, is a ligand for CD48. J Exp Med 1998; 188:2083–2090.

75. Tangye SG, Phillips JH, Lanier LL. The CD2-subset of the Ig superfamily of cell surface molecules: receptor-ligand pairs expressed by NK cells and other immune cells. Sem Immunol 2000; 12:149.

76. Sandrin MS, Henning MM, Lo MF, Baker E, Sutherland GR, McKenzie IF. Isolation and characterization of cDNA clones for Humly9: the human homologue of mouse Ly9. Immunogenetics 1996; 43:13–19.

77. Tangye SG, Lazetic S, Woollatt E, Suterland GR, Lanier LL, Phillips HJ. Human 2B4, an activating natural killer cell receptor, recruits the protein tyrosine phosphatase SHP-2 and the adaptor signaling protein SAP. J Immunol 1999; 162:6981–6985.

78. Sayos J, Martin M, Chen A, Simarro M, Howie D, Morra M. Cell surface receptors Ly-9 and CD84 recruit the X-linked lymphoproliferative gene product SAP. Blood 2001; 97:3867–3874.

79. Shlapatska LM, Mikhalap SV, Berdova AG, et al. CD150 association with either the SH2-containing inositol phosphatase or the SH2-containing protein tyrosine phosphatase is regulated by the adaptor protein SH2D1A. J Immunol 2001; 166:5480–5487.

80. Kishimoto T, Kikutani H, von demBore AEG, et al. Leukocyte Typing VI. New York: Garland Pub., 1997.

81. Aversa G, Carballido J, Punnonen J, et al. SLAM and its role in T-cell activation and Th cell responses. Immunol Cell Biol 1997; 75:202–205.

82. Polacino PS, Pinchuk LM, Sidorenko SP, Clark EA. Immunodeficiency virus cDNA synthesis in resting T lymphocytes is regulated by T-cell activation signals and dendritic cells. J Med Primatol 1996; 25:201–209.

83. Aversa G, Chang CC, Carballido JM, Cocks BG, deVries JE. Engagement of the signalling activation molecule (SLAM) on activated T-cells result in IL-2 independent, cyclosporin A sensitive T-cell proliferation and IFN-production. J Immunol 1997; 158:4036–4044.

84. Freeman RM Jr, Plutzky J, Neel BG. Identification of a human src homology 2-containing protein-tyrosine-phosphatase: a putative homolog of Drosophila corkscrew. Proc Natl Acad Sci USA 1992; 89:11,239–11,243.

85. Lechleider RJ, Sugimot S, Bennett AM, et al. Activation of the SH2-containing phosphotyrosine phosphatase SH-PTP2 by its binding site, phosphotyrosine 1009, on the human PDGF-R. J Biol Chem 1993; 268:21,478–21,480.

86. Pluskey S, Wandlass TJ, Walsh CT, Shoelson SE. Potent stimulation of SH-PTP2 phosphatase activity by simultaneous occupancy of both SH2 domains. J Biol Chem 1995; 270:2897–2900.

87. Eck M, Pluskey S, Trub T, Harrison SC, Shoelson SE. Spatial constraints on the recognition of phosphoproteins by the tandem SH2 domains of the phosphatase SH-PTP2. Nature 1996; 379:277–280.

88. Pei D, Wang J, Walsh CT. Differential functions of the two Src homology 2 domains in protein-tyrosine phosphatase SH-PTP1. Proc Natl Acad Sci USA 1996; 93:1141–1145.

89. Saxton TM, Henkemeyer M, Gasca S, et al. Abnormal mesoderm patterning in mouse embryos mutant for the SH2 tyrosine phosphatase Shp-2. EMBO 1997; 16:2352–2364.

90. Lamkin TD, Walk SF, Liu L, Damen JE, Krystal G, Ravichandran KS. Shc interaction with Src homology 2 domain containing inositol phosphatase (SHIP) in vivo requires the Shc-phosphotyrosine binding domain and two specific phosphotyrosines on SHIP. J Biol Chem 1997; 272:10,396–10,401.

91. Latchman Y, McKay PF, Reiser H. Identification of the 2B4 molecule as a counter-receptor for CD48. J Immunol 1998; 161:5809–5812.

92. Nakajima H, Cella M, Langen H, Friedlein A, Colonna M. Activating interactions in human NK cell recognition: the role of 2B4-CD48. Eur J Immunol 1999; 29:1676–1683.

93. Tangye SG, Phillips JH, Lanier LL, Nichols KE. Functional requirement for SAP in 2B4-mediated activation of human natural killer cells as revealed by the X-linked lymphoproliferative syndrome. J Immunol 2000; 165:2932–2936.

94. Benoit L, Wang X, Pabst HF, Dutz J, Tan R. Defective NK cell activation in X-linked lymphoproliferative disease. J Immunol 2000; 165:3549–3553.

95. Parolini S, Bottino C, Falco M, et al. X-linked lymphoproliferative disease: 2B4 molecules displaying inhibitory rather than activating function are responsible for the inability of natural killer cells to kill Epstein–Barr virus-infected cells. J Exp Med 2000; 192:337–346.

96. Wisniewski D, Strife A, Wojciechowicz D, Lambek C, Clarkson B. A 62 kilodalton tyrosine phosphoprotein constitutively present in primary chronic phase chronic myelogenous leukemia enriched lineage negative blast populations. Leukemia 1994; 8:688–693.

97. Carpino N, Wisniewski D, Strife A, et al. p62(dok): a constitutively tyrosine-phosphorylated, GAP-associated protein in chronic myelogenous leukemia progenitor cells. Cell Immunol 1997; 88:197–204.

98. Di Cristofano A, Carpino N, Dunant N, et al. Molecular cloning and characterization of p56dok-2 defines a new family of RasGAP-binding proteins. J Biol Chem 1998; 273:4827–4830.

99. Lemay S, Davidson D, Latou S, Veillette A. Dok-3, a novel adapter molecule involved in the negative regulation of immunoreceptor signaling. Mol Cell Biol 2000; 20:2743–2754.

100. Yamanashi Y, Tamura T, Kanamori T, et al. Role of the rasGAP-associated docking protein p62(dok) in negative regulation of B-cell receptor-mediated signaling. Gene Develop 2000; 14:11–16.

101. Koch CA, Moran M, Sadowski I, Pawson T. The common src homology region 2 domain of cytoplasmic signaling proteins is a positive effector of v-fps tyrosine kinase function. Mol Cell Biol 1989; 9:4131–4140.

102. Moran MF, Polakis P, McCormick F, Pawson T, Ellis C. Protein-tyrosine kinases regulate the phosphorylation, protein interactions, subcellular distribution, and activity of p21ras GTPase-activating protein. Mol Cell Biol 1991; 11:1804–1812.

103. Muller AJ, Young JC, Pendergast AM, et al. BCR first exon sequences specifically activate the BCR/ABL tyrosine kinase oncogene of Philadelphia chromosome-positive human leukemias. Mol Cell Biol 1991; 11:1785–1792.

104. Van der Geer P, Hunter T, Lindberg RA. Receptor protein-tyrosine kinases and their signal transduction pathways. Ann Rev Cell Biol 1994; 10:251–337.

105. Neet K, Hunter T. The nonreceptor protein-tyrosine kinase CSK complexes directly with GTP-ase-activating protein associated p62 protein in cells expressing v-Src or activated c-Src. Mol Cell Biol 1995; 15:4908–4920.

106. Moran MF, Koch CA, Anderson D, et al. Src homology region 2 domains direct protein-protein interactions in signal transduction. Proc Natl Acad Sci USA 1990; 87:8622–8626.

107. Tamir I, Stolpa JC, Helgason CD, et al. The RasGAP-binding protein p62dok is a mediator of inhibitory FcgammaRIIB signals in B-cells. Immunity 2000; 12:347–358.

108. Brauweiler AM, Tamir I, Cambier JC. Bilevel control of B-cell activation by the inositol 5-phosphatase SHIP. Immunol Rev 2000; 176:69–74.

109. Harriague J, Debre P, Bismuth G, Hubert P. Priming of CD20 induced p62Dok tyrosine phosphorylation by CD3 in Jurkat T-cells. Eur J Immunol 2000; 30:3319–3328.

110. Sylla BS, Murphy K, Cahir-McFarland E, Lane WS, Mosialos G, Kieff E. The X-linked lymphoproliferative syndrome gene product SH2D1A associates with p62dok (Dok1) and activates NF-kappa B. Proc Natl Acad Sci USA 2000; 97:7470–7475.

111. Latour S, Gish G, Helgason CD, Humphries RK, Pawson T, Veillette A. Regulation of SLAM-mediated signal transduction by SAP, the X-linked lymphoproliferative gene product. Nat Immunol 2001; 2:681–690.

112. Sylla BS, Wang O, Hayor D, Lathrop GM, Lenoir GM. Multipoint linkage mapping of the Xq25-q26 region in a family affected by the X-linked lymphoproliferative syndrome. Clin Genet 1989; 36:459–462.

113. Bolino A, Seri M, Casano R, et al. A new candidate region for the positional cloning of the XLP gene. Eur J Hum Genet 1998; 6:509–517.

114. Yin L, Ferrand V, Lavoue MJ, et al. SH2D1A mutation analysis for diagnosis of XLP in typical and atypical patients. Hum Genet 1999; 105:501–505.

115. Strahm B, Rittweiler K, Duffner U, et al. Recurrent B-cell non-Hodgkin's lymphoma in two brothers with X-linked lymphoproliferative disease without evidence for Epstein–Barr virus infection. Br J Haem 2000; 108:377–382.

116. Lappalainen I, Giliana S, Franceschini R, et al. Structural basis for SH2D1A mutations in X-linked lymphoproliferative disease. Biochem Biophys Res Commun 2000; 269:124–130.

117. Schuster V, Kreth HW. X-linked lymphoproliferative disease is caused by deficiency of a novel SH2 domain-containing signal transduction adaptor protein. Immunol Rev 2000; 178:21–28.

118. Morra M, Simarro-Grande M, Chen A, et al. Missense mutations that affect non-phospho-tyrosine interactions and stability of the SAP/SH2D1A SH2-domain in X-linked lymphoproliferative disease patients. J Biol Chem 2001; 276:36,809–36,816.

119. Maregere LE, Pawson T. Identification of residues in GTPase activating protein Src homology 2 domains that control binding to tyrosine phosphorylated growth factor receptors and p62. J Biol Chem 1992; 267:22,779–22,786.

120. Conley ME, Mathias D, Treadaway J, Minegishi Y, Rohrer J. Mutations in btk in patients with presumed X-linked agammaglobulinemia. Am J Hum Genet 1998; 62:1034–1043.

17

Diseases Possibly Associated with Epstein–Barr Virus

James F. Jones
Viral Exanthems and Herpesvirus Branch, Centers for Disease Control and Prevention, Atlanta, Georgia, and Department of Pediatrics, National Jewish Medical and Research Center, Denver, Colorado, U.S.A.

INTRODUCTION

With the ready availability of sophisticated laboratory procedures and inquiring physician minds, an increasing array of uncommon illnesses and diseases are being attributed to infection with Epstein–Barr virus (EBV). This is part of the expanding phenomenon and the advent of research programs supporting the evaluation of new and emerging infectious diseases. Just as the expanded scope of possible diseases attributed to EBV is unlikely to represent "new" illnesses, emerging infections are only likely to reflect pre-existing illnesses whose identification is made possible with advances in molecular epidemiology. The illnesses described in this chapter are putatively caused by EBV, but the principles that form the association can be applied to many infectious agents.

Infectious diseases are generally characterized by a pattern of recognizable symptoms and typical illness course (Table 1). Confirmation of the microbiologic etiology of a clinical diagnosis, however, requires corroborating laboratory evidence. Classical infectious mononucleosis is a prime example of the historical evolution of the understanding of a clinically distinct infectious disease. Infectious mononucleosis carried the moniker "infectious" based on its epidemiology, long before the viral etiology was known. EBV is now readily appreciated as the causative agent of almost all cases of the typical constellation of severe pharyngitis, cervical lymphadenopathy, a marked lymphocytosis with atypical lymphocytes, and the presence of heterophile antibodies. Without precise knowledge of the etiology and the defined spectrum of disease that has been proved to be caused by EBV, many infectious agents and non-infectious illnesses would have to be considered if cataloging all of the symptoms and signs of classical infectious mononucleosis, and many more etiologies if the myriad of uncommon manifestations that are not part of the classical syndrome were included.

Approaches to identifying infectious agents as causative factors of disease are to identify readily recognizable specific illness patterns and propose a definition of commonly reported symptoms, or to set criteria for detection of unexplained

Table 1 Spectrum of Illness Due to Infection

Host	Infectious agent expected	Altered
Expected	Classical disease[a]	Atypical disease
Altered[b]	Atypical disease	Atypical disease

[a]The prototype of "textbook" example.
[b]Altered host may result from human intervention or critical genetic variation.

illnesses or deaths and to explore their possible origins (1). Historically, application of Koch–Evans postulates (Table 2) is required to establish a cause-and-effect relationship between a microorganism and a disease (2). This set of criteria for causation of disease contains requirements in the areas of prevalence, exposure, incidence, timing of exposure, host responses, experimental reproduction of the disease, consequences of modification of the etiology, prevention, and biological plausibility. How these criteria are met in the era of molecular and genetic diagnosis remains to be determined. One additional component of many of the EBV-associated conditions is identification of a reactivated infection, a process not addressed in the Koch–Evans postulates, nor uniformly defined.

Besides deciding upon the method by which patients are identified, detection of diseases that are or may be caused by EBV requires selection and application of

Table 2 Koch–Evans Criteria for Causation: A Unified Concept

1. *Prevalence* of the disease should be significantly higher in those exposed to the putative cause than in cases controls not so exposed.[a]
2. *Exposure* to the putative cause should present more commonly in those with the disease than in controls without the disease when all risk factors are held constant.
3. *Incidence* of the disease should be significantly higher in those exposed to the putative cause than in those not so exposed as shown in prospective studies.
4. *Temporally*, the disease should *follow* exposure to the putative agent with a distribution of incubation periods on a bell shaped curve.
5. *A spectrum* of host responses should follow exposure to the putative agent along a logical biologic gradient from mild to severe.
6. *A measurable host response* following exposure to the putative cause should *regularly appear* in those lacking this before exposure (i.e., antibody and cancer cells) or should *increase* in magnitude if present before exposure; this pattern should not occur in persons so exposed.
7. *Experimental reproduction* of the disease should occur in higher incidence in animals or humans appropriately exposed to the putative cause than in those not so exposed; this exposure may be deliberate in volunteers, experimentally induced in the laboratory, or demonstrated in a controlled regulation of natural exposure.
8. *Elimination or modification* of the putative cause or of the vector carrying it should decrease the incidence of the disease (control of polluted water or smoke or removal of the specific agent).
9. *Prevention or modification* of the host's response on exposure to the putative cause should decrease or eliminate the disease (immunization, drug to lower cholesterol, and specific lymphocyte transfer factor in cancer).
10. The whole thing should make biologic and epidemiologic sense.

[a]The putative cause may exist in the external environment or in a defect in host response.
Source: From Ref. 2.

laboratory procedures that support the clinical suspicion. Methods by which this goal can be achieved include detection of isotype-specific antibodies by immunofluorescent techniques, enzyme-linked techniques, or Western blotting; detection of neutralizing antibodies using a neutralization assay based on interference of lymphocyte transformation; detection of viral proteins by immunohistochemical methods, by touch preps, or direct detection; the transformation assay, a time-consuming culture method involving growth of EBV-transformed naive B-lymphocytes, and virocyte assay, which is an endpoint dilution assay to estimate the number of virus-containing cells (virocytes) in peripheral blood; detection of viral RNA or viral DNA detection by dot blotting, Southern blotting, gene amplification, or in situ hybridization; and clonality assay to identify circular (episomal) and linear forms of EBV (3–7). The list of laboratory methods used for establishing a causal role of EBV has changed considerably from a similar list published in 1984 (8). These procedures may be applied to serum, plasma or other body fluids, isolated cells, and tissue samples. Fresh material is only required for examination of some types of viral gene expression. Noticeably missing from these approaches are conventional primary and secondary virus culture techniques because EBV cannot be cultured using standard virologic culture methods incorporating tissue monolayers. Use of nonspecific antibody responses, such as the heterophile antibody, does not establish causality because it does not identify EBV-specific proteins. These antibodies may be present in conditions in which EBV is not playing a pathogenic role. Use of EBV-specific antibodies to establish causality is problematic for EBV and other herpesvirus infections because these viruses establish lifelong infection in the host with enduring antigen exposure and lifelong detectable antibody responses.

Associations of illnesses or diseases with EBV are often initially based on the observation of individual or clustered clinical findings that may or may not occur in typical infectious mononucleosis. The pathways by which certain specific, uncommon manifestations were considered to be associated with EBV are often unclear, but these manifestations were frequently noted before or after identification of classical infectious mononucleosis. Because some clinical illnesses caused by infectious agents require a measured host response as well as the agent itself, host factors obviously play a role in illness expression. An important question to be asked of any manifestation attributed to EBV infection is whether a host factor affects the clinical illness as much or more than the virus itself. This issue is perhaps particularly important when a manifestation is rare, and most of the diagnostic procedures are designed to identify the infectious agent. The host immune responses associated with infectious mononucleosis are fairly well understood (see Chapters 4 and 5), but other than antibody levels directed against selected marker proteins, immune responses are not assayed in routine diagnostic testing. As more is learned about the genetics of the host response, for example, the Vβ repertoire expressed on T-cells during the different stages of ongoing EBV infections, application of such tools may be helpful in identifying true, active infection versus past exposure (9).

Determination of ongoing infection or the host response as the principal mechanism of causing symptoms is especially important from the standpoint of recommending specific antiviral treatment. If the infection produces new virions and the symptom is a direct consequence of the productive infection and the ongoing host response, interruption of active, productive replication is a reasonable goal, such as with an antiviral agent. Active host responses to an infection associated with new virion production may also be amenable to therapy. If the illness is simply associated with the presence of the virus in its latent state, it is important to query whether this state is influencing cell function and directly or indirectly contributing to the illness in question, such as with lymphoproliferative disease in the immunosuppressed host. In the latter case, it is uncertain if it is more important to try and affect the virus, the involved cell, or the process allowing uncontrolled growth of the cell. In the not so distant past, attribution of a disease to a specific virus was viewed as an academic exercise or as provision of epidemiologic information. The time for consideration of therapy of these diseases is now at hand.

LABORATORY DETECTION OF EBV INFECTION

Several recommended practices including characterization of antibody patterns, magnitude of the antibody response, and the presence and quantity of EBV in cells, tissues, serum, or plasma may greatly affect the determination of whether the virus is a participant in disease production. Interpretation of antibody patterns as determined by either the immunofluorescent antibody assay (IFA) technique or by identification of specific viral proteins on a solid base is based on the responses first observed by Henle et al. (10) utilizing IFA. The standard interpretation is that anti–viral capsid antigen (VCA) antibodies of the immunoglobulin M (IgM) class, with or without IgG anti-VCA, reflect acute, active infection. The presence of anti–early antigen (EA) antibodies, and simultaneous absence of anti–Epstein–Barr nuclear antigen (EBNA) antibodies, suggests and supports an active infection. Because anti-EBNA-2 antibodies precede anti-EBNA-1 antibodies, this pattern also suggests an early EBV infection (6).

Another assumption that affects the determination of disease causality is the magnitude of specific antibody levels. This concept for EBV infections is based on studies that utilized IFA titers as the measurement technique as applied to "severe active disease." However, the magnitude of such values, often expressed in geometric mean titers, does not seem to be of importance prognostically in the course of infectious mononucleosis, the disease in which their presence is of primary significance. Few studies have compared the current commonly used methods such as enzyme-linked immunosorbent assay (ELISA) to the IFA correlation; of those comparisons, the results are mixed (11).

Detection of either viral DNA or RNA by a variety of means is now a very important diagnostic tool. Two of the commonly used procedures rely upon the natural superabundance of certain viral genomic elements. The detection of RNA is frequently based on identification of EBV-encoded RNAs (EBERs), which are present in levels of up to 10^6 copies per cell, while *Bam*HI W (the large internal repeat) restriction fragments are repeated six to eight or more times in each EBV genome. EBERs are primarily, if not only, expressed when the virus is in one or all of its latent states (12). Viral DNA is obviously present in both the actively replicating form, with new virion production, and the latent form of infection. The prevailing assumption is that the EBV genome is in its latent form in tissue, and therefore identification by detection of EBERs or by the presence of proteins associated with latency, such as latent membrane protein 1 (LMP-1), will best identify the virus in all clinical specimens. There are two glaring exceptions to this approach—hairy cell leukoplakia and some EBV genome–bearing T-cell lymphomas (13,14). EBERs are not detected in these two conditions. Likewise, biopsy specimens of other tissues have been negative for these two markers in conditions where a clinical illness consistent with an active infection is present. Some of these conditions also lack diagnostic changes even in the presence of anti-EBV antibodies. Thus a number of observations suggest that if the primary purpose of performing these assays is detection of the virus, a sensitive system that allows detection of virus per se is desirable (15).

Examination of peripheral blood by polymerase chain reaction (PCR) is another tool that is being used increasingly in attempts to identify EBV infection. Quantitative techniques using whole blood are particularly helpful for the detection of cell-associated virus in lymphoproliferative diseases. Questions still remain whether quantitation of free viral DNA in serum or plasma is necessary to determine if an active infection, with new virion replication and release, is present. Free viral DNA is present during acute infection in plasma and serum and in cavity fluids containing EBV-associated malignant cells (16,17). Yamamoto et al. measured viral DNA by densitometry of Southern blots following PCR (18). The amount of virus varied in the following clinical diagnoses: infectious mononucleosis, fatal infectious mononucleosis, EBV-associated hemophagocytic syndrome, chronic active EBV, and healthy seronegativity and seropositivity in subjects. Only the plasma and serum of both seropositive and seronegative children were free of viral genomes. There was considerable overlap among the positive groups, and no statistical analyses were applied. Quantitative techniques based on competitive inhibition have also been described (19).

METHODOLOGICAL ISSUES AND THEIR APPLICATIONS

Gene amplification principles were in use prior to PCR techniques in detection of EBV DNA by exploiting the internal repeat in *Bam*HI W as the probe because of multiple copies of this repeat in each viral genome (3). The amplification technique using EBERs may be more sensitive but detects virus only in the latent state. Thus, the assumption that a very sensitive technique can be utilized in every circumstance without an understanding of the viral replicative state—latent or lytic— presents potential problems.

Another issue is to determine whether the pattern of antibody response or the reference level of specific antibodies is most meaningful in the establishment of a causal relationship between the virus and disease. For instance, are there factors that influence the magnitude of response in large segments of the population in which hypothesized disease relationships may be uncommon? For example, elevated anti-EA levels are seen in the elderly, in women in the latter stages of pregnancy, and in individuals with IgE-mediated allergy. Do these or other conditions contribute to the elevated titers seen in the populations under study?

CLINICAL ILLNESSES

A review of some of the illnesses that have been associated with EBV illustrates the application of various diagnostic tools to previously described illnesses. As of 1976 and 1980, reviews of diseases caused by EBV (20,21) discussed only Burkitt lymphoma, nasopharyngeal carcinoma (NPC), and infectious mononucleosis as being definitely associated with EBV. Of 11 possible conditions listed by Andiman (8) in 1984, seven illnesses were identified by serological means alone—Gianotti–Crosti syndrome, Guillain–Barré syndrome, virus-associated hemophagocytic syndrome, Kawasaki syndrome, selected lymphomas, postperfusion syndrome, and Reye's syndrome. The others, including acquired immunodeficiency syndrome in children, malignant histiocytosis, primary central nervous system lymphoma, Parinaud's oculoglandular syndrome, and pneumonia, were suspected on the basis of serologic and either molecular or virologic techniques. This expanded list of virus-associated diseases began to appear in 1979. Several of these entities continue to have tenuous associations with EBV, including Kawasaki syndrome, postperfusion syndrome, Reye's syndrome, and malignant histiocytosis. The remainder continues to share a close association.

Diseases of the Oral Cavity

Several of the possible associations of oral lesions with EBV are based on established observations. Benign salivary gland lesions in patients with and without human immunodeficiency virus (HIV) infection were evaluated only for EBERs. Only tissues from HIV-infected individuals were positive (22). Another study of oral lesions associated with HIV—oral hairy leukoplakia, pseudo-oral hairy leukoplakia, aphthous ulcers, and oral Kaposi sarcoma—found that Southern blot analysis for EBV replication was frequently negative in pseudohairy leukoplakia, aphthous ulcers, and Kaposi sarcoma, but DNA PCR was positive in all samples. The lack of specificity and extreme sensitivity of the procedures led the authors to conclude that contamination was responsible for the PCR findings (23).

A new association was proposed in the case of oral lichen planus. Patients with this condition were found to have a higher prevalence of anti-EA antibodies, but there was a negative correlation between duration of oral lichen planus symptoms and IgG anti-EA (24).

Molecular techniques have also been applied in some studies with apparent negative results. In an attempt to identify conditions leading to NPC in a geographic area of high prevalence, tissue specimens from workers in a newspaper-printing company who had chronic pharyngitis and sinusitis were evaluated. The presence of EBERs and colocalization with secretor protein were not found to predict NPC (25). Because EBERs are only expressed primarily during latency, the absence of EBERs may not exclude the absence of EBV in tissues.

Diseases of the Gastrointestinal Tract

Gastrointestinal involvement of EBV has been sought in variety of conditions. Recently, EBV was found in liver tissue by RT-PCR and in situ hybridization in a case of acute/chronic infection accompanied by vanishing bile duct syndrome in which anti-EBNA values were only 1:10, and cell-free EBV DNA was present in serum. The patient also had hemophagocytosis and perforations in the small bowel, but survived the illness (26). A very thorough review by Markin (27) in 1994 did not identify EBV involvement in diseases affecting the liver that are outside of known conditions.

Several reports identified EBV in involved tissue obtained from patients with Crohn's disease and ulcerative colitis. In one report, the virus was detected in DNA isolated from these diseased sites. EBV was more frequently seen in ulcerative colitis, but cytomegalovirus DNA and human herpesvirus type 6 (HHV-6) DNA were present only slightly less frequently. Control specimens were also positive, but less often than any of the patient samples. Virus-positive cells in peripheral blood were uncommon (28). This topic was addressed further by Yanai et al. (29) who performed in situ evaluation for EBERs and immunochemistry for cell identification. EBERs were found in B-cells or histiocyte-shaped cells in 60% of cases with each condition. The virus-containing cells were limited to diseased portions of the colon. Causality was not demonstrated in either report.

In another probative study, EBV was not found to be associated with either idiopathic megarectum or idiopathic megacolon (30).

Diseases of the Nervous System

Many of the cases of nervous system disease considered to be due to EBV have their counterparts in typical infectious mononucleosis (31,32). In some cases, only the central nervous system appears to be involved (see Chapter 8). Cerebellitis was identified clinically by severe headache, swollen hemispheres, and consequences of transforaminal herniation, but with an otherwise normal neurological examination. The association with EBV was based only on positive IgM anti-VCA antibodies at the time of admission to the hospital, with subsequently decreasing levels (33). Other cases are reported in conjunction with previously described central nervous system involvement. Two such instances accompanied meningoencephalitis. One was transient global amnesia and oscillopsia or jumbling phenomenon. In each instance, serological changes from acute to postinfection status were recorded (34). Optic neuritis has also been reported.

Several types of peripheral nerve involvement have been reported and include cranial nerve palsy, radiculopathy, plexopathy, and peripheral neuropathy. The cases are associated with either development of primary infectious mononucleosis or immediately follow the typical syndrome, with confirmation based on serological tests. The peripheral neuropathies per se consisted of subacute sensory neuropathy or inflammation of dorsal columns (35). This association was made based on simply the presence of an antibody pattern of past exposure.

A few cases of combined central and peripheral involvement have been identified using serological and molecular techniques. Myeloradiculitis and/or encephalomyeloradiculitis was identified by the presence of stiff neck, mental changes, weakness, and sensory loss. Two of the four cases had magnetic resonance image (MRI) abnormalities. The cerebrospinal fluid (CSF) demonstrated a pleocytosis and an increased total protein, but normal glucose levels. Diagnostic antibody changes were present in serum and CSF (36,37). Fisher syndrome, consisting of external ophthalmoplegia, ataxia, and areflexia, has also been associated with EBV. Eye findings included impaired vertical and horizontal movements, no pupillary reflexes, and enhanced ptosis (from a baseline of mild ptosis). Serology during an acute mononucleosis-like illness was positive for anti–EBV IgM that persisted until the Fisher complex appeared two months into the illness. No anti-EBNA was present initially, but IgG anti-VCA was present throughout the course (38).

Involvement of the autonomic nervous system is not commonly appreciated, but such an association was noted as early as 1972 based on serological tests (39). One form of presentation, as reported in an adult, is with burning pain, skin sensitivity, pupillary enlargement, trouble focusing visually, decreased taste sensation, prolonged urination, and constipation. The physical examination in this case identified decreased pinprick, allodynia, and vibration sense. Laboratory findings included EBV DNA in CSF and a serum antibody pattern that suggested remote infection. The authors queried a reactivated infection (40). Another case questioned a cause-and-effect relationship in a child with a previous history of persistent intestinal obstruction. After a febrile illness associated with pharyngitis, he developed an acute abdominal pain and underwent a laparotomy. He developed postoperative pancreatitis, hepatitis, orthostasis, altered consciousness, and seizures. He developed anti-EBNA antibodies in serum, and EBV was detected in the CSF by PCR. His peripheral B-cells underwent spontaneous transformation, and he was EBER-positive in mesenteric lymph nodes, appendix, and stomach. He was presumed to have a diagnosis of acquired hypoganglionosis. The histological evaluation did not show inflammation or preexisting obstruction. The authors were hesitant to label this situation as being caused by EBV (41).

Diseases of the Lungs

Pulmonary involvement in EBV-associated conditions appears to be quite diverse. The proposed illnesses can be divided into those with lymphoid cell infiltration or fibrosis. A case of interstitial lymphoid and granulomatous pneumonia was accompanied by acute serological changes (without anti-EBNA), the presence of EBNA protein in biopsy specimens, and the presence of DNA as observed by PCR and by Southern blot analysis. This patient also displayed presumed granulomatous lesions in the brain and genital ulcers, as observed using MRI. The patient was unable to inhibit outgrowth of EBV-infected autologous B-cells and had no spontaneous interferon (IFN) gamma production. Clinical resolution was associated with IFN gamma therapy (42).

Follicular bronchitis–bronchiolitis characterizes hyperplasia of the bronchus-associated lymphoid tissue and is considered to be part of the spectrum of lymphoid interstitial pneumonitis. The latter has been shown to be associated with EBV infection in HIV-infected patients and also in immunocompetent persons, whereas the follicular form has not been studied as a distinct entity (43,44).

Pulmonary lymphomatoid granulomatosis has been recognized as a pathological diagnosis for many years. Early studies in the 1980s questioned a role for EBV, but were based only on serologic testing. EBV DNA was found by Southern blot analysis and in situ hybridization, but the cells containing the virus were not identified. A T-cell origin of the infection was proposed. In a study that did double label cells in situ, the virus was found to reside solely in B-cells, but a marked T-cell response surrounded the granulomata. There were no serological studies in the report (45).

Pulmonary fibrosis identified on clinical grounds was associated with elevated IgG anti-VCA titers compared to controls. This study also found increased IgG anti-cytomegalovirus (CMV) and anti-herpes simplex virus (HSV) antibodies (46). In cryptogenic fibrosing alveolitis, an association had been made with serological and DNA findings. A second exploration of the question could not find a correlation with the presence of viral proteins, DNA, or EBERs in affected lung tissue. Similar amounts of viral proteins were identified in normal lungs and with other illnesses not thought to be associated with EBV (47).

Diseases of the Skin

Gianotti–Crosti syndrome continues to appear in the literature in conjunction with possible EBV infection. It begins with the acute onset of symmetrical, 2- to 3-mm flesh-colored or red papules on face and limbs, with truncal sparing. At least four other agents—*Mycoplasma pneumoniae*, cytomegalovirus, hepatitis B, and HIV—as well as measles and influenza immunizations have been associated with the syndrome. An outbreak of the syndrome was proposed in five out of twelve 13- to 15-month-old children in childcare. The authors identified both IgM anti-VCA and IgM anti-EBNA in all five affected children. Two healthy control children had only IgG anti-EBV (48).

Erythema multiforme frequently occurs in association with infections. An adult with chronic fatigue syndrome (CFS), itching, and erythema of hands and fingers 10 years ago had a diagnosis of infectious mononucleosis. Viral serologies had positive anti-VCA, EA, and low (1:2) anti-EBNA antibody titers. Several months into the illness, skin biopsies were positive by in situ hybridization utilizing a probe for *Bam*HI W. After a long course, the skin cleared following treatment with acyclovir (49). Cytophagic histiocytic panniculitis tissue during a nonmalignant infiltrative stage was EBER-negative. As the process evolved into a fatal, subcutaneous T-cell lymphoma, the samples became EBER-positive. No antibody testing was performed (50). Patients with chronic urticaria, as defined by urticaria of more than two months and no other explanations, had EBV with low to absent anti-EBNA (<1:40). Plasma or serum specimens were positive for EBV by PCR, and patients had a positive clinical response to antiviral therapy (Jones JF, unpublished).

Diseases of the Lower Genitourinary Tract

Genitourinary tract involvement with EBV is a relatively recent concept (51). Penile skin lesions as detected by application of acetic acid have a histological appearance similar to lesions associated with human papillomaviruses (HPV). PCR analysis for EBV and HPV yielded 15% of subjects with both viral DNAs, 45% with HPV DNA only, 5% (one case) with EBV DNA only, and 35% with the DNA of neither agent (52). EBV carriage detected by PCR in asymptomatic individuals was 28% on the cervix and 13% in the sulcus coronus in uncircumcised subjects (53). Two observed cases of genital ulcers in women and five in the literature were recently summarized (54). Five cases had IgM anti-VCA in the first week of illness; a tissue sample from the genital ulcers of one of the two cases was found to be positive for EBV by PCR. A systemic illness was present in all cases. A positive heterophile antibody and atypical lymphocytes were present in five subjects, but only two had pharyngitis. Painful ulcers were present in all cases. The ulcers had purple borders and were associated with distal lymphadenopathy. Resolution of the illness occurred after two to five weeks.

Association with urogenital tumors has been suggested. Vaginal malakoplakia and non-Hodgkin's lymphoma have been observed. Malakoplakia is an inflammatory disorder with histiocytes containing Michaelis–Gutman bodies. Two such cases with only the inflammatory lesions and a third with the inflammation and lymphoma containing immunoglobulin heavy chain gene rearrangements and EBV have been reported (55). Because the epidemiology of testicular tumors is similar to that of Hodgkin's disease, a study of untreated, stage 1 germ cell tumors compared antibody titers for EBV, CMV, hepatitis A, and hepatitis B. The tests showed that 80% of subjects were EBV seropositive with "elevated titers" (>1:128), compared to the laboratory mean values. Only 20% of control subjects' values were elevated (56).

Diseases of the Kidneys

Renal disease associated with EBV is a mixed story. Previous reports based on serology include IgA nephropathy, minimal change nephrotic syndrome, hemolytic-uremic syndrome, interstitial nephritis (most common in infectious mononucleosis), and post-transplant lymphoproliferative disorder (PTLD). A patient with mesangial disease had EBV in the blood and spleen, but there was no evaluation of renal parenchyma.

In addition, the patient was EBV seronegative, but had normal serum immunoglobulin levels. Another patient with PTLD did have virus in the transplanted kidney detected by both PCR and in situ hybridization, but also had negative serology (57).

Diseases of the Eyes

Descriptions of ophthalmologic disorders attributed to EBV appear to comprise a disproportionately high number of these reports. A retrospective review of intermediate uveitis described undocumented serological findings in a small patient population with only two of 83 patients with a history suggestive of EBV infection (58). Conjunctival lymphocytic infiltrates appear to have a specific relationship to EBV. One patient with pharyngitis, tender preauricular lymph node, and a bulbar conjunctival mass had both IgG and IgM antibodies (presumably anti-VCA). The excised mass was positive for B and T-cell markers and for EBV LMP-1 by immunocytochemistry. An eight-year-old patient with bilateral progressively enlarging conjunctival masses was found to have clonal B-cells by immunophenotyping and heavy chain PCR analysis. Cells in the masses were positive for LMP-1, but no antibody testing was performed. There was no recurrence after excision (59).

Two other conditions are based on antibody result alone. First, aqueous tear deficiency, with decreased tearing, was suggested with the only finding of importance being higher anti-VCA IgG and anti-EA than control subjects, though overlap for VCA titers was considerable. True Sjögren syndrome patients had a more severe reduction in tear production (60). Second, multifocal choroiditis and panuveitis, presenting with blurred vision, were suggested based on positive IgM anti-VCA or anti-EA, but all patients had anti-EBNA, thus suggesting old EBV infection. Eight control subjects with other eye diseases had no anti-EA antibodies (61).

Chronic Mononucleosis

In the early 1980s, there were several reports of "chronic mononucleosis" (62–64) that described prolonged clinical courses of mononucleosis-like illnesses. The clinical symptoms included fatigue, low-grade fever, myalgias, depression, headaches, recurrent pharyngitis, impaired cognition, sleep disorder, anxiety, lymphadenopathy, nausea, arthralgias, and paresthesias. The putative association was based on clinical symptoms and EBV serologies, particularly the presence of anti-EA in patients, but not in control subjects. Jones et al. (65) and Straus et al. (66) described similar patient cohorts and also based the relationship to EBV on the presence of anti-EA antibodies, but considered these patients to be having an active EBV infection in the absence of findings typical of classical infectious mononucleosis. Anti-EA antibodies of the IgG class with titers greater than 1:40 were considered to be abnormal if outside of the acute infection period, and consistent with an ongoing infection. In each of these reports the attribution of the illnesses was based on the clinical syndrome and an antibody pattern associated with active infection, therefore the name "chronic active EBV infection." Because such an illness was only thought to occur in an immune compromised host, immune function was tested, but was found to be normal. Other studies that questioned a relationship between this symptom complex and EBV soon followed (67).

A more severe form of chronic active EBV was proposed if IgG anti-VCA titers were greater than 1:10,000, anti-EA titers were greater than 1:640, and anti-EBNA titers were less than 1:40 (68). These individuals shared symptoms with the previously described group but were more apt to have altered hematological tests and immunoglobulin values (69). Some of this latter group was found to have elevated levels of anti-DNAase antibodies (70), T-cell lymphomas (3), and, more recently, elevated anti-gp350/220 antibodies (71).

The severe chronic form of EBV infection has remained an important clinical entity (72). Milder forms of chronic EBV infection per se appear to occur sporadically, but without definitive diagnostic criteria. Some of these individuals experienced a prolonged course of convalescence following typical infectious mononucleosis, while others present with hematological problems that subsequently are found to have EBV as their basis. An absence of anti-EBNA antibodies may herald this form of illness. Some individuals with such a process have been found to have circulating free viral DNA, utilizing a semiquantitative assay along with frequent positive spontaneous transformation (Xu JW, unpublished data).

Chronic Fatigue Syndrome

Many of the illnesses subsequently diagnosed as CFS were initially considered to be "chronic mononucleosis" or chronic active EBV. The chronic active infection concept was based on the presence of anti-EA titers that were above titers of 1:80. In the early 1980s, such levels were thought to be indicative of an active EBV infection. Not all patients with the syndrome had elevated anti-EA titers, however, and many normal control subjects demonstrate such levels (67). In addition, the concept that elevated anti-EA levels are indicative of active infection has been shown to be incorrect in longitudinal studies. This set of symptoms now falls under the name of CFS. This designation followed a number of studies that could not show a definite relationship between the symptom complex and EBV or other infectious agents (73). The 1988 version of the definition relied upon six months of fatigue, 50% reduction in activity, two of three signs and 6 of 11 symptoms or 8 symptoms in the absence of signs. Studies that identified patients on the basis of the syndromic criteria still found patients with elevated anti-EBV antibody titers compared to control populations (74). The definition was changed in 1994 to address concerns that the numbers of symptoms included in the 1988 version may identify subjects with somatizing disorders and the failure to substantiate the presence of the three signs (75). The emphasis was placed on fatigue in general as a morbid process, and no laboratory criteria were proposed. The 1994 version requires fatigue of greater than six months, no other medical or psychiatric diagnosis that might explain the fatigue, and four of the following eight problems accompanying the fatigue: pharyngitis, cervical or axillary lymph node swelling or pain, arthralgias, myalgias, sleep disturbance, cognitive problems, headache, or an increase in symptoms and malaise following exertion. It should be emphasized that CFS, in general, is not related to EBV or any other infectious agent. However, infectious agents (including EBV) may produce prolonged illnesses that can account for the symptoms seen in occasional patients that would otherwise fulfill criteria for CFS. The syndrome should only be considered if other disease processes have been excluded during a careful evaluation of the patient in question.

IDENTIFICATION OF EBV AS A POTENTIAL CAUSE OF AUTOIMMUNE DISEASE

Most studies have attempted to either identify EBV as the etiology of a clinical syndrome or link an uncommon manifestation with EBV using the laboratory or epidemiologic tools available at the time of the research, and the understanding generated by use of the available tools. Now those and newer tools are being used in attempts to link EBV with a myriad of other clinical presentations. Two of the conditions that are receiving renewed interest are systemic lupus erythematosus (SLE) and multiple sclerosis (MS).

The activation of B-cells and the potential for alteration of T-cell function that occurs in primary EBV infection are interesting prospects in the etiology of autoimmune diseases. The early questions positing a relationship between EBV and SLE began to appear in the 1970s (76). An excellent example is the onset of SLE during the course of infectious mononucleosis. A case described by Dror et al. (77) is instructive. The patient produced autoantibodies, had evidence of complement activation, and developed SLE nephritis with renal tissue that was positive for complement and EBV VCA protein. Only anti-VCA IgG and IgM antibodies were obtained, and both were positive. No molecular studies were obtained. This case is similar to another case before the advent of readily available molecular techniques (Jones JF, unpublished). In that case, a teenaged girl with typical infectious mononucleosis developed arthritis in both knees and skin lesions with malar and knee distribution that are typical of SLE. She continued to have elevated anti-EA titers and absence of anti-EBNA for many months, along with antinuclear antibody (ANA) titers greater than 1:1280. Her peripheral blood lymphocytes underwent spontaneous transformation, and she responded rapidly to a course of oral corticosteroids. SLE became the dominant disease.

Another set of observations is based on population studies. For example, serological and virological studies were performed on a group of adolescents previously diagnosed with SLE. All were EBV seropositive. Some had patterns considered to be primary or "active," with positive IgM anti-VCA or negative EBNA, while others had a "reactivated" pattern, with all EBV antibodies positive except VCA-IgM as determined by an ELISA system (78). The cells of two "reactive" subjects underwent spontaneous transformation, but no subjects' cells were found to be PCR positive using DNA probes.

A second autoimmune disease that has been associated with EBV is MS. This concept is also not new (79). Most early studies were based on antibodies to EBV in either serum or CSF. More recently, no viral genomes were found in the brain of MS subjects or control subjects by PCR (80). The serological data reviewed above showed 100% prevalence of EBV antibodies with higher anti-VCA and anti-EBNA-1 antibody levels in MS than in control persons. It also appeared that MS patients had a higher frequency of having had clinically apparent infectious mononucleosis. There also appeared to be an increased relative risk based on infection alone. In a recent prospective population study, the magnitude of antibody levels as compared between MS patients and healthy control persons continues to be used to support a relationship between the virus and MS (81). The apparent higher titers in MS were present before the onset of the neurological symptoms and findings. The authors interpreted these findings to show a specific response to EBV in patients and not a nonspecific response as a consequence of disease. However, no explanation is given for "why 'high' anti-EBV titers support a relationship to the pathogenesis of MS." High anti-EA titers are seen in a number of situations, and there are very few data regarding levels of anti-EBNA 2 antibodies in population-based studies.

Recent reports have hypothesized a link between infection and the pathophysiology of atherosclerosis (82). The list of agents includes *Chlamydia pneumoniae*, *Helicobacter pylori*, cytomegalovirus, herpes simplex virus, and EBV. Microorganism

DNA in plaques and serological evidence of inflammation by the presence of C-reactive protein support the concept of an infectious component in the development of atherosclerosis. Attempts to identify EBV in plaques has yielded conflicting results. One report suggests that antibody evidence of multiple infections, including EBV, is associated with vascular disease. The magnitude of the response to this virus alone, however, was not predictive (83).

SYNTHESIS

Deciphering the cause and effect of infectious diseases is a complex process. It is particularly difficult if the infectious agent remains in the host in a latent state but can undergo reactivation, as is the case for EBV and other herpesviruses. The host develops responses to each stage of infection.

Can these myriad observations of EBV and clinical manifestations be incorporated into Evans' modifications of Henle–Koch's postulates? For example, are different viral promoter regions (e.g., Fp, Qp, and Cp promoter use) expressed in tissue or lymphoid cells in identifiable clinical conditions (84)? Katz et al. (85) asked a similar question using the structure of EBV termini. Thus, not only would the genome be identifiable, but also its stage of replication would be of importance. Accompanying genome presence and stage of replication should be evidence of the host response to that process. Are there viral peptides that evoke a measurable response that is specific to the various stages of replication? Should we be evaluating antibody responses to these peptides as a means of identifying active infections? Measurements of EBV viral load using semiquantitative and quantitative techniques could be applied if they truly allow establishment of widely applicable criteria for recognition of disease (86,87).

Reactivation of EBV infection needs to be universally defined, and the definition needs to be applied uniformly. Should such a definition depend on identification of replicating virus? If so, where should replicating virus be sought? Because it is unusual to find free viral DNA in any body cavity in the absence of replication, free viral DNA detected quantitatively or semiquantitatively may be considered to be a component of such a definition. This concept does not include lymphoproliferative diseases in which there are an increased number of cells carrying latent state forms of the genome. The quantity of the latent viral genomes appears to be of importance here. In this case, is the clinical entity a reactivation of infection or is the problem purely secondary to diminished host responses or evolving tumor development? Which aspect of the host response might be the most important for tumor development?

Are there specific host responses that are important for discerning reactivation of infection? For example, loss or decrease of anti-EBNA-1 antibodies accompanies the presence of free viral DNA. The concept that reactivation of infection is accompanied by the reappearance of IgM anti-VCA antibodies is poorly documented, and is difficult to reconcile with the last of Koch–Evans postulates—the causation data make biologic and epidemiologic sense. Rather than assuming that the reappearance of such antibodies represents reactivation, acquisition of a different strain of EBV that expresses a different EBNA-1 protein is also possible. The presence of a different pattern of antibody responses as determined by Western blot analysis was seen in reactivated varicella infections (88). There do not appear to be any studies of the cell-mediated response as it pertains to differentiation between primary and reactivated responses.

The clinical examples vary widely as being supporting evidence of EBV being the causative agent in the various syndromes. These examples teach us that we must have purpose and rigor in the identification of EBV (or any infectious agent) in clinical settings. We must also have an understanding of the virus and its mode and timing of replication—its "life cycle"—along with knowledge of the host responses to infection. We must decide early in the course of the patient's evaluation whether we are seeking information to be used therapeutically in treating the infection, the host response, or both. We must be willing to rigorously apply widely accepted diagnostic criteria for the situation. We cannot assume that simply sending a specimen to the laboratory for the newest test will answer the question of causality.

REFERENCES

1. Hajjeh RA, Relman D, Cieslak PR, et al. Surveillance for unexplained deaths and critical illnesses due to possibly infectious causes, United States, 1995–1998. Emerg Infect Dis 2002; 8:145–153.
2. Evans AS. Causation and disease: Henle-Koch postulates revisited. Yale J 1976; 49:175–195.
3. Jones J, Shurin S, Abramowsky C, et al. T-cell lymphomas containing Epstein–Barr viral DNA in patients with chronic Epstein–Barr virus infections. N Engl J Med 1988; 318:733–741.
4. Jones JF, Streib J, Baker S, Herberger M. Chronic fatigue syndrome: I. Epstein–Barr virus immune response and molecular epidemiology. J Med Vir 1991; 33:151–158.
5. Ryon JJ, Hayward D, MacMahon EME, et al. In situ detection of lytic Epstein–Barr virus infection: Expression of the *Not*1 early gene and viral interleukin-10 late gene in clinical specimens. J Infect Dis 1993; 168:345–351.
6. Linde A. Diagnosis of Epstein–Barr virus-related diseases. Scand J Infect Dis 1996; 100:S83–S88.
7. Gulley M. Molecular diagnosis of Epstein–Barr virus-related diseases. J Mol Diag 2001; 3:1–10.
8. Andiman WA. Epstein–Barr virus-associated syndromes: a critical reexamination. Pediatr Infect Dis 1984; 84:198–203.
9. Smith T, Terada N, Robinson CC, Gelfand W. Acute infectious mononucleosis stimulates the selective expression/expansion of $V_\beta 6.1$–3 and $V_\beta 7$ T cells. Blood 1993; 81:1521–1526.
10. Henle W, Henle G, Horwitz CA. Epstein–Barr virus-specific diagnostic tests in infectious mononucleosis. Hum Pathol 1974; 5:551–565.
11. Rea TD, Ashley RL, Russo JE, Buchwald DS. A systematic study of Epstein–Barr virus serologic assays following acute infection. Am J Clin Pathol 2002; 117:156–161.
12. Ambinder R, Mann R. Epstein–Barr-encoded RNA in situ hybridization: diagnostic applications. Hum Pathol 1994; 25:602–605.
13. Gilligan K, Rajadurai P, Resnick L, Raab-Traub N. Epstein–Barr virus small nuclear RNAs are not expressed in permissively infected cells in AIDS-associated leukoplakia. Proc Natl Acad Sci USA 1990; 87:8790–8794.
14. Chen CL, Sadler RH, Walling DM, Su IJ, Hsieh HC, Raab-Traub N. Epstein–Barr virus (EBV) gene expression in EBV-positive peripheral T-cell lymphomas. J Virol 1993; 67:6303–6308.
15. Iwatsuki K, Xu Z, Ohtsuka M, Kaneko F. Cutaneous lymphoproliferative disorders associated with Epstein–Barr virus infection: a clinical overview. J Dermatol Sci 2000; 22:181–195.
16. Gan YJ, Sullivan JL, Sixbey JW. Detection of cell-free Epstein–Barr virus DNA in serum during acute infectious mononucleosis. J Infect Dis 1994; 170:436–439.

17. McClain KL, Leach CT, Jenson HB, et al. Association of Epstein–Barr virus with leiomyosarcomas in children with AIDS. N Engl J Med 1995; 332:12–18.

18. Yamamoto M, Kimura H, Hironaka T, et al. Detection and quantification of virus DNA in plasma of patients with Epstein–Barr virus-associated diseases. J Clin Microbiol 1995; 33:1765–1768.

19. Rowe DT, Qu L, Reyes J, et al. Use of quantitative competitive PCR to measure Epstein–Barr virus genome load in the peripheral blood of pediatric transplant patients with lymphoproliferative disorders. J Clin Microbiol 1997; 35:1612–1615.

20. de-The G. Epstein–Barr virus behavior in different populations and implications for control of Epstein–Barr virus-associated tumors. Cancer Res 1976; 36:692–695.

21. Henle W, Henle G. Epidemiologic aspects of Epstein–Barr virus (EBV)-associated diseases. Ann NY Acad Sci 1980; 80:326–331.

22. DiGiuseppe JA, Wu T-C, Corio RL. Analysis of Epstein–Barr virus-encoded small RNA 1 expression in benign lymphoepithelial salivary gland lesions. Mod Pathol 1994; 7: 555–559.

23. Raab-Traub N, Webster-Cyriaque J. Epstein–Barr virus infection and expression in oral lesions. Oral Dis 1997; 3:S164–S170.

24. Pedersen A. Abnormal EBV immune status in oral lichen planus. Oral Dis 1996; 2: 125–128.

25. Liu Y-H, Du C-L, Lin C-T, Chan C-C, Chen C-J, Wang J-D. Increased morbidity from nasopharyngeal carcinoma and chronic pharyngitis or sinusitis among workers at a newspaper printing company. Occup Environ Med 2002; 59:18–22.

26. Kikuchi K, Miyakawa H, Abe K, et al. Vanishing bile duct syndrome associated with chronic EBV infection. Digest Dis Sci 2000; 45:160–165.

27. Markin RS. Manifestations of Epstein–Barr virus-associated disorders in liver. Liver 1994; 14:1–13.

28. Wakefield AJ, Fox JD, Sawyerr AM, et al. Detection of herpesvirus DNA in the large intestine of patients with ulcerative colitis and Crohn's disease using the nested polymerase chain reaction. J Med Vir 1992; 38:183–190.

29. Yanai H, Shimizu N, Nagasaki S, Mitani N, Okita K. Epstein–Barr virus infection of the colon with inflammatory bowel disease. Am J Gastroenterol 1999; 94:1582–1586.

30. Gattuso JM, Debinski HS, Kangro HO, Jeffries D, Kamm MA. Evaluation of specific herpes DNA viruses in idiopathic megarectum and idiopathic megacolon. Int J Colorectal Dis 1998; 13:131–133.

31. Connelly KP, DeWitt LD. Neurologic complications of infectious mononucleosis. Pediatr Neurol 1994; 10:181–184.

32. Grose C, Henle W, Henle G, Feorino PM. Primary Epstein–Barr virus infections in acute neurologic diseases. N Engl J Med 1975; 292:392–395.

33. Gohlich-Ratmann G, Wallot M, Baethmann M, et al. Acute cerebellitis with near-fatal cerebellar swelling and benign outcome under conservative treatment with high dose steroids. Eur J Paediatr Neurol 1998; 2:157–162.

34. Mizutani T, Murashima A, Shiozawa R, Kamel S. Unusual neurologic manifestations associated with Epstein–Barr virus infection. Intern Med 1993; 32:36–38.

35. Rubin DI, Daube JR. Subacute sensory neuropathy associated with Epstein–Barr virus. Muscle Nerve 1999; 22:1607–1610.

36. Mereli E, Bedin R, Sola P, et al. Encephalomyeloradiculopathy associated with Epstein–Barr virus: primary infection or reactivation? Acta Neurol Scand 1997; 96:416–420.

37. Majid A, Galetta SL, Sweeney CJ, et al. Epstein–Barr virus myeloradiculitis and encephalomyeloradiculitis. Brain 2002; 125:159–165.

38. Ishikawa H, Wakakura M, Ishikawa S. Enhanced ptosis in Fisher's syndrome after Epstein–Barr virus infection. J Clin Neurol Ophthalmol 1990; 10:197–200.

39. Fujii N, Tabira T, Shibasaki H, Kuroiwa Y, Ohnishi A, Nagaki J. Acute autonomic and sensory neuropathy associated with elevated Epstein–Barr virus antibody titre. J Neurol Neruosurg Psych 1982; 45:656–661.

40. Bennett JL, Mahalingam R, Wellish MC, Gilden DH. Epstein–Barr virus-associated acute autonomic neuropathy. Ann Neurol 1996; 40:453–455.
41. Besnard M, Faure C, Fromont-Hankard G, et al. Intestinal pseudo-obstruction and acute pandysautonomia associated with Epstein–Barr virus infection. Am J Gastroenterol 2000; 95:280–284.
42. Andersson J, Isberg B, Christensson B, Veress B, Linde A, Bratel T. Interferon γ (IFN-γ) deficiency in generalized Epstein–Barr virus infection with interstitial lymphoid and granulomatous pneumonia, focal cerebral lesions, and genital ulcers: remission following IFN-γ substitution therapy. Clin Infect Dis 1999; 28:1036–1042.
43. Koss MN. Pulmonary lymphoid disorders. In: Seminars in Diagnostic Pathology. Philadelphia, PA: W.B. Saunders, 1995:158–171.
44. Fishback N, Koss M. Update on lymphoid interstitial pneumonitis. Curr Opin Pulmonary Med 1996; 2:429–433.
45. Guinee JD, Jaffe E, Kingma D, et al. Pulmonary lymphomatoid granulomatosis. Am J Surg Pathol 1994; 18:753–764.
46. Yonemaru M, Kasuga I, Kusumoto H, et al. Elevation of antibodies to cytomegalovirus and other herpes viruses in pulmonary fibrosis. Eur Respir J 1997; 10:2040–2045.
47. Wangoo A, Shaw RJ, Diss TC, Farrell PJ, du Bois RM, Nicholson AG. Cryptogenic fibrosing alveolitis: lack of association with Epstein–Barr virus infection. Thorax 1997; 52:888–891.
48. Baldara U, Monti A, Righini MG. An epidemic of infantile papular acrodermatitis (Gianotti–Crosti Syndrome) due to Epstein–Barr virus. Dermatology 1994; 188:203–204.
49. Drago F, Romagnoli M, Loi A, Rebora A. Epstein–Barr virus-related persistent erythema multiforme in chronic fatigue syndrome. Arch Dermatol 1992; 128:217–222.
50. Craig AJ, Cualing H, Thomas G, Lamerson C, Smith R. Cytophagic histiocytic panniculitis—a syndrome associated with benign and malignant panniculitis: case comparison and review of the literature. J Am Acad Dermatol 1998; 39:721–736.
51. Portnoy J, Ahronheim GA, Ghibu F, Clecner B, Joncas JH. Recovery of Epstein–Barr virus from genital ulcers. N Engl J Med 1983; 15:966–968.
52. Voog E, Ricksten A, Olofsson S, et al. Demonstration of Epstein–Barr virus DNA and human papillomavirus DNA in acetowhite lesions of the penile skin and the oral mucosa. Int J STD AIDS 1997; 8:772–775.
53. Nahwe H, Gissmann L, Freese UK, Petzoldt D, Helfrich S. Subclinical Epstein–Barr virus infection of both the male and female genital tract-indication for sexual transmission. J Invest Dermatol 1992; 98:791–793.
54. Taylor S, Drake SM, Dedicoat M, Wood MJ. Genital ulcers associated with acute Epstein–Barr virus infection. Sexual Transmission Infect 1998; 74:296–297.
55. Skinnider BF, Clement PB, MacPherson N, Gascoyne RD, Viswanatha DS. Primary non-Hodgkin's lymphoma and malakoplakia of the vagina: a case report. Hum Pathol 1999; 30:871–874.
56. Algood CB, Newell GR, Johnson DE. Viral etiology of testicular tumors. J Urol 1988; 139:308–310.
57. Nadasdy T, Park C-S, Peiper SC, Wenzl JE, Oates J, Silva FG. Epstein–Barr virus infection-associated renal disease: diagnostic use of molecular hybridization technology in patients with negative serology. J Am Soc Nephrol 1992; 2:1734–1742.
58. Boskovich SA, Lowder CY, Meisler DM, Gutman FA. Systemic diseases associated with intermediate uveitis. Cleveland Clin J Med 1993; 60:460–465.
59. Feinberg AS, Spraul CW, Holden JT, Grossniklaus HE. Conjunctival lymphocytic infiltrates associated with Epstein–Barr virus. Ophthalmology 2000; 107:159–163.
60. Pflugfelder SC, Tseng SCG, Pepose JS, Fletcher MA, Klimas N, Feuer W. Epstein–Barr virus infection and immunologic dysfunction in patients with aqueous tear deficiency. Ophthalmology 1990; 97:313–323.
61. Tiedeman JS. Epstein–Barr viral antibodies in multifocal choroiditis and panuveitis. Am J Ophthalmol 1987; 103:659–663.

62. DuBois RE, Seeley JK, Brus I, et al. Chronic mononucleosis syndrome. Southern Med J 1984; 77:1376–1382.
63. Tobi M, Ravid Z, Feldman-Weiss V, et al. Prolonged atypical illness associated with serological evidence of persistent Epstein–Barr virus infection. Lancet 1982:61–64.
64. Ballow M, Seeley JP, Purtilo DT, St Onge S, Sakamoto K, Rickles FR. Familial chronic mononucleosis. Ann Intern Med 1982; 97:821–825.
65. Jones JF, Ray CG, Minnich LL, Hicks MJ, Kibler R, Lucas DO. Evidence for active Epstein–Barr virus infection in patients with persistent, unexplained illnesses: elevated anti-early antigen antibodies. Ann Intern Med 1985; 102:1–7.
66. Straus SE, Tosato G, Armstrong G, et al. Persisting illness and fatigue in adults with evidence of Epstein–Barr virus infection. Ann Intern Med 1985; 102:7–16.
67. Buchwald DS, Sullivan JL, Komaroff AL. Frequency of "chronic active Epstein–Barr virus infection" in a general medical practice. JAMA 1987; 257:2303–2307.
68. Tobi M, Straus S. Chronic Epstein–Barr virus disease: a workshop held by the National Institute of Allergy and Infectious Diseases. Ann Intern Med 1985; 103:951–953.
69. Andersson J. Clinical and immunological considerations in Epstein–Barr virus-associated diseases. Scand Univ Press 1996; 100:S72–S82.
70. Jones J, Katz B. Epstein–Barr virus infections in normal and immunosuppressed patients. In: Jones JF, Glaser R, eds. Herpesvirus Infection. W.B. Saunders, 1994:187–226.
71. Xu J, Ahmad A, Blagdon M, et al. The Epstein–Barr virus (EBV) major envelope glycoprotein gp350/220-specific antibody reactivities in the sera of patients with different EBV-associated diseases. Int J Cancer 1998; 79:481–486.
72. Kawa K. Epstein–Barr virus-associated diseases in humans. Int J Hematol 2000; 71: 108–117.
73. Holmes GP, Kaplan JE, Stewart JA, Hunt B, Pinsky PF, Schonberger LB. A cluster of patients with a chronic mononucleosis-like syndrome Is Epstein–Barr virus the cause? JAMA 1987; 257:2297–2302.
74. Holmes GP, Kaplan JE, Gantz NM, et al. Chronic fatigue syndrome; a working case definition. Ann Intern Med 1988; 108:387–389.
75. Fukuda K, Straus SE, Hickie I, Sharpe MC, Dobbins JG, Komaroff A. The chronic fatigue syndrome: a comprehensive approach to its definition and study. International Chronic Fatigue Syndrome Study Group. Ann Intern Med 1994; 121:953–959.
76. Evan AS, Rothfield NF, Niederman JC. Raised antibody titers to EB virus in systemic lupus erythematosus. Lancet 1971:1.
77. Dror Y, Blachar Y, Cohen P, Livni N, Rosenmann E, Ashkenazi A. Systemic lupus erythematosus associated with acute Epstein–Barr virus infection. Am J Kidney Dis 1998; 32:825–828.
78. Katz BZ, Salimi B, Kim S, Nsiah-Kumi P, Wagner-Weiner L. Epstein–Barr virus burden in adolescents with systemic lupus erythematosus. Pediatr Infect Dis J 2001; 20:148–153.
79. Ascherio A, Munch M. Epstein–Barr virus and multiple sclerosis. Epidemiology 2000; 11:220–224.
80. Morré SA, van Beek J, De Groot DJA, et al. Is Epstein–Barr virus present in the CNS of patients with MS? Neurology 2001; 1:692.
81. Ascherio A, Munger KL, Lennette ET, et al. Epstein–Barr virus antibodies and risk of multiple sclerosis. JAMA 2001; 286:3083–3088.
82. Morré SA, Stooker W, Lagrand WK, van den Brude AJC, Niessen HWM. Microorganisms in the aetiology of atherosclerosis. J Clin Pathol: Mol Pathol 2000; 53:647–654.
83. Espinola-Klein C, Rupprecht HJ, Blankenberg S, et al. Impact of infectious burden on extent and long-term prognosis of atherosclerosis. Circulation 2002; 105:15–21.
84. Brink AATP, Meijer CJLM, Nicholls JM, Middeldorp JM, van den Brule AJC. Activity of the EBNA1 promoter associated with lytic replication (Fp) in Epstein–Barr virus associated disorders. J Clin Pathol: Mol Pathol 2001; 54:98–102.
85. Katz BZ, Raab-Traub N, Miller G. Latent and replicating forms of Epstein–Barr virus DNA in lymphomas and lymphoproliferative diseases. J Infect Dis 1989; 160:589–598.

86. Meerbach A, Gruhn B, Egerer R, Reischl U, Zintl F, Wutzler P. Semiquantitative PCR analysis of Epstein–Barr virus DNA in clinical samples of patients with EBV-associated diseases. J Med Virol 2001; 65:348–357.
87. Fan H, Gullery M. Epstein–Barr viral load measurement as a marker of EBV-related disease. Mol Diag 2001; 6:279–289.
88. Weigle K, Grose C. Molecular dissection of the humoral immune response to individual varicella-zoster viral proteins during chickenpox, quiescence, reinfection, and reactivation. J Infect Dis 1984; 149:741–749.

18

Treatment of Epstein–Barr Virus Infections: Chemotherapy, Antiviral Therapy, and Immunotherapy

Patrizia Comoli
Laboratorio Sperimentale di Immunologia e Trapianti, U.O. di Oncoematologia Pediatrica, IRCCS Policlinico S. Matteo, Pavia, Italy

Cliona Rooney
Department of Pediatrics, Center for Cell and Gene Therapy, Baylor College of Medicine, Houston, Texas, U.S.A.

INTRODUCTION

Epstein–Barr virus (EBV) has developed a relationship with its human host that allows it to persist throughout the life of the infected individual without pathology. However, disruptions of the highly evolved balance between the virus lytic and latent life cycles and host immune control result in a range of EBV-associated diseases involving B-cells, epithelial cells, T-cells, natural killer (NK) cells, or muscle. In the simplest case, iatrogenic immunosuppression occurring after stem cell or organ transplantation leads to the outgrowth of virus-transformed B-cells resulting in post-transplant lymphoproliferative disease (PTLD) (1). While PTLD clearly results from severe T-cell dysfunction, subtler and less well understood immune defects, such as cytokine imbalance, may also play a role in the etiology of PTLD (2,3). Loss of control of the lytic life cycle of EBV is associated with chronic active EBV (CAEBV) infection and oral hairy leukoplakia in AIDS patients. However, the immunological defects underlying these diseases are not understood, because less is known about the control of the lytic cycle of EBV than of its latent cycle. EBV may also cause disease by subverting the immune response, not directly as do other herpesviruses, but by interaction with the infected cell. For example, the malignant growth of EBV-infected germinal center B-cells in EBV-positive Hodgkin's disease (HD) occurs in individuals with no known preexisting immunological defect. EBV-infected malignant Hodgkin–Reed–Sternberg (HRS) cells secrete cytokines and chemokines that are inhibitory to the activation and function of cytotoxic T-lymphocytes (CTL) resulting in an ineffective immune response (4). The EBV latent membrane protein 1 (LMP1) that is expressed in EBV-positive HRS cells induces cytokine expression through activation of the NF-κB pathway and may have an important role in this

353

cytokine activation. However, because EBV-negative HRS cells also secrete inhibitory cytokines, the role of EBV is unclear (5). The cytokines produced by HRS cells are likely the cause of the generalized immune suppression seen in Hodgkin patients and may impede the efficacy of immunotherapies for this disease (6,7). Viral characteristics may also disrupt the virus–host balance, and much research has gone into identifying virological differences that might result in a more virulent virus. However, no clear association between virulence and genetic change has been found (5,8,9). EBV-associated diseases are generally difficult to treat because specific antiviral drugs influence only the lytic cycle (10,11). However, the viral antigens expressed in the involved cells provide target antigens against which immunotherapies and molecularly targeted drugs may be directed. Improved understanding of the defects, virological or immunological, underlying each disorder is key to developing rational and effective treatments. The immunological features of most of the diseases associated with EBV suggest that immunotherapeutic remedies may be appropriate, and it is the focus of this chapter to discuss possible immunological solutions.

EBV infection is controlled by both cellular and humoral immune responses. Virus-neutralizing antibodies control the spread of infectious virus particles and virus-specific CTL control virus-infected cells. CTL specific for viral latent cycle proteins prevent the outgrowth of cells latently infected with EBV, while CTL specific for the early lytic cycle proteins kill cells entering the lytic cycle before they are able to release infectious virus particles (12,13). B-cells transformed with EBV in vitro express at least nine latency-associated proteins, the virus nuclear antigens, EBV nuclear antigens (EBNAs) 1, 2, 3A, 3B, 3C, and leader protein (LP), and the membrane proteins, LMP1 and LMP2 as well as a protein product from the *Bam*HI A region of the genome (RK-BARF) (14,15). Of these proteins, EBNA3A, 3B, and 3C dominate the immune response in most normal individuals. Fewer CTL clones are directed against LMP2 and EBNA2, and CTL clones against the other proteins are undetectable in most individuals (12,16). Expression of all nine proteins has been termed type 3 latency and is highly immunogenic, and tumors expressing type 3 latency are found only in severely immunosuppressed individuals. Tumors that arise in normal individuals express a much more restricted array of less immunogenic proteins. Thus nasopharyngeal carcinoma (NPC) and HD express a type 2 latency in which only EBNA1, LMP1, LMP2, and RK-BARF are expressed, and Burkitt lymphoma (BL) and gastric carcinoma cells express the least immunogenic type 1 latency with only EBNA1 and RK-BARF being expressed. EBNA1 is not presented to the immune response by human leukocyte antigen (HLA) class I molecules because of its glycine/alanine repeat sequence that prevents its binding to the peptide transporter proteins required for peptide loading (17). RK-BARF–specific CTL can be generated in vitro, using peptides or vaccinia virus–expressed proteins, but they do not kill tumor cells that naturally express the protein (18). Thus while type 2 tumors may have intermediate immunogenicity, tumor cells expressing type 1 latency appear to be invisible to HLA class I–restricted complementarity determinant-8 (CD8) CTL. Recently, however, much interest in the role of virus-specific CD4 T-cells has been generated by observations that a high frequency of EBNA1-specific CD4 T-cells circulate in normal individuals and that CD4 T-cells are able to cause regression of lymphocyte cultures infected with EBV (19,20). As a result it has been postulated that EBNA1-specific CD4 T-cells may have some therapeutic potential against type 1 tumors. A high frequency of CTL with specificity against the early lytic cycle proteins of EBV has also been demonstrated, implying that killing of cells entering the lytic cycle plays an important role in virus control.

TREATMENT OF DISEASES ASSOCIATED WITH EBV INFECTION

Infectious Mononucleosis

When primary infection with EBV is delayed until adolescence, symptoms of infection may be more severe than those experienced in childhood, with 50% of infections resulting in infectious mononucleosis (IM) (see Chapter 6). In IM, replicative infection in oropharyngeal epithelial cells and/or B-cells results in infection of circulating B-cells expressing the full array of nine latency-associated genes, which in turn are responsible for a massive expansion of EBV-specific and nonspecific T-cells. The reason that primary infection sometimes results in IM is not understood, but may be related to the infecting virus dose or the maturity of the immune response, which is responsible for the symptoms. Thus, if a previous infection with an unrelated organism results in T-cell memory that cross-reacts with EBV antigens (molecular mimicry), then the cross-reactive response to EBV may be stronger or may interfere with the natural response to EBV, either resulting in IM. It has been suggested that the severity of disease may be controlled by the qualitative breadth of the T-cell repertoire elicited by primary infection, with a broad repertoire of T-cells being able to control disease more rapidly than a narrow repertoire (21).

The prognosis for IM is very favorable, and although a variety of acute complications, including rare life-threatening complications, may occur, most patients experience an uneventful and complete recovery (22,23). Consequently, the role of drug therapy for IM is limited, and treatment is mostly supportive.

Specific antiviral therapy with acyclovir, an inhibitor of viral replication, has been evaluated in double-blind, placebo-controlled studies for treatment of patients with acute IM (24–27). These studies showed that, although oropharyngeal shedding of EBV was significantly reduced during therapy, the effect was only transient. Moreover, no evidence was provided that acyclovir hastened the resolution of symptoms or prevented the development of complications, these being mostly the consequence of proliferation and activation of T-cells in response to infection rather than direct viral damage (22).

The anti-inflammatory effects of corticosteroids may shorten the duration of fever, oropharyngeal symptoms, and lymphadenopathy, although a study of combined therapy with prednisolone and acyclovir in uncomplicated IM showed that this treatment did not affect overall illness duration (26). However, use of corticosteroids in uncomplicated cases is not recommended, based on the consideration that its immunomodulatory effects during acute primary infection may prevent establishment of normal immune response and latency surveillance, and ultimately lead to the development of EBV-associated diseases (22). Thus, indications for corticosteroids are limited to severe complications of IM such as incipient upper airway obstruction, autoimmune hemolytic anemia or neutropenia, thrombocytopenia with hemorrhage, and neurologic complications (23).

Lymphoproliferative Disease

Lymphoproliferative disorders associated with EBV infection are seen in congenital or acquired immunodeficiency (see Chapters 9 and 16), and PTLD has emerged as a significant complication of both hematopoietic stem cell (HSC) and solid organ transplantation (see Chapter 12). The severe impairment of cellular immunity seen after transplantation allows uncontrolled proliferation of polyclonal B-cells latently infected with EBV. With time, isolated B-cell clones may acquire additional structural alterations leading to autonomous growth and escape from immune surveillance. The onset of PTLD is preceded by a preclinical phase characterized by elevated EBV-DNA titers in the peripheral blood as measured using the polymerase chain reaction (PCR) (28–30). EBV-DNA analysis represents a fundamental tool for early diagnosis and application of preemptive treatment. In addition, because successful treatment is associated with disappearance of detectable EBV DNA, the assessment of viral load by PCR is useful to monitor the response to treatment (31,32). However, while there is an unequivocal correlation between high viral load and PTLD in HSC transplant (HSCT) recipients, after solid organ transplantation, patients may persist with high viral loads for many months without developing PTLD, and not every case is associated with elevated EBV DNA (33). Further, it has been shown that disappearance of peripheral EBV DNA may not always reflect remission, and disappearance of virus DNA in peripheral blood may mask persistent disease in the brain, eye, or gut (our unpublished observations) (34).

The therapeutic options for PTLD are varied, ranging from reduction of immunosuppression to aggressive chemotherapy. Many reports are anecdotal, and case series vary considerably for diversity of pathologies included under the heading of PTLD, heterogeneity of treatments, response, and mortality rates. Given the lack of controlled trials, and difficulty in dissecting the respective role of therapeutic agents in the numerous combined-treatment series, it is difficult to define a standard approach to the treatment of established PTLD. In this section we will try to outline the available options for different clinical presentations and illustrate the latest advances in the treatment of PTLD.

Reduction of Immunosuppression

Reduction of immunosuppressive agents is the standard initial treatment for PTLD in the setting of solid organ transplantation. The reduction schedule generally applied consists of discontinuation of azathioprine or mycophenolate mofetil (in patients receiving a "triple" immunosuppressive regimen) followed by progressive reduction of calcineurin inhibitors. The reported response rates range from 10% to 80% according to the different case series (35–39). The probability of complete response rests mainly on the clinicopathologic features of PTLD: Patients with plasmacytic hyperplasia, polymorphic hyperplasia, and polymorphic lymphomas, presenting within the first year after transplantation, are more likely to respond. Conversely, diseases with B-cell or immunoblastic lymphoma morphology, usually presenting more than one year following allograft, often require additional therapy (37). Notwithstanding this general trend, disease behavior is unpredictable, and studies are warranted to identify predictors of response.

The extent and duration of immunosuppression reduction must balance "optimal" therapeutic effect with minimal risk of allograft rejection, and it is difficult to derive definitive answers from reported data. However, a schedule of progressive stepwise reduction, maintaining the lower therapeutic ranges of calcineurin inhibitors (e.g., tacrolimus, sirolimus, and cyclosporin A) and adjusting immunosuppressive drug dosage based on blood level monitoring, may avoid onset of acute rejection. Consequently, the low-level immunosuppressive regimen may be maintained for a longer time-span, to allow emergence of EBV-directed T-cell populations and recovery of specific T-cell function.

Antiviral Agents and Interferon-α

Virostatic drugs have not been evaluated in controlled clinical trials. Acyclovir, which inhibits the replication of linear EBV DNA and virion production but has no effect on the replication of EBV episomes in latently infected cells, is generally ineffective in PTLD (40). Regression of lymphoproliferation has been reported in a small number of cases, but reduction of immunosuppression and/or some other form of treatment were almost invariably associated, and therefore the role of acyclovir remains obscure (41,42). Anecdotal cases of complete response to PTLD with foscarnet or cidofovir treatment have also been reported (43,44). A recent clinical trial has evaluated the use of ganciclovir combined with arginine butyrate, a pharmacological inducer of the latent viral thymidine kinase (TK) gene and enzyme in tumor cells, to render them susceptible to antiviral therapy. Complete response was obtained in four of six patients, but adverse effects and toxicity were observed (45). Because PTLD in solid organ recipients almost always involves recipient B-cells and donor virus, there is clearly a phase in which productive replication in donor cells results in infection of recipient B-cells. This phase should be receptive to acyclovir derivatives and, indeed, the incidence of PTLD in pancreas recipients was dramatically reduced by acyclovir or ganciclovir.

Complete PTLD responses have been obtained with interferon-α, whose mechanism of action is yet undefined, but available data are limited. Stable remissions were obtained in both polyclonal and monoclonal lymphoproliferations occurring after HSCT (46). In a study of 14 solid organ transplantation recipients, eight patients treated with interferon-α experienced total regression of PTLD, although two had a subsequent relapse with a different neoplastic clone (47). However, reduction of immunosuppression was the associated first-line treatment in all patients and could have had a role in both induction of remission and onset of acute rejection (observed in four patients). Marrow suppression was an observed adverse effect, and infectious complications were one of the main causes of death in the treated cohort.

Surgical Resection, Radiotherapy, and Cytotoxic Chemotherapy

Surgical removal or irradiation of localized lymphoproliferative lesions has been employed and proved beneficial in certain cases, as first-line therapy or on residual lesions after reduction of immunosuppression (37,42). Debulking of extensive tumors may also be useful before application of other therapeutic agents.

Chemotherapy should be considered with caution for immunosuppressed patients, and has been viewed as the final option for patients with aggressive lymphoproliferations refractory to other first-line treatments. The mortality rates reported for standard combination chemotherapy regimens such as Children's Hospital of Philadelphia are very high (70%) and the response rate unsatisfactory (37,42,48). In a study conducted on heart transplant recipients, aggressive chemotherapy based on ProMACE-CytaBOM regimen was administered to eight patients unresponsive to reduction of immunosuppression and acyclovir, and results obtained were more encouraging: complete remission was obtained in 75% of treated patients, with no relapses at a median follow-up of 38 months; therapy-related mortality was 25% (36). The main toxicity observed was myelosuppression, responsible for the many episodes of neutropenic sepsis, and subclinical cardiac toxicity due to doxorubicin. Despite discontinuation of all immunosuppressive agents throughout the duration of chemotherapy, no treated patient experienced rejection episodes. A low dose chemotherapy regimen of cyclophosphamide ($600 \, \text{mg/m}^2$) and prednisone ($2 \, \text{mg/kg}$ per day for five days) given every three weeks for six cycles produced good results in children (49). The complete remission rate was 82%, with graft survival of 90% and a relapse rate of 22%.

In Vivo Use of Anti–B Cell mAbs

The initial in vivo experience with anti–B-cell monoclonal antibodies (mAbs) included 26 recipients of HSC or solid organ transplantation treated with a combination of murine antibodies, anti-CD21 (EBV receptor on B-cells), and anti-CD24 for PTLD (50). The indications that emerged from this early study suggested that the treatment was effective only in oligoclonal disease (89% of complete responses and 11% partial responses, compared with no response in the monoclonal lymphoproliferations) and in tumors not involving the central nervous system. These observations were extended in a larger update of the trial (51). Treatment of 58 patients (31 organ transplantation recipients and 27 HSCT recipients) presenting with aggressive PTLD resulted in 61% complete responses, with only 8% relapse and an overall survival of 46% at 61 months (HSCT 35% and organ transplant 55%). Most of the solid organ transplant recipients in this trial were first given reduction of immunosuppression, so that recovery of immune surveillance may have influenced the response rate. Factors that contributed to complete response were presentation less than one year, localized disease, polyclonal or oligoclonal process, and no central nervous system involvement.

More recently, a humanized monoclonal antibody directed against the B-cell antigen CD20 has been approved for the treatment of low-grade B-cell non-Hodgkin's lymphomas, and clinical trials have also started in the setting of PTLD. This antibody is able to fix human complement and has produced complete remissions of PTLD in both HSCT and solid organ recipients (52–54). A retrospective study conducted on 32 patients with PTLD (26 solid organ transplantation and six HSCT) receiving humanized anti-CD20 mAb after reduction of immunosuppressive treatment reported a response rate of 83% in HSCT patients and 65% in solid organ transplant (58% complete responses), with a relapse rate of 18%, higher than that observed in the CD21/CD24 trial (51,55). However, in a much larger cohort and with longer follow-up, the overall response rate was markedly lower, with a high percentage of additional patients either progressing or dying on study (56). Recently, it has been suggested that anti-CD20 mAb efficacy may augment with use as first-line treatment, and with a more prolonged treatment duration (57). Moreover, preliminary studies in the animal model seem to indicate that the Bcl-2 antisense oligonucleotide G3139 may potentiate the antitumor response of PTLD to rituximab in vivo and augment its antiproliferative and apoptotic effects in vitro (58). In addition, because it appears from studies on large patient cohorts that single-agent treatment with either chemotherapy or anti–B-cell mAbs does not result in a satisfying event-free patient and graft survival in the setting of disseminated monoclonal PTLD occurring after solid organ transplantation, efforts are currently underway to define new treatment protocols based on combination of the different available therapeutic agents, with the aim of augmenting efficacy while reducing overall toxicity and treatment-related adverse events by modulating therapy load. The preliminary results obtained in a pilot trial of chemoimmunotherapy including rituximab and cyclophosphamide/prednisone, with 83% disease-free survival at a median follow-up of 14 months, are encouraging, though they need to be confirmed in a controlled trial (59).

Toxicity does not seem to be a major concern with mAb treatment for early disease. However, with bulky tumors the decision to use an immunological method or a pharmacological method of tumor reduction is complicated, because a greater "cytokine storm" may be associated with the immunological method. Either way intensive care should be provided during the period of tumor lysis. It has been suggested that optimal results can be obtained by tumor debulking with chemotherapy or radiotherapy, followed by rituximab (60). Additional disadvantages of rituximab reported in the literature suggest that the B-cell depletion observed after rituximab therapy may be profound and prolonged in some patients, requiring substitutive immunoglobulin infusions (54,61). Moreover, severe IgM deficiency has been described following anti-CD20 mAb treatment (62). The risks of profound B-cell depletion in patients immunocompromised by transplant procedures are unknown, and require evaluation in studies with longer follow-up. Recently, cases of rituximab-associated immune myelopathy have also been described (63). In HSCT recipients endogenous immune responses usually recover before the return of B-cells and EBV, and therefore relapse may be uncommon. However, after solid organ transplant, improvement of EBV-specific immunity cannot be expected and when the B-cell compartment recovers, virus load frequently returns to pretreatment levels, sometimes accompanied by PTLD (Savoldo, unpublished observations). However, the four to six months of remission produced by rituximab may allow the preparation of EBV-specific CTL as therapy or consolidation (as described below).

Ex Vivo B Cell Depletion of Donor Marrow in HSCT Recipients

In stem cell recipients, the risk of PTLD is related to T-cell depletion of the donor marrow infusion used to prevent graft versus host disease in recipients of HLA-mismatched or unrelated stem cells. The more rigorous the T-cell depletion, the higher the risk for EBV lymphoma. However, if B-cells as well as T-cells are removed from the donor marrow, as occurs with the Campath 1 antibody for immunodepletion, the risk for PTLD is reduced to levels seen in patients who receive T-cell–replete marrow (64). This is because the major source of virus during the posttransplant period, even in EBV-carrying recipients, is the mature B-cell population carried with the donor stem cell product. Newer protocols to make the procedure of stem cell transplant (SCT) less toxic are currently in development (65). Some of these employ in vivo T- and B-cell depletion with antibodies, and chemotherapy may impart new risks for EBV lymphoma (66).

Cellular Immunotherapy

The use of cellular immunotherapy to prevent and/or treat herpesvirus-related complications is particularly attractive, as the primary defect contributing to the pathogenesis of progressive disease appears to be the inability to mount adequate virus-specific T-cell responses (67,68). There is ample evidence, derived from animal studies, and, more recently, from the first trials in humans, that adoptive transfer of the relevant antigen-specific T-cells can restore protective immunity and control established infection (69–72). Increased understanding of the mechanisms underlying the activation, targeting, and function of the cellular populations involved in the protective immune response to viruses, and the acquisition of expertise for cellular manipulation have led to significant achievements in cell-based virus-specific immunotherapy.

Because EBV-associated lymphoproliferative disease in immunocompromised hosts is unequivocally associated with a deficiency of virus-specific cytotoxic T-cells (12), it was reasonable to hypothesize that an adoptive immunotherapy approach with virus-specific T-lymphocytes could prevent lymphoproliferation and eradicate established disease. Because lymphoproliferative disease in HSCT is donor derived, therapeutic EBV-specific lymphocytes would most usefully be obtained from the donor. In 1994, the Memorial Sloan Kettering group first demonstrated remission of PTLD in five HSCT recipients after infusion of unselected donor leukocyte infusions (DLI) (71). However, this treatment was associated with graft-versus-host disease (GVHD) and two patients died of inflammatory-mediated lung damage, leading to respiratory failure. In an update of this study, 17 of 19 patients responded positively to DLI (73). However, other studies have been less successful and only four of 13 patients at the University of Indiana responded, and only two survived (74). To overcome the problem of alloreactivity-related complications, Bonini et al. adoptively transferred donor lymphocytes transfected with a retroviral vector encoding both a truncated nerve growth factor receptor and the herpes simplex suicide gene (75). The latter renders transduced cells susceptible to the cytotoxic effects of ganciclovir and the former allows for selection of transduced cells. After infusion of transduced cells, GVHD developed in three patients, and ganciclovir administration reversed the alloreactive response in two. The major concern of this approach relates to the immune response to the viral TK transgene, which developed in many of the patients and likely affected the longevity of transferred lymphocytes. More recently, suicide genes based on a chimeric Fas molecule linked to FK506-binding proteins in which Fas-mediated suicide can be induced by a dimerizing drug (76). Because both parts of this chimeric molecule are derived from human proteins, this offers a potentially nonimmunogenic alternative.

Further progress in this field was achieved by the first trial of adoptive immunotherapy with gene-marked EBV-specific CTL lines, reactivated from the peripheral blood of HSCT donors and infused as prophylaxis against EBV-PTLD in patients given T-cell depleted, HLA-disparate, unrelated HSCT (72,77). The infusion of these polyclonal CTL proved to be safe and effective in both prevention and treatment of EBV-related PTLD. This experience was confirmed in over 60 patients, none of whom developed PTLD after prophylactic CTL infusions, compared to seven out of 61 transplanted patients not receiving the prophylactic treatment (more recent unpublished data) (78). Moreover, three of three patients with early disease and two of three with aggressive disease who received CTL as treatment achieved complete remission after CTL therapy, with selective accumulation of gene-marked cells in tumor lesions. This experience showed that cellular immunotherapy with specific polyclonal CTL containing both CD4 and CD8 lymphocytes was effective in restoring antigen-specific long-term immunological memory. Indeed, gene-marking studies have shown the persistence of these donor-derived EBV-specific T-cells in patients' peripheral blood for up to six years after infusion. The re-expansion of marked T-cells during episodes of viral reactivation further emphasizes the importance of helper T-cell function for the persistence of transferred CD8 cells. A recent study confirmed the efficacy of EBV-specific CTL in reducing viral load in patients with high EBV-DNA levels early after HSCT (79).

Given the recipient origin of PTLD after solid organ transplantation, application of an immunotherapy approach in this setting at first appeared difficult, because an HLA-identical donor is rarely available, and it seemed unlikely that fully functional autologous CTL could be obtained from patients receiving pharmacological immunosuppression. The first attempt at immunotherapy for PTLD in solid organ transplant recipients was conducted with autologous lymphokine-activated killer

(LAK) lymphocytes (80). The seven patients treated in this trial had reduction of immunosuppression, followed by a single LAK-cell infusion (in the order of 10^9–10^{10} cells). In the four patients with EBV-associated PTLD, LAK infusion induced complete remission, but rejection was observed in two patients. The immunological effect of LAK cells requires infusion of high cell numbers, and the protection conferred is limited in time, because interleukin-2 (IL-2)–activated cells may not induce protective EBV-specific T-cell memory.

However, another strategy for treating PTLD in patients with solid organ transplants is to use partially HLA-matched allogeneic cytotoxic T-cells, because viral antigens may be presented—and recognized by T-cells—through a single HLA class I–matched allele. This is because the response to EBV has a very restricted pattern, and the single relevant epitope is presented by a single allele. Successful treatment of a PTLD with central nervous system presentation was achieved in a lung graft recipient with infusion of unmanipulated HLA-identical donor lymphocytes (81). Haploidentical or partially HLA-matched allogeneic EBV-specific CTL induced remission in a renal transplant and a small bowel and liver allograft recipient, respectively (82,83). However, the transient response in the former and failure to detect donor lymphocytes in the peripheral blood of the latter patient after CTL infusion suggest that allogeneic CTL did not survive long term in allograft recipients, probably due to a rapid immunological clearance of CTL secondary to allorecognition. Thus, regression of PTLD lesions in these patients may have been due to the direct effect of allogeneic CTL transiently homing at the tumor site, but a "helper" effect of allogeneic CTL lines on emergence of endogenous CTL populations cannot be entirely ruled out. These preliminary data were confirmed in a cohort of eight HSCT and solid organ transplant recipients with PTLD treated with partly HLA-matched allogeneic CTL (84).

Cell therapy with autologous in vitro generated EBV-specific CTL is a more appealing strategy in solid organ transplant patients, because PTLD in these patients is of recipient origin. Haque et al. reactivated virus-specific CTL from pretransplant blood samples of solid organ transplant recipients, which were effective in reconstituting specific immune function and controlling high virus loads posttransplant (85). Generation and storage of cytotoxic lines for each patient undergoing solid organ transplantation, however, require high levels of funding, extensive laboratory facilities, and a large workforce. Reactivation of autologous EBV-specific CTL after transplantation, from the peripheral blood of the patients at the time of PTLD diagnosis or, better, upon detection of increased EBV-DNA levels (the preemptive approach) is a more cost-effective strategy. The feasibility of the latter approach was supported by an early report that demonstrated how EBV-specific CTL could readily be generated from solid organ transplant recipients, even those with active PTLD, and that these CTL were effective in controlling EBV-DNA levels and inducing remission of clinical symptoms in three patients with evidence of PTLD (30,86). Khanna et al. generated an EBV-specific CTL line from a renal transplant patient with PTLD, and succeeded in inducing regression of the disease, though secondary PTLD developed at a different site 2.5 months after CTL infusion, reiterating concerns about the functional survival of CTL in patients (87). Autologous EBV-specific CTL have been recently used as prophylaxis of EBV-related lymphoproliferative disorders in seven solid organ transplant recipients, following a strategy of preemptive therapy guided by EBV-DNA levels (88). CTL transfer was well tolerated and none of the patients showed any evidence of rejection. An increase of EBV-specific immunity was observed after infusion, despite continuation of immunosuppressive therapy, and EBV-DNA levels decreased by 1.5 to 3 logs in five patients, whereas in the other two patients CTL transfer had no apparent stable effect on EBV load. These preliminary experiences underscore the possible requirement for a higher frequency of infusion in PTLD emerging after solid organ transplants, because it is not possible to discontinue immunosuppression in many of these patients, and CTL must persist and function in the presence of drugs specifically designed to suppress them.

The patients at highest risk of PTLD after SCT are seronegative children, who usually receive EBV with their graft and then must mount a primary immune response while receiving immunosuppression. While CTL infusions would be of most benefit for this group, standard methods have failed to generate EBV-specific CTL from seronegative individuals because of their low EBV-specific T-cell precursor frequency. Khanna et al. were able to generate CTL from transplant recipients shortly after seroconversion, but PTLD may occur and progress during the time taken to generate CTL lines (87). Savoldo et al. were able to generate EBV-specific CTL from seronegative children awaiting transplant by selecting CD25 T-cells on day 9 after stimulation of peripheral blood mononuclear cells (PBMCs) with autologous lymphoblastoid cell lines (LCL) (89). Interestingly, all of these CTL lines were composed predominantly of HLA class II–restricted CD4 CTL and while the efficacy of purely CD4 T-cells has not been demonstrated in vivo, CD4 CTL have been shown to be essential and sufficient for the regression of EBV-transformed B-cells after EBV infection of PBMC in vitro (20).

Failures in the treatment of established PTLD have been reported (78). The HSCT recipient who did not respond to CTL therapy and died of disease progression was shown to harbor in tumor cells a deletion in the EBNA3B gene that removed immunodominant epitopes, thereby inducing resistance to killing by CTL (90). Escape mutants such as the one described could represent a problem in patients with large tumor burden. In addition, danger of inducing massive inflammatory reactions argues for caution in the use of CTL therapy in patients with bulky disease (78,87).

Finally, cell culture protocols for EBV CTL reactivation and expansion are being implemented with new immunological techniques. The 10 to 12 weeks required to generate LCL/CTL precludes their use as standard treatment, and so there is great interest in the activation of CTL with professional antigen-presenting cells (dendritic cells) pulsed with relevant immunogenic peptides derived from virus-encoded latent proteins (12,91,92).

The occurrence of EBV-related lymphoproliferative disease is still associated with a high mortality rate, notwithstanding the use of specific therapeutic approaches. In the view of all data available, at the present time the optimal approach to PTLD management is clearly to prevent the development of overt lymphoproliferative disease through a preemptive therapeutic intervention. To this end, peripheral blood viral DNA monitoring is an essential part of patient management. As to the choice of therapeutic agent, those which have displayed minimal toxicity and fewer side effects are to be preferred, although all treatments may have toxicity in advanced disease. CTL are, when available, the more "physiologic" choice: their efficacy after HSCT is amply proven, while the encouraging data emerging in the setting of solid organ transplant need confirmation in larger trials. The benefits of anti-CD20 for prophylaxis must be weighed against the prolonged profound B-cell depletion and hypogammaglobulinemia that may exacerbate immunodeficiency in transplant recipients. Moreover, repeated use of rituximab may select a population of CD20-negative EBV-transformed proliferating B-cells. Gradual, controlled reduction of immunosuppression is a good option for prophylaxis of PTLD after solid organ allograft, but risks of inducing rejection must be counteracted by immunosuppressive agent dosage adjustments on the basis of peripheral blood virus load.

CAEBV Infection

Rarely, the symptoms of IM continue for many months or years. This heterogeneous syndrome varies in severity from mild to severe or fatal forms. In mild disease patients experience mild to debilitating fatigue accompanied by depression, low-grade fever, and myalgia. In these cases, CAEBV is difficult to diagnose but is characterized by the presence of high serum antibody titers to virus lytic cycle antigens [virus capsid antigen (VCA) and early antigen], the absence of antibodies to EBNA, and the presence of free virus in serum or other body fluids (93,94). The virus load in peripheral blood is often low or undetectable, suggesting that the disease is associated with lack of control of the lytic cycle rather than the latent cycle. In its more severe form, CAEBV may be associated with EBV genome–positive T and NK cell lymphomas and hemophagocytic syndrome. In these cases the latent virus load is also high and commonly associated with the T and NK cell compartments. This form of the disease is most common in Japan, but whether the cause is genetic or environmental is unknown. Lack of understanding of the immunologic basis of CAEBV hinders the development of appropriate treatments. For the milder forms, treatment is usually symptom driven, but for the severe forms, only allogeneic SCT is curative.

Antiviral or immunomodulating agents with acyclovir, ganciclovir, vidarabine (95), interferon-α (96), and recombinant IL-2 (97) have all been tried. Decrease of peripheral NK cells and viral DNA was observed after vidarabine therapy (98), while interferon-α seemed to restrain clonal proliferation of T-cells in one patient, without apparent effect on EBV genome load (96). These agents produced temporary improvement or resolution of symptoms, but relapses were observed soon after treatment discontinuation. A recent trial involving 17 patients with EBV-associated hemophagocytosis treatment with a combination of etoposide and corticosteroids succeeded in inducing complete remission in 15 patients, with only one relapse and two nonresponses (99).

NK/T-cell lymphomas developing in CAEBV patients show a very aggressive clinical course, and a recent report of 34 cases, mostly treated with chemotherapy based on CHOP, BACOP, or ProMACE-CytaBOM regimens, describes a mortality rate of 85% with very short median survival (100). Allogeneic HSCT has been performed in cases unresponsive to immunomodulatory agents or combined chemotherapy (101,102). However, despite success in inducing decrease of viral load in all patients and cure in some, HSCT represents a risk in these patients due to the high transplant-related mortality (102,103).

Adoptive transfer of virus-specific CTL is also an option in this setting. One patient with severe CAEBV was treated with allogeneic CTL from an HLA-identical sibling, and experienced a reduction of EBV-DNA levels accompanied by increase of virus-specific immunity (104). Unfortunately, the patient died of a streptococcal sepsis one month after the last infusion, and long-term efficacy could not be established. We have treated five patients with mild to severe disease using autologous EBV-specific CTL. These produced increases in the precursor frequency of EBV-specific CTL in peripheral blood, normalization of serological findings (decrease in VCA and reappearance of EBNA titers), decreases in virus load, and complete remission of symptoms in three patients and partial remissions in two (105). This included normalization of splenomegaly and lymphadenopathy in one patient and complete regression of oral and genital ulcers in the second. Confirmatory studies are warranted to assess the possibility of obtaining durable remissions with this approach.

Other Cancers Associated with EBV Infection

EBV infection is associated with a number of human malignancies including endemic BL, NPC, and HD. All three tumors are considered successes in the history of oncology, because they are characterized by a very favorable prognosis: Most patients in the first stages of disease are long-term survivors, and the percentage of cure for patients in advanced-stage disease reaches 70% to 75%. The most effective therapeutic approach for advanced-stage disease is intensive cyclophosphamide-based combination chemotherapy for BL and combined chemoradiotherapy regimens for NPC and HD (106–108). However, the prognosis for recurrent and refractory disease is generally poor, despite the efforts to prolong survival by means of high-dose regimens with or without autologous or allogeneic HSCT. Furthermore, a number of successfully treated patients develop severe late toxicities (106,108). Consequently, the current challenge is to delineate predictors of treatment failure to identify patients who require a novel or more intensive treatment approach and to develop therapies equally or more effective in rescuing refractory disease, but with less toxicity.

Novel strategies for the treatment of EBV-associated malignancies include the use of immunotherapeutic approaches such as antibody-directed cell targeting and development of CTL therapy. Phenotype-specific immunotoxins (109,110), NK cell–activating CD16/CD30 bispecific antibodies (111), or labeled anti-CD30 mAbs (112) are being developed, and both experimental results in animal models and early clinical trials have provided encouraging results.

Adoptive transfer of polyclonal CTL specific for viral latency antigens in the context of other EBV-associated malignancies is limited by the latency phenotypes displayed by tumor cells. Indeed, the immunodominant EBV-encoded antigens belong to the EBNA3 family, while CTL precursors (CTLps) to LMP2 are found with low frequency and to LMP1 are largely undetectable (12). Moreover, EBNA1 and LMP1 are not ideal targets for CTL therapy, as (*i*) EBNA1 cannot enter the HLA class I processing pathway because of its glycine–alanine (Gly–Ala) repeat, which inhibits its binding to the transporter associated with antigen processing (TAP) transporter proteins and (*ii*) frequent mutations of LMP1 have been described in EBV-related cancer patients (17,113). Thus, LMP2 may be the best available target for a CTL therapy in HD and NPC.

Another barrier to the function of infused CTL in immunocompetent hosts is the use of tumor-mediated immune evasion strategies. Thus tumors may downregulate molecules required for antigen processing and recognition, as found in BL (114,115), or inhibit antigen-presenting cell and T-cell function as in Hodgkin's lymphoma (4). The success of cell therapy–based treatments for these malignancies is dependent on the presentation of appropriate viral antigens by the type I MHC molecules of the tumor cells and the resistance of the infused cells to tumor-derived inhibitory molecules. It has been demonstrated that tumor cells in both HD and NPC show high levels of HLA class I alleles on the cell surface and have normal expression of the major histocompatibility complex (MHC)-encoded putative peptide transporters TAP-1 and TAP-2, as well as of other components of the class I processing pathway (116,117). These studies provided a rationale for focusing on cellular immunotherapy.

The first clinical trial of cell therapy for HD (118) demonstrated that polyclonal virus-specific CTL could be generated from most patients with EBV-positive HD, which displayed antiviral effect in vivo: two of the three patients treated with autologous EBV CTL had a temporary alleviation of stage B symptoms, while the third patient had an initial improvement and then a stabilization of the disease, before developing disease progression. Similar results in a total of 13 patients have since been observed with improved clinical responses to higher CTL doses. Although no complete responses were seen in patients with advanced disease, complete remission was produced in one patient whose disease was stabilized after receiving autologous CTL, allowing eventual allogeneic HSCT followed by donor-derived EBV-specific CTL. Further, CTL produced a remission in one patient with residual disease after autologous HSCT (unpublished data).

The encouraging data obtained with polyclonal CTL prompted further efforts aimed at expanding the subdominant component of the EBV-specific immune response directed toward LMP2, by stimulation with dendritic cells genetically modified to express the antigen (119–121). To improve the resistance of CTL to tumor-derived inhibitory cytokines, Bollard et al. have shown that EBV-specific CTL made transgenic for a dominant-negative transforming growth factor (TGF)-β receptor, in which the intracellular signaling domain is truncated, are rendered resistant to the devastating effects of TGF-β, secreted by Hodgkin's tumor cells (122,123). Thus CTL cultured in the presence of TGF-β fail to secrete cytokines and proliferate and lose their cytotoxic potential, while the transgenic CTL remain unaffected. Similar genetic modifications, tailored to the tumor type, may be necessary to allow functional persistence of CTL specific for the majority of human tumors that arise in immunocompetent individuals.

EBV-specific CTL were also used for the treatment of refractory NPC. A recent report showed an increase in EBV-specific CTLp frequency after infusion of autologous virus-specific CTL in three patients with NPC, but the lack of apparent clinical benefit may have been due to the advanced stage of disease (124). A patient with relapsed NPC refractory to conventional therapy was treated with polyclonal EBV-specific CTL from an HLA-matched sibling donor, and showed a partial regression of the intracranial tumor mass. The disease remained stable for a few months, but then progressed (125).

The phenotype expressed by BL tumor cells renders immunotherapeutic control of this malignancy particularly difficult. EBNA1, the only antigen expressed by BL cells, is devoid of class I CTL epitopes, and HLA molecules and TAP-1 and TAP-2 expression appear to be downregulated (126). Thus, immunotherapy strategies in BL have been directed toward reversing the phenotype to latency III tumor, by exploiting CD40 engagement (114,115). The cross-linking of CD40 was shown to upregulate expression of HLA molecules and TAP proteins, and though unable to cause presentation of endogenously processed viral antigens to CTL, it has succeeded in enhancing sensitivity to NK cells (127). An alternative approach is based on the finding of efficient processing function through the class II pathway in BL cells, which renders them susceptible to lysis by CD4 EBV-specific CTL (128). Munz et al. have demonstrated that HLA class II–restricted, EBNA1-specific CTL are able to kill BL cells in vitro and Nikiforow et al. have demonstrated the importance of CD4 killer cells in the inhibition of outgrowth of B-cells infected with EBV in vitro in the regression assay (19,20). Thus interest in immunotherapy of BL with CTL has been rekindled.

PREVENTION OF EBV INFECTION OR EBV-ASSOCIATED DISEASE

Prevention of the development of EBV-related complications (preemptive therapy) or prevention of EBV infection in seronegative individuals could be a safe and effective approach to reduce the risks of treatment for EBV-associated disorders.

Because EBV-related PTLD in recipients of HSCT is due to the outgrowth of donor B-cells, physical or pharmacological depletion of mature B-cells from the stem cell inoculum may reduce the incidence of lymphoproliferative disease in this group of patients. Hale et al. (129) demonstrated that the use of mAb Campath-1, which removes both T and B-cells, for T-cell depletion in unrelated or mismatched donor transplants was associated with a very low risk of developing PTLD. In HSCT recipients at risk, and who did not receive B-cell depleted transplant, the prophylactic or preemptive infusion of donor EBV-specific CTL is effective in preventing PTLD onset (78,79).

Data on preemptive antiviral treatment with acyclovir and ganciclovir in the setting of solid organ transplantation are conflicting. Some studies described a decrease in the incidence of PTLD after either acyclovir or ganciclovir preemptive therapy (130,131), while others did not find any significant benefit from the prophylactic treatment with antiviral agents (132). The efficacy of preemptive autologous EBV-specific CTL in this setting needs to be confirmed in a larger clinical trial (88). Relevant to PTLD prevention in allograft recipients is the demonstration of feasibility to generate a primary response in virus-naive solid organ transplant patients, who are at high risk of EBV-driven lymphoproliferation, through selective expansion of CD25-expressing T-cells, 9 to 11 days after activation with EBV-transformed LCL (89).

Vaccination against EBV might be an option for EBV-seronegative individuals at risk of developing EBV-associated complications, such as HSCT or solid organ allograft recipients, patients with X-linked lymphoproliferative disease, and people living in areas where BL or NPC is endemic. There are two approaches to EBV vaccine development currently under consideration (123,133): The first is based on the use of the major envelope glycoprotein gp350, the principal target of the virus-neutralizing antibodies, in various formulations as subunit antigen, or expressed from recombinant viral vectors (134). The alternative strategy is based on the development of a subunit vaccine that incorporates EBV CTL epitopes from latent antigens, with the aim of inducing EBV-specific CTL immunity (133). An overview of EBV vaccination strategies and clinical trials may be found in a separate chapter of this volume (see Chapter 19).

SUMMARY

In summary, the safety and efficacy of standard therapies for EBV-associated malignancies and diseases can be improved upon by targeting the unique viral proteins expressed using immune based or molecularly targeted therapies. This has been clearly demonstrated by the use of EBV-specific CTL in HSCT recipients. However, other diseases and malignancies provide more difficult challenges for immunotherapy, because the patient is receiving iatrogenic immunosuppression that may inhibit the survival and function of infused CTL, or the virus-infected cell secretes immunosuppressive factors that inhibit CTL function, or the immune defect underlying the disease is not understood. Genetic modification of T-cells offers an exciting challenge for the future, because CTL may be rendered resistant to immunosuppressive drugs and tumor-derived factors. Such CTL may have high specific activity and little toxicity. Molecular targeting of viral proteins is at an early stage, but the wealth of knowledge that has been gathered about the function of EBV genes provides an array of possible approaches. Modulation of virus gene expression in BL or HD to switch them from their poorly immunogenic type 1 or type 2 expression to an immunogenic type 3 expression or to induce viral kinases to render tumor cells sensitive to nucleoside analogs is already under consideration. Finally, increased understanding of the pathogenesis and immune control of EBV together with recently developed technology to harness the most potent antigen-presenting cells of the immune system should provide vaccine strategies, if not to protect against infection, then to protect against the diseases associated with EBV.

REFERENCES

1. Filipovich AH, Mathur A, Kamat D, Kersey JH, Shapiro RS. Lymphoproliferative disorders and other tumors complicating immunodeficiencies. Immunodeficiency 1992; 5:91–112.
2. Fassone L, Gaidano G, Ariatti C, et al. The role of cytokines in the pathogenesis and management of AIDS-related lymphomas. Leuk Lymphoma 2000; 38(5–6):481–488.
3. Mathur A, Kamat D, Filipovitch A, Steinbuch M, Shapiro R. Immunoregulatory abnormalities in patients with Epstein–Barr virus-associated B-cell lymphoproliferative disorders. Transplantation 1994; 57:1042–1045.
4. Poppema S, Potters M, Visser L, van den Berg AM. Immune escape mechanisms in Hodgkin's disease. Ann Oncol 1998; 9(suppl 5):S21–S24.
5. Dawson CW, Eliopoulos AG, Blake SM, Barker R, Young LS. Identification of functional differences between prototype Epstein–Barr virus-encoded LMP1 and a nasopharyngeal carcinoma-derived LMP1 in human epithelial cells. Virology 2000; 272(1):204–217.
6. Slivnick DJ, Ellis TM, Nawrocki JF, Fisher RI. The impact of Hodgkin's disease on the immune system. Semin Oncol 1990; 17:673–682.
7. Rooney CM, Aguilar LK, Huls MH, Brenner MK, Heslop HE. Adoptive immunotherapy of EBV-associated malignancies with EBV-specific cytotoxic T-cell lines. Curr Top Microbiol Immunol 2001; 258:221–229.
8. Zhang XS, Song KH, Mai HQ, et al. The 30-bp deletion variant: a polymorphism of latent membrane protein 1 prevalent in endemic and non-endemic areas of nasopharyngeal carcinomas in China. Cancer Lett 2002; 176(1):65–73.
9. Zhou XG, Sandvej K, Li PJ, et al. Epstein–Barr virus gene polymorphisms in Chinese Hodgkin's disease cases and healthy donors: identification of three distinct virus variants. J Gen Virol 2001; 82(Pt 5):1157–1167.
10. Colby BM, Shaw JE, Elion GB, Pagano JS. Effect of acyclovir [9-(2-hydroxyethoxymethyl) guanine] on Epstein–Barr virus DNA replication. J Virol 1980; 34:560–568.
11. Moore SM, Cannon JS, Tanhehco YC, Hamzeh FM, Ambinder RF. Induction of Epstein–Barr virus kinases to sensitize tumor cells to nucleoside analogues. Antimicrob Agents Chemother 2001; 45(7):2082–2091.
12. Rickinson AB, Moss DJ. Human cytotoxic T lymphocyte responses to Epstein–Barr virus infection. Ann Rev Immunol 1997; 15:405–431.
13. Steven NM, Annels NE, Kumar A, Leese AM, Kurilla MG, Rickinson AB. Immediate early and early lytic cycle proteins are frequent targets of the Epstein–Barr virus-induced cytotoxic T-cell response. J Exp Med 1997; 185(9):1605–1617.
14. Rickinson AB, Kieff E. Epstein–Barr virus. In: Fields BN, Knipe DM, Howley PM, eds. Fields Virology. Philadelphia: Lippincott-Raven, 1996:2397–2446.
15. Fries KL, Sculley TB, Webster Cyriaque J, Rajadurai P, Sadler RH, Raab-Traub N. Identification of a novel protein encoded by the Bam HI A region of the Epstein–Barr virus. J Virol 1997; 70:2490–2496.

16. Meij P, Leen A, Rickinson AB, et al. Identification and prevalence of CD8(+) T-cell responses directed against Epstein–Barr virus-encoded latent membrane protein 1 and latent membrane protein 2. Int J Cancer 2002; 99(1):93–99.

17. Levitskaya J, Sharipo A, Leonchiks A, Ciechanover A, Masucci MG. Inhibition of ubiquitin/proteasome-dependent protein degradation by the Gly-Ala repeat domain of the Epstein–Barr virus nuclear antigen 1. Proc Natl Acad Sci USA 1997; 94(23):12,616–12,621.

18. Kienzle N, Sculley TB, Greco S, Khanna R. Cutting edge: silencing virus-specific cytotoxic T-cell-mediated immune recognition by differential splicing: a novel implication of RNA processing for antigen presentation. J Immunol 1999; 162:6963–6966.

19. Munz C, Bickham KL, Subklewe M, et al. Human CD4(+) T lymphocytes consistently respond to the latent Epstein–Barr virus nuclear antigen EBNA1. J Exp Med 2000; 191:1649–1660.

20. Nikiforow S, Bottomly K, Miller G. CD4+ T-cell effectors inhibit Epstein–Barr virus-induced B-cell proliferation. J Virol 2001; 75:3740–3752.

21. Bharadwaj M, Burrows SR, Burrows JM, Moss DJ, Catalina M, Khanna R. Longitudinal dynamics of antigen-specific CD8+ cytotoxic T lymphocytes following primary Epstein–Barr virus infection. Blood 2001; 98:2588–2589.

22. Cohen JI. Epstein–Barr virus infection. N Engl J Med 2000; 343:481–492.

23. Jenson HB. Acute complications of Epstein–Barr virus infectious mononucleosis. Curr Opin Pediatr 2000; 12(3):263–268.

24. Andersson J, Britton S, Ernberg I, et al. Effect of acyclovir on infectious mononucleosis: a double-blind, placebo-controlled study. J Infect Dis 1986; 153(2):283–290.

25. van der HC, Joncas J, Ahronheim G, et al. Lack of effect of peroral acyclovir for the treatment of acute infectious mononucleosis. J Infect Dis 1991; 164(4):788–792.

26. Tynell E, Aurelius E, Brandell A, et al. Acyclovir and prednisolone treatment of acute infectious mononucleosis: a multicenter, double-blind, placebo-controlled study. J Infect Dis 1996; 174(2):324–331.

27. Torre D, Tambini R. Acyclovir for treatment of infectious mononucleosis: a meta-analysis. Scand J Infect Dis 1999; 31(6):543–547.

28. Savoie A, Perpete C, Carpentier L, Joncas J, Alfieri C. Direct correlation between the load of Epstein–Barr virus-infected lymphocytes in the peripheral blood of pediatric transplant patients and risk of lymphoproliferative disease. Blood 1994; 83:2715–2722.

29. Rooney CM, Loftin SK, Holladay MS, Brenner MK, Krance RA, Heslop HE. Early identification of Epstein–Barr virus-associated post-transplant lymphoproliferative disease. Br J Haematol 1995; 89:98–103.

30. Savoldo B, Goss J, Liu Z, et al. Generation of autologous Epstein Barr virus (EBV)-specific cytotoxic T-cells (CTL) for adoptive immunotherapy in solid organ transplant recipients. Transplantation 2001; 72(6):1078–1086.

31. Baldanti F, Grossi P, Furione M, et al. High levels of Epstein–Barr virus DNA in blood of solid-organ transplant recipients and their value in predicting posttransplant lymphoproliferative disorders. J Clin Microbiol 2000; 38:613–619.

32. Stevens SJ, Verschuuren EA, Pronk I, et al. Frequent monitoring of Epstein–Barr virus DNA load in unfractionated whole blood is essential for early detection of posttransplant lymphoproliferative disease in high-risk patients. Blood 2001; 97:1165–1171.

33. Rowe DT, Webber S, Schauer EM, Reyes J, Green M. Epstein–Barr virus load monitoring: its role in the prevention and management of post-transplant lymphoproliferative disease. Transpl Infect Dis 2001; 3:79–87.

34. Yang J, Tao Q, Flinn IW, et al. Characterization of Epstein–Barr virus-infected B-cells in patients with posttransplantation lymphoproliferative disease: disappearance after rituximab therapy does not predict clinical response. Blood 2000; 96:4055–4063.

35. Starzl TE, Naleskin MA, Porter KA, et al. Reversibility of lymphomas and lymphoproliferative lesions developing under cyclosporin-steroid therapy. Lancet 1984; 1:583.

36. Swinnen LJ, Mullen GM, Carr TJ, Costanzo MR, Fisher RI. Aggressive treatment for postcardiac transplant lymphoproliferation. Blood 1995; 86:3333–3340.

37. Armitage JM, Kormos RL, Stuart RS, et al. Posttransplant lymphoproliferative disease in thoracic organ transplant patients: ten years of cyclosporine-based immunosuppression. J Heart Lung Transpl 1991; 10(6):877–886.

38. Leblond V, Sutton L, Dorent R, et al. Lymphoproliferative disorders after organ transplantation: a report of 24 cases observed in a single center. J Clin Oncol 1995; 13:961–968.

39. Knowles DM, Cesarman E, Chadburn A, et al. Correlative morphologic and molecular genetic analysis demonstrates three distinct categories of posttransplantation lymphoproliferative disorders. Blood 1995; 85:552–565.

40. Cohen JI. Epstein–Barr virus lymphoproliferative disease associated with acquired immunodeficiency. Medicine 1991; 70:137–160.

41. Hanto DW, Frizzera G, Gajl-Peczalska KJ, et al. Epstein–Barr virus-induced B-cell lymphoma after renal transplantation: acyclovir therapy and transition from polyclonal to monoclonal B-cell proliferation. N Engl J Med 1982; 306(15):913–918.

42. Morrison VA, Dunn DL, Manivel JC, Gajl-Peczalska KJ, Peterson BA. Clinical characteristics of post-transplant lymphoproliferative disorders. Am J Med 1994; 97:14–24.

43. Oertel SH, Ruhnke MS, Anagnostopoulos I, et al. Treatment of Epstein–Barr virus-induced posttransplantation lymphoproliferative disorder with foscarnet alone in an adult after simultaneous heart and renal transplantation. Transplantation 1999; 67(5):765–767.

44. Hanel M, Fiedler F, Thorns C. Anti-CD20 monoclonal antibody (Rituximab) and Cidofovir as successful treatment of an EBV-associated lymphoma with CNS involvement. Onkologie 2001; 24(5):491–494.

45. Mentzer SJ, Perrine SP, Faller DV. Epstein–Barr virus post-transplant lymphoproliferative disease and virus-specific therapy: pharmacological re-activation of viral target genes with arginine butyrate. Transpl Infect Dis 2001; 3(3):177–185.

46. Shapiro RS, Chauvenet A, McGuire W, et al. Treatment of B-cell lymphoproliferative disorders with interferon alfa and intravenous gamma globulin. N Engl J Med 1988; 318(20):1334.

47. Davis CL, Wood BL, Sabath DE, Joseph JS, Stehman-Breen C, Broudy VC. Interferon-alpha treatment of posttransplant lymphoproliferative disorder in recipients of solid organ transplants. Transplantation 1998; 66:1770–1779.

48. Leblond V, Davi F, Charlotte F, et al. Posttransplant lymphoproliferative disorders not associated with Epstein–Barr virus: a distinct entity? J Clin Oncol 1998; 16:2052–2059.

49. Gross TG. Low-dose chemotherapy for children with post-transplant lymphoproliferative disease. Recent Results Cancer Res 2002; 159:96–103.

50. Fischer A, Blanche S, LeBidois J, et al. Anti-B-cell monoclonal antibodies in the treatment of severe B-cell lymphoproliferative syndrome following bone marrow and organ transplantation. N Engl J Med 1991; 324:1451–1456.

51. Benkerrou M, Jais JP, Leblond V, et al. Anti-B-cell monoclonal antibody treatment of severe posttransplant B-lymphoproliferative disorder: prognostic factors and long-term outcome. Blood 1998; 92:3137–3147.

52. Faye A, Van Den Abeele T, Peuchmaur M, Matheu-Boue A, Vilmer E. Anti-CD20 monoclonal antibody for post-transplant lymphoproliferative disorders. Lancet 1998; 352:1285.

53. Cook RC, Connors JM, Gascoyne RD, Fradet G, Levy RD. Treatment of post-transplant lymphoproliferative disease with rituximab monoclonal antibody after lung transplantation [letter]. Lancet 1999; 354:1698–1699.

54. Kuehnle I, Huls MH, Liu Z, et al. CD20 monoclonal antibody (rituximab) for therapy of Epstein–Barr virus lymphoma after hemopoietic stem-cell transplantation. Blood 2000; 95:1502–1505.

55. Milpied N, Vasseur B, Parquet N, et al. Humanized anti-CD20 monoclonal antibody (Rituximab) in post transplant B-lymphoproliferative disorder: a retrospective analysis on 32 patients. Ann Oncol 2000; 11(suppl 1):113–116.

56. Choquet S, Herbrecht R, Socie G, et al. Multicenter, open label, phase II trial to evacuate the efficacy and safety of treatment with rituximab in patients suffering from B-cell lymphoproliferative disorders (B-PTLD) (M39037 trial). Ann Oncol 2002; 13(suppl 2):37.

57. Berney T, Delis S, Kato T, et al. Successful treatment of posttransplant lymphoproliferative disease with prolonged rituximab treatment in intestinal transplant recipients. Transplantation 2002; 74:1000–1006.

58. Loomis R, Carbone R, Reiss M, Lacy J. Bcl-2 antisense (G3139, Genasense) enhances the in vitro and in vivo response of Epstein–Barr virus-associated lymphoproliferative disease to rituximab. Clin Cancer Res 2003; 9(5):1931–1939.

59. Orjuela M, Gross TG, Cheung Y, Alobeid B, Morris E, Cairo MS. A pilot study of chemoimmunotherapy (cyclophosphamide, prednisone, and rituximab) in patients with post-transplant lymphoproliferative disorder following solid organ transplantation. Clin Cancer Res 2003; 9:3945s–3952s.

60. Dotti G, Rambaldi A, Fiocchi R, et al. Anti-CD20 antibody (rituximab) administration in patients with late-occurring lymphomas after solid organ transplant. Haematologica 2001; 86(6):618–623.

61. Locatelli F, Zecca M, Rondelli R, et al. Graft versus host disease prophylaxis with low-dose cyclosporine-A reduces the risk of relapse in children with acute leukemia given HLA-identical sibling bone marrow transplantation: results of a randomized trial. Blood 2000; 95:1572–1579.

62. Lim SH, Zhang Y, Wang Z, Varadarajan R, Periman P, Esler WV. Rituximab administration following autologous stem cell transplantation for multiple myeloma is associated with severe IgM deficiency. Blood 2004; 103(5):1971–1972.

63. Papadaki T, Stamatopoulos K, Anagnostopoulos A, Fassas A. Rituximab-associated immune myelopathy. Blood 2003; 102(4):1557–1558.

64. Hale G, Waldmann H, for CAMPATH users. Risks of developing Epstein–Barr virus-related lymphoproliferative disorders after T-cell-depleted marrow transplants. Blood 1998; 91:3079–3083.

65. Slavin S, Nagler A, Naparstek E, et al. Nonmyeloablative stem cell transplantation and cell therapy as an alternative to conventional bone marrow transplantation with lethal cytoreduction for the treatment of malignant and nonmalignant hematologic diseases. Blood 1998; 91:756–763.

66. Chakraverty R, Robinson S, Peggs S, et al. Excessive T-cell depletion of peripheral blood stem cells has an adverse effect upon outcome following allogeneic stem cell transplantation. Bone Marrow Transplant 2001; 28(9):827–834.

67. Hanto DW, Frizzera G, Gajl-Peczalska KJ, Simmons RL. Epstein–Barr virus, immunodeficiency, and B-cell lymphoproliferation. Transplantation 1985; 39:461–472.

68. Shapiro RS, McClain K, Frizzera G, et al. Epstein–Barr virus associated B-cell lymphoproliferative disorders following bone marrow transplantation. Blood 1988; 71:1234–1243.

69. Reddehase MJ, Mutter W, Munch K, Buhring HJ, Koszinowski UH. CD8-positive T lymphocytes specific for murine cytomegalovirus immediate-early antigens mediate protective immunity. J Virol 1987; 61:3102–3108.

70. Riddell SR, Watanabe KS, Goodrich JM, Li CR, Agha ME, Greenberg PD. Restoration of viral immunity in immunodeficient humans by the adoptive transfer of T-cell clones. Science 1992; 257:238–241.

71. Papadopoulos EB, Ladanyi M, Emanuel D, et al. Infusions of donor leukocytes to treat Epstein–Barr virus-associated lymphoproliferative disorders after allogeneic bone marrow transplantation. N Engl J Med 1994; 330:1185–1191.

72. Rooney CM, Smith CA, Ng C, et al. Use of gene-modified virus-specific T lymphocytes to control Epstein–Barr virus-related lymphoproliferation. Lancet 1995; 345:9–13.

73. O'Reilly RJ, Lacerda JF, Lucas KG, Rosenfield NS, Small TN, Papadopoulos EB. Adoptive cell therapy with donor lymphocytes for EBV-associated lymphomas developing after allogeneic marrow transplants. In: DeVita VT, Hellman S, Rosenberg SA, eds. Important Advances in Oncology 1996. Philadelphia: Lippincott-Raven, 1996:149–166.

74. Lucas KG, Burton RL, Zimmerman SE, et al. Semiquantitative Epstein–Barr virus (EBV) polymerase chain reaction for the determination of patients at risk for EBV-induced lymphoproliferative disease after stem cell transplantation. Blood 1998; 91:3654–3661.

75. Bonini C, Ferrari G, Verzeletti S, et al. HSV-TK gene transfer into donor lymphocytes for control of allogeneic graft versus leukemia. Science 1997; 276:1719–1724.

76. Thomis DC, Marktel S, Bonini C, et al. A Fas-based suicide switch in human T cells for the treatment of graft-versus-host disease. Blood 2001; 97:1249–1257.

77. Heslop HE, Ng CYC, Li C, et al. Long-term restoration of immunity against Epstein–Barr virus infection by adoptive transfer of gene-modified virus-specific T lymphocytes. Nat Med 1996; 2:551–555.

78. Rooney CM, Smith CA, Ng CYC, et al. Infusion of cytotoxic T-cells for the prevention and treatment of Epstein–Barr virus-induced lymphoma in allogeneic transplant recipients. Blood 1998; 92:1549–1555.

79. Gustafsson A, Levitsky V, Zou JZ, et al. Epstein–Barr virus (EBV) load in bone marrow transplant recipients at risk to develop posttransplant lymphoproliferative disease: prophylactic infusion of EBV-specific cytotoxic T-cells. Blood 2000; 95:807–814.

80. Nalesnik MA, Rao AS, Furukawa H, et al. Autologous lymphokine-activated killer cell therapy of Epstein–Barr virus-positive and -negative lymphoproliferative disorders arising in organ transplant recipients. Transplantation 1998; 63:1200–1205.

81. Emanuel DJ, Lucas KG, Mallory GB, et al. Treatment of posttransplant lymphoproliferative disease in the central nervous system of a lung transplant recipient using allogeneic leucocytes. Transplantation 1997; 63:1691–1694.

82. O'Reilly RJ, Small TN, Papadopoulos E, Lucas K, Lacerda J, Koulova L. Adoptive immunotherapy for Epstein–Barr virus-associated lymphoproliferative disorders complicating marrow allografts. Springer Semin Immunopathol 1998; 20:455–491.

83. Haque T, Taylor C, Wilkie GM, et al. Complete regression of posttransplant lymphoproliferative disease using partially HLA-matched Epstein–Barr virus-specific cytotoxic T-cells. Transplantation 2001; 72:1399–1402.

84. Haque T, Wilkie GM, Taylor C, et al. Treatment of Epstein–Barr-virus-positive posttransplantation lymphoproliferative disease with partly HLA-matched allogeneic cytotoxic T-cells. Lancet 2002; 360:436–442.

85. Haque T, Amlot PL, Helling N, et al. Reconstitution of EBV-specific T-cell immunity in solid organ transplant recipients 2. J Immunol 1998; 160:6204–6209.

86. Comoli P, Locatelli F, Gerna G, Grossi P, Vigano M, Maccario R. Autologous EBV-specific cytotoxic T-cells to treat EBV-associated post-transplant lymphoproliferative disease (PTLD). Blood 1997; 90:249a.

87. Khanna R, Bell S, Sherritt M, et al. Activation and adoptive transfer of Epstein–Barr virus-specific cytotoxic T-cells in solid organ transplant patients with posttransplant lymphoproliferative disease. Proc Natl Acad Sci USA 1999; 96:10391–10396.

88. Comoli P, Labirio M, Basso S, et al. Infusion of autologous Epstein–Barr virus (EBV)-specific cytotoxic T-cells for prevention of EBV-related lymphoproliferative disorder in solid organ transplant recipients with evidence of active virus replication. Blood 2002; 99(7):2592–2598.

89. Savoldo B, Cubbage ML, Durett AG, et al. Generation of EBV-specific CD4(+) cytotoxic T-cells from virus naive individuals. J Immunol 2002; 168:909–918.

90. Gottschalk S, Ng CYC, Smith CA, et al. An Epstein–Barr virus deletion mutant that causes fatal lymphoproliferative disease unresponsive to virus-specific T-cell therapy. Blood 2001; 97:835–843.

91. Bakker ABH, Schreurs MWJ, de Boer AJ, et al. Melanocyte lineage-specific antigen gp100 is recognized by melanoma-derived tumor-infiltrating lymphocytes. J Exp Med 1994; 179:1005–1009.

92. Bharadwaj M, Sherritt M, Khanna R, Moss DJ. Contrasting Epstein–Barr virus-specific cytotoxic T-cell responses to HLA A2-restricted epitopes in humans and HLA transgenic mice: implications for vaccine design. Vaccine 2001; 19(27):3769–3777.

93. Miller G, Grogan E, Rowe D, et al. Selective lack of antibody to a component of EB nuclear antigen in patients with chronic active Epstein–Barr virus infection. J Infect Dis 1987; 156:26–35.

94. Jones JF, Streib J, Baker S, Herberger M. Chronic fatigue syndrome: I. Epstein–Barr virus immune response and molecular epidemiology. J Med Virol 1991; 33:151–158.

95. Hoshino Y, Kimura H, Tanaka N, et al. Prospective monitoring of the Epstein–Barr virus DNA by a real-time quantitative polymerase chain reaction after allogenic stem cell transplantation. Br J Haematol 2001; 115:105–111.

96. Sakai Y, Ohga S, Tonegawa Y, et al. Interferon-alpha therapy for chronic active Epstein–Barr virus infection: potential effect on the development of T-lymphoprolifera-tive disease. J Pediatr Hematol Oncol 1998; 20(4):342–346.

97. Kawa-Ha K, Franco E, Doi S, et al. Successful treatment of chronic active Epstein–Barr virus infection with recombinant interleukin-2. Lancet 1987; 1(8525):154.

98. Kimura H, Morita M, Tsuge I, et al. Vidarabine therapy for severe chronic active Epstein–Barr virus infection. J Pediatr Hematol Oncol 2001; 23(5):294–299.

99. Imashuku S, Hibi S, Ohara T, et al. Effective control of Epstein–Barr virus-related hemophagocytic lymphohistiocytosis with immunochemotherapy. Histiocyte Soc Blood 1999; 93(6):1869–1874.

100. Chan JK, Sin VC, Wong KF, et al. Nonnasal lymphoma expressing the natural killer cell marker CD56: a clinicopathologic study of 49 cases of an uncommon aggressive neoplasm. Blood 1997; 89(12):4501–4513.

101. Okamura T, Hatsukawa Y, Arai H, Inoue M, Kawa K. Blood stem-cell transplantation for chronic active Epstein–Barr virus with lymphoproliferation. Lancet 2000; 356(9225):223–224.

102. Fujii N, Takenaka K, Hiraki A, et al. Allogeneic peripheral blood stem cell transplanta-tion for the treatment of chronic active Epstein–Barr virus infection. Bone Marrow Transpl 2000; 26(7):805–808.

103. Kimura H, Hoshino Y, Kanegane H, et al. Clinical and virologic characteristics of chronic active Epstein–Barr virus infection. Blood 2001; 98(2):280–286.

104. Kuzushima K, Yamamoto M, Kimura H, et al. Establishment of anti-Epstein–Barr virus (EBV) cellular immunity by adoptive transfer of virus-specific cytotoxic T lympho-cytes from an HLA-matched sibling to a patient with severe chronic active EBV infec-tion. Clin Exp Immunol 1996; 103:192–198.

105. Savoldo B, Huls MH, Liu Z, et al. Autologous Epstein–Barr virus (EBV)-specific cytotoxic T-cells for the treatment of persistent active EBV infection. Blood 2002;100(12):4059–4066.

106. Sandlund JT, Downing JR, Crist WM. Non-Hodgkin's lymphoma in childhood. N Engl J Med 1996; 334(19):1238–1248.

107. Al Sarraf M, LeBlanc M, Giri PG, et al. Chemoradiotherapy versus radiotherapy in patients with advanced nasopharyngeal cancer: phase III randomized Intergroup study. J Clin Oncol 1998; 16(4):1310–1317.

108. Horwitz SM, Horning SJ. Advances in the treatment of Hodgkin's lymphoma. Curr Opin Hematol 2000; 7(4):235–240.

109. Uckun FM, Reaman GH. Immunotoxins for treatment of leukemia and lymphoma. Leuk Lymphoma 1995; 18(3–4):195–201.

110. Terenzi A, Bolognesi A, Pasqualucci L, et al. Anti-CD30 (BER=H2) immunotoxins containing the type-1 ribosome-inactivating proteins momordin and PAP-S (pokeweed antiviral protein from seeds) display powerful antitumour activity against CD30+ tumour cells in vitro and in SCID mice. Br J Haematol 1996; 92(4):872–879.

111. Hartmann F, Renner C, Jung W, et al. Anti-CD16/CD30 bispecific antibody treat-ment for Hodgkin's disease: role of infusion schedule and costimulation with cytokines. Clin Cancer Res 2001; 7(7):1835–1836.

112. Sforzini S, de Totero D, Gaggero A, et al. Targeting of saporin to Hodgkin's lymphoma cells by anti-CD30 and anti-CD25 bispecific antibodies. Br J Haematol 1998; 102(4):1061–1068.

113. Berger C, Rothenberger S, Bachmann E, McQuain C, Nadal D, Knecht H. Sequence polymorphisms between latent membrane proteins LMP1 and LMP2A do not correlate in EBV-associated reactive and malignant lymphoproliferations. Int J Cancer 1999; 81(3):371–375.

114. Khanna R, Cooper L, Kienzle N, Moss DJ, Burrows SR, Khanna KK. Engagement of CD40 antigen with soluble CD40 ligand up-regulates peptide transporter expression and restores endogenous processing function in Burkitt's lymphoma cells. J Immunol 1997; 159:5782–5785.
115. Frisan T, Zhang QJ, Levitskaya J, Coram M, Kurilla MG, Masucci MG. Defective presentation of MHC class I-restricted cytotoxic T-cell epitopes in Burkitt's lymphoma cells. Int J Cancer 1996; 68(2):251–258.
116. Sing AP, Ambinder RF, Hong DJ, et al. Isolation of Epstein–Barr Virus (EBV)-specific cytotoxic T lymphocytes that lyse Reed–Sternberg cells: implications for immune-medicated therapy of EBV Hodgkin's disease. Blood 1997; 89:1978–1986.
117. Khanna R, Busson P, Burrows SR, et al. Molecular characterization of antigen-processing function in nasopharyngeal carcinoma (NPC): evidence for efficient presentation of Epstein–Barr virus cytotoxic T-cell epitopes by NPC cells. Cancer Res 1998; 58(2):310–314.
118. Roskrow MA, Suzuki N, Gan Y-J, et al. EBV-specific cytotoxic T lymphocytes for the treatment of patients with EBV positive relapsed Hodgkin's disease. Blood 1998; 91:2925–2934.
119. Ranieri E, Herr W, Gambotto A, et al. Dendritic cells transduced with an adenovirus vector encoding Epstein–Barr virus latent membrane protein 2B: a new modality for vaccination. J Virol 1999; 73:10,416–10,425.
120. Gahn B, Siller-Lopez F, Pirooz AD, et al. Adenoviral gene transfer into dendritic cells efficiently amplifies the immune response to the LMP2A-antigen: a potential treatment strategy for Epstein–Barr virus-positive Hodgkin's lymphoma. Int J Cancer 2001; 93:706–713.
121. Su Z, Peluso MV, Raffegerst SH, Schendel DJ, Roskrow MA. The generation of LMP2a-specific cytotoxic T lymphocytes for the treatment of patients with Epstein–Barr virus-positive Hodgkin disease. Eur J Immunol 2001; 31:947–958.
122. Bollard CM, Rossig C, Calonge MJ, et al. Adapting a transforming growth factor beta-related tumor protection strategy to enhance antitumor immunity. Blood 2002; 99:3179–3187.
123. Wieser R, Attisano L, Wrana JL, Massague J. Signaling activity of transforming growth factor beta type II receptors lacking specific domains in the cytoplasmic region. Mol Cell Biol 1993; 13:7239–7247.
124. Chua D, Huang J, Zheng B, et al. Adoptive transfer of autologous Epstein–Barr virus-specific cytotoxic T-cells for nasopharyngeal carcinoma. Int J Cancer 2001; 94:73–80.
125. Comoli P, De Palma R, Siena S, et al. Adoptive transfer of allogeneic Epstein–Barr virus (EBV)-specific cytotoxic T-cells with in vitro antitumor activity boosts LMP2-specific immune response in a patient with EBV-related nasopharyngeal carcinoma. Ann Oncol 2004; 15(1):113–117.
126. Khanna R. Tumour surveillance: missing peptides and MHC molecules. Immunol Cell Biol 1998; 76:20–26.
127. Frisan T, Donati D, Cervenak L, Wilson J, Masucci MG, Bejarano MT. CD40 cross-linking enhances the immunogenicity of Burkitt's-lymphoma cell lines. Int J Cancer 1999; 83:772–779.
128. Khanna R, Burrows SR, Steigerwald-Mullen PM, Moss DJ, Kurilla MG, Cooper L. Targeting Epstein–Barr virus nuclear antigen 1 (EBNA1) through the class II pathway restores immune recognition by EBNA1-specific cytotoxic T lymphocytes: evidence for HLA-DM-independent processing. Int Immunol 1997; 9:1537–1543.
129. Hale G, Zhang MJ, Bunjes D, et al. Improving the outcome of bone marrow transplantation by using CD52 monoclonal antibodies to prevent graft-versus-host disease and graft rejection. Blood 1998; 92:4581–4590.
130. Darenkov IA, Marcarelli MA, Basadonna GP, et al. Reduced incidence of Epstein–Barr virus-associated posttransplant lymphoproliferative disorder using preemptive antiviral therapy. Transplantation 1997; 64(6):848–852.

131. McDiarmid SV, Jordan S, Kim GS, et al. Prevention and preemptive therapy of post-transplant lymphoproliferative disease in pediatric liver recipients. Transplantation 1998; 66(12):1604–1611.
132. Green M, Kaufmann M, Wilson J, Reyes J. Comparison of intravenous ganciclovir followed by oral acyclovir with intravenous ganciclovir alone for prevention of cytomegalovirus and Epstein–Barr virus disease after liver transplantation in children. Clin Infect Dis 1997; 6:1344–1349.
133. Khanna R, Moss DJ, Burrows SR. Vaccine strategies against Epstein–Barr virus-associated diseases: lessons from studies on cytotoxic T-cell-mediated immune regulation. Immunol Rev 1999; 170:49–64.
134. Jackman WT, Mann KA, Hoffmann HJ, Spaete RR. Expression of Epstein–Barr virus gp350 as a single chain glycoprotein for an EBV subunit vaccine. Vaccine 1999; 17(7–8): 660–668.

19

The Development of Epstein–Barr Virus Vaccines

Andrew J. Morgan and A. Douglas Wilson
Department of Cellular and Molecular Medicine, School of Medical Sciences,
University of Bristol, Bristol, U.K.

WHAT IS THE DEMAND FOR EBV VACCINES?

Epstein–Barr virus (EBV) is a ubiquitous human herpesvirus that is carried by more than 95% of the human population as a lifelong latent infection [reviewed in (1) and Chapter 3]. EBV immortalizes, or transforms, B-cells in vitro. A combination of six viral nuclear gene products and two membrane-associated viral proteins in transformed B-cells is primarily responsible for the changes in cell growth and phenotype. Expression of the growth-transformed phenotype has only been detected in the B-cell follicles of tonsils (2), while in peripheral blood, EBV is detected in a very small number of resting memory B-cells. EBV gene expression in these cells is restricted to, at most, one or two viral genes that are probably invisible to the immune system. A normal immune response appears to be essential in maintaining the asymptomatic carrier-state, as demonstrated by the occurrence of posttransplant lymphoproliferative disease (PTLD) in immunocompromised persons.

Primary infection usually occurs in the first few years of life and is asymptomatic (3). Symptomatic infectious mononucleosis (IM) arises in about half of individuals who have a primary infection during adolescence (4). While IM is uncommon in developing countries because primary infection invariably takes place early in childhood, it is common in the developed countries. Following primary infection, lifelong latent EBV infection in vivo is asymptomatic in the vast majority of individuals but is associated with a number of important cancers including undifferentiated nasopharyngeal carcinoma (NPC), endemic Burkitt lymphoma (BL), certain forms of Hodgkin's disease (HD), and PTLD. There are around 100,000 new cases of NPC annually, mainly in southern China and southeast Asia, making it a significant global health problem (5). HD is a common cancer in the Western world with an incidence of about 8000 cases annually in the United States. Vaccine approaches are being devised whereby the incidence of these EBV-associated cancers could be reduced.

The biology of EBV poses significant challenges in the development of EBV vaccines different to those faced in the successful development of more conventional vaccines such as for polio, measles, and smallpox. Almost the entire human population is infected with EBV, and for the vast majority there are no clinical manifestations. The long period of coevolution of primates and their respective γ-herpesviruses has led to stable host–virus relationships that, in the main, amount to a peaceful coexistence. It is not clear whether advantages are conferred to humans by lifelong EBV infection, but it seems possible that some immunological effects, such as bias of the T-cell receptor repertoire (6), are present on a population-wide basis. Any adverse effect arising from unselective mass vaccination of healthy individuals to prevent or modify EBV infection may affect this balance and cause more problems than it solves. The long period of coevolution, which probably preceded primate speciation, means that the interaction between virus and host has become very sophisticated in terms of the mechanisms deployed by the virus to evade innate and adaptive immune responses. EBV persists in the face of a range of antibody responses, some of which are virus-neutralizing in vitro (7), and a multitude of cell-mediated responses, including virus-specific CD8+ T-cells (8), CD4+ T-cells (9,10), and natural killer (NK) cells (11). EBV is now formally classified as a Grade 1 carcinogen (12), because several of its genes can independently transform certain cell types (13). The composition of an EBV vaccine for use in humans is therefore somewhat restricted because a licensed human vaccine can only contain viral elements that are nontransforming. However, this need not exclude nontransforming derivatives of virus-transforming gene products such as synthetic peptides. Because EBV infection is nonpermissive except under special circumstances, it is still not technically feasible to produce EBV on a scale large enough to support even a small vaccine trial using killed or attenuated forms.

The justification for developing EBV vaccines to prevent or ameliorate EBV-associated diseases is self-evident from the scope of the disease burden, including that of EBV-associated cancers. The development of EBV vaccines has been a long-term objective since its original suggestion more than 25 years ago (14). Since then, however, our understanding of EBV biology has been profoundly altered at both the molecular and cellular levels. Furthermore, vaccine development has always lagged behind scientific development for a variety of practical, commercial, and other nonscientific reasons, and the original rationale put forward in support of work on EBV vaccines must now be viewed from a different perspective. Initially, the apparent association between EBV and endemic BL (15,16) and undifferentiated NPC (17,18) led to the proposal that the development of a vaccine to prevent EBV primary infection should be the goal. A view was taken that whatever the complexities of the associations between EBV and BL or NPC, preventing infection would remove a link in the chain of events that gives rise to tumors. It has been clear for many years that EBV cannot be the single causal factor of NPC or BL. Holoendemic malaria has been identified as a probable cofactor for BL (19) but the cofactors involved in NPC remain unidentified (17). The absence of a clear immunological basis for EBV vaccine development, because of a limited understanding of the biology and immunology of the virus and less knowledge about immunological criteria that are important in preventing EBV-associated disease, has resulted in slow progress. Furthermore, the cost of developing an EBV vaccine together with the lack of a strong commercial incentive to produce a vaccine against BL and NPC has also delayed vaccine development. The increasing recognition of the significance of IM in the developed countries, offering greater commercial incentives for EBV vaccine development, gave rise to a renewed interest in this area (20). Any vaccine developed to prevent IM might also have more widespread application in the prevention of other EBV-associated diseases.

The early observation that serum EBV neutralizing antibodies largely recognized a major viral envelope glycoprotein, gp350 (7,21,22), set the scene for subsequent work over a number of years. This involved the characterization and purification of tractable quantities of the gp350 viral envelope glycoprotein from natural sources (23–25) and by recombinant DNA methods (26–30). These materials have been extensively evaluated in a primate model of EBV-induced B-cell lymphoma (31), and two derivatives of these experimental vaccines have entered small-scale human trials. Another approach using synthetic peptides based on the EBV latent antigen EBV nuclear antigen (EBNA)-3, to induce cell-mediated immune responses, has been developed in parallel and has been the subject of small-scale human trials (32).

PROGRESS WITH OTHER HUMAN HERPESVIRUS VACCINES

It is worthwhile to consider the progress made in the development of other human herpesvirus vaccines to ascertain if any lessons relevant to EBV vaccine development can be learned. One of the key shared characteristics of herpesvirus infection in humans is that despite there being widespread infection with herpes simplex virus (HSV), cytomegalovirus (CMV), and varicella zoster virus (VZV) in the human population, there is much less disease than might be expected. While the proportion of those who develop disease following infection may be small, the number of affected individuals is still substantial. Why some individuals develop herpesvirus disease and others do not is partly a consequence of the immune response. Altered immunity, by illness or treatment, may have serious clinical consequences with existing herpesvirus infections as well as newly acquired infections. That herpesvirus infections are normally controlled by the immune system suggests that vaccine-induced immune responses could be effective in preventing herpesvirus-associated disease. Apart from the relatively small group of immunocompromised persons, few other groups, if any, can be assigned a higher or lower risk of contracting herpesvirus disease except on a demographic basis. Modification of herpesvirus infection to prevent disease is clearly possible, as has been demonstrated with the varicella Oka strain vaccine (33). Furthermore, the validity of the concept that herpesvirus tumors can be prevented by vaccination was first demonstrated with Marek's disease of chickens (34) and *Herpes saimiri* in nonhuman primates (35). What is not clear is the immunological basis for disease prevention in these models. However, the herpesviruses each have quite different biological behaviors. It is very difficult to make generalizations from one herpesvirus to another that could contribute to the rational design of an EBV vaccine. The differences between the human herpesviruses in terms of host evasion mechanisms, portals of entry, target tissues for primary infection, cells in which latent infection is established, and gene products and mechanisms involved in establishing a latent infection are considerable.

Of all herpesvirus vaccines, HSV vaccines have probably received the greatest attention. A range of wild-type live HSV virus and inactivated HSV vaccines have been produced and tested in large numbers of individuals for their ability to reduce recurrent disease, but almost all of these trials have been inadequately controlled (36). A tentative conclusion from these studies might be that some short-term benefits can be achieved in terms of reducing the recurrence of HSV disease, but with no demonstrable long-term benefits. At the time when this type of HSV vaccine was being evaluated, it was perceived that genital HSV infection might be associated with cervical carcinoma, and the move toward using whole live or killed virus was abandoned in favor of subunit and other recombinant product vaccines. Despite showing promising results in animal models, subunit vaccine formulations using HSV envelope glycoproteins failed to protect human uninfected sexual partners from contracting genital HSV infections from their infected partners (37). Now that the perceived association between genital HSV infection and cervical carcinoma has receded, a renewed effort has been applied to developing live HSV vaccines. In general, live virus vaccines are more effective than killed virus vaccines because the vaccine virus replication is capable of generating a more broad-based immune response with a corresponding memory element. Clearly, a complication of using live herpesvirus vaccines is that they may infect persons other than those vaccinated and the live virus vaccine is also likely to establish a lifelong infection that can never be eradicated. Modern molecular genetics has allowed recombinant HSV to be produced in studies where genes important in neurovirulence, transformation in cell culture, primary infection, and reactivation can be deleted or attenuated (38). Other approaches have involved the production of a recombinant HSV from which the gH gene has been deleted. HSV gH is an essential viral envelope glycoprotein in the fusion of the HSV envelope with the target cell membrane (39). The HSV deletion mutant, otherwise known as a disabled infectious single cycle (DISC) virus, is propagated in a cell line that provides the gH gene *in trans*. On inoculation in humans or animals, the DISC virus is able to replicate only once and produces noninfectious progeny virus (40–42).

No CMV vaccines have been licensed for human use, and it may be some time before any are. Whether the presence of CMV antibodies reduces CMV disease or not is controversial (43). Passively administered antibodies appear to reduce CMV disease in renal transplant patients but not prevent CMV infection (44). The CMV Towne strain was created by extensive serial passage in culture to achieve attenuation prior to use as a live virus vaccine. However, inoculation of this strain into various groups of patients has yielded mixed results. CMV seronegative renal transplant patients were apparently protected against severe CMV disease although not against infection (45), while there was no evidence of protection among a group of healthy seronegative female adults of childbearing age (46). Recombinant subunit glycoprotein vaccine formulations based on the CMV gB glycoprotein and the oil-in-water adjuvant MF59 have been developed more recently (47,48). These preparations induce virus-neutralizing antibodies and proliferative T-cell responses in humans but results of phase II human trial have not yet been reported. Of particular interest has been the recent use of a murine CMV plasmid vaccine in conjunction with a formalin-inactivated murine CMV preparation in a prime-boost sequence (49), the plasmid being used to prime, and the inactivated virus used to boost immune responses. The plasmid expressed the murine homologue of human CMV pp65. Long-term and complete protection against a CMV challenge was achieved in a mouse model where antibody and cell-mediated immune responses were induced. It remains to be seen whether this vaccination boost strategy can prevent reactivation of latent CMV infection.

The most successful human herpesvirus vaccine to date is the VZV Oka strain vaccine (33), which is licensed for clinical use in children and adults in several countries. The Oka strain retains its ability to infect T lymphocytes but its ability to infect the skin is greatly impaired when compared to wild-type strains; this is the basis of its attenuation. From the experience of using other human herpesvirus vaccines, few definite conclusions can be drawn with respect to EBV vaccine development except that prevention of EBV infection itself is not a realistic objective, while prevention or reduction in disease probably is.

SEVERAL ALTERNATIVE OBJECTIVES FOR EBV VACCINATION

Three separate strategies for controlling EBV-associated disease by vaccination are under consideration. The first is to vaccinate with the major envelope glycoprotein, gp350, and/or other envelope glycoproteins, to modify EBV infection. A second approach would be to vaccinate at some time after infection has taken place, to modify the immune status of the individual with respect to EBV. It is envisaged that this postinfection approach could involve either envelope glycoproteins or latent antigen peptides or a combination of both. The third tactic is to use vaccination in a therapeutic mode to induce or enhance immune responses against the EBV-associated tumor cells. The antigens used in this strategy will depend on the tumor under consideration. BL cells only express EBNA1, while NPC and HD also express latent membrane protein (LMP)-2 and, in a proportion of cases, also LMP1. Effective vaccine-induced immune responses will be responses against which the virus has not necessarily evolved an evasion strategy. This would mean the balance of power is tipped in favor of the host immune response even though the virus itself may not be eliminated. A variety of approaches have been investigated in the development of EBV vaccines and have included a range of proteins, peptide antigens, adjuvants, live virus vectors, and even EBV "decoys" consisting of DNA-free EBV proteins condensed onto tin oxide particles (50).

   Any primary vaccination strategy to control EBV diseases must allow for the fact that most primary infection occurs in the first few years of life (51). For example, 95% of children in Hong Kong are infected with EBV before 12 years of age (3). It would seem impractical, although not impossible, to deliver an EBV vaccine to the very large numbers of children in populations in Africa and China where primary infection occurs during infancy and early childhood. Vaccination to prevent primary EBV infection could theoretically eliminate EBV-associated disease, completely. However, it seems unlikely that any vaccine could provide lifelong sterilizing immunity against EBV infection. Thus, the aim of EBV vaccination should be to prevent or minimize disease rather than to prevent or eliminate viral infection. Each EBV-associated disease arises for a complex set of different reasons and each is likely to require a different vaccination strategy.

   Primary EBV infection in infants is usually asymptomatic, whereas IM occurs in a proportion of individuals whose primary EBV infection has been delayed until adolescence. Of the remainder of this older group, a proportion seroconvert without symptoms, and some remain seronegative for life and are apparently never infected with the virus (52). Various hypotheses have been proposed to explain the age-restricted occurrence of IM. These have included a higher initial challenge dose of EBV and reduced primary immune responses as a consequence of stress. An alternative hypothesis proposes an altered balance between helper T-cell function and the activation of NK cells, by promoting the replication of virus-infected B-cells on one hand and by promoting cytotoxic antiviral T-cell responses on the other (53). An EBV vaccine to prevent IM will, therefore, be most effective if targeted at populations of seronegative adolescents in Western countries. Because achieving sterilizing immunity by vaccination against EBV seems an unlikely possibility, current aims will be limited to modifying primary infection. Perhaps only a small change in immune status caused by vaccination will be sufficient to prevent disease. Any EBV vaccine that could simply reduce the viral load on primary infection, or direct an appropriate T-cell immune response, may be sufficient to prevent manifestations of IM. It is, therefore, reasonable to conclude that vaccination with gp350 to modify primary EBV infection could prevent IM.

It is difficult to envisage how vaccine-induced responses could prevent the development of tumors such as NPC when the wide range of naturally occurring immune responses could not. One rationale for developing postinfection vaccines is based on the observation that a prognostic indicator of the onset of NPC is the rapid rise in the level of serum immunoglobulin (Ig)-A antibodies against lytic cycle antigens (54). This elevation in antibody presumably reflects an increase in virus production that is linked to the emergence of the tumor. This changed pattern of EBV replication may also reflect changes from Th1-type regulation to a mucosal-derived Th2-type response, in immune regulation of virus-infected cells. NPC in Chinese populations occurs in adults 40 years of age and older. Because a strategy of early childhood vaccination to prevent primary infection seems impractical, modification of infection by postinfection vaccination is feasible and potentially of much greater immediate value. Intervening by postinfection immunization with a gp350, or other type of vaccine, before the increase in EBV replication, signaling the onset of NPC, may well alter the immune balance at a crucial time and prevent NPC from developing. It should also be noted in this context that high titers of antibody against the viral capsid antigen (VCA) in Ugandan children are also prognostic with respect to the development of endemic BL (15). Immune responses to the vaccine antigen itself in persons already infected with EBV would have to be taken into account if this approach were adopted. Similar arguments may hold good in the case of endemic BL. Modification of primary infection by vaccination may itself be sufficient to provide additional control of virus load and replication. The success of such approaches will depend on whether the apparent reactivation of EBV is causally associated with the onset of NPC or is simply a consequence of tumor development.

Approximately 10% of seronegative children receiving solid organ transplants develop PTLD during the first year after transplant. The risk of developing significant morbidity or PTLD following primary EBV infection in seronegative transplant recipients is about 20 times greater than in seropositive transplant recipients. Primary EBV infection occurs in about 70% of all seronegative recipients during the first six months following organ transplantation (55,56). Immunization of seronegative patients before transplantation provides an opportunity to test whether the presence of antibody to the major EBV envelope glycoprotein gp350 will modify EBV infection and prevent or reduce disease, following transplantation and during the period of immunosuppression. A small trial of an EBV gp350 subunit vaccine in pediatric patients awaiting solid organ transplantation is in progress.

Thus far, two strategies have been followed in parallel in the development of EBV vaccines that might be used to modify primary EBV infection. The first is based on the major envelope glycoprotein, gp350, and the second strategy is based on the identification of latent antigen peptide epitopes recognized by cytotoxic T lymphocytes (CTLs) in a major histocompatablity complex (MHC) class I context. EBV infection in otherwise healthy seropositive persons is controlled to some extent by CTLs specific to particular immunodominant epitopes in the latency nuclear protein, EBNA3. The two approaches are considered in more detail below.

GP350 VACCINES

The major EBV envelope glycoprotein gp350 was originally selected as a candidate subunit vaccine to prevent EBV infection on the basis that antibodies raised against this molecule are virus-neutralizing in vitro (22,24,57). It is worth noting that human monoclonal antibody Fab fragments have now been produced in a recombinant phage system (58), but it is not yet known whether these can neutralize the virus in vitro. Of particular relevance to gp350 vaccine development is the observation that there is very little sequence variation in gp350 genes taken from various EBV isolates around the world (59). EBV gp350 contains up to 50% carbohydrate, much of which is O-linked (60,61). Very little is yet known about the contribution that carbohydrate may make to the immunological profile of gp350. Although at least 20 open-reading frames in the EBV genome can potentially code for glycoproteins, only a few of these have been identified and characterized and their possible role in making an effective EBV vaccine has not received serious consideration to date.

What has been established recently is that gp350 is not an absolute requirement for EBV infection to occur. A recombinant EBV in which the gp350 gene had been deleted was found to be able to infect a range of B-cell lines and epithelial cells, albeit at a lower efficiency (62). Based on these results alone it would seem most unlikely that a gp350 vaccine, which acts by the induction of neutralizing antibodies, would be able to prevent infection. However, these results do not rule out an EBV gp350 vaccine being effective. A simple modification of infection may be all that is needed to prevent or alleviate disease. Infection of epithelial cells in vitro may take place by both gp350-dependent and -independent pathways (63). It was found that EBV infection of an epithelial cell line, AGS, was not inhibited by the presence of soluble gp350 but was inhibited by soluble gp25, the EBV homologue of herpes simplex gL. A third EBV membrane component, gp42, binds to MHC class II molecules on the surface of B-cells (64,65). One EBV variant that has a 16-kb deletion containing the gp350 and EBNA3A genes and the amino terminal region of EBNA3B has been isolated. This variant apparently cannot transform primary B-cells in culture, and replication is not induced by the presence of phorbol esters (66).

EBV gp350 binds to the host cell complement receptor CD21 (67,68). Cross-linking of CD21 by gp350 induces the synthesis of interleukins (IL)-1 to 6 (69) and can modulate IL-1 and tumor necrosis factor synthesis (70). CD21 is part of a membrane signaling complex involved in the activation of B-cell immune responses, and cross-linking by gp350 may be an important early event in driving infected B-cells into the cell cycle prior to immortalization (71). Indeed, it might be expected that gp350 could affect any cell expressing CD21, which includes dendritic cells, T-cells, monocytes, epithelial cells, and other cells. These gp350 effects could be both advantageous and disadvantageous in vaccination, but it has not yet been possible to evaluate the potential effects of gp350 vaccines in these respects.

Some work has been performed in identifying gp350 B and T-cell epitopes with the view of producing a gp350 peptide vaccine. However, because of the discontinuous or conformation-dependent nature of the B-cell epitopes, little progress has been made and no peptides have been tested in any of the animal models (72–75). At least two T-helper cell epitopes in the gp350 amino acid sequence have been identified in the amino terminal region (76). More recently, gp350-specific CTL epitopes have been identified (77). It has now become apparent that CTL responses in the blood of IM patients are mainly against lytic cycle antigens, while CTL responses in healthy seropositive persons can be directed at lytic cycle antigens as well as latent antigens (78–81). Whether these responses to lytic antigens serve to control viral infection or merely reflect acute viral replication remains to be determined.

GP350 VACCINES AND A PRIMATE MODEL OF EBV LYMPHOMA

Malignant lymphoma can be induced in the New World primate, the cottontop tamarin, by injection of large doses of EBV, and the tumors induced have been studied in some detail. The lymphoid lesions generated by the virus in this animal are clearly genuine tumors because they are monoclonal or oligoclonal, and arise independently at different sites in the injected animal (82). One further reason for selecting this animal model was that it was believed at the time that γ-herpesviruses were not present in New World primates. However, a naturally occurring γ-herpesvirus, CalHV-3, is found in the common marmoset (*Callithrix jaccus*) and in naturally occurring B-cell tumors from these animals (83). It seems likely that cottontop tamarins will also carry indigenous γ-herpesviruses. A number of EBV vaccines based on the envelope glycoprotein gp350 have been evaluated in the cottontop tamarin (31). As is the case with most animal models, the cottontop tamarin is less than ideal. First, the tamarin is not infectable by the oral route and does not appear to sustain a persistent infection, at least not at the same level as in humans. It has been shown that the tamarin can sustain latent infection because small numbers of EBV-positive B-cells have been detected in animals that had been immunized and protected against challenge with a lymphomagenic dose of EBV (84). Furthermore, the tamarin has a very restricted MHC class I polymorphism and expresses MHC alleles G, F, and E, which are associated primarily with NK cell function, but not A, B, and C, which are associated with antigen-specific CTLs (85). Nevertheless, analysis of the immune responses in this model indicated that both cytotoxic CD4+ and CD8+ T-cells participate (86), and that their activity was markedly enhanced following gp350 vaccination (87).

The first subunit vaccine was based on gp350 purified from bulk cultures of EBV-infected cells. The purified antigen was initially made by preparative sodium dodecyl sulfate–polyacrylamide gel electrophoresis, and was incorporated into artificial liposomes. This vaccine formulation induced virus-neutralizing antibodies and a protective immune response in the cottontop tamarin model of EBV lymphoma. Subsequently, a number of different EBV vaccines based on gp350 were developed and evaluated in the tamarin model. The gp350 gene has been expressed in a variety of mammalian cell expression systems where glycosylation and posttranslational modifications, which are closely similar to those found on the natural product, occur (26,88,89). It has not been possible to distinguish between these products and the natural product gp350 in terms of their ability to induce virus-neutralizing antibodies, bind a range of monoclonal antibodies, induce protective immunity in the tamarin, and in some studies, stimulate the proliferation of gp350-specific T-cells. In most cases, the C-terminal membrane anchor sequence has been removed from the gene allowing secretion of the expressed eukaryotic product into the culture medium. These techniques offer major advantages in the large-scale preparation of a defined product that is relatively easy to purify.

Most proteins or glycoproteins are weakly immunogenic when inoculated alone into animals, and gp350 is no exception. An adjuvant is invariably required to stimulate the immune response to the subunit antigen (90). Successful protection studies in the tamarin lymphoma model with gp350 subunit vaccines have so far used artificial liposomes (22,91), threonyl muramyl dipeptide (92), or immunostimulating complexes (ISCOMs). Iscoms are supramolecular structures containing immunologically active plant triterpenoids (93). Iscoms that have chemically defined and pure triterpenoid components, and predictable immunomodulatory properties without deleterious adverse effects, are now being produced (94,95). However, the only adjuvants currently licensed for general human use are aluminium salts. An alum adjuvant was tested in the tamarin lymphoma model with a recombinant gp350 subunit and was found to induce protective immunity in three out of five animals (96). The choice of adjuvant can profoundly affect the outcome of vaccination, and the selection of an adjuvant for any gp350 subunit vaccine human trial could make the difference between success and failure.

A plasmid vector containing the gene for gp350 has been shown to induce effective immune responses against the antigen in mice (97). The gp350 DNA–vaccine induced gp350-specific antibodies, mainly of the IgG1 isotype, and could mediate antibody-dependent cellular cytotoxicity (ADCC) against cells expressing gp350. Furthermore, the gp350 plasmid induced a gp350-specific precursor T-cell population and gp350-specific CTLs. Both the qualitative and quantitative responses associated with DNA immunization in the mouse may prove to be advantageous in the prevention or modification of EBV infection in humans.

EBV gp350 has been expressed in recombinant vaccinia (98), adenovirus (99), and varicella (88). Recombinant vaccinia viruses expressing gp350 have been derived from the relatively virulent Western Reserve (WR) strain and the more attenuated Wyeth vaccine strain and both have been tested in the tamarin lymphoma model (100). The key observation in these experiments was that the more virulent WR strain derivative gave protective immunity but did not induce antibodies to gp350. Antibodies against vaccinia proteins were induced by both vaccinia strains. Clearly, in this case, protective immunity arises from some form of gp350-specific cell-mediated immune response. Replication of the M81 EBV strain in a group of common marmosets vaccinated with a gp350 vaccinia recombinant was decreased as compared to that in control groups (101). Further work needs to be done in developing effective vaccinia recombinants that strike the correct balance between attenuation and immunogenicity. Progress to this end could be made with the Copenhagen strain vaccinia derivative (102), canarypox recombinants (103), or the modified Ankara vaccine (104).

Recombinant adenovirus expressing gp350 has been tested in the tamarin model (99). Several features of adenovirus have made them attractive for vaccine antigen delivery. First, adenoviruses types 4 and 7 have already been used on a large scale in the U.S. Armed Forces to prevent respiratory disease and have a good safety record (105). Second, the adenovirus can be given orally following encapsulation. Mucosal immunity is induced in the respiratory tract, although primary immune contact is in the gut lymphoid tissue. Though these may prove to be important factors in the future, it is possible that the induction of mucosal immunity in the form of IgA antibodies will enhance infection by EBV (106,107). When protective immunity was induced in the tamarin lymphoma model using replication-defective adenovirus expressing gp350, antibodies against gp350 were induced but they did not have the capacity to neutralize EBV in vitro (99). In contrast, when high titers of neutralizing antibody against gp350 were generated by immunization with purified gp350 incorporated in liposomes, protective immunity was not always induced (108). These results suggest that cellular responses are important in protective immunity in the tamarin lymphoma model but antibody responses may still be required in preventing or controlling EBV infection in humans. In the common marmoset model of the EBV-induced mononucleosis-like syndrome, protective immunity did not correlate with the presence of serum virus-neutralizing antibodies following immunization with gp350 and alum (109).

Some developmental work has been carried out on the generation of a recombinant VZV vaccine vector for the delivery of EBV genes. VZV recombinants which are able to express EBV gp350 were produced (88,110). It may be timely to explore this option further given the success of the Oka VZV vaccine strain and its incorporation into national vaccine programs in the United States, Japan, and elsewhere. A large body of health and safety information has now been accumulated over the past two decades of use of the VZV Oka strain in humans (33). VZV is the only human herpesvirus in which vaccination has been successful in preventing or modifying disease, both in the modification of primary infection and reactivation phenomena (111).

PEPTIDE VACCINES

The use of EBV latent antigen peptides representing MHC class I–restricted CTL epitopes in EBNA3 to induce CTL memory by vaccination has been reviewed thoroughly elsewhere (112). EBV infection of B-cells mainly gives rise to latent infection and only switches to productive infection under certain circumstances. Eleven EBV genes, including EBNAs 1 to 6 and LMPs 1, 2A, and 2B are expressed in latent infection. It is believed that the numbers of EBV infected cells expressing the whole panel of EBNA and LMP latent genes in the circulation of human seropositive persons is very low and that this low level is largely maintained by CTLs specific for EBNA3. One approach to EBV vaccination has been based on these factors, and epitopes recognized by CD8+ CTLs against particular MHC backgrounds have been documented. Peptide vaccines based on these epitopes could be used to vaccinate a significant proportion of a given population provided the distribution of particular MHC restrictions is known. The stated aim of this strategy is not to prevent infection but to reduce the number of virus-infected cells that develop on infection, and thereby reduce the incidence of disease. Human trials of an EBNA3 peptide that is restricted through the human leukocyte antigen (HLA) B8 allele are in progress, although no results have been reported other than that the peptide vaccine and adjuvant, Montanide ISA 720, are well tolerated. These vaccines could elicit T-cell memory that would be activated on natural EBV challenge to produce specific CTLs. However, the central problems remain the same with this strategy as with the approach using gp350. How does the virus persist in the face of an apparently healthy and effective cellular and humoral immune response? How does a certain population of latently infected B-cells escape immunosurveillance? What kind of cellular and humoral immune response will be required to prevent primary infection, or at least modify primary infection? One important observation that has implications for EBV vaccine design using epitopes, whether they come from latent or lytic antigens, is that epitopes assembled in a polypeptide chain or "polytope" are effective immunogens. The "string of beads" epitope immunogen can induce T-cell responses to all the epitopes in the string and is apparently not adversely affected by the presence of adjacent epitopes of different MHC class I restriction (113) or MHC class II restriction (114).

OTHER ANIMAL MODELS

Animal models are of variable use in evaluating vaccines when the infectious agent has a different pathogenesis in the experimental host, as is usually the case. However, it is necessary that the immunogenicity and possible induction of adverse effects by new vaccines be evaluated in laboratory animals such as mice and rabbits. Two primate model systems—the cottontop tamarin (*Saguinus oedipus oedipus*) (82) and the common marmoset (*C. jaccus*)—have been used in EBV vaccine research (115–117). No satisfactory animal model of human EBV infection exists and the inevitable shortcomings of the tamarin and marmoset models must be taken into account when interpreting results obtained. Inoculation of EBV into the common marmoset can give rise to a poorly defined mononucleosis-like syndrome. EBV infection in the common marmoset with the M81 strain of EBV gives rise to the long-term maintenance of antibodies to viral antigens without clinical disease. The presence of EBV DNA can be demonstrated in tissues and oral fluids using polymerase chain reaction (PCR) analysis. When infected common marmosets were paired with uninfected animals, the uninfected animals seroconverted within four to six weeks (116). Results obtained in this particular model may be difficult to interpret reliably because it was discovered that another virus similar to EBV is endemic in at least some captive populations of the common marmoset.

A rodent γ2-herpesvirus that infects mice, designated murine γ-herpesvirus 68 (MHV68) (118), was isolated some years ago and has subsequently been developed into a sophisticated model of γ-herpesvirus infection (119,120). Although MHV68 is a γ2-herpesvirus, clear similarities with EBV include the establishment of a lytic infection of respiratory epithelium that is rapidly cleared by CD8+ and other T-cells, and latent infection of splenic B-cells. The capacity to induce B-cell proliferation is another common feature but no evidence for oncogenicity has been found for MHV68. One important observation is that CD4+ T-cells were found to be essential in the control of MHV68 infection and disease (121). The central role for CD4+ T-cells in the regulation of EBV is supported by data obtained using the cottontop tamarin as discussed above. This may have implications in the design of a human EBV vaccine where the role of CD4+ T-cells in the control of EBV infection has been somewhat neglected. The use of both latent and lytic MHV68 antigens as vaccines has been explored. The MHV68 analogue of EBV gp350 is gp150 (122) which has been used to vaccinate mice prior to intranasal infection with MHV68 (123). The characteristic lytic infection was dramatically lowered in lung respiratory epithelium, as was the MHV68 IM-like disease. Nevertheless the virus still established latent infection. Other studies show that priming lytic protein–specific CD8+ T-cells by immunizing mice with the D^b-restricted p56 epitope of MHV68 also abrogates lytic replication in lung epithelium (124,125). However, the number of persistently infected cells in the spleens of vaccinated animals was the same as in controls after three weeks, and the characteristic MHV68-associated IM-like disease still developed, albeit much later than in controls. Similar results were obtained in another study where MHV68-specific CD8+ T-cells were generated in mice immunized with dendritic cells pulsed with MHV68 (126). Vaccination with the MHV68 M2 latency protein in this model failed to reduce lytic replication in the lung but did reduce the latently infected cell load in the early stages of latent infection, when M2 is expressed (127,128). Further work on this model is likely to be informative.

A greater understanding of the relationships between γ-herpesviruses in different primates has come about because of the work of Wang et al. (129). γ-herpesviruses closely related to EBV have been known, for some time, to infect Old World monkeys, and are classified in the *Lymphocryptovirus* (LCV) genus. This group of viruses shares a similar biology and has a common genetic identity with many shared genes. The greatest similarities are found between EBV and rhesus macaque LCV, and it has been proposed that this model would be useful in analyzing pathogenesis of infection and, possibly, vaccination strategies (129). Rhesus macaques can be infected with LCV by the oral route (130), support persistent asymptomatic peripheral blood infection, shed virus in saliva, and develop B-cell lymphoma when immunosuppressed (131). A gp350 homologue has been identified in rhesus macaque LCV and is likely to use the same receptor, the rhesus CD21 equivalent. Experiments with this model are likely to be very expensive. No results of vaccination studies have been published to date.

Inoculation of lymphocytes from human EBV-positive donors into severe combined immunodeficient mice frequently gives rise to B-cell lymphoproliferative disease. This animal model has been used extensively (56,132) in the study of EBV lymphoma but not in vaccine development. In the absence of a satisfactory animal system it seems reasonable to directly progress to human trials with rationally designed candidate vaccines, after initial immunogenicity and toxicity evaluation has been carried out in animals.

HUMAN TRIALS

A recombinant form of the major EBV envelope glycoprotein gp350 has been expressed in Chinese hamster ovary cells (30) and has been evaluated in human phase I trials (133). Ultimately, the first target population for this vaccine will be matriculating college or university students. A proportion of these students will not have been infected with EBV but many of them will become infected with EBV during their college years, and about half of the newly infected group will develop IM. This susceptible population is well defined and accessible for properly controlled human trials. Early studies (134) indicated that the incidence of IM in the United States is 65 cases per 100,000, which is greater than that of all reportable diseases, except gonorrhea. There are no reasons to suppose that this frequency of IM is significantly different in Western Europe. The high incidence of IM therefore provides a strong incentive for the development of an EBV vaccine initially for use in the West not only because of a well defined and accessible target population, but also because the results of such trials could be known in a relatively short time. The above factors, among others, have led to a limited commercial interest in EBV vaccine development. A trial using this population would have endpoints of EBV seroconversion, development or otherwise of IM, and changes in a range of immunological parameters such as virus-neutralizing antibodies. Any further progress in EBV vaccine development will depend heavily on the outcome of such trials.

Another much smaller target population exists in the form of immunosuppressed pediatric transplant patients. Children undergoing stem cell transplant and solid organ transplants are often EBV seronegative and become seropositive either through natural infection during their treatment or by infection transmitted by the transplanted organ itself. The risk of developing PTLD is high in these patients because of immunosuppression. Trial of a gp350 vaccine is planned in these patients to determine whether gp350 vaccination offers some protection against PTLD. There appears to be a correlation between viral load, as judged by quantitative PCR, and the development of PTLD. Is this increased viral load a cause or an effect of PTLD? If it is a cause then a reduction in viral replication by vaccination may have some effect on the emergence of PTLD.

The observations that the onset of NPC is accompanied by a rise in serum IgA antibodies against lytic cycle antigens (135,136) and that high anti-VCA titers in Ugandan children are prognostic for the development of endemic BL (15,137) also indicate a potential role for intervention with a gp350 vaccine. Answers to the above questions will not be obtained until candidate vaccines have been evaluated in human trials. These trials of postinfection vaccination are not currently planned.

Probably the most significant results obtained in EBV vaccine trials to date with gp350 are with a recombinant derivative of the Chinese vaccinia strain (Tien Tan) expressing gp350 that was used to vaccinate a small group of both seronegative and seropositive children in southern China (138). It was reported that antibody levels to gp350 were increased in those subjects who were already seropositive, and were induced in those who were seronegative at the beginning of the trial. Six out of nine vaccinated children who were seronegative for EBV at the time of vaccination remained seronegative for at least three years after vaccination. This particular vaccinia recombinant used in this trial would probably not be acceptable for large-scale use because of safety considerations.

FURTHER CONSIDERATIONS IN EBV VACCINE DESIGN

It has been suggested that persistent and/or excessive replication of EBV, as reflected in serum IgA anti-VCA levels at the onset of NPC, is itself the basis for development of the disease. Mechanistic explanations may involve EBV-induced cell fusion (139) or IgA-mediated infection (107) of atypical target cells for EBV along with insufficient clearance of the infected target cells. Such a scenario is consistent with the persistently high antibody titers to EBV replicative antigens among populations at risk, and high levels of IgA antibodies against the same antigens marking the onset, and preceding, the clinical detection of NPC. The masking of ADCC by IgA antibodies has been another suggested mechanism (140) but the rise in IgA may also reflect an alteration in CD4+ T-cell function. If these, or other mechanisms, are involved, then a postexposure vaccine that could better control the lytic cycle of EBV could be expected to have beneficial effects. Stimulation of CTL responses and modulation of the humoral responses could be the levels at which a postexposure vaccine might act by changing the quality and quantity of specific IgG and IgA antibodies, respectively.

The rational design of an EBV vaccine depends on an understanding of the EBV life cycle and the natural immune responses generated by the virus in vivo in humans. Current evidence suggests that a small subset of latently infected B-cells in the circulation or bone marrow escape immune detection because their EBV gene expression is limited to EBNA1, a molecule resistant to MHC class I–restricted antigen processing and presentation (141,142), and/or LMP2 (143). The presence or absence of EBV in epithelial cells in the oropharyngeal epithelium has been controversial (17). How the virus moves from the latently infected B-cell in the circulation to the epithelium, and whether this involves lytic replication in B-cells at any stage is unknown. Consequently, the development of EBV vaccines and their mode of action continue to be speculative because EBV biology is not understood well enough. Immune control of the virus certainly exists because immunocompromised persons demonstrate increased shedding of virus in the saliva and are predisposed to EBV

B-cell lymphomas (144,145). Immune responses to EBV include the generation of virus-neutralizing antibodies against envelope glycoproteins (96), MHC class I–restricted CTLs recognizing latent antigens (8), ADCC against cells carrying surface gp350 (146), and MHC class II–restricted T-cell responses (76,96,147–149). Primary MHC class II–restricted CTLs have been found in seronegative people (150). More recently, an EBV superantigen activity that stimulates Vβ 13 CD4+ T-cells from cord blood has been discovered (151), but this activity may be the result of EBV activation of an endogenous retrovirus (152).

CD4+ T-cells can regulate the growth of EBV-infected human B-cells in vitro. These T-cells induce apoptosis of autologous lymphoblastoid cell lines (LCLs) as well as heterologous LCLs and certain other tumor cell targets. Further, it was established that such control is, in part, via antigen-independent Fas/Fas ligand–mediated apoptosis (9). EBV gp350-reactive cells induced in the tamarin by gp350 vaccination may act to control EBV-infected cells by similar mechanisms (86,87). Interestingly, CD4+ T-cells specific for EBV can be detected in EBV-seronegative individuals (153), and primary responses to EBV include CD4+ T-cells and NK cells that inhibit EBV transformation in vitro (53).

Patients with IM have some circulating B-cells expressing lytic cycle antigens (154), but acyclovir treatment has no effect on the course or symptoms of the disease, although virus shedding is reduced (155). Detection of B-cells expressing the growth program of EBV in vivo has only been demonstrated in B-cell follicles in the tonsil of healthy individuals (2). CD8+ CTLs that are frequently cited as being important in the control of EBV-infected cells may have limited access to the B-cell follicle because it has been shown that EBV specific CD8+ T-cells lack homing receptors for lymphoid sites of infection (156). CD4+ T-cells are detectable at low frequencies within B-cell follicles and may, therefore, interact directly with EBV-infected B-cells at this site. It is possible that CD4+ T-cells primed by gp350 vaccination would become reactivated on viral challenge. Such cells could influence the course of IM by inducing apoptosis of EBV-infected B-cells within infected lymph nodes and by downregulating the large monoclonal or oligoclonal populations of CD8+ T-cells that account for much of the lymphocytosis that is symptomatic of IM (157).

POSSIBLE THERAPEUTIC VACCINATION

Therapeutic vaccination will aim to enhance the immune response against EBV-associated tumors, and strategies involving the few EBV latent genes such as EBNA1, LMP1, and LMP2 that may be expressed in the tumors themselves, would be most appropriate (158–160). Certain LMP2 CTL epitopes are restricted through HLA alleles that are common in the Chinese and southeast Asian populations (161). Therapeutic vaccination with defined antigens is a quite distinct approach from other therapeutic interventions using T-cells or dendritic cells grown ex vivo prior to infusion into the patient.

How do NPC and BL escape immune detection and destruction? NPC cells express normal levels of TAP1/2 and HLA class I molecules, and are able to process and present some EBV antigens normally. On these grounds, it can be argued that NPC does not escape immune detection because of a failure in T-cell recognition (162). However, there are many other elements of the CTL recognition and destruction process that have not yet been evaluated for NPC cells. These could include the expression of coreceptors and adhesion molecules, production of cytokines that provide an inappropriate milieu for CTLs, production of T-cell inhibitory receptors such as Fas, and alteration in proteasome function and other tumor cell-specific factors. There is a deficit in peripheral $\gamma\delta$ T-cells in NPC patients when compared to healthy persons and those in clinical remission suggesting a role for this cell type in the defense against NPC (163).

One aspect that is likely to be significant is that EBNA1 is not processed for MHC class I epitope presentation because the internal glycine–alanine repeat blocks normal proteasome processing (141). Dendritic cells are able to process and present exogenous EBNA1, and bystander presentation may explain the presence of EBNA1-specific CD8+ memory T-cells that are refractory to stimulation by autologous LCLs (164). It seems that NPC cells are not recognized by CTLs that have EBNA1 specificities in vivo and it is not clear how EBNA1 could be used as a vaccine antigen for this purpose. LMP2 expression levels in NPC are extremely low, although sufficient to prime small numbers of CD8+ memory T-cells in vivo. One possibility is that, like EBNA1, the EBV LMPs are not processed appropriately for MHC class I antigen presentation in tumor cells because of altered proteasome interactions or other related mechanisms. EBV NPC cells have normal levels of TAP1 and 2, and of proteasome components Lmp2 and Lmp7 indicating that, in these respects at least, antigen processing should be normal (162). The NPC lines C15 and C666.1 are able to process and present EBNA3 peptides to CTLs, but this has not been established for LMP1 and LMP2 in this cell line (165). Although MHC class 1–restricted CTLs that recognize LMP1 and LMP2 can be detected in healthy persons, and LMP2-specific CTLs can be detected in NPC patients they appear to be relatively uncommon (165–167). LMP1 can be ubiquitinated and degraded through a proteasome pathway (168), so it is not understood, at present, why LMP1-specific CTLs are absent or very rare. Similarly, the degradation and processing pathways for LMP2 are unknown. However, it is known that MHC class I–restricted antigen presentation of LMP2 is unusual in one respect. Some, but not all, LMP2 epitopes are presented independently of TAP (169). The subdominance or absence of appropriate CTL activities against LMP1 and LMP2 on NPC or HD tumor cells may be a factor in the establishment of these tumors.

A novel method of enhancing CTL responses to LMP1 and LMP2 using a nontoxic, recombinant B-subunit of Escherichia coli heat-labile enterotoxin (EtxB) has recently been devised (170). EtxB and its counterpart, the cholera toxin B-subunit, are being investigated by a number of groups for their capacity to induce mucosal immune responses. EtxB undergoes rapid aggregation and internalization following binding to its ganglioside receptor GM1 found within glycosphingolipid-rich rafts on mammalian cell membranes. On EBV-infected LCL, both EBV LMP1 and LMP2 are also found within the rafts that are enriched for GM1 (171,172). EtxB reacts with GM1 and colocalizes with LMP1 and LMP2 on the cell surfaces of EBV-positive LCLs. Both EtxB and the LMPs undergo capping and internalization following binding of EtxB to GM1. This phenomenon gives rise to a substantial increase in HLA class I–mediated killing of EtxB-treated LCL targets by CD8+ CTL lines specific for known LMP1 and LMP2 epitopes. These effects are proteosome-dependent and limited to raft-associated viral antigens. Enhanced CTL responses are found against both TAP-dependent and TAP-independent LMP2 epitopes. These findings demonstrate potential therapeutic applications for EtxB in NPC and HD. Furthermore, EtxB, being a well-characterized mucosal adjuvant (173,174), may have a particular application to NPC in the induction of LMP2-specific CTLs in the nasopharynx.

CONCLUSIONS AND FUTURE OBJECTIVES

NPC was the first malignant tumor of humans where a close association with a virus was substantiated by the repeated demonstration of the presence of EBV DNA sequences in the tumor cells (18). The factors determining the odd geographical clustering of NPC in North Africa, Greenland, and particular regions of southern China are not understood (175–179), and the suggested pivotal role of EBV can only be proven by effective vaccination. The rationale for a prophylactic EBV vaccine to control NPC must allow for the fact that most primary infection occurs in the first few years in life and almost the entire population is eventually infected. The modification of EBV infection would perhaps be worth attempting in these regions. In other areas where NPC is far less frequent, and also for those who are already infected, the possibility of postinfection and therapeutic vaccination should be given serious consideration. The correlates of protective immunity in humans that either prevent EBV infection or provide resistance against EBV-associated diseases are not known. Virus infection persists for life in the face of what appear to be considerable humoral and cell-mediated immune responses. Until human trials have taken place, it is unlikely that any correlates of protective immunity against either infection or disease will become known. The success of gp350-based EBV vaccines depends on the role of gp350 and lytic replication in infection and disease. Primary infection of B-cells in the oropharynx is mediated by gp350 in the viral envelope, but it appears that gp350 is not absolutely required for this essential stage in the infectious cycle. Vaccine-induced mucosal IgA against gp350 could well act at this level, controlling, to some extent, but probably not preventing infection (180). IgA may also enhance infection in some circumstances (107). It is impossible to say at this stage what effects gp350 vaccine–induced mucosal or systemic immune responses might have on primary EBV infection or existing EBV infection. Once latency has been established, will immune responses in the vaccinee be more effective in preventing EBV disease than in a healthy unvaccinated seropositive person? Ultimately, successful EBV vaccines, either therapeutic or postinfection, will be made up of a number of EBV components derived from lytic cycle envelope glycoproteins and latent antigens. The conducting of properly controlled human trials to evaluate the options set out above is clearly the first priority, and little further progress can be expected until they take place.

REFERENCES

1. Rickinson AB, Kieff E. Epstein–Barr virus. In: Knipe DM, Howley PM, eds. Fields Virology. Philadelphia: Lippincott-Raven, 2001:2575–2627.
2. Babcock GJ, Thorley-Lawson DA. Tonsillar memory B cells, latently infected with Epstein–Barr virus, express the restricted pattern of latent genes previously found only in Epstein–Barr virus-associated tumors. Proc Natl Acad Sci USA 2000; 97:12,250–12,255.
3. Kangro HO, Osman HK, Lau YL, Heath RB, Yeung CY, Ng MH. Seroprevalence of antibodies to human herpesviruses in England and Hong Kong. J Med Virol 1994; 43:91–96.
4. Henle G, Henle W, Diehl V. Relation of Burkitt's tumor-associated herpes-type virus to infectious mononucleosis. Proc Natl Acad Sci USA 1968; 59:94–101.
5. Parkin DM, Pisani P, Ferlay J. Estimates of the worldwide incidence of 25 major cancers in 1990. Int J Cancer 1999; 80:827–841.
6. Rickinson AB, Callan MF, Annels NE. T-cellmemory: lessons from Epstein–Barr virus infection in man. Philos Trans R Soc Lond B Biol Sci 2000; 355:391–400.

7. Pearson G, Dewey F, Klein G, Henle G, Henele W. Relation between neutralization of Epstein–Barr virus and antibodies to cell membrane antigens induced by the virus. J Nat Cancer Inst 1970; 45:989–995.

8. Rickinson AB, Moss DJ. Human cytotoxic T lymphocyte responses to Epstein–Barr virus infection. Annu Rev Immunol 1997; 15:405–431.

9. Wilson AD, Redchenko I, Williams NA, Morgan AJ. CD4+ T-cells inhibit growth of Epstein–Barr virus-transformed B-cells through CD95-CD95 ligand-mediated apoptosis. Int Immunol 1998; 10:1149–1157.

10. Munz C, Bickham KL, Subklewe M, et al. Human CD4(+) T lymphocytes consistently respond to the latent Epstein–Barr virus nuclear antigen EBNA1. J Exp Med 2000; 191:1649–1660.

11. Parolini S, Bottino C, Falco M, et al. X-linked lymphoproliferative disease. 2B4 molecules displaying inhibitory rather than activating function are responsible for the inability of natural killer cells to kill Epstein–Barr virus-infected cells. J Exp Med 2000; 192:337–346.

12. Ablashi D, Bornkamm GW, Boshoff C, et al. Epstein–Barr virus and Kaposi's sarcoma herpesvirus/human herpesvirus. IARC Monographs on the evaluation of carcinogenic risks to humans. IARC, Lyon, 1997; 70:497.

13. Kieff E, Rickinson AB. Epstein–Barr virus and its replication. In: Knipe DM, Howley PM, eds. Fields Virology. Philadelphia: Lippincott Williams and Wilkins, 2001:2511–2573.

14. Epstein MA. Epstein–Barr virus—is it time to develop a vaccine program? J Natl Cancer Inst 1976; 56:697–700.

15. de-The G, Geser A, Day NE, et al. Epidemiological evidence for causal relationship between Epstein–Barr virus and Burkitt's lymphoma from Ugandan prospective study. Nature 1978; 274:756–761.

16. Rao CR, Gutierrez MI, Bhatia K, et al. Association of Burkitt's lymphoma with the Epstein–Barr virus in two developing countries. Leuk Lymphoma 2000; 39:329–337.

17. Niedobitek G. Epstein–Barr virus infection in the pathogenesis of nasopharyngeal carcinoma. Mol Pathol 2000; 53:248–254.

18. Wolf H, zur Hausen H, Becker V. EB viral genomes in epithelial nasopharyngeal carcinoma cells. Nat New Biol 1973; 244:245–247.

19. Whittle HC, Brown J, Marsh K, Blackman M, Jobe O, Shenton F. The effects of *Plasmodium falciparum* malaria on immune control of B lymphocytes in Gambian children. Clin Exp Immunol 1990; 80:213–218.

20. Spring SB, Hascall G, Gruber J. Issues related to development of Epstein–Barr virus vaccines. J Natl Cancer Inst 1996; 88:1436–1441.

21. Thorley-Lawson DA, Poodry CA. Identification and isolation of the main component (gp350-gp220) of Epstein–Barr virus responsible for generating neutralizing antibodies in vivo. J Virol 1982; 43:730–736.

22. North JR, Morgan AJ, Thompson JL, Epstein MA. Purified Epstein–Barr virus Mr 340,000 glycoprotein induces potent virus-neutralizing antibodies when incorporated in liposomes. Proc Natl Acad Sci USA 1982; 79:7504–7508.

23. Morgan AJ, North JR, Epstein MA. Purification and properties of the gp340 component of Epstein–Barr virus membrane antigen in an immunogenic form. J Gen Virol 1983; 64(Pt 2):455–460.

24. Randle BJ, Morgan AJ, Stripp SA, Epstein MA. Large-scale purification of Epstein–Barr virus membrane antigen gp340 with a monoclonal antibody immunoabsorbent. J Immunol Meth 1985; 77:25–36.

25. David EM, Morgan AJ. Efficient purification of Epstein–Barr virus membrane antigen gp340 by fast protein liquid chromatography. J Immunol Meth 1988; 108:231–236.

26. Madej J, Conway MJ, Morgan AJ, et al. Purification and characterization of Epstein–Barr virus gp340/220 produced by a bovine papillomavirus vector system. Vaccine 1992; 10:777–782.

27. Conway M, Morgan A, Mackett M. Expression of Epstein–Barr virus membrane antigen gp340/220 in mouse fibroblasts using a bovine papillomavirus vector. J Gen Virol 1989; 70(Pt 3):729–734.

28. Motz M, Deby G, Jilg W, Wolf H. Expression of the Epstein–Barr virus major membrane proteins in Chinese hamster ovary cells. Gene 1986; 44:353–359.

29. Schultz LD, Tanner J, Hofmann KJ, et al. Expression and secretion in yeast of a 400-kDa envelope glycoprotein derived from Epstein–Barr virus. Gene 1987; 54:113–123.

30. Jackman WT, Mann KA, Hoffmann HJ, Spaete RR. Expression of Epstein–Barr virus gp350 as a single chain glycoprotein for an EBV subunit vaccine. Vaccine 1999; 17:660–668.

31. Morgan AJ. Epstein–Barr virus vaccines. Vaccine 1992; 10:563–571.

32. Khanna R, Moss DJ, Burrows SR. Vaccine strategies against Epstein–Barr virus-associated diseases: lessons from studies on cytotoxic T-cell-mediated immune regulation. Immunol Rev 1999; 170:49–64.

33. Takahashi M. 25 years' experience with the Biken Oka strain varicella vaccine: a clinical overview. Paediatr Drugs 2001; 3:285–292.

34. Churchill AE, Payne LN, Chubb RC. Immunization against Marek's disease using a live attenuated virus. Nature 1969; 221:744–747.

35. Laufs R and Steinke H. Vaccination of non-human primates against malignant lymphoma. Nature 1975; 253:71–72.

36. Meignier B. Vaccination against herpes simplex virus infections. In: Roizman B, Lopez C, eds. The herpesvirus: Immunology and Prophylaxis of Human Herpesvirus Infection. New York: Plenum, 1985:265–296.

37. Corey L, Langenberg AG, Ashley R, et al. Recombinant glycoprotein vaccine for the prevention of genital HSV-2 infection: two randomized controlled trials. Chiron HSV Vaccine Study Group. JAMA 1999; 282:331–340.

38. Spector FC, Kern ER, Palmer J, et al. Evaluation of a live attenuated recombinant virus RAV 9395 as a herpes simplex virus type 2 vaccine in guinea pigs. J Infect Dis 1998; 177:1143–1154.

39. Desai PJ, Schaffer PA, Minson AC. Excretion of non-infectious virus particles lacking glycoprotein H by a temperature-sensitive mutant of herpes simplex virus type 1: evidence that gH is essential for virion infectivity. J Gen Virol 1988; 69(Pt 6):1147–1156.

40. Ali SA, Lynam J, McLean CS, et al. Tumor regression induced by intratumor therapy with a disabled infectious single cycle (DISC) herpes simplex virus (HSV) vector, DISC/HSV/murine granulocyte-macrophage colony-stimulating factor, correlates with antigen-specific adaptive immunity. J Immunol 2002; 168:3512–3519.

41. Rees RC, McArdle S, Mian S, et al. Disabled infectious single cycle-herpes simplex virus (DISC-HSV) as a vector for immunogene therapy of cancer. Curr Opin Mol Ther 2002; 4:49–53.

42. McLean CS, Ni Challanain D, Duncan I, Boursnell ME, Jennings R, Inglis SC. Induction of a protective immune response by mucosal vaccination with a DISC HSV-1 vaccine. Vaccine 1996; 14:987–992.

43. King SM. Immune globulin versus antivirals versus combination for prevention of cytomegalovirus disease in transplant recipients. Antiviral Res 1999; 40:115–137.

44. Snydman DR, Werner BG, Heinze-Lacey B, et al. Use of cytomegalovirus immune globulin to prevent cytomegalovirus disease in renal-transplant recipients. N Engl J Med 1987; 317:1049–1054.

45. Plotkin SA, Smiley ML, Friedman HM, et al. Towne-vaccine-induced prevention of cytomegalovirus disease after renal transplants. Lancet 1984; 1:528–530.

46. Adler SP, Starr SE, Plotkin SA, et al. Immunity induced by primary human cytomegalovirus infection protects against secondary infection among women of childbearing age. J Infect Dis 1995; 171:26–32.

47. Pass RF, Duliege AM, Boppana S, et al. A subunit cytomegalovirus vaccine based on recombinant envelope glycoprotein B and a new adjuvant. J Infect Dis 1999; 180:970–975.

48. Frey SE, Harrison C, Pass RF, et al. Effects of antigen dose and immunization regimens on antibody responses to a cytomegalovirus glycoprotein B subunit vaccine. J Infect Dis 1999; 180:1700–1703.
49. Morello CS, Cranmer LD, Spector DH. Suppression of murine cytomegalovirus (MCMV) replication with a DNA vaccine encoding MCMV M84 (a homolog of human cytomegalovirus pp65). J Virol 2000; 74:3696–3708.
50. Kossovsky N, Gelman A, Sponsler E, Millett D. Nanocrystalline Epstein–Barr virus decoys. J Appl Biomater 1991; 2:251–259.
51. Chan KH, Tam JS, Peiris JS, Seto WH, Ng MH. Epstein–Barr virus (EBV) infection in infancy. J Clin Virol 2001; 21:57–62.
52. Ternak G, Szucs G, Uj M. The serological signs of the Epstein–Barr virus (EBV) activity in the elderly. Acta Microbiol Immunol Hung 1997; 44:133–140.
53. Wilson AD, Morgan AJ. Primary immune responses by cord blood CD4+ T-cells and NK cells inhibit Epstein–Barr Virus B-celltransformation in vitro. J Virol 2002; 76:5071–5081.
54. Zeng Y. Seroepidemiological studies on nasopharyngeal carcinoma in China. Adv Cancer Res 1985; 44:121–138.
55. Hopwood P, Crawford DH. The role of EBV in post-transplant malignancies: a review. J Clin Pathol 2000; 53:248–254.
56. Crawford DH. Biology and disease associations of Epstein–Barr virus. Philos Trans R Soc Lond B Biol Sci 2001; 356:461–473.
57. North JR, Morgan AJ, Epstein MA. Observations on the EB virus envelope and virus-determined membrane antigen (MA) polypeptides. Int J Cancer 1980; 26:231–240.
58. Bugli F, Bastidas R, Burton DR, Williamson RA, Clementi M, Burioni R. Molecular profile of a human monoclonal antibody Fab fragment specific for Epstein–Barr virus gp350/220 antigen. Hum Immunol 2001; 62:362–367.
59. Lees JF, Arrand JE, Pepper SD, Stewart JP, Mackett M, Arrand JR. The Epstein–Barr virus candidate vaccine antigen gp340/220 is highly conserved between virus types A and B. Virology 1993; 195:578–586.
60. Morgan AJ, Smith AR, Barker RN, Epstein MA. A structural investigation of the Epstein–Barr (EB) virus membrane antigen glycoprotein, gp340. J Gen Virol 1984; 65(Pt 2):397–404.
61. Serafini-Cessi F, Malagolini N, Nanni M, et al. Characterization of N- and O-linked oligosaccharides of glycoprotein 350 from Epstein–Barr virus. Virology 1989; 170:1–10.
62. Janz A, Oezel M, Kurzeder C, et al. Infectious Epstein–Barr virus lacking major glycoprotein BLLF1 (gp350/220) demonstrates the existence of additional viral ligands. J Virol 2000; 74:10142–10152.
63. Maruo S, Yang L, Takada K. Roles of Epstein–Barr virus glycoproteins gp350 and gp25 in the infection of human epithelial cells. J Gen Virol 2001; 82:2373–2383.
64. Wang X, Hutt-Fletcher LM. Epstein–Barr virus lacking glycoprotein gp42 can bind to B-cells but is not able to infect. J Virol 1998; 72:158–163.
65. Li Q, Spriggs MK, Kovats S, et al. Epstein–Barr virus uses HLA class II as a cofactor for infection of B lymphocytes. J Virol 1997; 71:4657–4662.
66. Lee W, Hwang YH, Lee SK, Subramanian C, Robertson ES. An Epstein–Barr virus isolated from a lymphoblastoid cell line has a 16-kilobase-pair deletion which includes gp350 and the Epstein–Barr virus nuclear antigen 3A. J Virol 2001; 75:8556–8568.
67. Tanner J, Whang Y, Sample J, Sears A, Kieff E. Soluble gp350/220 and deletion mutant glycoproteins block Epstein–Barr virus adsorption to lymphocytes. J Virol 1988; 62:4452–4464.
68. Tanner JE, Alfieri C, Chatila TA, Diaz-Mitoma F. Induction of interleukin-6 after stimulation of human B-cell CD21 by Epstein–Barr virus glycoproteins gp350 and gp220. J Virol 1996; 70:570–575.
69. D'Addario M, Ahmad A, Morgan A, Menezes J. Binding of the Epstein–Barr virus major envelope glycoprotein gp350 results in the upregulation of the TNF-alpha gene

expression in monocytic cells via NF-kappaB involving PKC, PI3-K and tyrosine kinases. J Mol Biol 2000; 298:765–778.

70. Gosselin J, Flamand L, D'Addario M, et al. Modulatory effects of Epstein–Barr, herpes simplex, and human herpes-6 viral infections and coinfections on cytokine synthesis. A comparative study. J Immunol 1992; 149:181–187.

71. Sinclair AJ, Farrell PJ. Host cell requirements for efficient infection of quiescent primary B lymphocytes by Epstein–Barr virus. J Virol 1995; 69:5461–5468.

72. Pither RJ, Nolan L, Tarlton J, Walford J, Morgan AJ. Distribution of epitopes within the amino acid sequence of the Epstein–Barr virus major envelope glycoprotein, gp340, recognized by hyperimmune rabbit sera. J Gen Virol 1992; 73(Pt 6):1409–1415.

73. Pither RJ, Zhang CX, Shiels C, Tarlton J, Finerty S, Morgan AJ. Mapping of B-cell epitopes on the polypeptide chain of the Epstein–Barr virus major envelope glycoprotein and candidate vaccine molecule gp340. J Virol 1992; 66:1246–1251.

74. Qualtiere LF, Decoteau JF, Hassan Nasr-el-Din M. Epitope mapping of the major Epstein–Barr virus outer envelope glycoprotein gp350/220. J Gen Virol 1987; 68(Pt 2):535–543.

75. Zhang PF, Klutch M, Armstrong G, Qualtiere L, Pearson G, Marcus-Sekura CJ. Mapping of the epitopes of Epstein–Barr virus gp350 using monoclonal antibodies and recombinant proteins expressed in *Escherichia coli* defines three antigenic determinants. J Gen Virol 1991; 72(Pt 11):2747–2755.

76. Wallace LE, Wright J, Ulaeto DO, Morgan AJ, Rickinson AB. Identification of two T-cell epitopes on the candidate Epstein–Barr virus vaccine glycoprotein gp340 recognized by CD4+ T-cell clones. J Virol 1991; 65:3821–3828.

77. Khanna R, Sherritt M, Burrows SR. EBV structural antigens, gp350 and gp85, as targets for ex vivo virus-specific CTL during acute infectious mononucleosis: potential use of gp350/gp85 CTL epitopes for vaccine design. J Immunol 1999; 162:3063–3069.

78. Tan LC, Gudgeon N, Annels NE, et al. A re-evaluation of the frequency of CD8+ T-cells specific for EBV in healthy virus carriers. J Immunol 1999; 162:1827–1835.

79. Yang J, Lemas VM, Flinn IW, Krone C, Ambinder RF. Application of the ELISPOT assay to the characterization of CD8(+) responses to Epstein–Barr virus antigens. Blood 2000; 95:241–248.

80. Pepperl S, Benninger-Doring G, Modrow S, Wolf H, Jilg W. Immediate-early transactivator Rta of Epstein–Barr virus (EBV) shows multiple epitopes recognized by EBV-specific cytotoxic T lymphocytes. J Virol 1998; 72:8644–8649.

81. Bharadwaj M, Sherritt M, Khanna R, Moss DJ. Contrasting Epstein–Barr virus-specific cytotoxic T-cell responses to HLA A2-restricted epitopes in humans and HLA transgenic mice: implications for vaccine design. Vaccine 2001; 19:3769–3777.

82. Cleary ML, Epstein MA, Finerty S, et al. Individual tumors of multifocal EB virus-induced malignant lymphomas in tamarins arise from different B-cell clones. Science 1985; 228:722–724.

83. Cho Y, Ramer J, Rivailler P, et al. An Epstein–Barr-related herpesvirus from marmoset lymphomas. Proc Natl Acad Sci USA 2001; 98:1224–1229.

84. Niedobitek G, Agathanggelou A, Finerty S, et al. Latent Epstein–Barr virus infection in cottontop tamarins. A possible model for Epstein–Barr virus infection in humans. Am J Pathol 1994; 145:969–978.

85. Cadavid LF, Mejia BE, Watkins DI. MHC class I genes in a New World primate, the cotton-top tamarin (*Saguinus oedipus*), have evolved by an active process of loci turnover. Immunogenetics 1999; 49:196–205.

86. Wilson AD, Shooshstari M, Finerty S, Watkins P, Morgan AJ. Virus-specific cytotoxic T cell responses are associated with immunity of the cottontop tamarin to Epstein–Barr virus (EBV). Clin Exp Immunol 1996; 103:199–205.

87. Wilson AD, Lovgren-Bengtsson K, Villacres-Ericsson M, Morein B, Morgan AJ. The major Epstein–Barr virus (EBV) envelope glycoprotein gp340 when incorporated into

Iscoms primes cytotoxic T-cell responses directed against EBV lymphoblastoid cell lines. Vaccine 1999; 17:1282–1290.

88. Whang Y, Silberklang M, Morgan A, et al. Expression of the Epstein–Barr virus gp350/220 gene in rodent and primate cells. J Virol 1987; 61:1796–1807.

89. Hessing M, van Schijndel HB, van Grunsven WM, Wolf H, Middeldorp JM. Purification and quantification of recombinant Epstein–Barr viral glycoproteins gp350/220 from Chinese hamster ovary cells. J Chromatogr 1992; 599:267–272.

90. Schijns VE. Induction and direction of immune responses by vaccine adjuvants. Crit Rev Immunol 2001; 21:75–85.

91. Epstein MA, Morgan AJ, Finerty S, Randle BJ, Kirkwood JK. Protection of cottontop tamarins against Epstein–Barr virus-induced malignant lymphoma by a prototype subunit vaccine. Nature 1985; 318:287–289.

92. Morgan AJ, Allison AC, Finerty S, Scullion FT, Byars NE, Epstein MA. Validation of a first-generation Epstein–Barr virus vaccine preparation suitable for human use. J Med Virol 1989; 29:74–78.

93. Morgan AJ, Finerty S, Lovgren K, Scullion FT, Morein B. Prevention of Epstein–Barr (EB) virus-induced lymphoma in cottontop tamarins by vaccination with the EB virus envelope glycoprotein gp340 incorporated into immune-stimulating complexes. J Gen Virol 1988; 69(Pt 8):2093–2096.

94. Hu KF, Lovgren-Bengtsson K, Morein B. Immunostimulating complexes (ISCOMs) for nasal vaccination. Adv Drug Deliv Rev 2001; 51:149–159.

95. Morein B, Villacres-Eriksson M, Ekstrom J, Hu K, Behboudi S, Lovgren-Bengtsson K. ISCOM: a delivery system for neonates and for mucosal administration. Adv Vet Med 1999; 41:405–413.

96. Finerty S, Mackett M, Arrand JR, Watkins PE, Tarlton J, Morgan AJ. Immunization of cottontop tamarins and rabbits with a candidate vaccine against the Epstein–Barr virus based on the major viral envelope glycoprotein gp340 and alum. Vaccine 1994; 12:1180–1184.

97. Jung S, Chung YK, Chang SH, et al. DNA-mediated immunization of glycoprotein 350 of Epstein–Barr virus induces the effective humoral and cellular immune responses against the antigen. Mol Cells 2001; 12:41–49.

98. Mackett M, Arrand JR. Recombinant vaccinia virus induces neutralising antibodies in rabbits against Epstein–Barr virus membrane antigen gp340. EMBO J 1985; 4:3229–3234.

99. Ragot T, Finerty S, Watkins PE, Perricaudet M, Morgan AJ. Replication-defective recombinant adenovirus expressing the Epstein–Barr virus (EBV) envelope glycoprotein gp340/220 induces protective immunity against EBV-induced lymphomas in the cottontop tamarin. J Gen Virol 1993; 74(Pt 3):501–507.

100. Morgan AJ, Mackett M, Finerty S, Arrand JR, Scullion FT, Epstein MA. Recombinant vaccinia virus expressing Epstein–Barr virus glycoprotein gp340 protects cottontop tamarins against EB virus-induced malignant lymphomas. J Med Virol 1988; 25:189–195.

101. Mackett M, Cox C, Pepper SD, et al. Immunisation of common marmosets with vaccinia virus expressing Epstein–Barr virus (EBV) gp340 and challenge with EBV. J Med Virol 1996; 50:263–271.

102. Taylor J, Weinberg R, Tartaglia J, et al. Nonreplicating viral vectors as potential vaccines: recombinant canarypox virus expressing measles virus fusion (F) and hemagglutinin (HA) glycoproteins. Virology 1992; 187:321–328.

103. Tartaglia J, Cox WI, Taylor J, et al. Highly attenuated poxvirus vectors. AIDS Res Hum Retroviruses 1992; 8:1445–1447.

104. Stittelaar KJ, Wyatt LS, de Swart RL, et al. Protective immunity in macaques vaccinated with a modified vaccinia virus Ankara-based measles virus vaccine in the presence of passively acquired antibodies. J Virol 2000; 74: 4236–4243.

105. Top FH Jr, Buescher EL, Bancroft WH, Russell PK. Immunization with live types 7 and 4 adenovirus vaccines II. Antibody response and protective effect against acute respiratory disease due to adenovirus type 7. J Infect Dis 1971; 124:155–160.

106. Sixbey JW, Yao QY. Immunoglobulin A-induced shift of Epstein–Barr virus tissue tropism. Science 1992; 255:1578–1580.

107. Gan YJ, Chodosh J, Morgan A, Sixbey JW. Epithelial cell polarization is a determinant in the infectious outcome of immunoglobulin A-mediated entry by Epstein–Barr virus. J Virol 1997; 71:519–526.

108. Epstein MA, Randle BJ, Finerty S, Kirkwood JK. Not all potently neutralizing, vaccine-induced antibodies to Epstein–Barr virus ensure protection of susceptible experimental animals. Clin Exp Immunol 1986; 63:485–490.

109. Emini EA, Schleif WA, Silberklang M, Lehman D, Ellis RW. Vero cell-expressed Epstein–Barr virus (EBV) gp350/220 protects marmosets from EBV challenge. J Med Virol 1989; 27:120–123.

110. Lowe RS, Keller PM, Keech BJ, et al. Varicella-zoster virus as a live vector for the expression of foreign genes. Proc Natl Acad Sci USA 1987; 84:3896–3900.

111. Arvin AM. Varicella-Zoster virus. In: Knipe DM, Howley PM, eds. Fields Virology. Philadelphia: Lippincott Williams and Wilkins, 2001:2731–2767.

112. Moss DJ, Burrows SR, Silins SL, Misko I, Khanna R. The immunology of Epstein–Barr virus infection. Philos Trans R Soc Lond B Biol Sci 2001; 356:475–488.

113. Thomson SA, Khanna R, Gardner J, et al. Minimal epitopes expressed in a recombinant polyepitope protein are processed and presented to CD8+ cytotoxic T-cells: implications for vaccine design. Proc Natl Acad Sci USA 1995; 92:5845–5849.

114. Thomson SA, Burrows SR, Misko IS, Moss DJ, Coupar BE, Khanna R. Targeting a polyepitope protein incorporating multiple class II-restricted viral epitopes to the secretory/endocytic pathway facilitates immune recognition by CD4+ cytotoxic T lymphocytes: a novel approach to vaccine design. J Virol 1998; 72:2246–2252.

115. Wedderburn N, Edwards JM, Desgranges C, Fontaine C, Cohen B, de The G. Infectious mononucleosis-like response in common marmosets infected with Epstein–Barr virus. J Infect Dis 1984; 150:878–882.

116. Cox C, Chang S, Karran L, Griffin B, Wedderburn N. Persistent Epstein–Barr virus infection in the common marmoset (*Callithrix jacchus*). J Gen Virol 1996; 77(Pt 6):1173–1180.

117. Emini EA, Luka J, Armstrong ME, Banker FS, Provost PJ, Pearson GR. Establishment and characterization of a chronic infectious mononucleosis like syndrome in common marmosets. J Med Virol 1986; 18:369–379.

118. Blaskovic D, Stancekova M, Svobodova J, Mistrikova J. Isolation of five strains of herpesviruses from two species of free living small rodents. Acta Virol 1980; 24:468.

119. Doherty PC, Christensen JP, Belz GT, Stevenson PG, Sangster MY. Dissecting the host response to a gamma-herpesvirus. Philos Trans R Soc Lond B Biol Sci 2001; 356:581–593.

120. Nash AA, Dutia BM, Stewart JP, Davison AJ. Natural history of murine gamma-herpesvirus infection. Philos Trans R Soc Lond B Biol Sci 2001; 356:569–579.

121. Stevenson PG, Cardin RD, Christensen JP, Doherty PC. Immunological control of a murine gammaherpesvirus independent of CD8+ T-cells. J Gen Virol 1999; 80(Pt 2):477–483.

122. Stewart JP, Janjua NJ, Pepper SD, et al. Identification and characterization of murine gammaherpesvirus 68 gp150: a virion membrane glycoprotein. J Virol 1996; 70:3528–3535.

123. Stewart JP, Micali N, Usherwood EJ, Bonina L, Nash AA. Murine gamma-herpesvirus 68 glycoprotein 150 protects against virus-induced mononucleosis: a model system for gamma-herpesvirus vaccination. Vaccine 1999; 17:152–157.

124. Stevenson PG, Belz GT, Altman JD, Doherty PC. Changing patterns of dominance in the CD8+ T-cell response during acute and persistent murine gamma-herpesvirus infection. Eur J Immunol 1999; 29:1059–1067.

125. Stevenson PG, Belz GT, Castrucci MR, Altman JD, Doherty PC. A gamma-herpesvirus sneaks through a CD8(+) T-cell response primed to a lytic-phase epitope. Proc Natl Acad Sci USA 1999; 96:9281–9286.

126. Liu L, Flano E, Usherwood EJ, Surman S, Blackman MA, Woodland DL. Lytic cycle T-cell epitopes are expressed in two distinct phases during MHV-68 infection. J Immunol 1999; 163:868–874.

127. Usherwood EJ, Ward KA, Blackman MA, Stewart JP, Woodland DL. Latent antigen vaccination in a model gammaherpesvirus infection. J Virol 2001; 75: 8283–8288.

128. Usherwood EJ, Roy DJ, Ward K, et al. Control of gammaherpesvirus latency by latent antigen-specific CD8(+) T-cells. J Exp Med 2000; 192:943–952.

129. Wang F, Rivailler P, Rao P, Cho Y. Simian homologues of Epstein–Barr virus. Philos Trans R Soc Lond B Biol Sci 2001; 356:489–497.

130. Moghaddam A, Rosenzweig M, Lee-Parritz D, Annis B, Johnson RP, Wang F. An animal model for acute and persistent Epstein–Barr virus infection. Science 1997; 276:2030–2033.

131. Habis A, Baskin G, Simpson L, Fortgang I, Murphey-Corb M, Levy LS. Rhesus lymphocryptovirus infection during the progression of SAIDS and SAIDS-associated lymphoma in the rhesus macaque. AIDS Res Hum Retroviruses 2000; 16:163–171.

132. Johannessen I, Crawford DH. In vivo models for Epstein–Barr virus (EBV)-associated B-cell lymphoproliferative disease (BLPD). Rev Med Virol 1999; 9:263–277.

133. Gilbert K. Mountain View, CA, U.S.A.: Aviron Press Release, 1999.

134. Evans AS. Epstein–Barr vaccine: use in infectious mononucleosis. In: Turz T, Pagano JS, Ablashi DV, De The G, Lenoir G, Pearson GS, eds. The Epstein–Barr Virus and Associated Diseases. London: Libby, 1993:593–598.

135. Zeng Y, Zhong JM, Li LY, et al. Follow-up studies on Epstein–Barr virus IgA/VCA antibody-positive persons in Zangwu County, China. Intervirology 1983; 20:190–194.

136. Zeng J, Gong CH, Jan MG, Fun Z, Zhang LG, Li HY. Detection of Epstein–Barr virus IgA/EA antibody for diagnosis of nasopharyngeal carcinoma by immunoautoradiography. Int J Cancer 1983; 31:599–601.

137. Geser A, de The G, Lenoir G, Day NE, Williams EH. Final case reporting from the Ugandan prospective study of the relationship between EBV and Burkitt's lymphoma. Int J Cancer 1982; 29:397–400.

138. Gu SY, Huang TM, Ruan L, et al. First EBV vaccine trial in humans using recombinant vaccinia virus expressing the major membrane antigen. Dev Biol Stand 1995; 84:171–177.

139. Bayliss GJ, Wolf H. Epstein–Barr virus-induced cell fusion. Nature 1980; 287:164–165.

140. Jilg W, Bogedain C, Mairhofer H, Gu SY, Wolf H. The Epstein–Barr virus-encoded glycoprotein gp 110 (BALF 4) can serve as a target for antibody-dependent cell-mediated cytotoxicity (ADCC). Virology 1994; 202:974–977.

141. Levitskaya J, Coram M, Levitsky V, et al. Inhibition of antigen processing by the internal repeat region of the Epstein–Barr virus nuclear antigen-1. Nature 1995; 375:685–688.

142. Levitskaya J, Sharipo A, Leonchiks A, Ciechanover A, Masucci MG. Inhibition of ubiquitin/proteasome-dependent protein degradation by the Gly-Ala repeat domain of the Epstein–Barr virus nuclear antigen 1. Proc Natl Acad Sci USA 1997; 94:12,616–12,621.

143. Babcock GJ, Hochberg D, Thorley-Lawson AD. The expression pattern of Epstein–Barr virus latent genes in vivo is dependent upon the differentiation stage of the infected B-cell. Immunity 2000; 13:497–506.

144. Thomas JA, Allday MJ, Crawford DH. Epstein–Barr virus-associated lymphoproliferative disorders in immunocompromised individuals. Adv Cancer Res 1991; 57:329–380.

145. Preiksaitis JK, Diaz-Mitoma F, Mirzayans F, Roberts S, Tyrrell DL. Quantitative oropharyngeal Epstein–Barr virus shedding in renal and cardiac transplant recipients: relationship to immunosuppressive therapy, serologic responses, and the risk of posttransplant lymphoproliferative disorder. J Infect Dis 1992; 166:986–994.

146. Khyatti M, Stefanescu I, Blagdon M, Menezes J. Epstein–Barr virus gp350-specific antibody titers and antibody-dependent cellular cytotoxic effector function in different

groups of patients: a study using cloned gp350-expressing transfected human T-cell targets. J Infect Dis 1994; 170:1439–1447.

147. Ulaeto D, Wallace L, Morgan A, Morein B, Rickinson AB. In vitro T-cell responses to a candidate Epstein–Barr virus vaccine: human CD4+ T-cell clones specific for the major envelope glycoprotein gp340. Eur J Immunol 1988; 18:1689–1697.

148. Lee SP, Wallace LE, Mackett M, et al. MHC class II-restricted presentation of endogenously synthesized antigen: Epstein–Barr virus transformed B-cell lines can present the viral glycoprotein gp340 by two distinct pathways. Int Immunol 1993; 5:451–460.

149. White CA, Cross SM, Kurilla MG, et al. Recruitment during infectious mononucleosis of CD3+CD4+CD8+ virus-specific cytotoxic T-cells which recognise Epstein–Barr virus lytic antigen BHRF1. Virology 1996; 219:489–492.

150. Misko IS, Pope JH, Hutter R, Soszynski TD, Kane RG. HLA-DR-antigen-associated restriction of EBV-specific cytotoxic T-cell colonies. Int J Cancer 1984; 33:239–243.

151. Sutkowski N, Palkama T, Ciurli C, Sekaly RP, Thorley-Lawson DA, Huber BT. An Epstein–Barr virus-associated superantigen. J Exp Med 1996; 184:971–980.

152. Sutkowski N, Conrad B, Thorley-Lawson DA, Huber BT. Epstein–Barr virus transactivates the human endogenous retrovirus HERV-K18 that encodes a superantigen. Immunity 2001; 15:579–589.

153. Savoldo B, Cubbage ML, Durett AG, et al. Generation of EBV-specific CD4+ cytotoxic T-cells from virus naive individuals. J Immunol 2002; 168:909–918.

154. Anagnostopoulos I, Hummel M, Kreschel C, Stein H. Morphology, immunophenotype, and distribution of latently and/or productively Epstein–Barr virus-infected cells in acute infectious mononucleosis: implications for the interindividual infection route of Epstein–Barr virus. Blood 1995; 85:744–750.

155. Tynell E, Aurelius E, Brandell A, et al. Acyclovir and prednisolone treatment of acute infectious mononucleosis: a multicenter, double-blind, placebo-controlled study. J Infect Dis 1996; 174:324–331.

156. Chen G, Shankar P, Lange C, et al. CD8 T-cells specific for human immunodeficiency virus, Epstein–Barr virus, and cytomegalovirus lack molecules for homing to lymphoid sites of infection. Blood 2001; 98:156–164.

157. Callan MF, Steven N, Krausa P, et al. Large clonal expansions of CD8+ T-cells in acute infectious mononucleosis. Nat Med 1996; 2:906–911.

158. Rickinson AB. Immune intervention against virus-associated human cancers. Ann Oncol 1995; 6(suppl 1):69–71.

159. Ambinder RF, Robertson KD, Moore SM, Yang J. Epstein–Barr virus as a therapeutic target in Hodgkin's disease and nasopharyngeal carcinoma. Semin Cancer Biol 1996; 7:217–226.

160. Moss DJ, Schmidt C, Elliott S, Suhrbier A, Burrows S, Khanna R. Strategies involved in developing an effective vaccine for EBV-associated diseases. Adv Cancer Res 1996; 69:213–245.

161. Lee SP, Tierney RJ, Thomas WA, Brooks JM, Rickinson AB. Conserved CTL epitopes within EBV latent membrane protein 2: a potential target for CTL-based tumor therapy. J Immunol 1997; 158:3325–3334.

162. Khanna R, Busson P, Burrows SR, et al. Molecular characterization of antigen-processing function in nasopharyngeal carcinoma (NPC): evidence for efficient presentation of Epstein–Barr virus cytotoxic T-cell epitopes by NPC cells. Cancer Res 1998; 58:310–314.

163. Zheng BJ, Ng SP, Chua DT, et al. Peripheral gammadelta T-cell deficit in nasopharyngeal carcinoma. Int J Cancer 2002; 99:213–217.

164. Blake N, Lee S, Redchenko I, et al. Human CD8+ T-cell responses to EBV EBNA1: HLA class I presentation of the (Gly-Ala)-containing protein requires exogenous processing. Immunity 1997; 7:791–802.

165. Lee SP, Chan AT, Cheung ST, et al. CTL control of EBV in nasopharyngeal carcinoma (NPC): EBV-specific CTL responses in the blood and tumors of NPC patients and the antigen-processing function of the tumor cells. J Immunol 2000; 165:573–582.

166. Redchenko IV, Rickinson AB. Accessing Epstein–Barr virus-specific T-cell memory with peptide-loaded dendritic cells. J Virol 1999; 73:334–342.

167. Khanna R, Burrows SR, Nicholls J, Poulsen LM. Identification of cytotoxic T-cell epitopes within Epstein–Barr virus (EBV) oncogene latent membrane protein 1 (LMP1): evidence for HLA A2 supertype-restricted immune recognition of EBV-infected cells by LMP1-specific cytotoxic T lymphocytes. Eur J Immunol 1998; 28:451–458.

168. Aviel S, Winberg G, Massucci M, Ciechanover A. Degradation of the Epstein–Barr virus latent membrane protein 1 (LMP1) by the ubiquitin-proteasome pathway Targeting via ubiquitination of the N-terminal residue. J Biol Chem 2000; 275:23,491–23,499.

169. Lee SP, Thomas WA, Blake NW, Rickinson AB. Transporter (TAP)-independent processing of a multiple membrane-spanning protein, the Epstein–Barr virus latent membrane protein 2. Eur J Immunol 1996; 26:1875–1883.

170. Ong KW, Wilson AD, Hirst TR, Morgan AJ. The subunit of Escherichia coli heat-labile enterotoxin enhances CD8+ cytotoxic-T-lymphocyte killing of Epstein–Barr Virus–infected cell lines. J Virol 2003; 77(7):4298–4305.

171. Rothenberger S, Rousseaux M, Knecht H, Bender FC, Legler DF, Bron C. Association of the Epstein–Barr virus latent membrane protein 1 with lipid rafts is mediated through its N-terminal region. Cell Mol Life Sci 2002; 59:171–180.

172. Clausse B, Fizazi K, Walczak V, et al. High concentration of the EBV latent membrane protein 1 in glycosphingolipid-rich complexes from both epithelial and lymphoid cells. Virology 1997; 228:285–293.

173. Richards CM, Aman AT, Hirst TR, Hill TJ, Williams NA. Protective mucosal immunity to ocular herpes simplex virus type 1 infection in mice by using Escherichia coli heat-labile enterotoxin B subunit as an adjuvant. J Virol 2001; 75:1664–1671.

174. Williams NA, Hirst TR, Nashar TO. Immune modulation by the cholera-like enterotoxins: from adjuvant to therapeutic. Immunol Today 1999; 20:95–101.

175. Griffin BE. Epstein–Barr virus (EBV) and human disease: facts, opinions and problems. Mutat Res 2000; 462:395–405.

176. van den Bosch C, Griffin BE, Kazembe P, Dziweni C, Kadzamira L. Are plant factors a missing link in the evolution of endemic Burkitt's lymphoma? Br J Cancer 1993; 68:1232–1235.

177. Raab-Traub N. Epstein–Barr virus and nasopharyngeal carcinoma. Semin Cancer Biol 1992; 3:297–307.

178. Ohigashi H, Koshimizu K, Tokuda H, Hiramatsu S, Jato J, Ito Y. Epstein–Barr virus-inducing activity of Euphorbiaceae plants commonly grown in Cameroon. Cancer Lett 1985; 28:135–141.

179. Mizuno F, Koizumi S, Osato T, Kokwaro JO, Ito Y. Chinese and African Euphorbiaceae plant extracts: markedly enhancing effect on Epstein–Barr virus-induced transformation. Cancer Lett 1983; 19:199–205.

180. Yao QY, Rowe M, Morgan AJ, et al. Salivary and serum IgA antibodies to the Epstein–Barr virus glycoprotein gp340: incidence and potential for virus neutralization. Int J Cancer 1991; 48:45–50.

Index

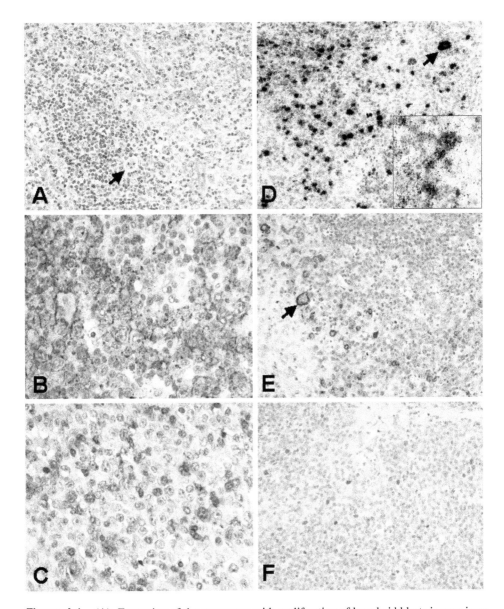

Figure 4-1 (**A**) Expansion of the paracortex with proliferation of lymphoid blasts is seen in an infectious mononucleosis tonsil (H and E). Note occasional Reed-Sternberg-like cells (*arrow*). (**B**) Immunohistochemistry reveals expression of the CD20 B-cell antigen in most lymphoid blasts (red membrane staining). (**C**) There are also numerous admixed CD3-positive T-cells, including larger, activated cells (red membrane staining, *arrows*). (**D**) In situ hybridization with radiolabeled EBER-specific probes reveals numerous EBV-positive cells in the paracortex (black labeling), including multinucleated Reed-Sternberg-like cells (*arrow*). (D, inset) A proportion of these cells express the CD30 activation antigen as shown by double labeling (inset red staining). (**E**) Variable proportions of lymphoid cells express LMP1 (red membrane staining). Note a LMP1-positive Reed-Sternberg-like cell (*arrow*). (**F**) Variable proportions of lymphoid cells express EBNA2 [red nuclear labeling (*arrows*)]. *Abbreviations:* EBNA, Epstein-Barr nuclear antigen; EBER, EBV encoded RNA; EBV, Epstein-Barr virus; LMP, latent membrane protein. (*See page 61.*)

(A)　　　　　　　　**(B)**

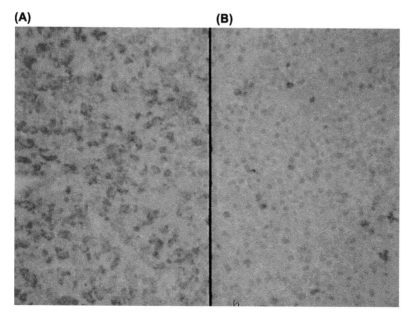

Figure 8-6 Primary CNS lymphoma in an AIDS patient. Same patient as in Figure 5 (Chapter 8). **(A)** Stained for L26, a B lymphocyte marker. **(B)** Stained for CD3, a T lymphocyte marker. This shows that the neoplastic cells are B lymphocytes, in accord with the known tropism of EBV. *Source:* Courtesy of Dr. William Kupsky, Division of Neuropathology, Harper University Hospital, Detroit, Michigan. (*See page 160.*)

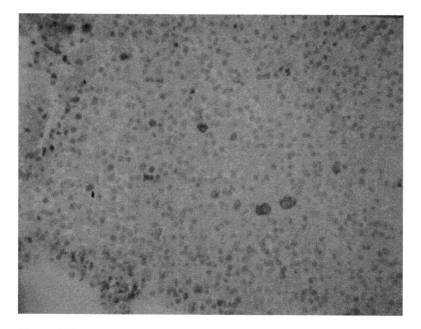

Figure 8-7 Primary CNS lymphoma in an AIDS patient. Same patient as in Figure 6 (Chapter 8). Immunostained for the EBV-antigen, LMP-1, which is a marker of latent infection. Note expression in the cytoplasm of the neoplastic cells. *Source:* Courtesy of Dr. William Kupsky, Division of Neuropathology, Harper University Hospital, Detroit, Michigan. (*See page 161.*)

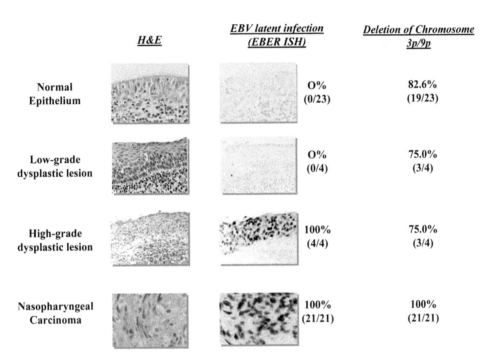

	H&E	EBV latent infection (EBER ISH)	Deletion of Chromosome 3p/9p
Normal Epithelium		0% (0/23)	82.6% (19/23)
Low-grade dysplastic lesion		0% (0/4)	75.0% (3/4)
High-grade dysplastic lesion		100% (4/4)	75.0% (3/4)
Nasopharyngeal Carcinoma		100% (21/21)	100% (21/21)

Figure 14-1 Expression of EBER in premalignant nasopharyngeal epithelium carrying allelic deletion of chromosomes 3p and 9p. Note the expression of EBER in the high-grade precancerous lesion but its absence in the low-grade precancerous lesion. Allelic deletion of chromosomes 3p (at locus D3S1076) and 9p (at loci IFNA and DS9161) could be detected in both high- and low-grade precancerous lesions of nasopharyngeal epithelium, suggesting that the deletions occur before EBV infection. *Abbreviations:* EBER, Epstein-Barr virus encoded ribonucleic acids; EBV, Epstein-Barr virus. (*See page 277.*)

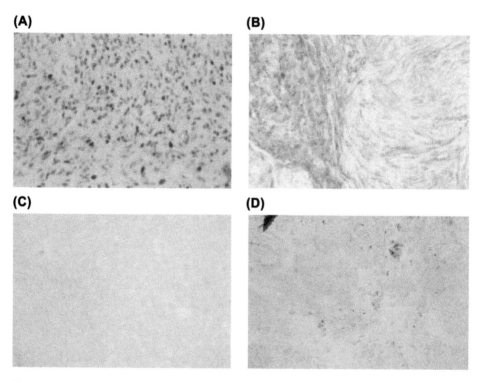

Figure 15-1 Photomicrographs of tumor specimens studied to detect EBV. Panel **(A)** (630) shows in situ hybridization of a leiomyosarcoma specimen from an HIV-positive patient (Patient 1). When tested with the EBER probe, the sample shows bright-red nuclear staining, indicating prominent hybridization of the biotinylated probe. Panel **(B)** (250) shows immunoperoxidase staining of the tissue from Patient 1 with antibody to the EBV receptor (CD21). The golden-brown precipitate observed on staining with DAB peroxidase reveals masses of tumor cells that bound the CD21 antibody. Under identical conditions, a pan-B cell antibody, CD20, did not react with the tissue. Panel **(C)** (630) shows in situ hybridization of a leiomyoma specimen from an HIV-negative patient (Patient 10). When this sample was tested with the EBER probe as in Panel A, there was no detectable hybridization of the probe. Panel **(D)** (250) shows immunoperoxidase staining of the tissue from Patient 10 with antibody to CD21. There are moderate numbers of golden-brown precipitates in the muscle fibers on staining with DAB peroxidase. Abbreviations: DAB, 3,30-diaminobenzidine; EBV, Epstein- Barr virus; EBER, EBV-encoded ribonucleic acid; HIV, human immunodeficiency virus. *Source:* From Ref. 51. (*See page 300.*)